MEDICAL RADIOLOGY
Diagnostic Imaging

Editors:
A. L. Baert, Leuven
K. Sartor, Heidelberg

Springer-Verlag Berlin Heidelberg GmbH

Fred E. Avni (Ed.)

Perinatal Imaging

From Ultrasound to MR Imaging

With Contributions by

F. E. Avni · M. Cassart · C. Christophe · T. Cos · C. Devalck · C. Donner · J. Dubois
J. Estroff · D. Eurin · L. Garel · A. Grignon · M. Hall · A. Massez · Y. Robert · F. Rypens
P. Sonigo · G. Vaksmann · N. Vanregemorter · F. Ziereisen

Foreword by

A. L. Baert

With 389 Figures in 615 Separate Illustrations, 14 in Color and 31 Tables

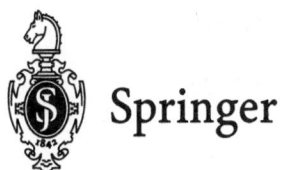 Springer

FRED E. AVNI, MD, PhD
Professor, Service d'imagerie pédiatrique
Hôpital Universitaire des Enfants Reine Fabiola
Avenue J. J. Crocq 15
1020 Bruxelles
Belgium

MEDICAL RADIOLOGY · Diagnostic Imaging and Radiation Oncology
Series Editors: A. L. Baert · L. W. Brady · H.-P. Heilmann · F. Molls · K. Sartor

Continuation of
Handbuch der medizinischen Radiologie
Encyclopedia of Medical Radiology

ISBN 978-3-642-63143-6   ISBN 978-3-642-56402-4 (eBook)
DOI 10.1007/978-3-642-56402-4

CIP data applied for

Die Deutsche Bibliothek – CIP-Einheitsaufnahme
Perinatal imaging : from ultrasound to MR imaging / Fred E. Avni (ed.). With contributions by F. E. Avni ... Foreword by
Albert L. Baert. – Berlin ; Heidelberg ; New York ; Barcelona ; Hong Kong ; London ; Milan ; Paris ; Singapore ; Tokyo :
Springer, 2002
    (Medical radiology)

http//www. springer.de
© Springer-Verlag Berlin Heidelberg 2002
Ursprünglich erschienen bei Springer-Verlag Berlin Heidelberg New York 2002
Softcover reprint of the hardcover 1st edition 2002

The use of general descriptive names, trademarks, etc. in this publication does not imply, even in the absence of a specific
statement, that such names are exempt from the relevant protective laws and regulations and therefore free for general
use.

Product liability: The publishers cannot guarantee the accuracy of any information about dosage and application contained
in this book. In every case the user must check such information by consulting the relevant literature.

Cover-Design and Typesetting: Verlagsservice Teichmann, 69256 Mauer

SPIN: 107 607 91   21/3130 – 5 4 3 2 1 0

This book is dedicated

to all our teachers,

To my wife
Jacqueline,

To my children
Sarah, Fanny and Nathan

Foreword

Fetal and perinatal medicine is a rapidly expanding field, and noninvasive imaging by means of ultrasonography and MRI is playing a major role in refining diagnosis and therapy. Recent technological advances in these imaging modalities now allow unprecedented morphological depiction of the fetus and excellent insight into complex pathologic conditions, as well as yielding superior guidance for therapeutic fetal interventions.

I am very pleased that Professor F. Avni , a leading international pediatric radiologist, was prepared to take on the challenging task of preparing and editing this comprehensive and up-to-date overview of our knowledge in the area of fetal and perinatal imaging. He has been successful in engaging well-known experts with outstanding qualifications in fetal imaging to join him in this venture. I would like to congratulate Professor Avni and all contributing authors most sincerely for their excellent work.

I am confident that this outstanding volume will meet with great interest not only from general as well as specialized pediatric radiologists but also from neonatologists and pediatricians. I trust it will enjoy the same success as many previous volumes in this series.

Leuven   ALBERT L. BAERT

Preface

Fetal and perinatal medicine would not have developed without the extensive use of obstetric ultrasound (US).

In order to be efficient, the examination has to be performed very carefully and by sonologists fully conversant with the normal and abnormal development of the fetus.

Various factors are leading to improvements in obstetric US. Better equipment with high-resolution transducers has become widely available; color Doppler and endo-cavitary transducers are also facilitating the evaluation of the embryo and fetus. Three-dimensional imaging of the fetus is another step forward in the global evaluation of pregnancy.

On the other hand, recent years have seen the increasing use of fetal magnetic resonance (MR) imaging. Newer machines provide better images with faster acquisition. MR imaging is revolutionary in that it provides fetal anatomical details never previously visualized.

Therefore, it seemed to be a good time to describe through the present book the status of techniques for the assessment of both the normal and abnormal fetus. One goal is to underline in what ways various techniques are complementary. Our second aim is to transmit the general philosophy of the authors regarding perinatal imaging. We wish to illustrate the continuity from in-utero to postnatal imaging and to help all physicians dealing with perinatology in their decisions. It is our hope to make diagnosis more accurate and counseling of the parents easier.

Brussels   FRED E. AVNI

Contents

1 Routine Obstetrical Ultrasound Examination in the Second and Third Trimester
FRED E. AVNI, FRANÇOISE RYPENS, CATHERINE DONNER 1

2 Abnormal Fetal Growth
CATHERINE DONNER and FRED E. AVNI 13

3 Placenta and Fetal Surroundings
JOSÉE DUBOIS, LAURENT GAREL, ANDRÉE GRIGNON 25

4 Perinatal Diagnosis of Central Nervous System, Face and Neck Anomalies
FRED E. AVNI, TERESA COS, PASCALE SONIGO, CATHERINE CHRISTOPHE 39

5 The Fetal Chest
FRANÇOISE RYPENS, ANDRÉE GRIGNON, FRED E. AVNI 77

6 Heart Disease in the Fetus – Diagnosis and Management
GUY VAKSMAN and YANN ROBERT 103

7 Abdomen (Digestive Tract, Wall and Peritoneum)
JOSÉE DUBOIS and ANDRÉE GRIGNON 125

8 Perinatal Approach in Anomalies of the Urinary Tract, Adrenals,
and Genital System
FRED E. AVNI, LAURENT GAREL, MICHELLE HALL, FRANÇOISE RYPENS 153

9 Perinatal Diagnosis of Musculoskeletal Anomalies
FRANÇOISE RYPENS, FRANCE ZIEREISEN, FRED E. AVNI 197

10 The Evaluation of Twin Pregnancy
ANDRÉE GRIGNON and JOSÉE DUBOIS 227

11 Ultrasound and Perinatal Infection
CATHERINE DONNER, FRANÇOISE RYPENS, FRED E. AVNI 245

12 Fetal Chromosomal Anomalies
FRED E. AVNI, JUDY ESTROFF, ANNE MASSEZ, NICOLE VANREGEMORTER 255

13 Fetal Tumors and Pseudotumors
FRED E. AVNI, MARIE CASSART, CHRISTINE DEVALCK, DANIÈLE EURIN 267

14 Fetal Hydrops
FRANÇOISE RYPENS 285

Subject Index 295

List of Contributors 303

1 Routine Obstetrical Ultrasound Examination in the Second and Third Trimester

Fred E. Avni, Françoise Rypens, Catherine Donner

CONTENTS

1.1   General Considerations *1*
1.1.1 Safety of US Examinations *1*
1.1.2 "To Routine or Not to Routine" *1*
1.1.3 The Pregnant Woman *2*
1.1.4 The Fetus *2*
1.2   To Date the Pregnancy *2*
1.2.1 Dating on the Basis of a Previous US Examination *2*
1.2.2 Dating on the Basis of the LMP *2*
1.2.3 Dating Without LMP and Without Previous US *2*
1.3   US Technique *2*
1.4   Routine Second Trimester Examination: The "Morphologic Examination" *2*
1.4.1 Fetal Biometry *3*
1.4.1.1 Measurements Verifying GA and Fetal Growth *3*
1.4.1.2 Measurements of Fetal Organs *4*
1.4.2 Verifying the Fetal Anatomy *4*
1.4.2.1 Central Nervous System *4*
1.4.2.2 Fetal Spine *5*
1.4.2.3 Face and Neck *5*
1.4.2.4 Chest *5*
1.4.2.5 Abdomen *6*
1.4.2.6 Extremities *7*
1.4.2.7 Fetal Sex *7*
1.4.3 The Placenta and Fetal Environment *7*
1.4.3.1 Amniotic Membrane and Fluid Volume *7*
1.4.3.2 Placenta and Umbilical Cord *7*
1.4.3.3 Uterus and Adnexa *7*
1.4.4 Fetal Well-being *8*
1.4.5 Conclusion of the Second Trimester Examination *8*
1.5   Third Trimester Examination: "The Growth Control" Examination *8*
1.5.1 Fetal Lie *8*
1.5.2 Measurements *8*
1.5.3 Anatomy *9*
1.5.3.1 Central Nervous System *9*
1.5.3.2 Spine and Spinal Canal *9*
1.5.3.3 Face and Neck *9*
1.5.3.4 Chest *9*
1.5.3.5 Abdomen *9*
1.5.3.6 Extremities *10*
1.5.3.7 Fetal Sex *10*
1.5.4 Placenta and Adnexa *10*
1.5.4.1 Placenta and Cord *10*
1.5.4.2 Amniotic Fluid Volume *10*
1.5.5 Fetal Well-being *10*
1.5.6 Cervical Length *10*
1.5.7 Conclusion of the Third Trimester Examination *11*
1.6   The Use of Doppler During Pregnancy *11*
1.7   Medical Report and Iconography *11*
1.8   The Transition from Antenatal to Postnatal Management *11*
       References *11*

F. E. Avni, MD, PhD
Department of Pediatric Imaging, University Children's Hospital, Avenue J. J. Crocq 15, 1020 Brussels, Belgium
F. Rypens, MD
Department of Medical Imaging, Sainte Justine Hospital, 3175 Côte-Sainte-Catherine, Montréal, Québec H3T 1C5, Canada
C. Donner, MD, PhD
Department of Obstetrics and Gynecology, University Clinic of Brussels, Erasme Hospital, Route de Lennik 808, 1070 Brussels, Belgium

1.1 General Considerations

1.1.1 Safety of US Examinations

Since the beginning of a more systematic use of medical ultrasound in the 1970s, a lot of scientific material has been collected, and to date there is no evidence that obstetrical US is harmful to the fetus (Reece et al.1990, Wagber and Calhoun1998). Even Doppler, which had raised lots of concerns, is now considered sufficiently safe. Yet, still, the equipment must be adapted to the type of examination and US settings must be optimized. It seems wise to use color Doppler during the first trimester only in cases with significant clinical indications.

1.1.2 "To Routine or Not to Routine"

Whether each pregnant woman should undergo systematic obstetrical US survey during her pregnancy is still controversial and attitudes vary from country to country. The yield of a systematic examination has been questioned by some studies; none of them is entirely convincing due to bias in patient selection. In Belgium, three examinations are performed during the pregnancy: one during each trimester. Most obstetricians feel that this systematic follow-up helps them in their practice and decreases the neonatal morbidity (SEEDS 1996, WAGBER and CALHOUN 1998, DOOLEY 1999, EIK-NES et al. 2000, ANTSALKIS 1998).

1.1.3
The Pregnant Woman

Before starting the US examination, the sonologist must question the pregnant woman in order to determine whether any circumstance may alter the normal course of the pregnancy. Any particular family history, genetic diseases, consanguinity, previous abnormal pregnancy and the age of the patient may influence the development of the pregnancy and should be noted.

1.1.4
The Fetus

The US examination represents a direct contact between the mother and the baby to be. It encompasses many of symbols for the future parents. The sonologist has a double role: on the one hand he or she is able to show a representation of the fetus to the parents, while on the other, he or she has to watch carefully in order to depict any anomaly. It is important to make the parents understand that a normal US examination does not mean absence of chromosomal abnormality and is not a 100% "health certificate".

1.2
To Date the Pregnancy

Dating of the pregnancy can be based on the last menstrual period (LMP) or on a previous US examination. The gestational age (GA) must be expressed in weeks LMP.

1.2.1
Dating on the Basis of a
Previous US Examination

If a previous US examination had been performed between 8 and 12 weeks LMP, the GA calculated on this basis becomes the "official" age and the end of the pregnancy can be estimated on this basis too. The measurement of the crown-rump length at this stage provides the best approximation of the GA with an error <1 week. After this period, the accuracy of the US estimation weakens.

1.2.2
Dating on the Basis of the LMP

If there was no previous US examination, the GA must be calculated on the basis of the LMP.

1.2.3
Dating Without LMP and Without Previous US

In cases of no previous US examination and without knowledge of the LMP, dating must be based on the fetal biometry (see below). There must be a balance between the estimation of the GA obtained by the various measurements. Some among them will provide more accurate evaluation than others (BENSON and DOUBILET 1991). For instance, the abdominal circumference measured before 28 weeks gives a good evaluation of the GA, considering the 50th centile.

1.3
US Technique

The examination must be performed the patient lying relatively flat in order to avoid contraction of the muscles of the lower abdomen. The bladder must be partially filled so that the cervix can be verified. Curvilinear 3.5–7 MHz transducers are best adapted to the pregnant abdomen. Endovaginal probes should be used whenever fetal position obscures the evaluation of some specific areas or whenever the cervical region of the uterus has to be investigated (TIMOR-TRISCH and MONTEAGUDO 1996).

1.4
Routine Second Trimester Examination:
The "Morphologic Examination"

The routine midtrimester examination is ideally performed at between 18 and 22 weeks. At this stage it is already possible to measure and to evaluate the anatomy of most fetal structures. The examination includes measurements, anatomical survey, and evaluation of the fetal well-being and environment (amniotic fluid, placenta and membranes). As for each examination, the number of fetuses, the type of chorionicity and fetal viability must first be assessed.

1.4.1
Fetal Biometry

Every measurement must be performed as accurately and precisely as possible, referring to well established standards. Ideally, the normative curve must adapted to the population studied (LHEI and WHEN 1998). Each measurement must be plotted against curves showing the normal evolution of the specific measurement throughout pregnancy. The result must be expressed as a centile of the normal values.

1.4.1.1
Measurements Verifying GA and Fetal Growth

During the second trimester, GA and fetal growth are assessed through the systematic measurements of the biparietal diameter (BPD), of the abdominal circumference (AC) and of the femoral shaft length (F). The *BPD* is measured on a symmetric transverse scan of the fetal head that includes the falx cerebri, the cerebral peduncles, the third ventricle and the upper part of the posterior fossa. This diameter is measured from the outer edge of one parietal bone to the inner edge of the other (Fig. 1.1). Whenever the skull presents an usual form (dolicho- or brachycephaly), it is advisable to measure the cephalic perimeter (outer margins) or combine BPD and fronto-occipital diameter (Fig. 1.1). The *AC* is measured on a transverse scan of the fetal abdomen that includes the liver, a horizontal segment of the umbilical vein and the stomach (Fig. 1.2). Most equipment provides the value of the AC once the circumference is drawn on the screen (on the outer margins of the abdomen). It can also be calculated by the sum of two orthogonal abdominal diameters multiplied by 1.57. The *femoral shaft* must be measured on a scan that includes both cartilaginous epiphyses; only then can one be sure that the entire length of the femur is measured (Fig. 1.3). If possible both femurs must be measured. Evaluation of the fetal weight can be performed at the end of the second trimester in a similar way to the methods used during the third trimester (see below). These are based on the three major biometric

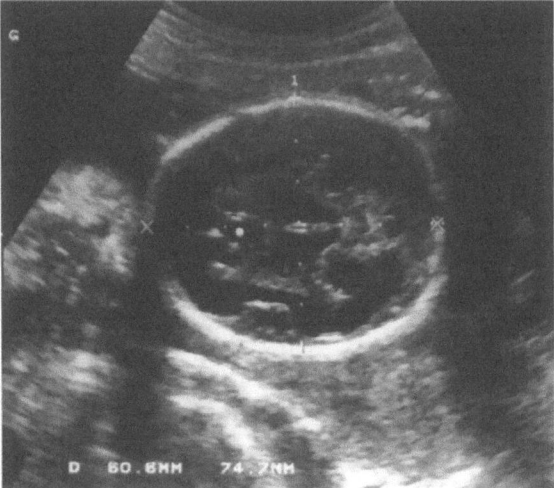

Fig. 1.1. Biparietal scan. Second trimester. Transverse scan of the head at the level of the third ventricle (*arrow*), the cerebral peduncles (*p*) and the septum pellucidum (*). The biparietal and fronto-occipital diameters are measured and limited by *crosses*

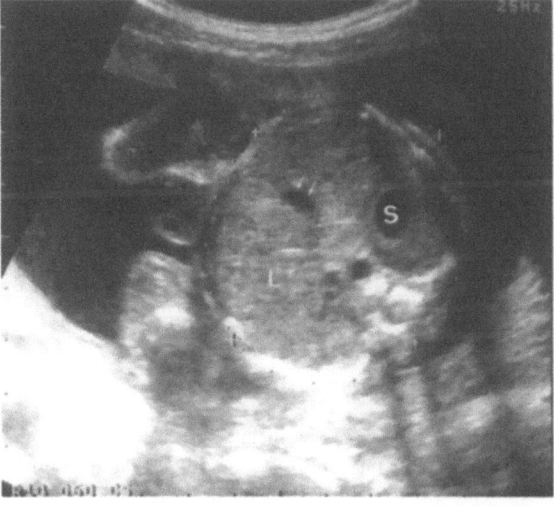

Fig. 1.2. Abdominal circumference measured on a transverse scan at the level of the stomach (*S*), liver (*L*) and umbilical vein (*arrows*). *Sp* spine

measurements and the result must be plotted against a normative curve.

Besides these systematic measurements, other may be of some help in order to confirm the GA. For instance, the transverse diameter of the cerebellum measured in millimeters before 23 weeks provides a good evaluation of the GA expressed in weeks (Fig. 1.4). (SNIJDERS and NICOLAIDES 1994, KURZ and NEEDLEMAN 1998, KURMANAVICIUS et al. 1999).

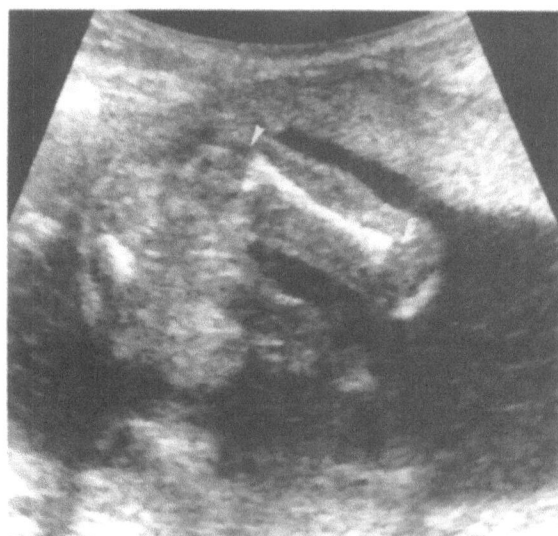

Fig. 1.3. Femur. Second trimester. The femoral diaphyseal shaft is well visualized as well as the hypoechoic cartilaginous epiphyses (*arrowheads*)

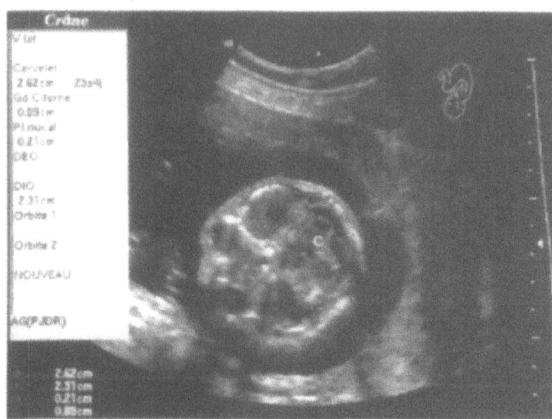

Fig. 1.4. Posterior fossa view includes measurements of the cerebellum (*c*), the posterior fossa and the nuchal skin thickness, and of the interorbital distance

1.4.1.2
Measurements of Fetal Organs

Curves are available in order to evaluate the growth of almost every fetal organ and structure. These measurements help to confirm the normal anatomical development and growth of the fetus (see under specific organs). These measurements should be performed whenever a specific problem or doubt exists. Some ratios are also interesting since they provide supplementary evidence for assessing normal development: for instance, the ratio between the fetal foot

and the femoral shaft equals 1, during the entire pregnancy (Hata and Deter 1992).

1.4.2
Verifying the Fetal Anatomy

Most fetal structures can be verified at this stage. The anatomical survey must be rigorous and systematic as if a checklist has to be completed. This is a good method to minimize omissions or mistakes. For each structure, it should be noted whether the organ has or has not been correctly evaluated and whether it appears normal, abnormal or of some variant form (Rebaud and Rebaud 1989, Filly 2000).

1.4.2.1
Central Nervous System

Several landmarks of the fetal skull must be systematically verified in all three planes whenever possible:
- The ossified skull.
- The midline, falx cerebri.
- The third ventricle and at that level the symmetric cerebral peduncles.
- On the midline, above the third ventricle, the cyst of the septum pellucidum that provides indirect evidence for the presence of the corpus callosum. The corpus callosum itself should be visualized on a mid-sagittal scan of the fetal brain.
- The lateral ventricles: the atrium of the lateral ventricles should measure less than 10 mm (Fig. 1.5).
- The choroid plexus within the lateral ventricles.
- The sylvian fissures, symmetrically shaped.

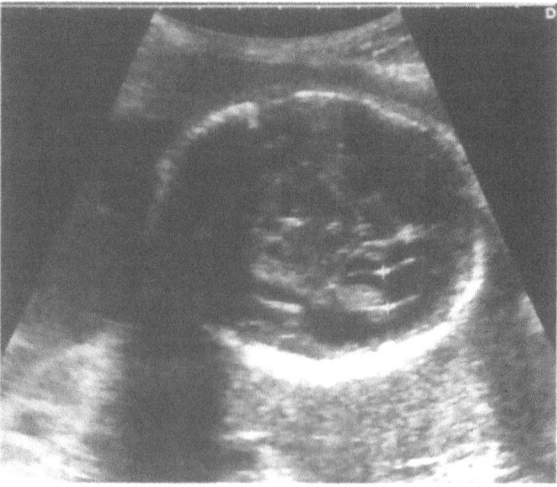

Fig. 1.5. Atrium of lateral ventricles (10 mm between *crosses*)

- The posterior fossa: cerebellum lobes, the hyper-echoic vermis, the fourth ventricle, the cisterna magna that should be septated by subarachnoid folds and measure 2–10 mm (GUSHIKEN and GOLDSTEIN 1999). Nuchal skin thickness must be measured at this level (under 5 mm) (Fig. 1.4).

1.4.2.2
Fetal Spine

The ossification of the fetal spine is progressive. The sacrum starts to be ossified around the 16th week, the coccyx ending the process after birth. The vertebrae ossify through three centers, one (composed of two ossification centers that fuse rapidly) for the body and two for the lateral processes (Fig. 1.6). Therefore in order to verify the correct ossification, the examination must include coronal, transverse and sagittal-oblique scans. The integrity of the dorsal skin must be part of the evaluation (FILLY 2000).

1.4.2.3
Face and Neck

The examination of the face and neck must include the visualization of:
- Orbits and lens: symmetric size, movements, hyaloid artery.
- Nose, nostrils and the length of the nasal bone.
- Upper and lower lips, mouth movements, tongue.
- Bony maxillary and mandible.
- The fetal profile.

1.4.2.4
Chest

Verifying the chest must include the chest wall and the chest contents (Fig. 1.7).
- The upper limit is represented by the neck and clavicles.
- The lower limit is the diaphragm, appearing as a hypoechoic thick line (Fig. 1.8).
- The outer limit is represented by the skeleton, which includes the ribs, the partially ossified sternum and the scapulae.

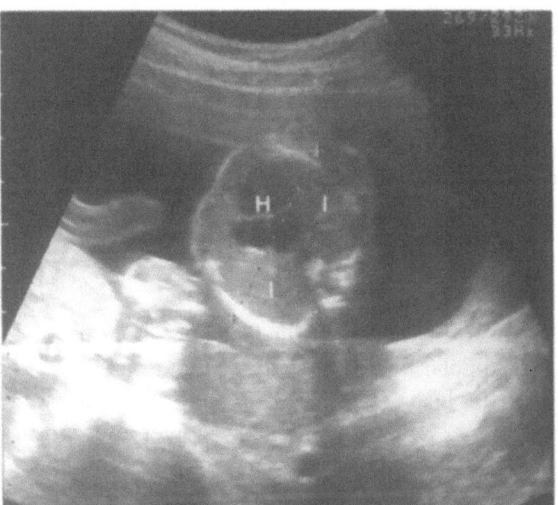

a

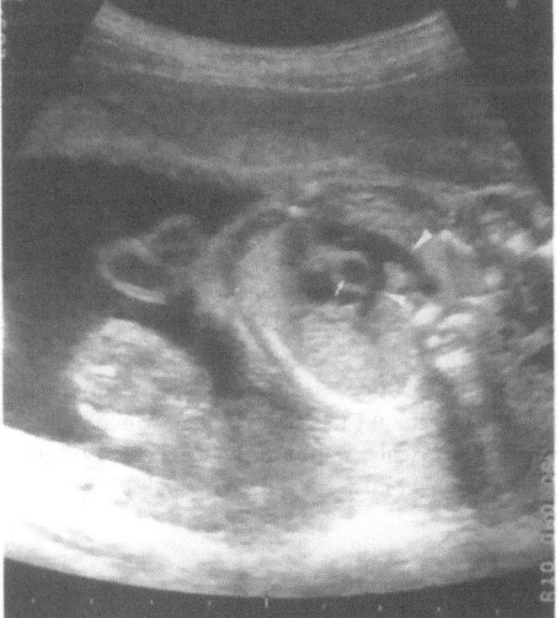

b

Fig. 1.7a, b. Chest. Transverse scan. a Four-chamber view. *H* heart, *l* lungs. b Aorto-pulmonary crossing view. *Arrow* aorta, *arrowheads* pulmonary arteries

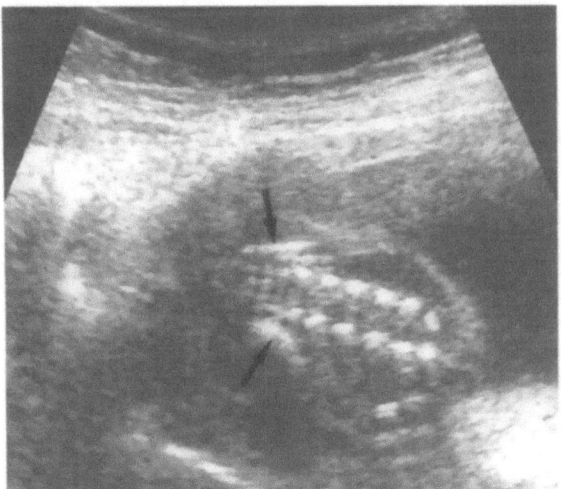

Fig. 1.6. Spine. Frontal view. The lateral ossification centers are visible as well as the iliac wings (*arrows*)

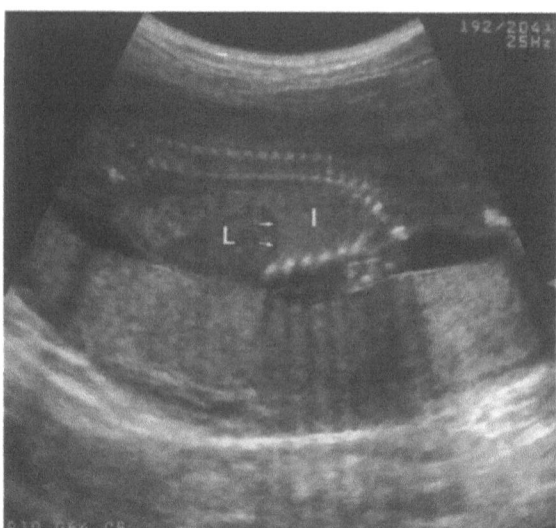

Fig. 1.8. Pulmonary abdominal limit. Sagittal scan of the trunk. *l* lung, *L* liver, *arrows* diaphragm

– On a transverse scan, the fetal lungs appear as two triangular finely echogenic structures at each side of the heart (Figs. 1.7, 1.8). Lung vascularization can be evaluated with color Doppler and appears as a branching tree starting from the hilum.

The US study of the heart begins with the identification of the position of the heart in the chest. The tip of the heart is rotated towards the left side within the mediastinum; it must be on the same side as the stomach. A normal four-chambered heart, obtained in semi-axial thoracic plane, shows a symmetrical size of the two ventricles, normal inter-auricular and interventricular septa, a normal foramen of Botal, and normally positioned atrioventricular valves (Fig. 1.7a). Routine US survey should also include the study of the emergence of the great vessels and the crossing between the aorta and the pulmonary artery (Fig. 1.7b). The aortic arch must be followed on a sagittal scan. The other vessels of the mediastinum can be followed thanks to color Doppler, which helps to verify the vascular nature of any structure (McGAHAN 1991, MAY et al. 1993, BROWN et al. 1993).

1.4.2.5
Abdomen

The analysis of the fetal abdomen should include both the abdominal wall and the abdominal contents.

– Both the fluid-filled and solid organs must be evaluated
– The stomach lies in the left hypochondrium, at the same side as the tip of the heart. It may be filled with echogenic material. The small bowel is relatively empty at this stage and may appear under a hyperechoic pseudomass (Fig. 1.9). The colon is empty.
– The liver appears homogeneous and triangular-shaped (Figs. 1.2, 1.8). The gallbladder is easily identified; its size may vary. The vascular network of the liver may also be easily identified. The spleen is harder to visualize; on a transverse scan it appears as a hypoechoic triangular mass behind the stomach.
– The bladder is filled with urine starting at the 10th week; filling and emptying of the bladder can be monitored throughout pregnancy. At the beginning of the second trimester, the kidneys are somewhat more echogenic that the liver. Their echogenicity will diminish progressively. They are located in the lumbar areas. At the end of the second trimester a corticomedullary differentiation will appear. The renal pelvis is easily visible and on a transverse scan the anteroposterior diameter should measure less than 4 mm. Normal ureters and urethra are not visible. The adrenals are relatively large and hypoechoic at the top of the kidneys.
– The aorta and inferior vena cava must be identified and they can be studied with color Doppler.

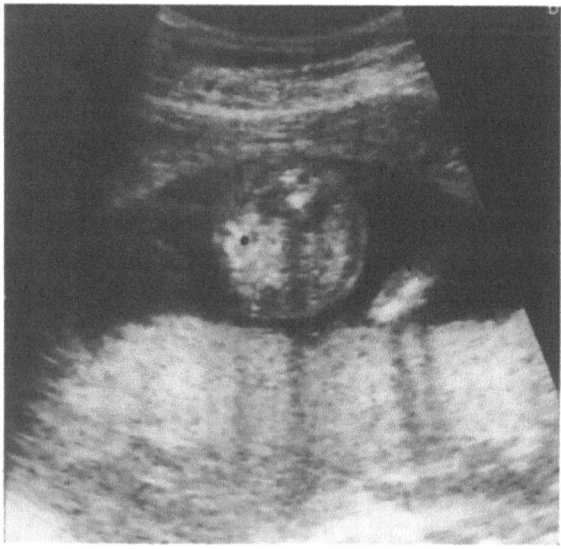

Fig. 1.9. Intestinal hyperechoic pseudomass (*). Transverse scan of the abdomen

– The integrity of the fetal abdominal wall must be verified as well as the course of the umbilical vessels: the vein courses between the stomach and the gallbladder; the arteries down the pelvis lateral to the bladder (HERZBERG 1998, ANTGUADO 1999).

1.4.2.6
Extremities

– Examination of the upper extremities must start at the shoulder and end at the end of the fingers, if possible with the hand unrolled (Fig. 1.10).
– Examination of the lower extremities starts at the hip and ends at the end of the toes (Fig. 1.11).
– The axis of the feet in relation with the legs must be checked

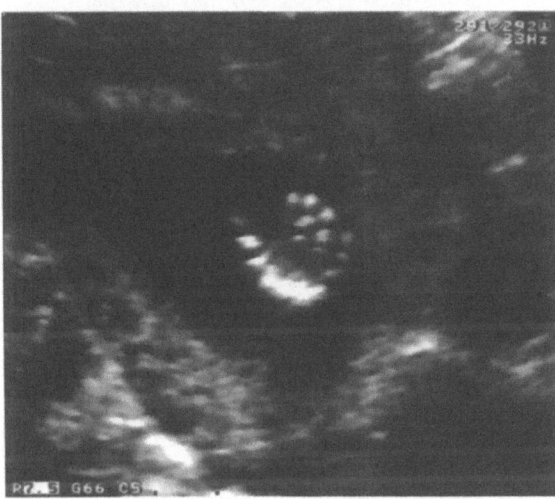

Fig. 1.10. Hand. Palmar view

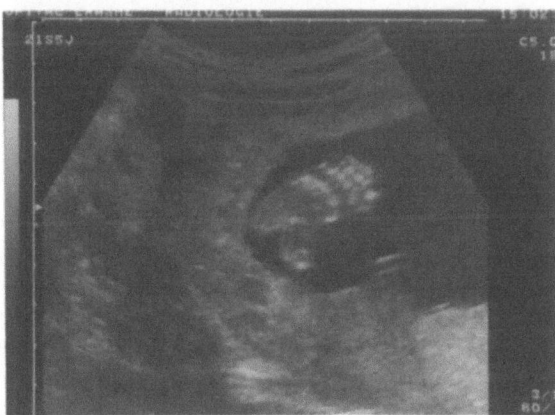

Fig. 1.11. Foot. Plantar view

1.4.2.7
Fetal Sex

The determination of fetal sex is theoretically easy at this stage unless the legs are folded in front of the fetal pelvis. The determination of male sex is based upon visualization of the penis. Absence of visualization of a penis is not sufficient to determine female sex; identification of a vulva is necessary.

1.4.3
The Placenta and Fetal Environment

1.4.3.1
Amniotic Membrane and Fluid Volume

A separate amniotic membrane can be visualized up to the 16th week; it fuses with the placental surface thereafter (WILLIAMS 1993).

The amniotic fluid is relatively abundant during the second trimester. This can be evaluated subjectively or objectively. For the latter, the pregnant abdomen can be divided into four quadrants; in each one, the depth of the pocket of fluid without fetal structure is measured. The sum of the four quadrant pockets determines a value that is plotted against the graph of normal values determining the amniotic fluid index (HALLAK et al. 1993).

1.4.3.2
Placenta and Umbilical Cord

The placenta must be localized even though its insertion relative to the cervix has not reached its final location; this final location may change with the growth of the inferior segment of the uterus during the third trimester. Therefore, one should not diagnose a previa insertion before the third trimester (KUHLMAN and WARSOF 1996). Low placental location during the second trimester should induce an US survey of the placental location and a search for vasa previa at the third trimester. The number of vessels (two arteries and one vein) as well as the insertion of the umbilical cord must also be assessed (HILL et al. 1987).

1.4.3.3
Uterus and Adnexa

A survey of the uterus and adnexa is useful in order to detect possible masses. The most frequent are fibromas. Their location and size must be recorded. At this stage, cervical length and morphology must already be verified by transvaginal or abdominal approach. A cervix length under 20 mm at 24 weeks is a good predictor of preterm delivery (KUSHNIR et al. 1990).

1.4.4
Fetal Well-being

Fetal well-being is determined thanks to the monitoring of fetal heart rate (normal=120–160/min) and through observation of fetal activities. It is noteworthy that transitory bradycardia can be observed around 18–20 weeks, usually without any consequence. During the second trimester the fetus presents passive and active movements of the body and of the extremities. Specific eyes movements can be monitored. The fetus is alternating active and slow motion periods. With time, the movements will diminish in number but increase in complexity (JAMES 1997).

1.4.5
Conclusion of the Second Trimester Examination

The conclusion of the second trimester examination should include comments on every aspect of the fetus that was evaluated in accordance with the GA. Any feature that remains undetermined should be controlled during a subsequent examination.

1.5
Third Trimester Examination: "The Growth Control" Examination

Before starting this examination it is mandatory to obtain the conclusions of the previous one. It is also important to inquire about the clinical evolution of the pregnancy. The way this examination is conducted is very similar to that of the second trimester. Several aspects become more important: the fetal lie, evaluation of the fetal weight or the development of the various organs.

1.5.1
Fetal Lie

Classically the fetus will be in cephalic presentation; it should be interesting to locate its face. In the case of a breech presentation it must be recorded whether it is complete (feet down) or incomplete (feet up). A

transverse lie should prompt a control examination of the placental insertion, which may be too low.

1.5.2
Measurements

The evaluation of fetal growth is based upon the same measurements as during the second trimester: BPD (Fig. 1.12), AC (Fig. 1.13) and F. Precise measurements may be more difficult to obtain due to the limited transducer opening compared with the size of the pregnant abdomen. Estimation of fetal weight can be calculated using various formulae that include BPD, F and/or AC. Whatever the formula, the error is always around 10–15% and therefore it will be greater in heavier babies than in small for gestational age

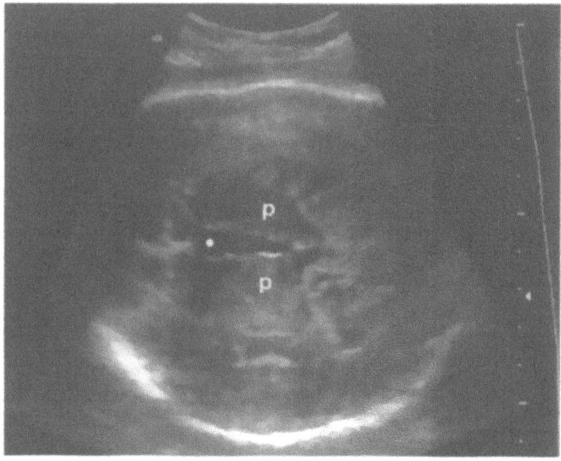

Fig. 1.12. Biparietal view. Third trimester. Symmetric view. *p* cerebral peduncles, *asterisk* septum pellucidum

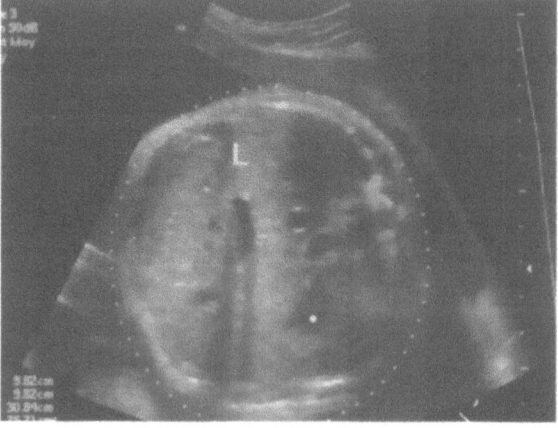

Fig. 1.13. Abdominal circumference. Third trimester. *Asterisk* stomach, *L* liver

fetuses (PRESSMAN et al. 2000, MIELKE et al. 1995, McLAREN et al. 1995).

1.5.3
Anatomy

At this stage two aspects of the anatomy must be verified: (1) the presence and normal size of each anatomical structure; (2) the normal development of each organ in relation to the GA.

1.5.3.1
Central Nervous System

The main difference in the nervous system in comparison with the second trimester examination is the progressive development of the cerebral sulci starting from the peri-rolandic sulcus during the seventh month. The progressive operculation of the sylvian fissures is another significant step in normal development that can be assessed during the eighth month (Fig. 1.12).

1.5.3.2
Spine and Spinal Canal

The spine is now ossified up the first coccygeal vertebra. The spinal cord and cauda equina are clearly visible within the spinal canal; the end of the cord is located at its almost final level (L1–L2).

1.5.3.3
Face and Neck

At this stage, more details of the eyes, lips and nose (Fig. 1.14) can be visualized as well as the emerging teeth. At the level of the neck it must be possible to demonstrate the thyroid and the trachea.

1.5.3.4
Chest

The same verifications of structures in the chest have to be performed as during the second trimester. Within the heart, more details are seen of the valves and muscular cords can be identified.

1.5.3.5
Abdomen

The main difference in the abdomen in comparison with the second trimester is the progressive filling of

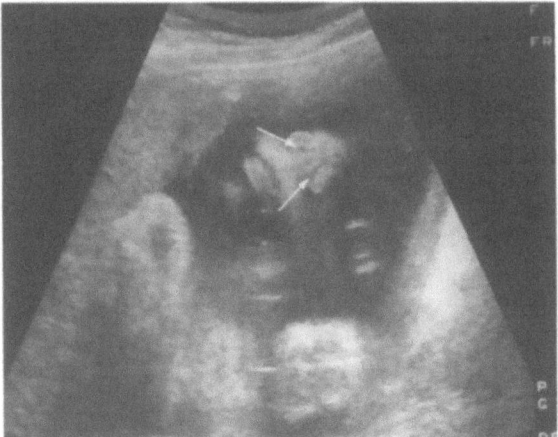

Fig. 1.14. Face. Frontal view. Nose, nostrils (*arrows*) and lips are visible

the small bowel loops with fluid; intestinal peristalsis can now be observed on real-time US. The colon fills with hypoechoic meconium. The diameter of the transverse colon may reach up to 2 cm (Fig. 1.15).

Important evolution can be observed at the level of the kidneys as they grow progressively to reach their neonatal size of around 4 cm. As mentioned above, their global echogenicity diminishes, and a corticomedullary differentiation appears (Fig. 1.16). The final US appearance is reached by 27 weeks. There is a slowing of the cycles of filling and emptying of the bladder towards the end of the pregnancy; this slowing is more marked in girls, explaining the frequent observation of a large bladder in female fetuses at the end of pregnancies.

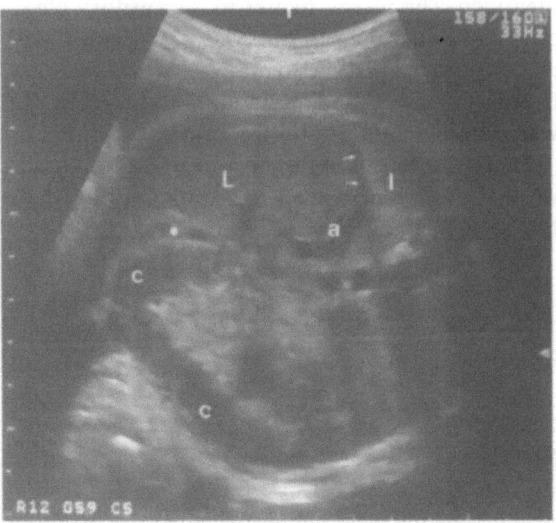

Fig. 1.15. Abdominal contents. Transverse scan. *L* liver, *asterisk* gallbladder, *c* colon, *a* adrenal, *l* lung, *arrow* diaphragm

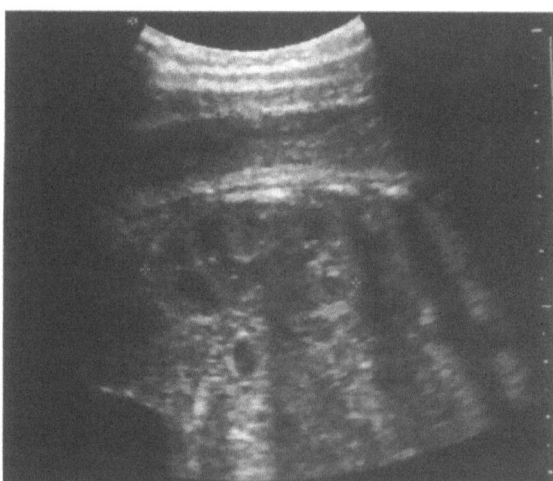

Fig. 1.16. Kidney (between *crosses*). Third trimester sagittal scan. Corticomedullary differentiation is present

1.5.3.6
Extremities

Muscles, tendons, bones and cartilage are easily identified. A progressive ossification of the epiphyses can be monitored. The calcaneum is first to ossify around 23 weeks, then the talus at 25 weeks, the distal femoral epiphysis at 32 weeks, the proximal tibial epiphysis at 34 weeks and the proximal humeral epiphysis at 38 weeks (MAHONNY et al. 1986).

1.5.3.7
Fetal Sex

In the female, the outer and inner sex structures are identified. The uterus, thanks to a transitory physiological hypertrophy, appears as a pear-shaped mass on a sagittal scan similar to the postnatal appearance. It appears as a round mass on a transverse scan, which should not be mistaken for a pelvic tumor.

In the male, the testes may already be located within the scrotum and a small amount of free fluid is usually observed.

1.5.4
Placenta and Adnexa

1.5.4.1
Placenta and Cord

At this time the placental insertion has its final location and the distance to the internal os of the cervix should be verified (>2.5 cm). Signs of placental matu-

ration may start to develop; progressive fibrosis and calcifications of the cotyledons will appear as hyperechoic foci with or without acoustic shadowing.

The placental and umbilical insertions of the cord should be checked (Fig. 1.17). A velamentous insertion must be excluded (KUHLMAN and WARSOF 1996).

1.5.4.2
Amniotic Fluid Volume

The volume of amniotic fluid tends to diminish towards the end of the pregnancy. Its echogenicity increases due to debris and to meconium cells.

1.5.5
Fetal Well-being

Fetal well-being is evaluated on the basis of heart rate, movements, amniotic fluid volume and reaction to stimuli. Growth and evolution of the fetal anatomy between successive examinations are also relevant factors. Pseudo-respiratory movements are observed.

1.5.6
Cervical Length

The length of cervix decreases normally during the third trimester: from a mean of 35 mm at 30 weeks to a mean of 22 mm at term; this can be checked endovaginally whenever necessary (BRIEGER et al. 1997).

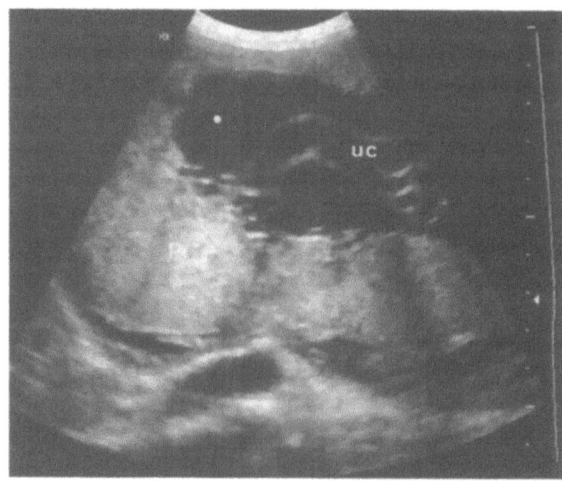

Fig. 1.17. Placenta (*P*), amniotic fluid (*) and umbilical cord (*oc*)

1.5.7
Conclusions of the Third Trimester Examination

Conclusions of the third trimester examination should include a commentary on the growth, the anatomical development and on fetal well-being.

1.6
The Use of Doppler During Pregnancy

Doppler US is a complementary tool. It is not useful to perform systematic pulsed Doppler study of the umbilical, cerebral and uterine arteries in each patient. Conversely, pulsed Doppler may be useful in selected circumstances. During the second trimester, uterine Doppler might help to identify, among a population at risk, patients susceptible to developing eclampsia. During the third trimester of pregnancy, Doppler US may be indicated in the case of various maternal clinical conditions (hypertension, pre-eclampsia, maternal coagulopathy, etc.), in the case of abnormal previous pregnancy histories, or in the case of intrauterine growth retardation. Doppler examination is also useful in multiple pregnancies and in cases of suspected vascular malformations (Fortunato 1996).

1.7
Medical Report and Iconography

The medical report must be standardized and adjustable. The quality and possible limits of the US examination must be clearly stated. The report must be structured and address clearly the three different parts of the fetal US study (biometry, anatomy, environment and well-being). It should include a conclusion and, if necessary, recommendations for follow-up and management. The iconography provided varies according to the local legislation and practice. An ideal attitude does not exist and depends on the local context. However, it seems advisable to provide pictures of the most significant parts of the examination.

The medical report is an informative document and is a reflection of the quality of the US examination. It is very important in the case of prenatal or postnatal follow-up of an anomaly. This document is also likely to be used in cases of suspected malpractice.

1.8
The Transition from Antenatal to Postnatal Management

The aim of routine obstetrical US is to ascertain the normal development of the fetus, to detect fetal anomalies and to prevent perinatal complications. The conclusion of the examination has to be transmitted to the obstetrician and to any physician who might take care of the fetus or the newborn.

> Routine fetal US must be a systematic and standardized examination. It must include measurements, verification of fetal anatomy and evaluation of fetal environment and well-being. Its conclusions must be transmitted to the physician managing the fetus before and after birth.

References

Antguado TL, Collins HB, Quirk JG (1999) The fetal G-U tract. Semin Roentgenol 14:13–28

Antsaklis AJ (1998) Debate about US screening policies. Fetal Diagn Ther13:209–215

Benson CB, Doubilet PM (1991) Sonographic prediction of gestational age. AJR Am J Roentgenol 157:1275–1277

Brieger GM, Ning XH, Dawkins RR, et al (1997) Transvaginal US assessment of cervical dynamics during the third trimester of normal pregnancy. Acta Obstet Gynecol Scand 76:118–122

Brown DL, Di Salvo DN, Frates MC, et al (1993) Sonography of the fetal heart. AJR Am J Roentgenol 160:1251–1255

Dooley SL (1999) Routine US in pregnancy. Clin Obstet Gynecol42:737–748

Eik-Nes SH, Salvesen KA, Okland O, Vatten JL (2000) Routine US fetal examination in pregnancy: the Alesund randomized controlled trial. Ultrasound Obstet Gynecol 15:473–478

Filly RA (2000) US evaluation of normal fetal anatomy. In: Callen (ed) US in obstetrics and gynecology. WB Saunders, Philadelphia, pp 221–276

Fortunato SJ (1996) The use of color Doppler and power Doppler angiography in fetal imaging. Am J Obstet Gynecol174:1828–1833

Gushiken BJ, Goldstein RB (1999) Practical approach to evaluating the fetal neural axis. Semin Roentgenol 14:5–12

Hallak M, Kirshon B, Smith EO, Cotton DB (1993) Amniotic fluid index–gestational age: specific values for normal human pregnancy. J Reprod Med 38:853–856

Hata T, Deter RL (1992) A review of fetal organ measurements obtained with US: normal growth. J Clin Ultrasound20:155–174

Herzberg BS (1998) The fetal GI tract. Semin Roentgenol 13:360–368

Hill LM, Kislak S, Rumo C (1987) An US view of the umbilical cord. Obstet Gynecol Surv 42:82–88

James A (1997) Fetal behaviour. Curr Obstet Gynecol 7:30–35

Kuhlman RS, Warsof S (1996) US of the placenta. Clin Obstet Gynecol 3:519–534

Kurmanavicius J, Wright EM, Royston P, et al (1999) Fetal US biometry. 1. Head reference values. Br J Obstet Gynecol 106:126–135

Kurmanavicius J, Wright EM, Royston P, et al (1999) Fetal US biometry. 2. Abdomen and femur length reference values. Br J Obstet Gynaecol 106:136–143

Kurz AB, Needleman L (1998) ACR standards: obstetrical measurements. Semin Roentgenol 33:309–332

Kushnir O, Vigil DA, Isquierdo L, et al (1990) Transvaginal US assessment of cervical length changes during normal pregnancy. Am J Obstet Gynecol 162:991–993

Lhei H, When SW (1998) Sonographic examination of IUGR for multiple fetal dimensions in a Chinese population. Am J Obstet Gynecol 178:916–921

McGahan JP (1991) US of the fetal heart. AJR Am J Roentgenol 156:547–563

McLaren R, Puckett JL, Chanhan SP (1995) Estimators of birth weight in pregnant women requiring insulin. Obstet Gynecol 85:565–569

Magann EF, Martin JN. Amniotic fluid volume assessment in singleton and twin pregnancies. Obstet Clin North Am 26:579–593

Mahonny BS, Bowie JD, Killam AP (1986) Epiphyseal ossification centers in the assessment of fetal maturity. Radiology 159:521–554

May DA, Barth RA, Yeager S, et al (1993) Perinatal and postnatal chest sonography. Radiol Clin North Am 31:499–516

Mielke G, Pietch Breifeld B, Sahwash, et al (1995) A new formula for prenatal US weight estimation in extremely preterm fetuses. Obstet Gynecol Invest 40:84–88

Pressman EK, Bienstock JL, Blakemore KJ, et al (2000) Prediction of birth weight by US in the 3rd trimester. Obstet Gynecol 95:502–506

Rebaud A, Rebaud MF (1989) L'échographie des 2ème et 3èmetrimestres. Rev Fr Gynecol Obstet 84:571–587

Reece EA, Assimakopoulos E, Zhang X, et al (1990) The safety of obstetric US: concern for the fetus. Obstet Gynecol 76:139–146

Seeds HW (1996) The routine or screening obstetrical US examination. Clin Obstet Gynecol 39:814–830

Snijders RJM, Nicolaides KH (1994) Fetal biometry at 14–40 weeks gestation. Ultrasound Obstet Gynecol 4:34–48

Timor-Tritsch IE, Monteagudo A (1996) Scanning techniques in obstetrics and gynecology. Clin Obstet Gynecol 39:167–174

Wagber RK, Calhoun BC (1998) The routine obstetric US examination. Obstet Clin North Am 25:451–463

Wilfe HM, Zadir IE, Bottoms SR, et al (1993) Trends in US fetal organ visualization. Ultrasound Obstet Gynecol 3:97–99

Williams K (1993) Amniotic fluid assessment. Obstet Gynecol Survey 48:795–800

2 Abnormal Fetal Growth

Catherine Donner, Fred E. Avni

CONTENTS

2.1   Intrauterine Growth Restriction 13
2.1.1   Introduction 13
2.1.2   Definition 14
2.1.3   Ultrasound Assessment 14
2.1.3.1 Ultrasound Biometry 14
2.1.3.2 Amniotic Fluid 15
2.1.3.3 Placental Morphology 15
2.1.3.4 Doppler Ultrasound 15
2.1.3.5 Biophysical Profile Score 18
2.1.4   Multiparameter Approach
        in Perinatal Management 18
2.2   Macrosomia 18
2.2.1   Introduction 18
2.2.2   Definition and Etiological Factors 18
2.2.3   Ultrasound Evaluation 19
2.2.4   Maternal and Clinical Estimates
        of Birth Weight 20
2.2.5   Perinatal Management 20
        References 20

2.1
Intrauterine Growth Restriction

2.1.1
Introduction

Fetal growth restriction (FGR) is an important cause of increased morbidity and mortality during the perinatal period (e.g., stillbirth, prematurity, asphyxia and neonatal complication) and in childhood (e.g., growth failure, neurological impairment and behavioral disorders) (SCHAUSEIL-ZIPF et al. 1989, Allen 1984, WIENERROITHER et al. 2001). Fur-

C. DONNER, MD, PhD
Department of Obstetrics and Gynecology, University Clinic of Brussels, Erasme Hospital, Route de Lennik 808, 1070 Brussels Belgium
F. E. AVNI, MD, PhD
Department of Pediatric Imaging, University Children's Hospital Queen Fabiola, Avenue J. J. Crocq 15, 1020 Brussels, Belgium

thermore, during recent years, several large-scale epidemiological studies in England and in Sweden have tended to suggest a relation between low birth weight and several diseases in adulthood (so-called Barker's theory) (BARKER et al. 1990, WILLIAMS et al. 1992, BAKER et al. 1993). In studies exploring these associations, the trends in coronary heart disease, hypertension and non-insulin-dependent diabetes mellitus were significantly higher in low-birth-weight infants. To date, the most widely accepted explanation of this would be an adaptation of the fetus to a limited supply of nutrients. In doing so, the fetus would permanently change its physiology and metabolism and accelerate its postnatal growth as a result of good living conditions, but this may lead to excessive demand on limited cell mass (ERIKSSON 2000).

The diagnosis of FGR begins with the identification of maternal risk factors (smoking, previous growth-restricted infant, hypertension, etc.). FGR can also arise because of different conditions such as chromosome defects, infection, uteroplacental insufficiency, severe pre-eclampsia or drugs. Despite the diversity of causes of FGR, they all have as consequence that the fetus will not achieve its optimal growth. By contrast, the concept of the small for gestational age (SGA) fetus is purely statistical (i.e., less than the 10th centile for the gestational age). SGA fetuses are caused by genetic factors and are probably appropriately nourished in utero.

Every small fetus should have a detailed anatomical assessment, as the early recognition of a cause of FGR could help in adequate management of the pregnancy. The next step is to distinguish between fetuses affected by hypoxemia and those normally oxygenated. This is possible by analyzing by Doppler the fetoplacental circulation; the benefit of Doppler measurements in the umbilical artery in a high-risk population, is well documented (ALFIREVIC and NEILSON 1995).

The aim of this chapter is to better define FGR and to discuss the role of the obstetrical ultrasound in optimizing its management.

2.1.2
Definition

Until recent years, the diagnosis of FGR and SGA was postnatal. A birth weight below the 10th centile for gestational age is associated with an increased risk of poor outcome. Yet, approximately 70% fetuses with a birth weight below the 10th percentile are constitutionally small (SGA) (OTT 1988). Furthermore, there is no agreement as to which cut-off point should be used (the 10th, 5th or 3rd centile) for the diagnosis (SEEDS 1984, VARMA 1984). As FGR does not affect all fetal organs equally, a ponderal index (PI) was added (weight/length) (LUBCHENCO 1966). While the concept of PI might be appropriate in the neonatal period, it does not help the obstetricians in charge of the antenatal management.

Routine pregnancy dating by ultrasound has been practiced in developed countries for more than 20 years. Ultrasound obstetrical biometry is now the key examination for assessing fetal age, size and growth. Among all the parameters studied, fetal weight correlates most closely with the abdominal size (SMITH et al. 1997). Yet, the estimation of fetal weight by US carries a 10–15% error. Still, the abdominal circumference (AC) is the most appropriate criterion for the evaluation of fetal growth. Serial ultrasound measurements are needed to distinguish SGA from FGR fetuses. Growth is a dynamic process and at least two measurements are required (ideally ≥2 weeks apart) to assess growth rate. On the other hand, no single ultrasound parameter can be used to establish the diagnosis of utero-placental insufficiency and to fulfill all the criteria of FGR. The following data have to be evaluated: elevated resistance index (RI) in the umbilical arteries, reduced amniotic fluid, elevated head/abdomen circumference ratio, coexisting maternal pre-eclampsia, elevated RI/diastolic notches in the proximal uterine arteries (KINGDOM and SMITH 2000).

2.1.3
Ultrasound Assessment

The obstetrical ultrasound examination provides information about the size of the fetus, its morphology, its environment and its well-being.

2.1.3.1
Ultrasound Biometry

Biparietal diameter (BPD), head circumference (HC), abdominal circumference (AC) and femur length (FL) are commonly measured for the assessment of fetal size. Fetal growth is a complex phenomenon that is not necessarily linear, and each fetus has an individualized profile of growth. Furthermore, there are differences in fetal growth between countries, sexes and ethnic groups. This means that a standardized growth curve cannot be used invariably in every population and specific charts for different communities should be used whenever possible (DEGANI 2001). Unfortunately, this has not been applied on a large series of fetuses and the clinical yield of such curves has still to be determined. Therefore, several authors have started to determine customized growth curves. A ratio of head to abdominal size is proposed to detect asymmetrical growth of fetuses which represent almost 70% of FGR. The ratio is presumed to reflect the "brain sparing effect" related to the capacity of the fetus to adapt and redistribute its cardiac output in favor of vital organs (GOLDENBERG and CLIVER 1997, LIN and SAMBOYA-FORGAS 1998). Contradictory results are obtained concerning whether or not HC/AC ratios improve the accuracy of the diagnosis of FGR (DASHE et al. 2000, OTT 2001). Furthermore, fetuses with symmetrical and asymmetrical FGR have similar acid-base status results as tested by cordocentesis (BLACKWELL et al. 2001).

The efficacy of ultrasound biometry to predict a small fetus or infant depends upon the definition of "smallness" (cut-off values, e.g., AC < 5th centile), and the prevalence of the condition. Very wide ranges of sensitivity (11–94%) and positive predictive value (17–92%) were found in studying various antenatal and neonatal biometric criteria in different populations (SECHER et al. 1987). AC offers the best sensitivity (95%) but lower positive prediction (36%) (BROWN et al. 1987).

As the "classical measurements" do not discriminate well between SGA and FGR fetuses, other measurements have been proposed . The growth of the transverse cerebellar diameter (TCD) seems less affected by FGR and the TCD/AC ratio could be a good method for detecting FGR. This theory has been questioned by some and a prospective large-scale study has to confirm this hypothesis (GOLDENBERG et al. 1989, TONSONG et al. 1999).

Evaluation of the subcutaneous adipose tissue and other soft tissues has been extensively studied. Unfortunately, there is a wide overlap between FGR and non-retarded fetuses (HILL et al. 1992, GARDEIL et al. 1999).

Recently, fetal hepatic size or volume have been evaluated for the detection of FGR., The preliminary results are contradictory (CHANG et al. 1997, ROBERTS et al. 1999). Measurements of the fetal organ volumes using techniques such as magnetic resonance imaging (MR imaging) might help in fetal assessment (BAKER et al. 1995).

The combination of fetal biometry with serial measurements and Doppler enhances the detection of FGR. The best method of diagnosis seems to couple AC or estimated fetal weight with umbilical artery Doppler evaluation (OTT 1999, CRAIGO et al. 1996).

2.1.3.2
Amniotic Fluid

Oligohydramnios is frequently associated with FGR but is not related to a poorer prognosis (LIN et al. 1990, MCCURDY and SEEDS 1993). The ultrasound assessment of amniotic fluid volume is performed by measuring the deepest pool or by calculating the amniotic fluid index (AFI) (PHELAN et al. 1987). The measurement of amniotic fluid pockets has been shown to be of some value when included in the biophysical score (MANNING et al. 1980).

2.1.3.3
Placental Morphology

The placental morphology has been extensively studied in relation to FGR; the placenta tends to be smaller in FGR fetuses and its maturation tends to be more advanced according to the Grannum classification (GRANNUM and HOBBINS 1979). One study suggested a reduction in perinatal mortality when obstetricians were informed of a Grannum's grade 3 placenta (PROUD and GRANT 1987). However, to date this method has not been established as a potential screening tool for FGR. It is noteworthy that in Baker's theory, low-birth-weight neonates with a thick placenta presented the highest risk for long-term complications (BARKER et al. 1990).

2.1.3.4
Doppler Ultrasound

After a careful ultrasonic evaluation of the fetal anatomy and fetal biometry, the next step is to evaluate the risk of hypoxemia and/or acidemia. Fetal oxygenation is best assessed by Doppler ultrasound. Several factors may lead to uteroplacental insufficiency, including deficient peripheral villous development, accelerated trophoblast apoptosis, placental infarcts and decreased trophoblast invasion. These can all lead to hemodynamic changes, with increased resistance to flow in both fetal (umbilical arteries) and maternal (uterine arteries) vessels. This phenomenon leads to decreased velocity in the arteries, especially during diastole. Angle-independent parameters such as the pulsatility index (PI) or the resistance index (RI) are obtained from peripheral arteries and veins and reflect downstream blood flow resistance (GOSLING and KING 1975, POURCELOT 1974). In cases of hypoxemia, the fetus shows sequential progression from adaptation to decompensation. First, a peripheral vasoconstriction is observed while cerebral vessels show a reduction of PI or RI values due to vasodilatation (the "brain sparing effect"). At the level of the umbilical arteries, diastolic flow can be absent or even reversed. Venous flow can also be modified by hypoxemia (SENAT et al. 2000).

Therefore, Doppler velocity flow studies are important both for diagnosis and for management of FGR.

2.1.3.4.1
Umbilical Artery

In FGR, PI or RI can be increased. The absence of or reversed end-diastolic flow (A/REDF) is associated with significant placental structural damage and fetal compromise (Figs. 2.1, 2.2). ARED carries a 36% risk of perinatal death (NEILSON and ALFIREVIC 1997). Moreover absent or reversed end-diastolic flow velocity associated with FGR is followed by an increased risk of intellectual impairment, neurodevelopmental delay and mental retardation when compared with appropriate-for-gestational-age preterm infants of the same gestational age (WIENERROITHER et al. 2001, VOSSBECK et al. 2001).

Several randomized controlled trials have been carried out concerning the use of umbilical artery Doppler velocimetry in high-risk pregnancies. They all conclude that the use of this technique reduces perinatal morbidity and mortality (DIVON and FERBER 2001).

In a recent study BASCHAT and WEINER (2000) observed in a population of SGA fetuses that no fetus with normal Doppler flow measurement had metabolic acidemia at birth. They even suggested that antenatal surveillance is unnecessary in fetuses with SGA and normal umbilical artery Doppler indices. This opinion has been contradicted by others (MCCOWAN et al. 2000), who demonstrated that the perinatal outcome of small fetuses with normal Doppler findings is not always benign. Further studies are needed.

In low-risk pregnancies, the systematic use of Doppler studies has no statistically detectable effects

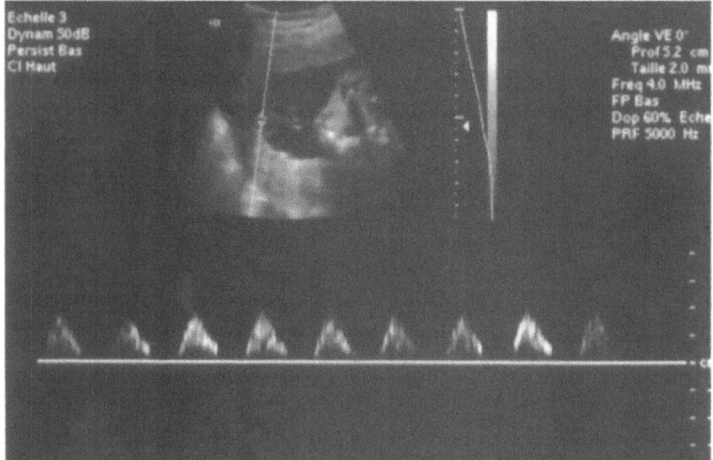

Fig. 2.1. Doppler of the umbilical artery in a growth-restricted fetus demonstrating absent diastolic flow

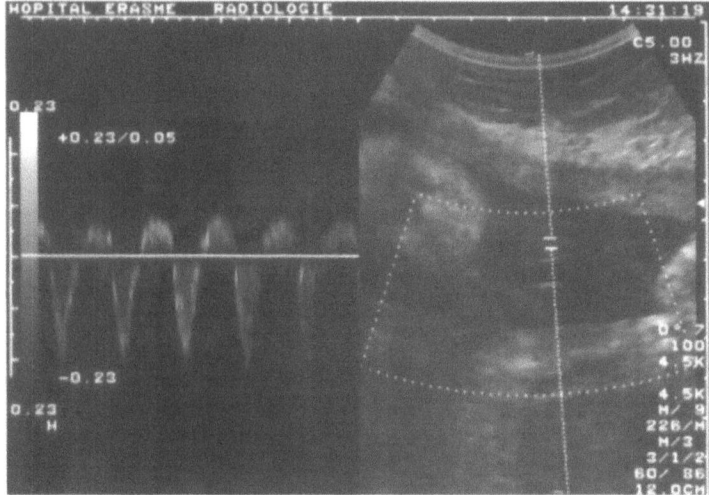

Fig. 2.2. Doppler of the umbilical artery in fetal growth restriction (FGR) with reversed diastolic flow

on perinatal mortality and does not seem to be beneficial (GOFFINET et al. 1997).

2.1.3.4.2
Cerebral Circulation

The middle cerebral artery (MCA) is the most commonly studied fetal vessel. The diastolic blood flow in the MCA increases with gestational age, particularly through the third trimester (MARI and DETER 1992b). Thus, increased diastolic blood flow may be a more useful test in the preterm than the term fetus. In FGR fetuses there is a redistribution of blood flow to the cerebral circulation with increasing flow and low MCA resistance index (Fig. 2.3) (WOO et al. 1987). Cerebroplacental ratios have been studied, for instance the ratio between the resistance indices of the middle cerebral artery and the umbilical artery (UA). This ratio remains constant throughout pregnancy but decreases in fetuses with FGR (GRAMELLINI et

al. 1992). Several studies have shown significant differences in the neonatal outcome when these ratios are abnormal (OTT 1991, ARIAS 1994, STERNE et al. 2001) and suggest that the MCA/UA ratio has the best sensitivity in predicting neonatal outcome in FGR fetuses (GUZMAN et al. 1995). A sudden rise in resistance or pulsatility index of the MCA Doppler velocimetry in FGR fetuses with blood flow redistribution has been suggested to be predictive of a poor prognosis (MARI and DETER 1992a). This phenomenon is called "reversal of adaptation" and can show daily variation (MARI and DETER 1992b). In the case of an abnormal UA Doppler velocimetry and a persistent fall in volume flow of the MCA (i.e., the MCA PI increases by more than 20–30% of its value for gestational age over a 48h period) delivery should be considered (KONJE et al. 2001). Recently the observation of absence or reversal of end-diastolic velocity in the aortic isthmus has been proposed as a simple and indirect index of cerebral oxygenation and pos-

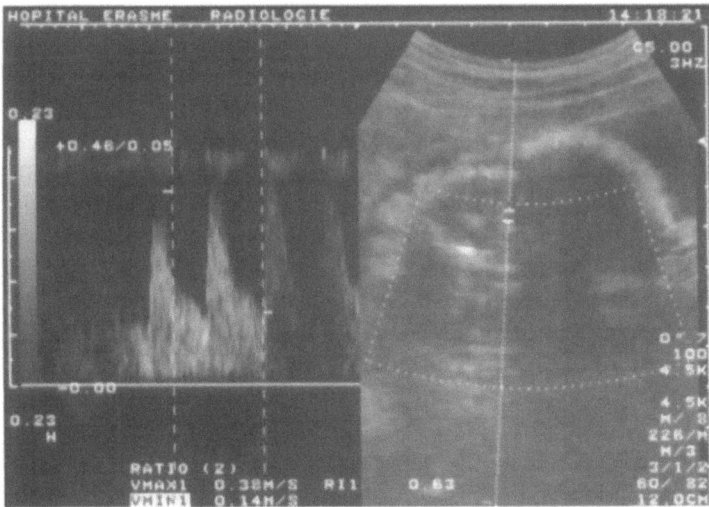

Fig. 2.3. Doppler study of a cerebral artery demonstrating increased diastolic flow in FGR (sparing effect)

sible correlation with fetal cerebral hypoxic damage (BRANTBERG et al. 1999, FOURON et al. 2001).

2.1.3.4.3
Other Vessels

Doppler studies on smaller arteries such as the renal artery have been performed. Correlation has been found between PI values and the fetal arterial pO_2 and the quantity of amniotic fluid in FGR fetuses (VYAS et al. 1989, ARDUINI and RIZZO 1991). This concept of increased renal vascular resistance in FGR fetuses was not confirmed by more recent studies, suggesting that urine production is reduced because of reduced kidney size (STIGTER et al. 2001).

The venous system and cardiac activity can also be influenced by hypoxemia. Several Doppler indices have been studied at the level of the vena cava, the ductus venosus, the umbilical vein and the heart. In the final stages of placental insufficiency, cardiac dysfunction can be observed. Cardiac dysfunction elevates central venous pressure, which is reflected by increasing venous indices, reverse flow in the vena cava and the ductus venosus, and finally venous pulsations in the umbilical vein (SEVERI et al. 2000, SENAT et al. 2000, BASCHAT et al. 2001). The perinatal outcome is significantly poorer in the latter cases.

2.1.3.4.4
Screening by Uterine Artery Velocimetry

In theory, placental "insufficiency" could be detected by Doppler studies in the uterine arteries. Doppler PI or RI have been studied during the entire pregnancy and the presence or absence of an early diastolic notch has been observed (Fig. 2.4). An association

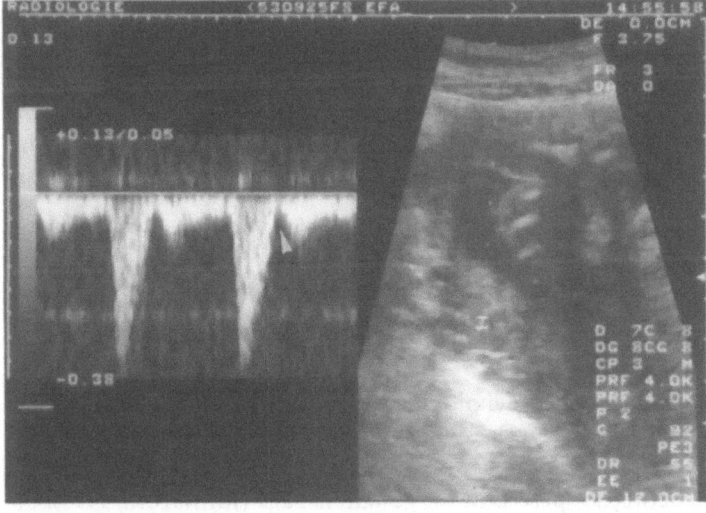

Fig. 2.4. Doppler study of a uterine artery. A protodiastolic notch is present (*arrowhead*)

was demonstrated between waveform alteration in the uterine artery and pre-eclampsia (Campbell et al. 1983), perinatal death, FGR and abruptio placentae (Jacobson et al. 1990, Bewley et al. 1991). High positive predictive values are not achieved in all studies, reflecting the differences in prevalence of obstetric complications in each studied population. In a low-risk population, screening by Doppler of the uterine artery does not seem to be justified (Irion et al. 1998). This concept was confirmed in a recent study of screening by uteroplacental artery Doppler flow velocity. The test was performed between 20 and 24 weeks' gestation in low-risk pregnant women followed by the prescription of low-dose aspirin in cases with an abnormal result. The incidence of FGR or pre-eclampsia was not reduced. The authors plead for future studies assessing predictive tests early in pregnancy (Goffinet et al. 2001).

2.1.3.5
Biophysical Profile Score

The most commonly used scoring system is that of Manning et al. (1980). The BPS determines fetal well-being using biophysical variables (breathing, movements, tone, amniotic fluid volume, fetal heart rate). Each of these variables is assigned a score of 2 (normal) or 0 (abnormal). A normal BPS is reassuring; the risk of fetal death within 7 days of a normal BPS is 0.6/1000 and a normal BPS excludes acidemia (Manning 1997). The likelihood of developing fetal distress with an abnormal score (0–4/10) is 67%. However, sequential alterations of arterial and venous flow usually precede the appearance of an abnormal BPS. It has been demonstrated that 63% of FGR fetuses delivered for abnormal BPS (≤4/10) had deterioration of venous flow 1 or 2 days earlier (Baschat et al. 2001).

2.1.4
Multiparameter Approach in Perinatal Management

FGR is a complex multisystem disorder, and the combination of Doppler velocity waveform analysis and the ultrasonic estimation of fetal growth (fetal weight, abdominal circumference) is the best choice to diagnose the disease and to evaluate the fetal compromise. When a diagnosis of FGR is made, serial examinations have to be proposed including fetal growth evaluation, Doppler velocity waveform studies and biophysical testing. The interval between successive examinations has not been standardized, and depends on which test is used and the clinical situation. To prevent perinatal mortality and morbidity, the optimal time for delivery has to be defined; there must be a balance between premature delivery and the risk of continuing the pregnancy with FGR. This decision depends not only on the results of the antenatal testing but also on the individual clinical situation (Harrington 2000). Prolonging a gestation with intensive fetal monitoring may be beneficial or harmful depending on gestational age, severity of FGR and maternal condition (hypertension, etc.). The results of the GRIT (Growth Restriction Intervention Trial) study, which is a randomized trial of timed delivery for preterm FGR fetuses, may provide data regarding the value of an obstetrical multiparameter approach. The results are to be published in 2003 and the endpoint is pediatric neurodevelopment at ≥2 years old (Grit Study Group 1996).

2.2
Macrosomia

2.2.1
Introduction

The concept of macrosomia has been recognized for a long time. In the sixteenth century François Rabelais told the story of the birth of a " giant baby" – Pantagruel – who was "so amazingly large and heavy that he could not come into the world without suffocating his mother". Delivery of a big baby is associated with many maternal and fetal complications: prolonged labor, operative vaginal delivery, cesarean section, shoulder dystocia, birth asphyxia, brachial nerve palsy, clavicular fracture and meconium aspiration (Mocanu et al. 2000).

Macrosomia is a multifactorial condition, and no single diagnostic method has yet been validated. The purpose of this section is to review the most commonly used tests and their implication in the perinatal management.

2.2.2
Definition and Etiological Factors

The definition of macrosomia varies in the literature. The classic definition of a large-for-gestational-age (LGA) fetus is a birth weight larger than the 95th percentile for gestational age (Johnstone 1996); the use of this definition includes a substantial proportion of normal babies. Other studies define macrosomia as a birth weight greater than 4000 g, 4100 g, 4500 g or 4536 g (GOLDITCH 1978, MONDALOU et al. 1980).The ACOG definition of macrosomia is a birth weight of more than 4500 g (ACOG 1991, 2001). In the United States about 10% of newborns weigh more than 4000 g.

The growth and the development of the fetus depend on several factors: the maternal environment, the placenta, genetic and hormonal factors. Certain factors such as multiparity, macrosomia antecedents, maternal height and weight, and postdated pregnancy have been associated with macrosomia (UDALL et al. 1978, CHEVERNAK et al. 1989). The size, the weight or the percentile do not permit the categorization of a large fetus as a functionally normal fetus or an abnormally large one in a pregnancy complicated by diabetes. The risk of perinatal morbidity and mortality is higher in the second category. Some fetal syndromes are also associated with abnormal accelerated growth, including Beckwith-Wiedemann syndrome, Weaver syndrome, Sotos syndrome, Simpson-Golabi-Behmel syndrome and congenital hyperinsulinemia (LANGER 2000).

2.2.3
Ultrasound Evaluation

An AC greater than the 90th percentile during the third trimester is associated with fetal macrosomia. Different ratios have been calculated: head to chest ratio (WLADIMIROFF et al. 1978), FL/AC (HADLOCK et al. 1985a), AC/FL (BRACERO et al. 1985). The sensitivities for detecting a LGA fetus are between 45% and 80%. An AC of 35 or 38 cm has been proposed as a predictor of macrosomia (GILBY et al. 2000). The interval from the ultrasound study to delivery was about 21/2 days. If the cut-off was AC +35 cm, the reported sensitivity to predict an infant weighing more than 4500 g was 98.5%, the negative predictive value was 99% but the false-positive rate was 34%. A cut-off at 38 cm was associated with a lower sensitivity of 53% and a greater specificity of 96%. The AC was a better predictor of a birth weight >4500 g than >4000 g. In view of these results, the best use of the AC would be in the exclusion of macrosomia; the risk of a macrosomic infant was <1% with an AC <35 cm.

Many formulas have been applied in fetal weight estimation. The detection rate of macrosomia (birth weight greater than 4000 g or 4500 g) is between 33% and 82%, with a specificity of 70–100%, a positive

predictive value of 40–83% and a negative predictive value of 68–92% (DEGANI 2001). Moreover, the accuracy of estimating fetal weight decreases with increasing birth weight (DUDLEY 1995). Recently, SOKOL et al. analyzed retrospectively the data of 4831 cases with estimated fetal weight obtained 14 days before delivery. The authors used a new computerized formula and compared it with the formula of HADLOCK et al. (1985b). They used the traditional measurements of AC, FL and HC. Of 4831 newborns, 308 (6.4%) had a birth weight >4000 g, and 56 (1.2%) had a birth weight >4500 g. In 154 pregnancies complicated by diabetes mellitus, 26 (16.9%) infants weighted more than 4000 g, and 5 (3.2%) more than 4500 g. They found that AC had a greater reliability than HC or FL in estimation of fetal weight. They improved the performance of ultrasound detection of macrosomia by taking into account that different groups of patients (maternal height, weight, the presence of diabetes mellitus) need different equations, although this approach still needs to be validated (SOKOL et al. 2000).

Another method of investigation is the measurement of soft tissue. It was shown that although neonatal fat mass represents only 14% of birth weight, it accounts for 46% of its variation (CATALANO et al. 1992). Different measurements have been proposed: cheek-to-cheek diameter (ABRAMOWICZ et al. 1991), humeral, shoulder, femoral, abdominal subcutaneous tissue thickness (SOOD et al. 1995, MINTZ et al. 1989, ROTMENSCH et al. 1999, PETRIKOVSKI et al. 1997). These measurements used as independent predictors of macrosomia or integrated in a fetal weight estimation formula do not really improve the detection rate compared with using AC alone (O'REILLY-GREEN and DIVON 2000, CHAUHAN et al. 2000). The optimal cut-off for abdominal subcutaneous tissue thickness as a predictor of birth weight +4000 g was a thickness +11 mm (PETRIKOVSKI et al. 1997).

Three-dimensional (3D) volume ultrasound has been proposed for the estimation of fetal weight (ZELOP 2000). Upper arm, thigh and abdominal volumes have been measured. In a recent study, a new 3D formula was tested for estimating fetal weight (SCHILD et al. 2000). This showed a better accuracy than conventional 2D fetal weight estimation by including soft tissue volume. However, 3D ultrasound is more time-consuming than 2D and the authors conclude that further studies are needed to estimate the value the method at the extremes of fetal weight.

MR imaging has recently been used to take shoulder measurements of fetuses with suspected macrosomia (TUKEVA et al. 2001). This technique was evaluated in eight fetuses of diabetic pregnant women and the first results show a statically significant correlation between the MR imaging measurements and the actual shoulder width.

2.2.4
Maternal and Clinical Estimates of Birth Weight

In one study, multiparous women were asked intrapartum to predict the birth weight of their fetus. They were asked whether the fetus felt bigger or smaller than in their previous pregnancy. The mothers' estimates were better than clinical or sonographic ones (70% of maternal estimates were within 10% of birth weight) (CHAUHAN et al. 1992).

Clinical estimates of birth weight (palpation and symphysial fundal height measurements) have wide variations in sensitivity (24–97%) and specificity (82–98%) (O'REILLY-GREEN AND DIVON 2000). To predict a birth weight more than 4500 g, sensitivities reported are between 10% and 100% and the specificities from 92% to 100%. In comparison with the commonly sonographic methods, clinical examination performs equally well or better.

2.2.5
Perinatal Management

The incidence of fetal macrosomia has been reported to be increasing (GOLDENBERG et al. 1983, BAKER et al. 1992) and perinatal management of these pregnancies is still controversial. Many complications can be associated with "big" babies, shoulder dystocia that can produce brachial plexus injury, hypoxia and even death being some of the most studied. The incidence of shoulder dystocia increases with birth weight and about 50% of shoulder dystocia occurs with a birth weight >4000 g (LANGER et al. 1991). The reported incidence of shoulder dystocia is 3–13% when the birth weight is >4000 g (ACKER et al. 1985). This emphasizes the need to diagnose the macrosomic fetus; however, as has been seen in this chapter, the value of fetal biometry in predicting fetal macrosomia is not clinically useful. Moreover, no obstetrical measure has been validated to date; induced labor for fetal macrosomia does not reduce the cesarean delivery rate (HORRIGAN 2001), the estimation of fetal weight is not useful in the prediction of shoulder dystocia (SACKS and CHEN 2000) and the low incidence of shoulder dystocia and its complications does not

justify elective cesarean section for suspected macrosomia (MOCANU et al. 2000).

References

Abramowicz JS, Sherer DM, Bar-Tov E, Woods JR (1991) The cheek-to-cheek diameter in the ultrasonographic assessment of fetal growth. Am J Obstet Gynecol 165:846-852
Acker DB, Gregory KD, Sachs BP, Friedman ED (1988) Risk factors for shoulder dystocia. Obstet Gynecol 66:762-768
Alfirevic A, Neilson JP (1995) Doppler ultrasonography in high-risk pregnancies: systematic review with meta-analysis. Am J Obstet Gynecol 172:1379-1387
Allen MC (1984) Developmental outcome and follow-up of the small for gestational age infant. Semin Perinatol 8:123-156
ACOG (2001) American College of Obstetricians and Gynecologists issues guidelines on fetal macrosomia. Am Fam Physician 64:169-170
Arduini A, Rizzo G (1991) Fetal renal artery velocity waveforms and amniotic fluid volume in growth retarded and post-term fetuses. Obstet Gynecol 77:370-373
Arias F (1994) Accuracy of the middle cerebral-to-umbilical artery resistance index ratio in the prediction of neonatal outcome in patients at high risk for fetal and neonatal complication. Am J Obstet Gynecol 171:1541-1545
Baker DJP, Gluckman PO, Godfrey KM, et al (1993) Fetal nutrition and cardiovascular disease in adult life. Lancet 341:938-941
Baker P, Lever P, Gorton E (1992) An increasing incidence of fetal macrosomia. J Obstet Gynecol 12:281
Baker PN, Johnson IR, Gowland PA, Hykin J, Adams V, Mansfield P, et al (1995) Measurement of fetal liver, brain and placental volumes with echo-planar magnetic resonance imaging. Br J Obstet Gynecol 102:35-39
Barker DJP, Bull AR, Osmond C, Simmonds SJ (1990) Fetal and placental size and risk of hypertension in adult life. BMJ 301:259-262
Baschat AA, Weiner CP (2000) Umbilical artery Doppler screening for detection of the small fetus in need of antepartum surveillance. Am J Obstet Gynecol 182:154-158
Baschat AA, Gembruch U, Weiner CP, et al (2001) In severe growth restriction (IUGR), Doppler deteriorates before biophysical parameters worsen (abstract). Am J Obstet Gynecol 184:102
Bewley S, Cooper D, Campbell S (1991) Doppler investigation of uteroplacental blood flow resistance in the second trimester: a screening study for pre-eclampsia and intrauterine growth retardation. Br J Obstet Gynaecol 98:871-879
Blackwell SC, Moldenhauer J, Redman M, Hassan SS, Wolfe M, Berry L (2001) Relationship between sonographic pattern of intrauterine growth restriction and acid-base status at the time of cordocentesis. Arch Gynecol Obstet 264:191-193
Bracero LA, Baxi LV, Rey HR, et al (1985) Use of ultrasound in antenatal diagnosis of large for gestational age infants in diabetic gravid patients. Am J Obstet Gynecol 152:43-47
Brantberg A, Schwarzler P, Alcais A, et al (1999) Central arterial hemodynamics in small-for gestational-age fetuses

before and during maternal hyperoxygenation: a Doppler velocimetric study with particular attention to the aortic isthmus. Ultrasound Obstet Gynecol 14:237–243

Brown HL, Miller JM, Gabert HA, et al (1987) Ultrasonic recognition of the small-for gestational-age fetus. Obstet Gynecol 69:631–635

Campbell S, Diaz-Racasens J, Griffin D, Cohen-Overbeek RE, Pearce JM, Wilson K (1983) New Doppler technique for assessing uteroplacental blood flow. Lancet I: 675–679

Catalano PM, Tyzbir ED, Allen SR, McBean JH, McAuliffe TL (1992) Evaluation of fetal growth by estimation of neonatal body composition. Obstet Gynecol 79:46–50

Chang FM, Hsu K, Ko H, et al. (1997) 3D US assessment of fetal liver volume in normal pregnancies. Ultrasound Med Biol 23:381–389

Chauhan SP, Lutton PM, Bailey KJ, Guerrieri JP, Morrison JP (1992) Intrapartum clinical, sonographic, and parous patient' estimates of newborn birth weight. Obstet Gynecol 79:956–958

Chauhan SP, West DJ, Scardo JA, Boyd JM, Joiner J, Hendrix NW (2000) Antepartum detection of macrosomic fetus: clinical versus sonographic, including soft-tissue measurements. Obstet Gynecol 95:639–642

Chevernak JL, Divon MY, Hirsch J, et al (1989) Macrosomia in postdate pregnancy: Is routine sonographic screening indicated? Am J Obstet Gynecol 161:753

Craigo SD, Beach ML, Harvey-Wilkes KB, D'Alton ME (1996) Ultrasound predictors of neonatal outcome in intrauterine growth restriction. Am J Perinatol 13:465–471

Dashe JS, McIntire DD, Lucas MJ, Leveno KJ (2000) Effects of symmetric and asymmetric fetal growth on pregnancy outcomes. Obstet Gynecol 96:321–327

Degani S (2001) Fetal biometry: clinical, pathological and technical considerations. Obstet Gynecol Surv 56:159–167

Divon M, Ferber A (2001) Umbilical artery Doppler velocimetry: an update. Semin Perinatol 25:44–47

Dudley NJ (1995) Selection of appropriate ultrasound methods for the estimation of fetal weight. Br J Radiol 68:385–388

Eriksson J, Forsen T, Tuomilehto J, Osmond C, Barker D (2000) Fetal and childhood growth and hypertension in adult life. Hypertension 36:790–794

Fouron JC, Gosselin J, Amiel-Tison C, Infante-Rivard C, Fouron C, Skoll A, Veilleux A (2001) Correlation between prenatal velocity waveforms in the aortic isthmus and neurodevelopmental outcome between the ages of 2 and 4 years. Am J Obstet Gynecol 184:630–636

Gardeil F, Greene R, Stuart B, Turner MJ (1999) Subcutaneous fat in fetal abdomen as a predictor of growth restriction. Obstet Gynecol 94:209–212

Gilby JR, Williams MC, Spellacy WN (2000) Fetal abdominal circumference measurements of 35 and 38 cm as predictors of macrosomia: a risk factor for shoulder dystocia. J Reprod Med 45:936–938

Goffinet F, Paris-Llado J, Nisand I, et al (1997) Umbilical artery Doppler velocimetry in unselected and low risk pregnancies: a review of randomized controlled trials. Br J Obstet Gynaecol 104:425–430

Goffinet F, Aboulker D, Paris-Llado J, Bucourt M, Uzan M, Papiernik E, Bréart G (2001) Screening with a uterine doppler in low risk pregnant women followed by low dose aspirin in women with abnormal results: a multicenter randomised controlled trial. Br J Obstet Gynaecol 108: 510–518

Goldenberg RL, Cliver SP (1997) Small for gestational age and IUGR: definitions and standards. Clinic Obstet Gynecol 40: 704–714

Goldenberg RL, Humphrey JL, Hale CB, et al (1983) Neonatal deaths in Alabama, 1970–1980: an analysis of birth weight and race-specific neonatal mortality rates. Am J Obstet Gynecol 145:545–555

Goldenberg RL, Cutter GR, Hoffman HJ, et al (1989) IUGR: standards for diagnosis. Am J Obstet Gynecol 161:271–277

Golditch IM (1978) The large fetus: management and outcome. Obstet Gynecol 52:26–30

Gosling RG, King DH (1975) Ultrasonic angiology. In: Harcus AW, Adamson L (eds) Arteries and veins. Edinburgh: Churchill-Livingstone, pp 61–98

Gramellini D, Folli MC, Raboni S, et al (1992) Cerebral umbilical Doppler ratio as a predictor of adverse perinatal outcome. Obstet Gynecol 79:416–420

Grannum PA, Hobbins JC (1979) The ultrasound changes in the maturing placenta and their relationship to fetal pulmonic maturity. Am J Obstet Gynecol 133:915–922

GRIT Study Group (1996) When do obstetricians recommend delivery for high-risk preterm growth-retarded fetus? Eur J Obstet Gynecol Reprod Biol 67:121–126

Guzman E, Vintzileos A, Martins M (1995) Relationship between middle cerebral artery velocimetry, computer fetal heart rate assessment and degree of academia at birth in intrauterine growth restricted fetuses. Am J Obstet Gynecol 172:337

Hadlock FP, Harrist RB, Fearneyhough TC, et al (1985a) Use of femur length/abdominal circumference ratio in detecting the macrosomic fetus. Radiology 154:503–505

Hadlock FP, Harrist RB, Sharman RS, et al (1985b) Estimation of fetal weight with the use of head, body, and femur measurements: a prospective study. Am J Obstet Gynecol 151:333–337

Harrington KF (2000) Making best and appropriate use of fetal biophysical and Doppler ultrasound data in the management of the growth restricted fetus. Ultrasound Obstet Gynecol 16:399–401

Hill IM, Guzick D, Doyles D, et al (1992) Subcutaneous tissue thickness can not be used to distinguish abnormalities of fetal growth. Obstet Gynecol 80:268–271

Horrigan TJ (2001) Physicians who induce labor for fetal macrosomia do not reduce cesarean delivery rates. J Perinatol 21:93–96

Irion O, Massé J, Forest JC, Moutquin JM (1998) Prediction of pre-eclampsia, low birthweight for gestation and prematurity by uterine artery velocity waveform analysis in low risk nulliparous women. Br J Obstet Gynaecol 105:422–429

Jacobson SL, Imhof R, Manning N, et al (1990) The value of Doppler assessment of the uteroplacental circulation in predicting preeclampsia or intrauterine growth retardation. Am J Obstet Gynecol 162:110–114

Johnstone FD, Prescott RJ, Steel JM, Mao JH, Chambers S, Muir N (1996) Clinical and ultrasound prediction of macrosomia in diabetics pregnancy. Br J Obstet Gynaecol 103: 747–754

Kingdom J, Smith G (2000) Diagnosis and management of IUGR. In: Kingdom J, Baker P (eds) Intrauterine growth restriction. Springer, Berlin Heidelberg New York, pp 257–273

Konje JC, Bell S, Taylor DJ (2001) Abnormal doppler velocimetry and blood flow volume in the middle cerebral artery in severe intrauterine growth restriction: Is the occurrence of reversal of compensatory flow too late? Br J Obstet Gynaecol 108:973–979

Langer O (2000) Fetal macrosomia: etiologic factors. Clin Obstet Gynecol 43:283–297

Langer O, Berkus MD, Huff RW, Samueloff A (1991) Shoulder dystocia: should the fetus weighing greater than or equal to 4000 grams be delivered by cesarean section? Am J Obstet Gynecol 165:831–837

Lin CC, Samboya-Forgas z (1998) Current concepts of FGR. Obstet Gynecol 92:1044–1055

Lin CC, Sheikh Z, Lopata R (1990) The association between oligohydramnios and IUGR. Obstet Gynecol 76:1100–1104

Lubchenco LO, Hansman C, Boyd E (1966) Intrauterine growth in length and head circumference as estimated from live births at gestational age from 26–42 weeks. Pediatrics 37:403

Manning FA (1997) Fetal biophysical profile: a critical appraisal. Fetal Matern Med Rev 9:103–123

Manning FA, Platt LD, Sipos L (1980) Antepartum fetal evaluation: the development of fetal biophysical profile score. Am J Obstet Gynecol 136:187–195

Mari G, Deter RL (1992a) Middle cerebral flow velocity waveform and fetal compromise. Am J Obstet Gynecol 168:1336

Mari G, Deter RL (1992b) Middle cerebral artery flow velocity waveforms in normal and small-for-gestational-age fetuses. Am J Obstet Gynecol 166:1262–1270

McCowan LM, Harding JE, Stewart EW (2000) Umbilical artery studies in small for gestational age babies reflect disease severity. Br J Obstet Gynaecol 107:916–925

McCurdy CM, Seeds JW (1993) Oligohydramnios. Semin Perinatol 17:183–196

Mintz MC, Landon MB, Gabbe SG, et al (1989) Shoulder soft tissue width as a predictor of macrosomia in diabetic pregnancies. Am J Perinatol 6:240

Mocanu E, Greene R, Byrne M, Turner M (2000) Obstetric and neonatal outcome of babies weighing more than 4.5 kg: an analysis by parity. Eur J Obstet Gynaecol 92:229–233

Mondalou HD, Dorchester WL, Thorosian A, et al (1980) Macrosomia: maternal, fetal, and neonatal complication. Obstet Gynecol 55:420

Neilson JP, Alfirevic Z (1997) Doppler ultrasound in high risk pregnancies. Cochrane Library, issue 4

O'Reilly-Green C, Divon M (2000) Sonographic and clinical methods in the diagnosis of macrosomia. Clin Obstet Gynecol 43:309–320

Ott WJ (1988) The diagnosis of altered fetal growth. Obstet Gynecol 15:237–263

Ott WJ (1991) Value of fetal umbilical artery and carotid doppler flow studies in the evaluation of suspected IUGR. J Matern Fetal Invest 1:185–190

Ott WJ (1999) Altered fetal growth. In: Ott WJ (ed) Clinical obstetrical ultrasound. Wiley-Liss, New York, pp 229–262

Ott WJ (2001) The ultrasonic diagnosis and evaluation of intrauterine growth restriction. Ultrasound Rev Obstet Gynecol 1:205–215

Pattinson RC, Odendaal HJ, Kisten G (1993) The relationship between absent end-diastolic velocities of the umbilical artery and perinatal mortality and morbidity . Early Hum Dev 33:61–9

Petrikovski BM, Oleschuk C, Lesser M, Gelertner N, Gross B (1997) Prediction of fetal macrosomia using sonographically measured abdominal subcutaneous tissue thickness. J Clin Ultrasound 25:378–382

Phelan JP, Ahn MO, Smith CV, Rutherford SE, Anderson E (1987) Amniotic fluid index measurements during pregnancy. J Reprod Med 32:601–604

Pourcelot L (1974) Application clinique de l'examen Doppler transcutané. In: Peronneau P (ed) Velocimetric ultrasonore Doppler. INSERM, Paris, pp 213–240

Proud J, Grant AM (1987) Third trimester placental grading by ultrasonography as a test of fetal wellbeing. BMJ 294:1641–1644

Roberts AB, Mitchell JM, McCowan LM, Barker S (1999) US measurements in the SGA fetus. Am J Obstet Gynecol 180:634–638

Rotmensch S, Celentano C, Liberati M, et al (1999) Screening efficacy of the subcutaneous tissue width/femur length ratio for fetal macrosomia in the nondiabetic pregnancy. Ultrasound Obstet Gynecol 13:340–344

Sacks DA, Chen W(2000) Estimation of fetal weight in the management of macrosomia. Obstet Gynecol Surv 55:229–239

Schauseil-Zipf U, Hamm W, Stenzel B, Bolte A, Gladtke E (1989) Severe intrauterine growth retardation: obstetrical management and follow-up studies in children born between 1970 and 1985. Eur J Obstet Gynecol Reprod Biol 30:1–9

Schild RL, Fimmers R, Hansmann M (2000) Fetal weight estimation by three-dimensional ultrasound. Ultrasound Obstet Gynecol 16:445–452

Secher NJ, Kern Hansen P, Lenstrup C, Sindberg Eriksen P, Morsing GA (1987) A randomized study of fetal abdominal diameter and fetal weight estimation for detection of light-for-gestation infants in low risk pregnancies. Br J Obstet Gynaecol 94:105–109

Seeds JW (1984) Impaired fetal growth: definition and clinical diagnosis. Obstet Gynecol 64:415–422

Senat MV, Schwarzler P, Alcais A, et al (2000) Longitudinal changes in the ductus venosus, cerebral transverse sinus and cardiotogram in fetal growth restriction. Ultrasound Obstet Gynecol 16:19–24

Severi FM, Rizzo G, Bocchi C, D'Antona D, Verzuri MS, Arduini D (2000) Intrauterine growth retardation and fetal cardiac function. Fetal Diagn Ther 15:8–19

Smith GC, Smith MF, McNay MB, Fleming JE (1997) The relation between fetal abdominal circumference and birthweights: findings in 3512 pregnancies. Br J Obstet Gynaecol 104:186–190

Sokol RJ, Chik L, Dombrowski MP, Zador I (2000) Correctly identifying the macrosomic fetus: improving ultrasonography-based prediction. Am J Obstet Gynecol 182:1489–1496

Sood AK, Yancey M, Richards D (1995) Prediction of fetal macrosomia using humeral soft tissue thickness. Obstet Gynecol 85:937–940

Sterne G, Shields LE, Dubinsky TJ (2001) Abnormal fetal cerebral and umbilical Doppler measurements in fetuses with intrauterine growth restriction predicts the severity of perinatal morbidity. J Clin Ultrasound 29:146–151

Stigter RH, Mulder EJH, Bruinse HW, Visser GHA (2001) Doppler studies on the fetal renal artery in the severely growth-restricted fetus. Ultrasound Obstet Gynecol 18: 141–145

Tonsong T, Wanapirek C, Thongpaduroy T (1999) US diagnosis of IUGR by transverse cerebellar (TCD)/ abdominal circumference (AC) ratio. Int J Gynaecol 180:634–638

Tukeva TA, Salmi H, Poutanen VP, Karjalainen PT, Hytinantti T, Paavonen J, Teramo KA, Aronen HJ (2001) Fetal shoulder measurements by fast and ultrafast MRI techniques. J Magn Reson Imaging 13:938–942

Udall JN, Harrison GG, Vaucher Y, et al (1978) Interaction of maternal and neonatal obesity. Pediatrics 62:17

Varma TR (1984) Low birth weight babies. The small-for-gestational age: a review of current management. Obstet Gynecol Surv 39:616–631

Vossbeck S, Kraus de Camargo O, Grab D, Bode H, Pohlandt F (2001) Neonatal and neurodevelopmental outcome in infants born before 30 weeks of gestation with absent or reversed end-diastolic flow velocities in the umbilical artery. Eur J Pediatr 160:128–134

Vyas S, Nicolaides KH, Campbell S (1989) Renal artery flow-velocity waveforms in normal and hypoxemic fetuses. Am J Obstet Gynecol 161:168–172

Wienerroither H, Steiner H, Tomaselli J, Lobendanz M, Thun-Hohenstein L (2001) Intrauterine blood flow and long-term intellectual, neurologic, and social development. Obstet Gynecol 97:449–453

Williams H, St George IM, Silva PA (1992) IUGR and blood pressure at age 7 and 18. J Clin Epidemiol 45:1257–1263

Wladimiroff JW, Bloesma CA, Wallenburg HCS (1978) Ultrasonic diagnosis of large for dates infants. Obstet Gynecol 52:285–288

Woo JK, Liang ST, Chan FY (1987) Middle cerebral artery doppler flow velocity waveforms. Obstet Gynecol 70:613–616

Zelop CM (2000) Prediction of fetal weight with the use of three-dimensional ultrasonography. Clin Obstet Gynecol 43:321–325

3 Placenta and Fetal Surroundings

Josée Dubois, Laurent Garel, Andrée Grignon

CONTENTS

3.1   The Placenta 25
3.1.1   Development 25
3.1.2   Placental Shape 25
3.1.2.1 Normal 25
3.1.2.2 Circumvallate 26
3.1.2.3 Succenturiate 26
3.1.3   Placental Size 27
3.1.3.1 Normal 27
3.1.3.2 Thin Placenta Versus Placentomalacia 27
3.1.3.3 Thick Placenta Versus Placentomegaly 27
3.1.4   Abnormalities 28
3.1.4.1 Calcifications 28
3.1.4.2 Hypoechoic Areas 29
3.1.4.3 Placental Infarct 29
3.1.5   Placental Position 30
3.1.5.1 Normal 30
3.1.5.2 Low-lying Placenta 30
3.1.5.3 Marginal and Partial Placenta Previa 30
3.1.5.4 Placenta Previa 30
3.1.5.5 Placenta Accreta 30
3.1.6   Retroplacental Area 31
3.1.6.1 Normal 31
3.1.6.2 Subchorionic or Marginal Hematoma 32
3.1.6.3 Retroplacental Hematoma
        or Abruptio Placentae 32
3.1.6.4 Tumors 33
3.2   The Umbilical Cord 34
3.2.1   Anatomy 34
3.2.2   Number of vessels 34
3.2.2.1 Single Umbilical Artery 34
3.2.2.2 Persistence of the Right Umbilical Vein 34
3.2.2.3 Multivessel Cord 34
3.2.3   Cord Length 34
3.2.3.1 Normal 34
3.2.3.2 Short Umbilical Cord 34
3.2.3.3 Long Umbilical Cord 34
3.2.3.4 Nuchal Cord 35
3.2.3.5 Cord Prolapse 35
3.2.3.6 Coiling 35
3.2.3.7 Wharton's Jelly Anomaly 35
3.2.3.8 Enlarged Cord 35
3.2.4   Cord Insertion and Attachment 35
3.2.4.1 Central 35
3.2.4.2 Eccentric Insertion 36
3.2.4.3 Velamentous Insertion 36
3.2.4.4 Vasa Previa 36
3.2.4.5 Cord Cysts and Masses 36
3.2.4.6 Membranes 37
        References 37

3.1
The Placenta

The investigation of the placenta should be routinely performed during obstetrical sonograms. Often forgotten, this organ provides essential information, especially in patients presenting with bleeding or with fetal growth anomalies. The placenta is vital for fetal survival: the transfer site for oxygen, carbon dioxide and nutrition, it also synthesizes hormones and prostaglandins. The placenta remains mysterious regarding its vascularization, synthesis and functions. There is a growing interest in research concerning these unknowns. In this chapter, we will principally define a practical approach to anomalies of the placenta and umbilical cord.

3.1.1
Development

The placenta cannot be well visualized before 10–12 weeks of gestation. True maternal blood flow is not established until 12 weeks of gestation. Plasma flow occurs in the intervillous spaces.

3.1.2
Placental Shape

3.1.2.1
Normal (Figs. 3.1–3.3)

At 10 weeks, the placenta is seen as a thickening of the hyperechoic rim of tissue around the gestational sac. At 12–13 weeks, intervillous blood is easily visualized by color or power Doppler. At 14–15 weeks, the placenta is well-defined as a discoid organ. The retroplacental complex is composed of the decidua, myo-

J. Dubois, MD; L. Garel, MD; A. Grignon, MD
Department of Medical Imaging, Sainte-Justine Hospital, 3175 Côte-Sainte-Catherine, Montréal, Québec H3T 1C5, Canada

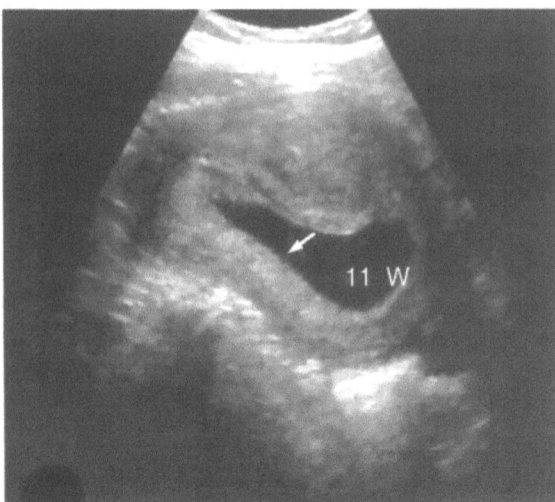

Fig. 3.1. Eleven weeks gestation. Twin pregnancy. Identification of the posterior placenta (*arrow*)

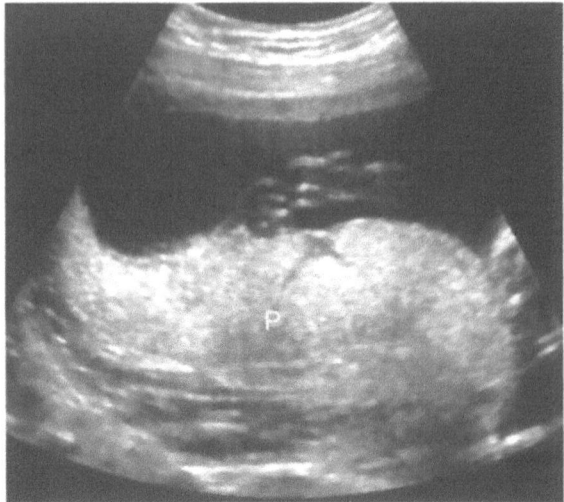

Fig. 3.3. Eighteen weeks gestation. Normal echo texture of the placenta (*P*), homogeneous and hyperechogenic at this stage. Cord insertion is well seen

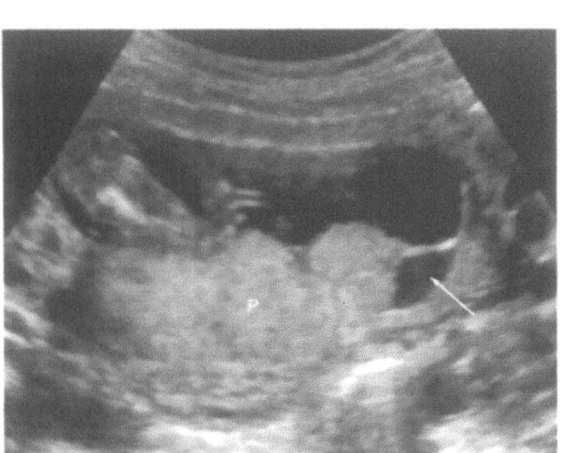

Fig. 3.2. Eighteen weeks gestation. Normal placenta (*P*). Normal marginal sinus (*arrow*)

metrium and uterine vessels. At 16–18 weeks, small intraplacental arteries may be demonstrated by color or power Doppler. During the third trimester, the placenta is richly vascularized.

3.1.2.2
Circumvallate

Definition: This is an abnormality of placental shape in which the chorioamniotic membrane is inserted away from the placental edge towards the center. It may be partial, which is 10–20 times more frequent (ZIEL 1963), or complete.

US Findings: These criteria include an irregular edge, uplifted margin, placental sheet or shelf. In a study of 62 patients, HARRIS et al. (1997) reported that the accuracy of prenatal sonographic detection is poor.

Significance: A partial circumvallate placenta has no association with any fetal problem, but the complete form involving 100% of the placental circumference has a higher incidence of abruptio placentae, preterm labor, intrauterine growth restriction (IUGR), fetal anomalies or perinatal death.

3.1.2.3
Succenturiate (Fig. 3.4)

Definition: An accessory lobe of the placenta present in 0.5–1% of pregnancies (BENIRSCHKE and KAUFMANN 1999).

US Findings: A placenta with an accessory lobe is connected by a sheet. Color Doppler helps to visualize the vessels running between the two lobes (CHIARA et al. 2000).

Significance: It is associated with a higher incidence of placental infarction and velamentous insertion of the umbilical cord. Complications are not seen except in the case of vasa previa, in which the accessory lobe with umbilical vessels may be compressed or ruptured by the presenting parts at the onset of labor.

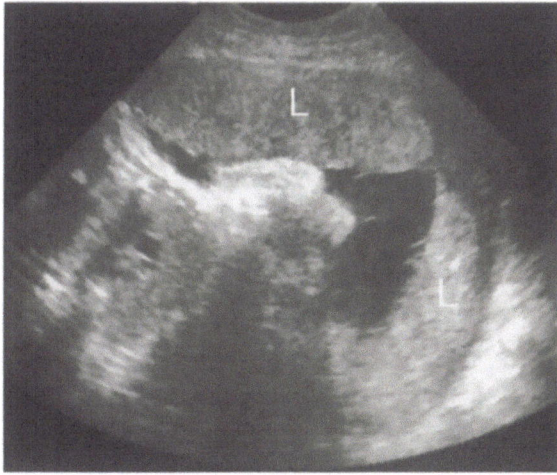

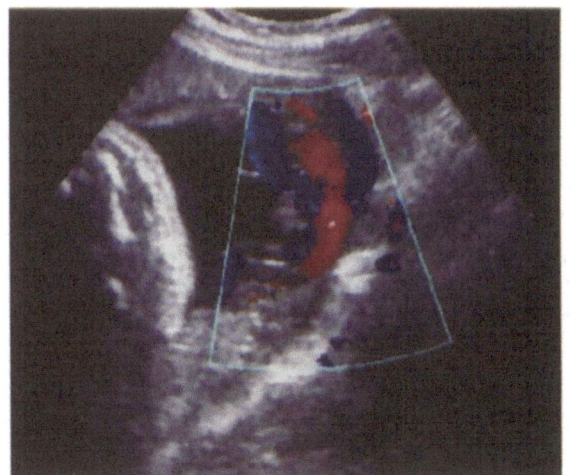

a   b

Fig. 3.4a, b. Thirty-three weeks gestation. Succenturiate placenta. **a** Two lobes (*L*) are displayed, connected by a sheet of tissue. **b** Color Doppler ultrasonography shows the vessels running between the lobes

3.1.3
Placental Size

3.1.3.1
Normal (Fig. 3.5)

The thickness of the placenta is 3 cm before 20 weeks of gestation, and between 4 and 5 cm up to 40 weeks. It should be approximately equal in thickness (mm) to gestational age in weeks ±10 mm. Most placentas are not thicker than 4 cm (HODDICK et al. 1985).

3.1.3.2
Thin Placenta Versus Placentomalacia (Fig. 3.6)

In the presence of a thin placenta, one should look for signs of IUGR, chromosomal anomalies, severe uterine infection, insulin-dependent diabetes mellitus and placenta-induced hypertension. Be cautious in the case of polyhydramnios, which may cause apparent thinning of the placenta.

3.1.3.3
Thick Placenta Versus Placentomegaly
(Figs. 3.7–3.10)

Some complications are associated with homogeneous placentomegaly: diabetes mellitus, anemia, hydrops, infection, aneuploidy or rhesus isoimmunization. Heterogeneous placentomegaly occurs in molar pregnancy, triploidy, placental hemorrhage, uteroplacental insufficiency and mesenchymal dysplasia (JAUNIAUX et al. 1997).

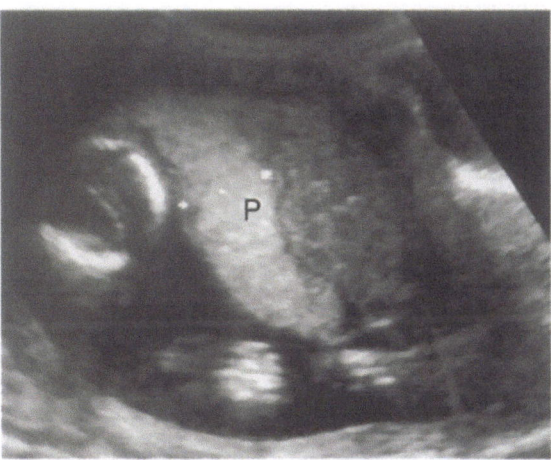

Fig. 3.5. Twenty weeks gestation. The placenta (*P*) measured 2 cm (normal for the gestational age)

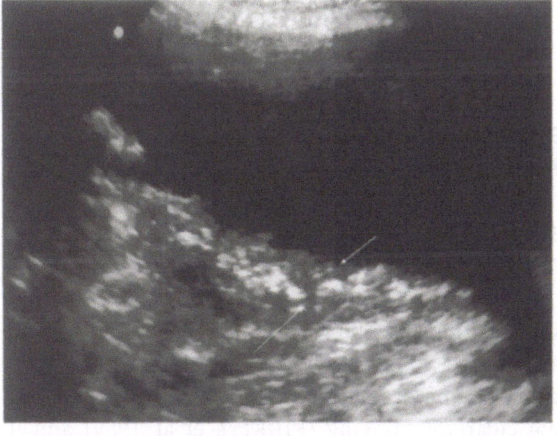

Fig. 3.6. Second trimester pregnancy. Primary placental insufficiency with a thin and very mature placenta (*arrows*)

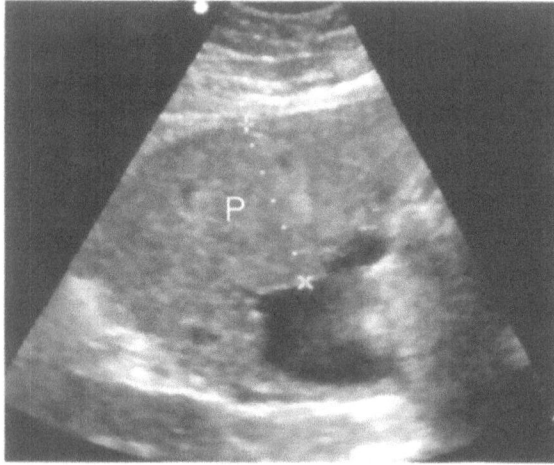

Fig. 3.7. Twenty-six weeks gestation. Placentomegaly (6 cm) in a normal pregnancy. Placenta (*P*)

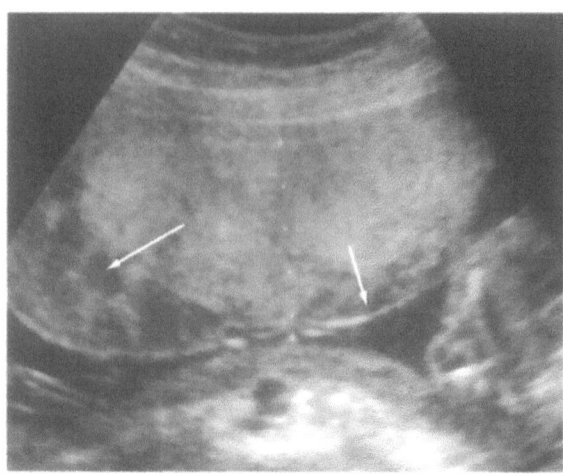

Fig. 3.9. Twenty-two weeks gestation. Placentomegaly. Numerous subchorionic lakes (*arrows*). Normal evolution of the pregnancy

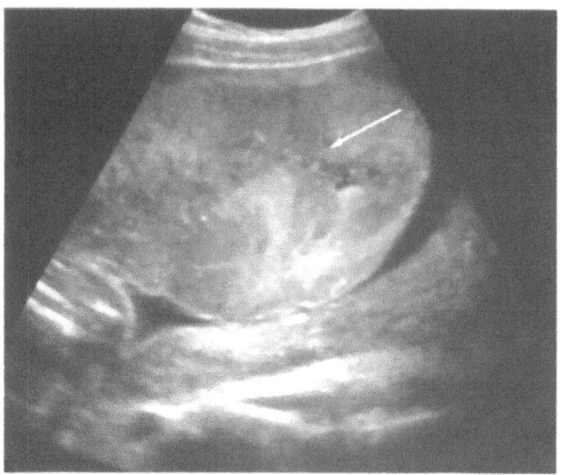

Fig. 3.8. Twenty-seven weeks gestation. Patient with high blood pressure and uteroplacental insufficiency. Thick and heterogeneous placenta (6 cm anteroposterior diameter) (*arrow*)

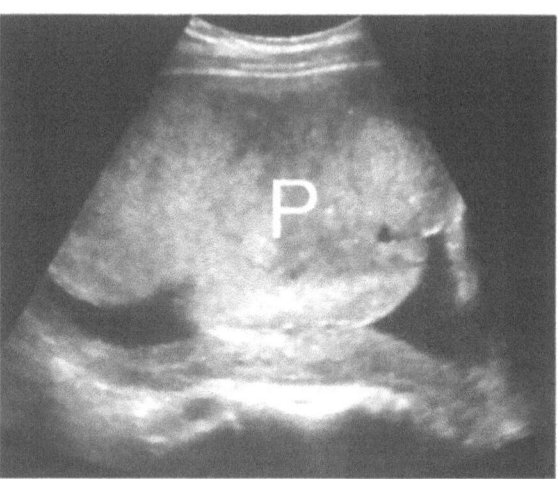

Fig. 3.10. Twenty-eight weeks gestation. Patient with high blood pressure, and uteroplacental insufficiency demonstrated at Doppler sonography. Hydropic and heterogeneous placenta (*P*)

3.1.4
Abnormalities

3.1.4.1
Calcifications (Figs. 3.11, 3.12)

Calcifications can be seen with placental aging and are graded accordingly; this has no clinical significance. Premature calcifications can occur with maternal cigarette smoking (PINETTE et al. 1989) and if mothers with thrombotic disorders have been placed on heparin or aspirin prophylaxis.

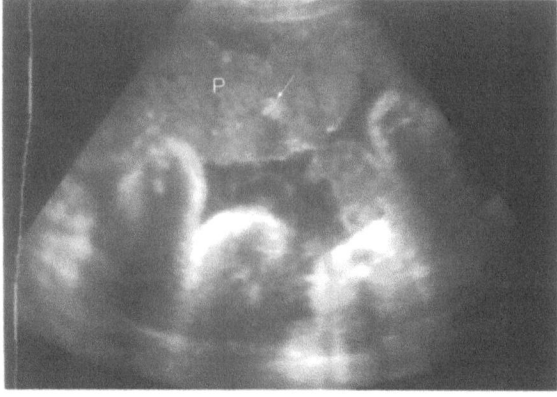

Fig. 3.11. Third trimester pregnancy. Slightly heterogeneous placenta (*P*) with calcifications (*arrow*)

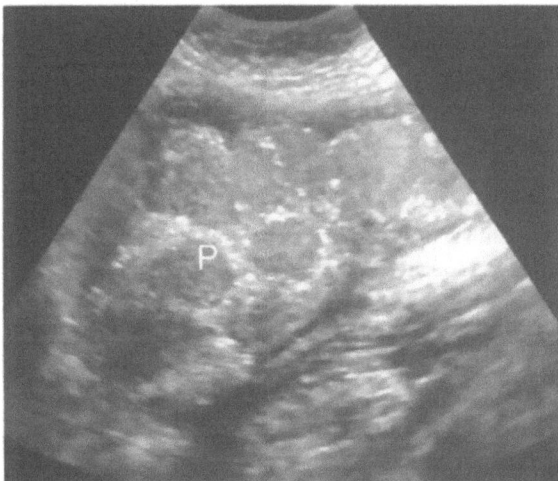

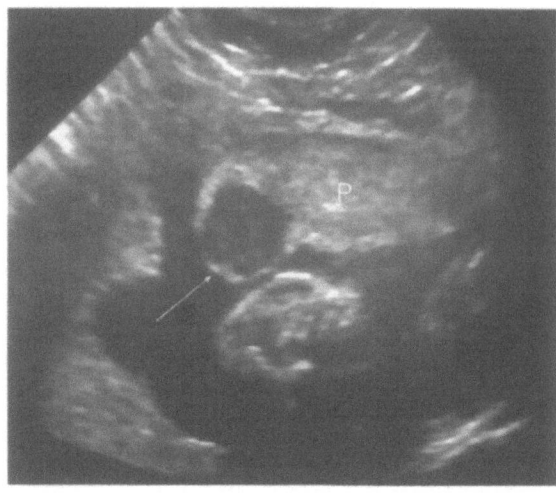

Fig. 3.12. Thirty-two weeks gestation. Highly mature placenta (*P*), grade 3, in a patient who smoked

Fig. 3.13. Eighteen weeks gestation. Venous lake (*arrow*) mimicking a mass effect. Placenta (*P*)

3.1.4.2
Hypoechoic Areas (Figs. 3.13, 3.14)

Frequently seen in the third trimester, the differential diagnosis for hypoechoic areas includes decidual septal cysts, fibrin deposition or intervillous thrombosis without infarct. The hypoechoic areas seen on ultrasound consist of fibrin or blood. Most of them have no clinical significance. They are seen more frequently at the periphery or under the chorion. The presence of more than five areas and/or a diameter greater than 2–3 cm may be associated with rhesus incompatibility or elevated maternal serum alpha-fetoprotein (AFP).

3.1.4.3
Placental Infarct (Figs. 3.15, 3.16)

Placental infarct is an area of ischemic villous necrosis related to the blood supply distribution of a uteroplacental artery. Infarct is more common at the periphery of the placenta with a triangular base along the basal plate near the decidua. Most infarcts are not seen at ultrasonography. HARRIS et al. (1990) reported that ultrasonography is insensitive for the detection of placental infarction. Small areas of infarcts involving less than 5% of the villous parenchyma are seen in as many as 25% of normal pregnancies and are not clinically significant (Fox 1987). Infarcts involving more than 10% of the villous parenchyma have been associated with fetal hypoxia, IUGR and fetal death (Fox 1987). The

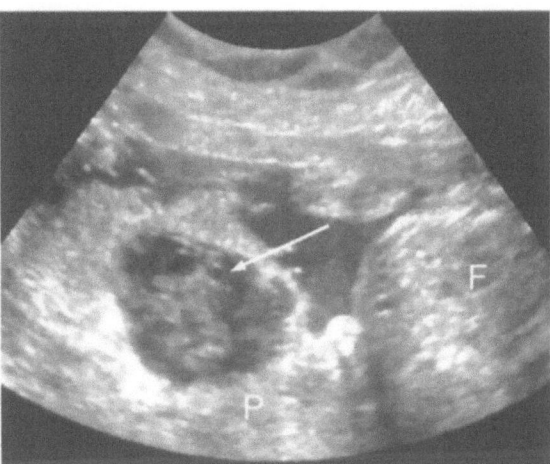

Fig. 3.14. Twenty-five weeks gestation. Fetus (*F*). Placenta (*P*). Intervillous thrombosis (*arrow*)

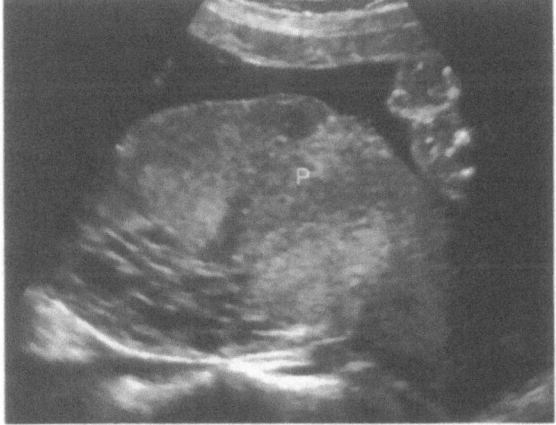

Fig. 3.15. Twenty-eight weeks gestation. Very heterogeneous placenta (*P*). Numerous infarct zones were demonstrated at pathology

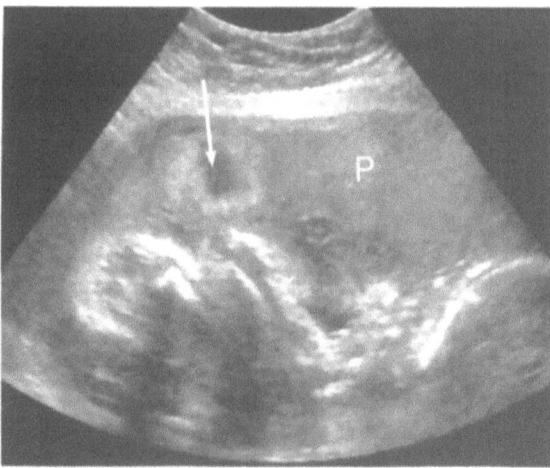

Fig. 3.16. Twenty-eight weeks gestation. Placenta (*P*). Incidentally demonstrated infarct (*arrow*)

prevalence increases in patients with advanced maternal age and in those with diabetes, hypertension, pre-eclampsia or systemic lupus erythematosus (HARRIS et al. 1990).

3.1.5
Placental Position

3.1.5.1
Normal

OPPENHEIMER et al., in a prospective study, suggested that the critical distance of the lower placental edge from the cervical os was 2 cm (OPPENHEIMER et al. 1991, 2001).

3.1.5.2
Low-lying Placenta

A low-lying placenta is one in which the placental edge is within 2 cm of the internal cervical os but not covering any significant portion of it. It is common in the second trimester, but only a small minority persists into the third trimester (1–5%).

3.1.5.3
Marginal and Partial Placenta Previa

Marginal and partial placenta previa is defined as placental tissue at the edge of or encroaching into the cervical os.

3.1.5.4
Placenta Previa

Complete placenta previa occurs when the cervical os is totally covered by the placenta. It is the primary cause of third trimester bleeding. The incidence is 0.5–1% and increases with maternal age, multiparity, previous cesarean section and prior abortion. Placenta previa is weakly associated with maternal smoking history.

US Findings: The translabial or transvaginal approach improves the diagnosis if there is less interposing tissue and less acoustic shadow. Also, these approaches avoid artifacts from an overdistended bladder or uterine contraction resulting in a false-positive diagnosis of placenta previa. Uterine contraction or fibroid is suggested if the thickness of the myometrium is over 2 cm. It is important to remember that locating a placenta 2 cm or less from the internal cervical os near term (at transabdominal sonography) places the patient at risk for placenta previa and may require cesarean section for delivery (OPPENHEIMER et al. 1991).

3.1.5.5
Placenta Accreta (Fig. 3.17)

Placenta accreta is defined as an abnormal adherence of the placenta to the uterus myometrium with subsequent failure to separate after delivery of the fetus secondary to a deficiency of the decidua basalis. It is subcategorized as:

- Placenta accreta vera: Attached to the myometrium but does not invade the muscle.
- Placenta increta: Villi invade the muscle.
- Placenta percreta: Villi penetrate the uterus and often the bladder or rectum (Fox 1997).

The prevalence is 1 in 2,500 pregnancies, and the association with placenta previa is 10%. Independent risk factors are advanced maternal age, previous cesarean section and race (Thai, Chilean, New Guinean). The previous maternal mortality rate of 10–25% is nowadays lower thanks to the accurate detection of placenta accreta by ultrasonography, magnetic resonance imaging (MRI) and maternal serum AFP screening (abnormally elevated). O'BRIEN et al. (1996) reported a series of 109 placenta percreta resulting in eight maternal deaths from major hemorrhage and 10 perinatal deaths.

US Findings: MEGIER et al. (1999), using ultrasound reported the following features on gray-scale ultra-

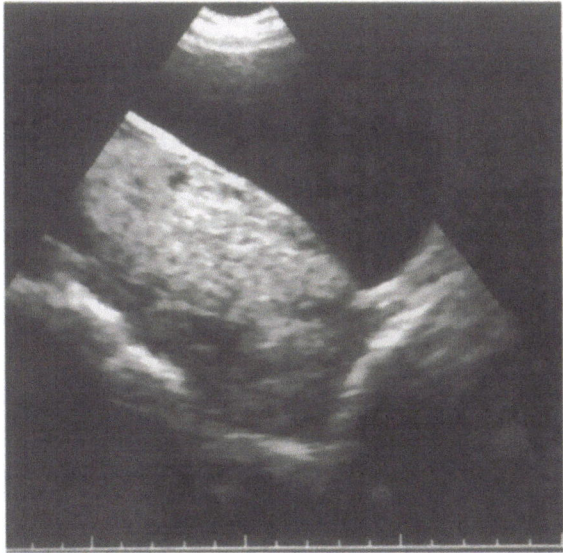
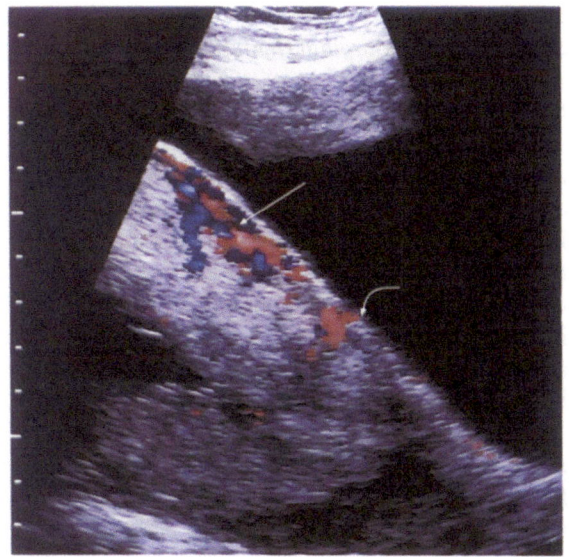

a   b

Fig. 3.17a, b. Thirty-one weeks gestation. Previous history of cesarean delivery. **a** Placenta previa. **b** The loss of hypoechoic myometrium suggests the coexistence of placental increta. Normal subplacental vessels (*arrow*). Abnormal vessels suggest a placenta increta (*curved arrow*)

sound: loss of the normal hypoechoic retroplacental myometrial zone (<2 mm), focal disruption of the uterine serosa and surrounding tissues, and the presence of intraplacental lacunae. On color Doppler, arterial vessels had a diastolic flow value less than that of a spiral artery behind the placenta, arterial vessels were seen crossing from the placenta to surrounding tissues, and there were intraplacental lacunae with arterial flow. Often prominent multiple hypoechoic-anechoic spaces in the placenta with marked periplacental vascularity are seen on color Doppler imaging.

MEGIER et al. (1999) reported that gray-scale ultrasonography for abnormal adherence of the placenta is the reference technique. Color Doppler is helpful but may give false negatives.

MRI: MRI is especially valuable in depicting posterior placenta accreta.

Management: In cases of placenta percreta, profuse bleeding is responsible for the maternal morbidity and mortality because it is impossible to completely remove the placenta after delivery without en bloc resection of the uterus and adherent organs in the case of extrauterine extension. To reduce the intraoperative blood loss, peroperative balloon occlusion of the internal iliac arteries is recommended to decrease the morbidity and mortality (DUBOIS et al. 1997).

3.1.6
Retroplacental Area

3.1.6.1
Normal (Fig. 3.18)

In the retroplacental area, the most common finding is a large retroplacental hypoechoic complex composed of uteroplacental vessels, predominantly veins and myometrium. The veins appear as parallel hypoechoic channels between the placenta and myometrium.

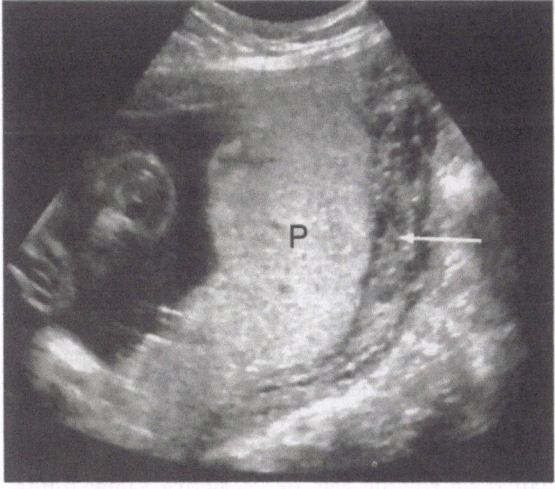

Fig. 3.18. Twenty-four weeks gestation. Normal placenta (*P*). Normal subplacental caducous reaction (*arrow*)

3.1.6.2
Subchorionic or Marginal Hematoma (Fig. 3.19)

Subchorionic or marginal hematoma is defined as an echogenic-free area located between the membranes and the uterine wall. Physiologically, this represents a separation of the chorionic plate from the underlying decidua secondary to rupture of the uteroplacental veins. The incidence is reported to be 2%. Most common with inferior implantation of the placenta, it is associated with preterm delivery or miscarriage, autoimmune reaction, coumadin use and hematological factor deficiency (KURJAK et al. 1996).

3.1.6.3
Retroplacental Hematoma or Abruptio Placentae (Figs. 3.20, 3.21)

Retroplacental hematoma or abruptio placentae is defined as an echogenic-free area separating the uterine wall and basal plate. The incidence is 0.5–1% with a 3-fold increase in pre-eclampsia (RASMUSSEN et al. 1996, ABU-HEIJA et al. 1998). It is due to the rupture of a decidual arteriole, often leading to basal plate necrosis and villous infarction. Associations include maternal hypertension/pre-eclampsia, obstruction of venous drainage of the placenta, cocaine abuse, cigarette smoking, anticardiolipin antibodies, blunt trauma and chorioamnionitis.

US Findings: The retroplacental complex should never exceed 2 cm in thickness. The sensitivity of ultrasound in visualizing hemorrhaging is approximately 50% (SHOLL 1987). The hematoma is hyperechoic for 0–48 h, followed by an isoechoic appearance for 3–7 days and a hypoechoic appearance for 1–2 weeks. Color Doppler is necessary to confirm the hematoma because, on occasion, the echo-free area looks like vessels which turn out to be highly vascularized placental sites.

Significance: The impact depends on gestational age, and the size and site of the hematoma. If the hematoma is not subplacental, no adverse consequence is observed, compared with subplacental hematoma where the pregnancy is compromised. Smaller hematomas have a more negative impact on early pregnancy (less than 20 weeks of gestation). KURJAK et al. (1996) showed that in the first trimester the location of subchorionic hematomas rather than their volume was of predictive value: fundal or corpus hematomas had a worse prognosis than supracervical hematomas. Larger hematomas have a

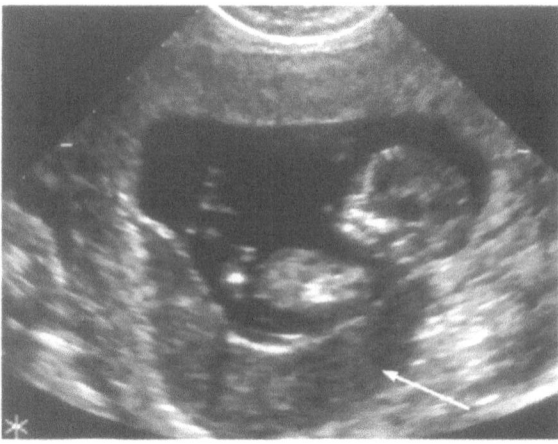

Fig. 3.19. First trimester pregnancy. Sagittal section of the fetus (*F*). Large chorionic hematoma (*arrow*)

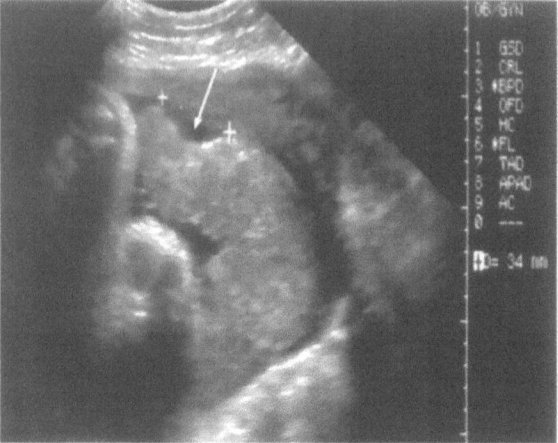

Fig. 3.20. Third trimester pregnancy. Retroplacental hematoma (*arrow*, between calipers)

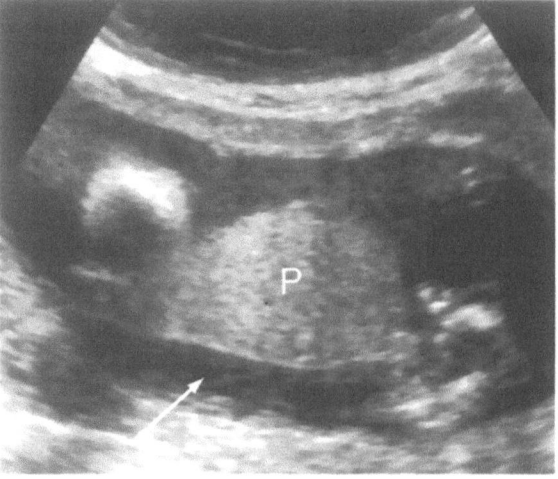

Fig. 3.21. Twenty weeks gestation. Placenta (*P*). Detachment of the placenta (*arrow*)

more significant impact but must separate 30–40% of the placenta away from the myometrium to be significant in the third trimester.

3.1.6.4
Tumors

Chorioangioma (Fig. 3.22): Chorioangioma is the most common benign vascular mass arising from chorionic tissue. It remains clinically insignificant until it exceeds 5 cm in diameter (PRAPAS et al. 2000). The incidence at pathology is 1%. It is reported to increase with fetal alcohol syndrome (THOMAS et al. 1992). However, when the tumor is larger than 5 cm, fetal or maternal complications occur in 30% of cases: polyhydramnios, fetal heart failure, fetal death, preterm labor, IUGR, placenta previa and abruptio placentae, pre-eclampsia, anemia and congenital anomalies (SEPULVEDA et al. 2000a).

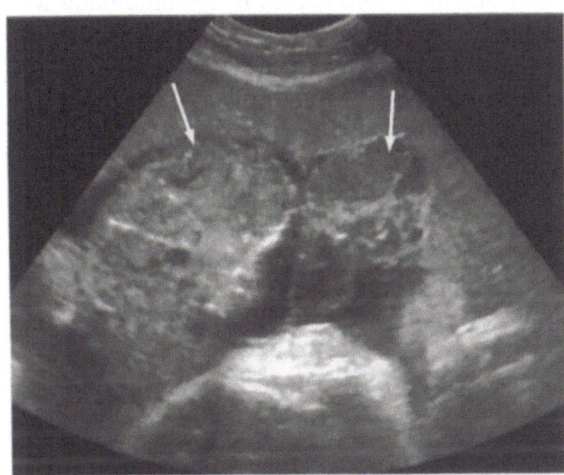

a

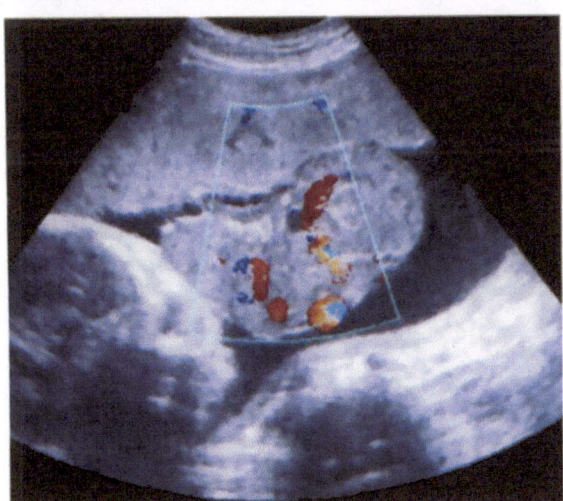

b

Fig. 3.22a, b. a Chorioangioma (*arrows*). **b** Color Doppler shows high flow lesion

US Findings: Chorioangiomas appear as well-circumscribed, rounded hypoechoic lesions near the chorionic surface and adjacent to the cord insertion. Calcification is rare. A hyperechoic region can be seen secondary to hemorrhage or postinfarct fibrosis. Color Doppler shows typically increased blood flow within the mass (SEPULVEDA et al. 2000a,b, ZOPPINI et al. 1997). However, some placental chorioangiomas may present with undetectable flow, because thrombosis may occur spontaneously.

Outcome: Weekly follow-up of this tumor is recommended owing to its unpredictable growth rate and progression (PRAPAS et al. 2000).

Differential Diagnoses: The differential diagnoses are (a) hematoma: avascular; (b) subchorionic fibrin: avascular; (c) partial mole or hydropic degeneration: poorly defined, thick, vascular areas; (d) degenerating fibroid: hypovascular; (d) placental teratoma: cystic and solid masses with calcification.

Hydatidiform Mole (Fig. 3.23): The incidence of hydatidiform mole ranges from 1 in 2,000 in the UK to 1 in 200 in Hong Kong. The clinical signs include vomiting, vaginal bleeding and pregnancy-induced hypertension.

US Findings: On ultrasonography hydatidiform mole appears as a snowstorm-like mass with multiple hypoechoic areas and lack of fetal parts. If the fetus is present, a partial mole with triploidy is common.

Non-trophoblastic Tumors: These are rare and consist of secondary deposits from malignant maternal melanoma or fetal neuroblastoma.

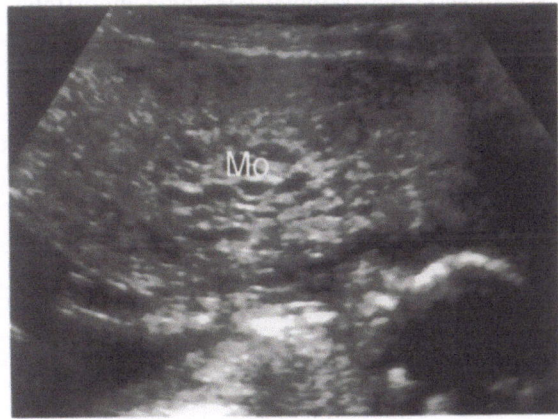

Fig. 3.23. Placenta with molar degeneration (*Mo*)

3.2
The Umbilical Cord

3.2.1
Anatomy

The umbilical cord consists of a central umbilical vein with two umbilical arteries seen spiraling around it. These arteries arise from the internal iliac arteries in the fetus, and carry deoxygenated blood to the placenta. They pass laterally to the fetal urinary bladder. The umbilical vein carries oxygenated blood, enters the falciform ligament, and joins the left portal vein. The vein perfuses the liver, while the remainder of the flow is directed to the inferior vena cava and right atrium through the ductus venosus.

3.2.2
Number of Vessels

3.2.2.1
Single Umbilical Artery

Single umbilical artery occurs in 0.2–1% of pregnancies (NYBERG and FINDBERG 1990, BYRNE and BLANC 1985, NYBERG et al. 1991). A single umbilical artery may be associated with malformation of major organ systems (e.g., genitourinary system), with chromosomal anomalies, the most commonly reported being trisomy 13 and trisomy 18 (NYBERG et al. 1991), and with IUGR, with a reported incidence of 30–60%. A higher frequency of velamentous cord insertion is also reported (NYBERG and FINDBERG 1990).

US Findings: Color Doppler imaging demonstrates the presence of a single artery at the fetal end of the cord. Examination of the fetal pelvis will demonstrate only one umbilical artery lateral to the bladder in its course toward the umbilical cord (JEANTY 1989). The transverse diameter of a single umbilical artery is usually greater than 4 mm between 20 and 36 weeks, as determined by PERSUTTE and LENKE (1994).

3.2.2.2
Persistence of the Right Umbilical Vein

Persistence of the right umbilical vein is rare and associated with a high risk of fetal anomaly (RICHARDS and BENNETT 1998).

3.2.2.3
Multivessel Cord

Multivessel cord is rare and associated with congenital anomalies and conjoined twins.

3.2.3
Cord Length

3.2.3.1
Normal

The normal umbilical cord is 50–60 cm long and may coil as many as 40 times, usually to the left.

3.2.3.2
Short Umbilical Cord (Fig. 3.24)

Short umbilical cord occurs in the limb-body wall complex, with decreased fetal movement secondary to central nervous system and skeletal problems, and with an increased incidence of congenital anomalies, oligohydramnios and breech presentation. Complications can arise from cord compression, abruptio placentae and decreased fetal movement.

3.2.3.3
Long Umbilical Cord

The cord knots in less than 1% of pregnancies. Predisposing factors are polyhydramnios, small fetus and monoamniotic twins (NYBERG and FINDERG 1990, JEANTY 1989). Knots are mostly loose and not clinically significant. Tight knots can induce significant hypoxia or anoxia with frequent fetal demise. They are rarely detected on antenatal US.

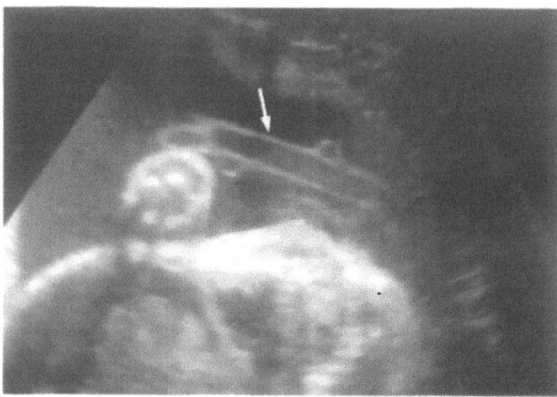

Fig. 3.24. Two vessels (*arrow*) present in a rectilinear and stretched cord

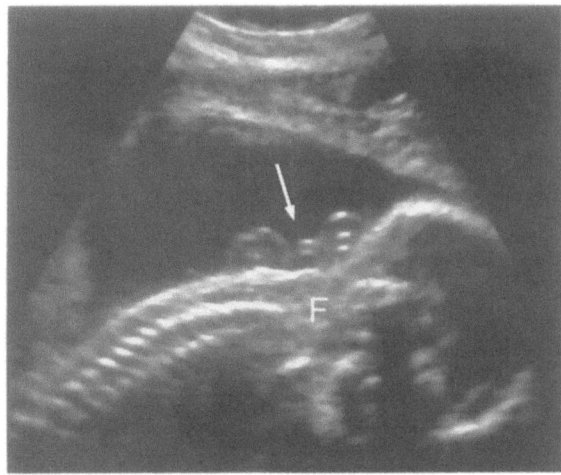

Fig. 3.25. Twenty-four weeks gestation. Fetus (*F*). Circular cord (*arrow*)

3.2.3.4
Nuchal Cord (Fig. 3.25)

The cord encircles the fetal neck in 25% of cases (MISER 1992) and is associated with increased cord length, small fetuses, vertex presentation and polyhydramnios (NYBERG and FINDERG 1990, MISER 1992). Two or more tight nuchal loops are more likely to be associated with increased fetal mortality (NYBERG and FINDERG 1990). Signs of fetal distress are: bradycardia, variable deceleration, and depressed 1-min Apgar score. There are no predictors of nuchal cord in the second trimester.

US Findings: One or more loops of cord are seen encircling the fetal neck. Color Doppler is useful for the diagnosis.

3.2.3.5
Cord Prolapse

Cord prolapse occurs at delivery in 0.5% of cases in association with high perinatal mortality secondary to cord compression (SHEINER et al. 2000). The predisposing factors are nonvertex fetal presentation, polyhydramnios, cephalopelvic disproportion, multiple gestations and increased umbilical cord length. The baby should be delivered by cesarean section.

3.2.3.6
Coiling

Absent coiling of the cord is seen in 4% of fetuses, with an increased incidence of perinatal mortality

and morbidity (LACRO et al. 1987, STRONG et al. 1993), especially trisomy 21, velamentous cord insertion, coarctation of the aorta, intrauterine death and preterm delivery (STRONG et al. 1993).

3.2.3.7
Wharton's Jelly Anomaly (Fig. 3.26)

Wharton's jelly varies in amount. It is decreased in IUGR, and increased in hydrops, polyhydramnios and diabetes.

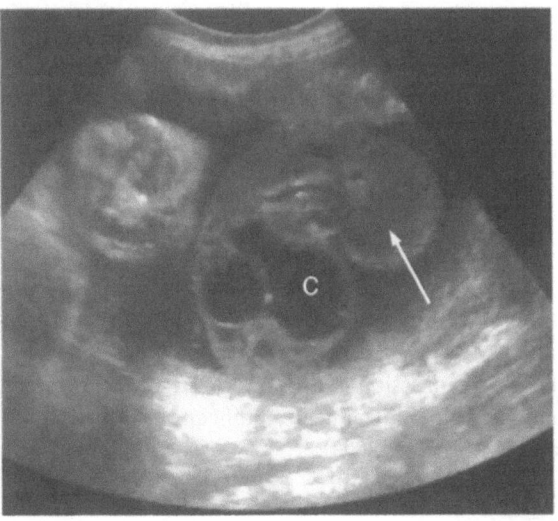

Fig. 3.26. Twenty-eight weeks gestation. Cysts (*C*) of the cord associated with a localized thickness of Wharton's jelly (*arrow*)

3.2.3.8
Enlarged Cord

Enlarged cord is seen in diabetes, hydrops, hematoma and twin-twin transfusion.

3.2.4
Cord Insertion and Attachment

3.2.4.1
Central (Fig. 3.27)

Cord insertion is initially central. Trophotropism (BENIRSCHKE and KAUFMANN 1990) is the process resulting in the final insertion of the cord in relation to the preferential growth of the placenta in areas of adequate perfusion.

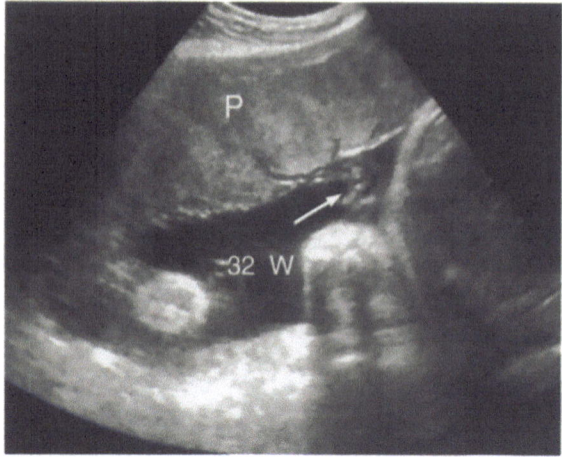

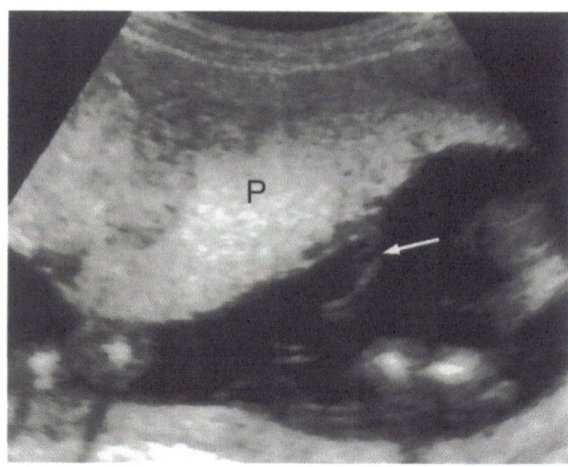

Fig. 3.27. Thirty-two weeks gestation. Central insertion of the cord (*arrow*). Normal aspect of the placenta (*P*) with a slight heterogeneity and hypoechogenicity

Fig. 3.28. Nineteen weeks gestation. Eccentric cord insertion (*arrow*). Normal placenta (*P*)

3.2.4.2
Eccentric Insertion (Fig. 3.28)

Eccentric insertion of the cord occurs in 7% of pregnancies with no clinical significance (BENIRSCHKE and KAUFMANN 2000).

3.2.4.3
Velamentous Insertion (Fig. 3.29)

In 1% of pregnancies, the cord inserts beyond the placental edge into the free membranes of the placenta. Velamentous insertion of the cord may be complicated by rupture and thrombosis of the umbilical vessels because they are not protected by Wharton's jelly (BENIRSCHKE and KAUFMANN 1990, BENIRSCHKE and KAUFMANN 2000). IUGR increases as a result of diminished blood flow and nutrition. Velamentous insertion of the cord is associated with multiple gestations, uterine anomalies and the presence of an intrauterine contraceptive device (NYBERG and FINDERG 1990).

3.2.4.4
Vasa Previa

In vasa previa the umbilical cord crosses the internal os in front of the presenting part. The cord may rupture with hemorrhage and fetal death. It occurs in two settings: velamentous cord insertion and succenturiate lobe on the opposite site of the internal os from the main placental structure.

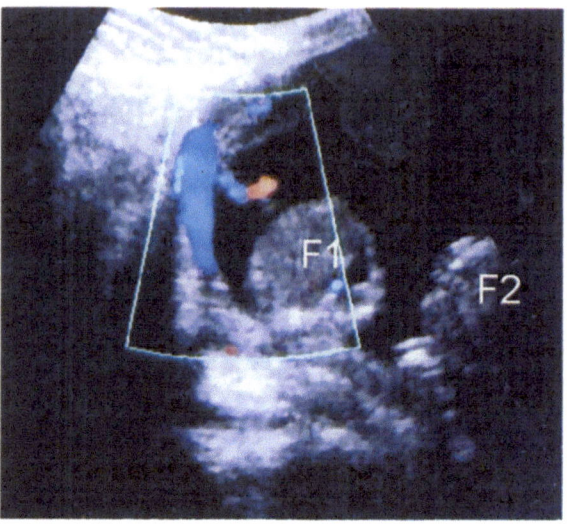

Fig. 3.29. Twin pregnancy (*F1* fetus 1, *F2* fetus 2). Velamentous insertion of the cord in fetus 1

US Findings: Echogenic linear or tubular structures are seen near the internal cervical os. Color or power Doppler can be useful to confirm the diagnosis (NELSON et al. 1990, HSIEH et al. 1991).

Outcome: There is 50–100% fetal mortality.

3.2.4.5
Cord Cysts and Masses (Figs. 3.30, 3.31)

Cysts are associated with fetal anomalies and aneuploidy in up to 50% of cases (WEISSMAN et al. 1994, SKIBO et al. 1992, RAMIREZ et al. 1995, JAUNIAUX et

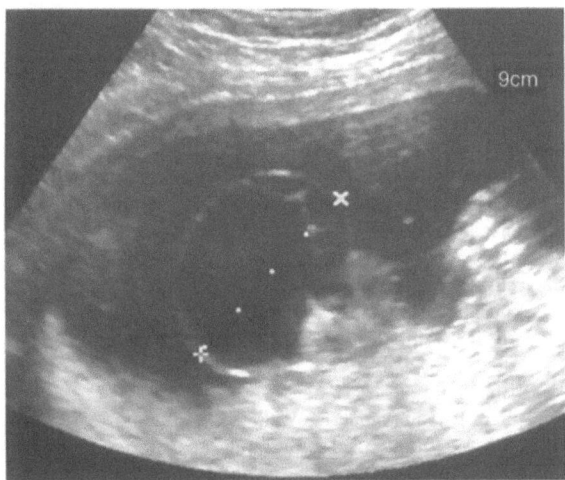

Fig. 3.30. Eighteen weeks gestation. Septated cyst of the cord (4.2 cm)

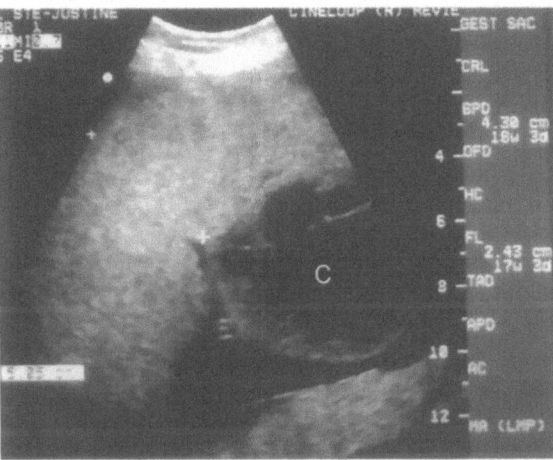

Fig. 3.31. Seventeen weeks gestation. Cyst of the cord (C)

al. 1988). Fetal karyotyping is recommended. In the first trimester, the cysts can be a normal finding and most of them resolve. Fetal anomalies increase if the cysts are situated near the placental or fetal end and if they are eccentric (WEISSMAN et al. 1994). Remnant cysts originate from the omphalomesenteric or allantoic ducts. Toward the fetal end of the umbilical cord they are associated with anomalies of the gastrointestinal and genitourinary tracts, omphalocele, patent urachus, obstructive uropathy (FINK and FILLY 1983, FRAZIER et al. 1992), cardiac defects and trisomy 18 (HEIFETZ and RUEDA-PEDRAZA 1983, SEPULVEDA et al. 1995, ROSENBERG et al. 1986, SACHS et al. 1982, FRAZIER et al. 1992).

Pseudocysts are secondary to focal edema within Wharton's jelly or focal absence of Wharton's jelly (RAMIREZ et al. 1995).

Hemangiomas and teratomas are the most common differential diagnosis of cord masses.

3.2.4.6
Membranes

Chorioamniotic separation is a normal findings in the first 16 weeks. Separation after this time is of no significance. Chorioamniotic elevation occurs with hematoma and in conjunction with retroplacental hematoma.

References

Abu-Heija A, al-Chalabi J, el-Iloubani N (1998) Abruptio placentae: risk factors and perinatal outcome. J Obstet Gynecol 24:141–144

Benirschke K, Kaufmann P (1990) Pathology of the human placenta, 2nd edn. Springer, Berlin Heidelberg New York, p 31, p 319

Benirschke K, Kaufmann P (2000) Pathology of the human placenta, 4th edn. Springer, Berlin Heidelberg New York, pp 335–398

Byrne J, Blanc WA (1985) Malformations and chromosome anomalies in spontaneously aborted fetuses with single umbilical artery. Am J Obstet Gynecol 151:340–342

Chiara H, Otsubo Y, Ohta Y, Araki T (2000) Prenatal diagnosis of succenturiate lobe by ultrasonography and color Doppler imaging. Arch Gynecol Obstet 263:137–138

Dubois J, Garel L, Grignon A, Lemay M, Leduc L (1997) Placenta percreta: balloon occlusion and embolization of the internal iliac arteries to reduce intraoperative blood losses. Am J Obstet Gynecol 176:723–726

Fink IJ, Filly RA (1983) Omphalocele associated with umbilical cord allantoic cyst: sonographic evaluation in utero. Radiology 149:473–476

Fox H (1987) General pathology of the placenta. In: Fox H (ed) Obstetrical and gynaecological pathology, 3rd edn. Churchill Livingstone, Edinburgh, , pp 978–979

Fox H (1997) Abnormalities of placentation. In: Fox H (ed) Pathology of the placenta, 2nd edn. WB Saunders, Philadelphia, p 54

Frazier HA, Guerrieri JP, Thomas RL, Christenson PJ (1992) The detection of a patent urachus and allantoic cyst of the umbilical cord on prenatal ultrasonography. J Ultrasound Med 11:117–120

Harris RD, Simpson WA, Pet LR, Marin-Padilla M, Crow HC (1990) Placental hypoechoic-anechoic areas and infarction: sonographic-pathologic correlation. Radiology 176:75–80

Harris RD, Wells WA, Black WC, et al (1997) Accuracy of prenatal sonography for detecting circumvallate placenta. AJR Am J Roentgenol 168:1603–1608

Heifetz SA, Rueda-Pedraza ME (1983) Omphalomesenteric duct cysts of the umbilical cord. Pediatr Pathol 1:325–335

Hoddick WK, Mahoney BS, Callen PW, Filly RA (1985) Placental thickness. J Ultrasound Med 4:479–482

Hsieh F, Chen H, Ko T, Hsieh CY, Chen HY (1991) Antenatal diagnosis of vasa previa by color-flow mapping. J Ultrasound Med 10:397–399

Jauniaux E, Donner C, Thomas C, Francotte J, Rodesch F, Avni FE (1988) Umbilical cord pseudocyst in trisomy 18. Prenat Diagn 8:557–563

Jauniaux E, Nicolaides KH, Hustin J (1997) Perinatal features associated with placental mesenchymal dysplasia. Placenta 18:701–706

Jeanty P (1989) Fetal and funicular vascular anomalies: identification with prenatal US. Radiology 173:367–370

Kurjak A, Schulman H, Zudenigo D, Kupesic S, Kos M, Goldenberg M (1996) Subchorionic hematomas in early pregnancy: clinical outcome and blood flow patterns. J Maternal-Fetal Med 5:41–44

Lacro RV, Jones KL Benirschke K (1987) The umbilical cord twist: origin, direction and relevance. Am J Obstet Gynecol 157:833–838

Levine D, Hulka CA, Ludmir J, Li W, Edelman RR (1997) Placenta accreta: evaluation with color Doppler US, power Doppler US, and MR imaging. Radiology 205:773–776

Megier P, Gorin V, Desroches, A (1999) Placentas bas insérés échographiquement au 3e trimestre de la grossesse: recherche de signes de placenta accreta/percreta et de vaisseaux pravia. J Gynecol Obstet Biol Reprod 28:239–244

Miser WF (1992) Outcome of infants born with nuchal cords. J Fam Pract 34:441–445

Nelson L, Melone PJ, King M (1990) Diagnosis of vasa previa with transvaginal and color flow Doppler ultrasound. Obstet Gynecol 76:506–509

Nyberg DA, Findberg JH (1990) The placenta, placental membranes, and umbilical cord. In: Nyberg DA, Mahony BS, Pretorius D (eds) Diagnostic ultrasound of fetal anomalies: text and atlas. Year Book Medical Publishers, Chicago, pp 635–659

Nyberg DA, Mahony BS, Luthy D, Kapur R (1991) Single umbilical artery: prenatal detection of concurrent anomalies. J Ultrasound Med 10:247–253

O'Brien JM, Barton JR, Donaldson ES (1996) The management of placenta percreta: conservative and operative strategies. Am J Obstet Gynecol 175:1632–1638

Oppenheimer LW, Farine D, Ritchie JW, Lewinsky RM, Telford J, Fairbanks LA (1991) What is a low-lying placenta? Am J Obstet Gynecol 165:1036–1038

Oppenheimer L, Holmes P, Simpson N, Dabrowski A (2001) Diagnosis of low-lying placenta: can migration in the third trimester predict outcome? Ultrasound Obstet Gynecol 18:100–102

Persutte WH, Lenke RR (1994) Transverse umbilical arterial diameter: technique for the prenatal diagnosis of single umbilical artery. J Ultrasound Med 13:763–766

Pinette MG, Loftus-Brault K, Nardi DA, Rodis JF (1989)

Maternal smoking accelerated placental maturation. Obstet Gynecol 73:379–382

Ramirez P, Haberman S, Baxi L (1995) Significance of prenatal diagnosis of umbilical cord cyst in a fetus with trisomy 18. Am J Obstet Gynecol 173:955–957

Prapas N, Liang RI, Hunter D, Copel JA, Lu LC, Pazkash V, Mari G (2000) Color Doppler imaging of placental masses: differential diagnosis and fetal outcome. Ultrasound Obstet Gynecol 16:559–563

Rasmussen S, Irgens LM, Bergsjo P, Dalaker K (1996) The occurrence of placental abruption in Norway. Acta Obstet Gynecol Scand 75:222–228

Richards DS, Bennett BB (1998) Prenatal ultrasound diagnosis of massive subchorionic thrombohematoma. Ultrasound Obstet Gynecol 11:364–366

Rosenberg JC, Chervenak FA, Walker BA, Chitkara U, Berkowitz RL (1986) Antenatal sonographic appearance of omphalomesenteric duct cyst. J Ultrasound Med 5:719–720

Sachs L, Fourcroy JL, Wenzel DJ, Austin M, Nash JD (1982) Prenatal detection of umbilical cord allantoic cyst. Radiology 145:445–446

Sepulveda W, Bower S, Dhillon HK, Fisk NM (1995) Prenatal diagnosis of congenital patent urachus and allantoic cyst: the value of color flow imaging. J Ultrasound Med 14:47–51

Sepulveda W, Aviles G, Carstens E, Corral E, Perez N (2000a) Prenatal diagnosis of solid placental masses: the value of color flow imaging. Ultrasound Obstet Gynecol 16:554–558

Sepulveda W, Aviles G, Carstens E, Corral E, Perez N (2000b) Placental choriangioma. Ultrasound Obstet Gynecol 16:597–598

Sheiner E, Hallak M, Shoham-Vardi I, Goldstein D, Mazor M, Katz M (2000) Determining risk factors for intrapartum fetal death. J Reprod Med 45:499–424

Sholl JS (1987) Abruptio placentae: clinical management in nonacute cases. Am J Obstet Gynecol 156:40–51

Skibo LK, Lyons EA, Levi CS (1992) First-trimester umbilical cord cysts. Radiology 182:719–722

Strong TH Jr, Elliott JP, Radin TG (1993) Non-coiled umbilical blood vessels: a new marker for the fetus at risk. Obstet Gynecol 81:409–411

Thomas D, Makhoul J, Muller C (1992) Fetal growth retardation due to massive subchorionic thrombohematoma: report of two cases. J Ultrasound Med 11:245–247

Weissman A, Jacobi P, Bronshtein M, Goldstein I (1994) Sonographic measurements of the umbilical cord and vessels during normal pregnancies. J Ultrasound Med 13:11–14

Ziel H (1963) Circumvallate placenta, a cause of antepartum bleeding, premature delivery, and perinatal mortality. Obstet Gynecol 22:798–802

Zoppini C, Acaia B, Lucci G, Pugni L, Tassis B, Nicolini U (1997) Varying clinical course of large placental chorioangiomas. Report of 3 cases. Fetal Diagn Ther 12:61–64

4 Perinatal Diagnosis of Central Nervous System, Face and Neck Anomalies

Fred E. Avni, Teresa Cos, Pascale Sonigo, Catherine Christophe

CONTENTS

4.1   Central Nervous System   39
4.1.1   Normal US Technique and Anatomy   39
4.1.2   MR Imaging of the Fetal Brain: Technique
          and Normal Anatomy   42
4.1.3   Measurements of Fetal Cerebral Structures   44
4.1.4   Congenital CNS Anomalies   44
4.1.4.1   Ventriculomegaly   44
4.1.4.2   Neural Tube Defects   45
4.1.4.3   Microcephaly and Disorders of Neuronal
          Proliferation   47
4.1.4.4   Infections Affecting the CNS   50
4.1.4.5   Intracranial Hemorrhage and Ischemia   52
4.1.4.6   Organogenesis Anomalies   52
4.1.4.7   CNS Tumors and Vascular Malformations   57
4.2   Face   59
4.2.1   Normal Facial Anatomy   62
4.2.1.1   Lips and Maxillae   63
4.2.1.2   Nose   64
4.2.1.3   Eyes   64
4.2.1.4   Ears   65
4.2.1.5   Fetal Profile   65
4.2.2   Facial Anomalies   65
4.2.2.1   Cleft Lip and Palate   65
4.2.2.2   Macroglossia   65
4.2.2.3   Nasal Malformation   67
4.2.2.4   Eye Anomalies   67
4.2.2.5   Micrognathia   67
4.3   Fetal Neck   67
4.3.1   Posterior Masses   69
4.3.1.1   Cystic Hygroma   69
4.3.1.2   Meningo-encephalocele   69
4.3.1.3   Fetal Scalp Cyst   69
4.3.2   Lateral Masses   69
4.3.3   Anterior Masses   69
          References   71

F. Avni, MD, PhD, C. Christophe, MD
Department of Radiology, University Children's Hospital
Queen Fabiola, Avenue J. J. Crocq 15, 1020 Brussels, Belgium
T. Cos, MD
Department of Obstetrics and Gynecology, Brugmann Hospital,
4 Place van Gehuchten, 1090 Brussels, Belgium
P. Sonigo, MD
Department of Pediatric Imaging, Enfants Malades Hospital,
Rue de Sèvres 149, 75743 Paris Cedex, France

4.1 Central Nervous System

4.1.1 Normal US Technique and Anatomy

The fetal central nervous system (CNS) has to be evaluated considering two perspectives: one is the careful, systematic analysis of all structures visualized; the second, equally important, is to compare the appearance of each structure with the expected stage of development.

During the first trimester, transvaginal sonography (TVS) defines most clearly and precisely the structures of the early developing fetal CNS. For instance, the fetal rhombencephalon is easily demonstrated around 7 weeks of gestation as is the developing fourth ventricle. Other structures that may be visualized at this stage include the falx cerebri, the lateral ventricles and the choroid plexus. The spine appears as two echogenic lines (Fig. 4.1) (Blaas et al. 1995, Cyr et al. 1988, Kushnir et al. 1989, Pilu 2000, Timor-

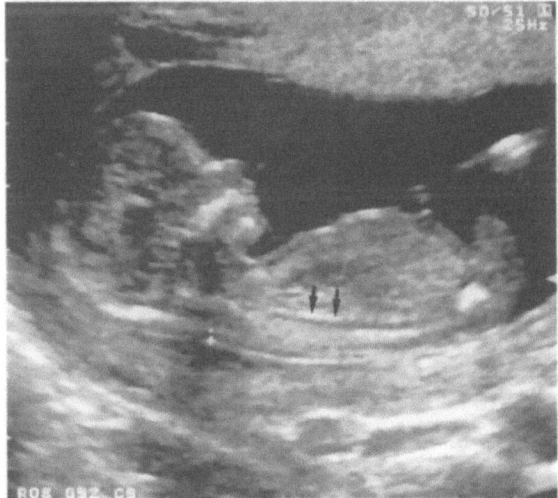

Fig. 4.1. Head and spine. First trimester. Sagittal scan of the fetus. Fetal profile is visible. The spine is partially ossified (*arrows*)

TRISCH et al. 1991, TIMOR-TRISCH and MONTEAGUDO 1996b).

During the second and third trimesters, transabdominal US (TAS) remains the primary tool for the evaluation of the brain and neural axis. TVS may complement or enhance the examination in the case of difficult presentation or maternal obesity. The axial (transverse) scan of the head is the most classical and useful plane; it is usually easily obtained, whatever the fetal lie (Fig. 4.2). Most measurements and anatomical information are visible with TAS (COHEN 1994, PILU et al. 2000, TIMOR-TRISCH and MONTEAGUDO 1996a). Fetal ventricles, midline structures, thalami, posterior fossa, cerebral sulci, sylvian fissures and the bony

structures are among those well demonstrated thanks to the currently available high-resolution transducers. Among the structures visualized, the most important seem to be the atria of the lateral ventricles (their size should not exceed 12 mm), the cisterna magna (it should measure between 2 and 10 mm) and the cavum of the septum pellucidum. The presence and size of these normal structures help to exclude most congenital anomalies (BAUMEISTER et al. 1994, FILLY et al. 1989, KNUTZON et al. 1991). Complementary sagittal or coronal scans may be obtained in order to visualize specific structures such as the corpus callosum (Figs. 4.3, 4.4) (as early as the 18th week) or the vermis of the cerebellum (Fig. 4.5) (BROMLEY

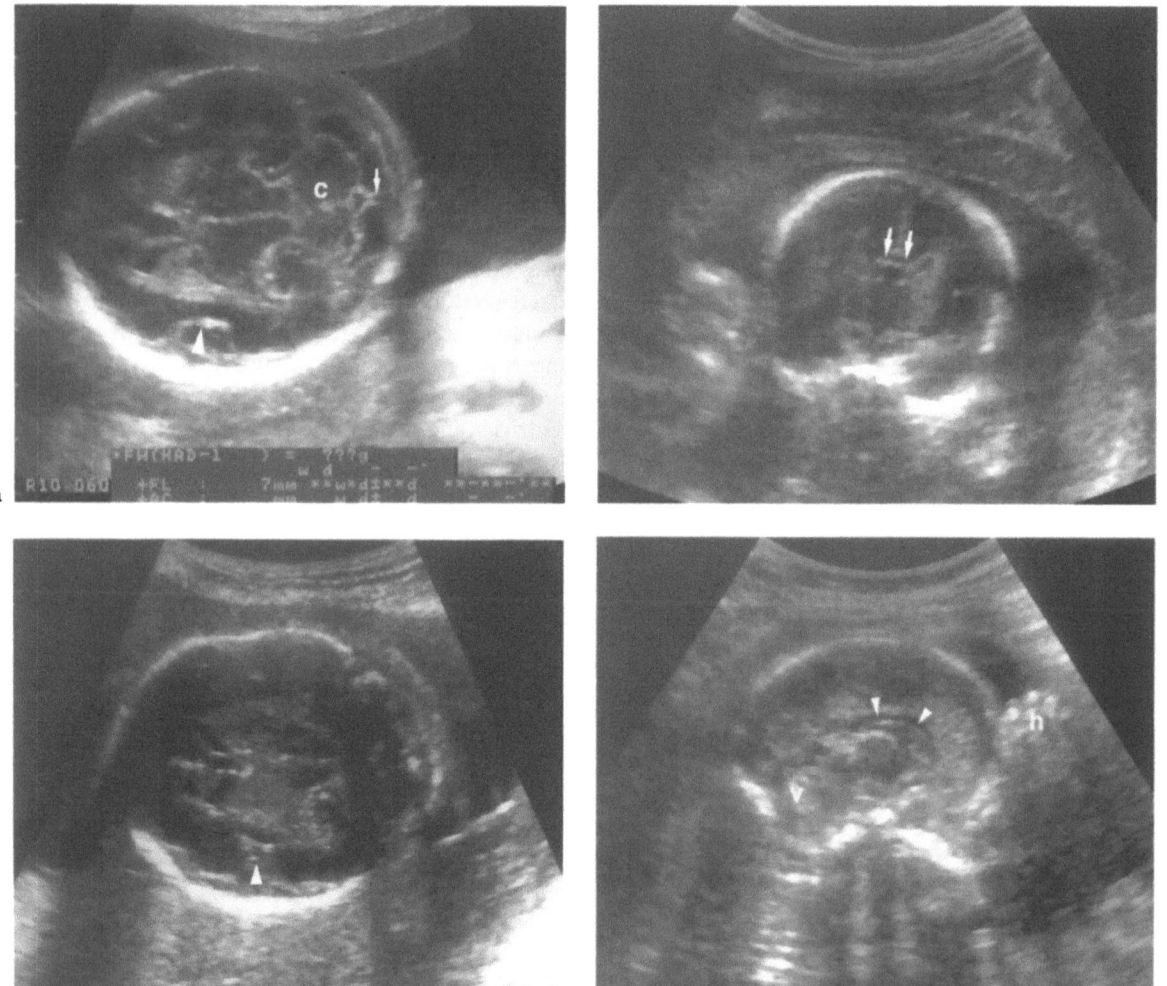

Fig. 4.2a, b. Biparietal view. Second and third trimester. **a** Second trimester. Symmetrical transverse view that includes the cerebellum (*c*) and cisterna magna with normal arachnoid folds within it (*arrow*). The sylvian fissure starts to operculate (*arrowhead*). **b** Third trimester. Transverse view. Operculation of the sylvian fissure has progressed (*arrowhead*)

Fig. 4.3a, b. Corpus callosum. Second trimester. **a** Frontal view, 22 weeks. The corpus callosum (*arrows*) interrupts the falx cerebri. **b** Sagittal view. The hypoechoic corpus callosum (*arrowheads*) can be followed from its anterior to its posterior part. *v* vermis, *h* hand

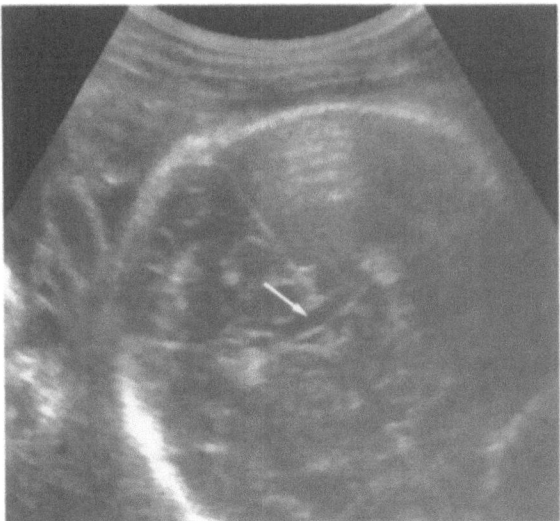

Fig. 4.4. Corpus callosum. Third trimester. Frontal view. The thick hypoechoic corpus callosum is clearly visible (*arrow*)

et al. 1994, MALINGER and ZAKU 1993). These planes may be harder to obtain using TAS than with TVS, especially when the fetus is in the vertex position. The images obtained on TVS resemble those obtained during scanning of the neonatal brain using the anterior fontanelle (COHEN and HALLER 1994, PILU et al. 2000, TIMOR-TRISCH and MONTEAGUDO 1996b).

In order to visualize the fetal spine, axial coronal and sagittal planes are mandatory as each vertebra develops from three ossification centers (a central one for the body and two posterior for the laminae). The ossified centers appear as echogenic foci within hypoechoic cartilage. TVS may be useful in the case of

breech presentation or oligohydramnios (BUDORICK et al. 1991, 1995, DE ELEJADE and DE ELEJADE 1985).

As mentioned above, it is mandatory to compare the appearance of each structure with its expected stage of development. The lateral ventricles, the cerebellum, the cerebral sulci and the spine demonstrate important variations throughout gestation that can be followed by US (or MR imaging) and that should not be considered as abnormal (BABCOOK et al. 1996a). For instance, early in the second trimester, the lateral ventricle is composed predominantly of the frontal horn, body and atrium. The frontal horns appear globular, the temporal and occipital horns are rudimentary. Later, the temporal and occipital bones and their respective ventricular horns grow rapidly and the shape of the ventricle resembles its adult configuration. Also, early in development the choroid plexus occupies most of the ventricle and appears relatively huge. During the second trimester, its size relative to the ventricle diminishes (FILLY et al. 1991).

More and more, thanks to better equipment and experience, it has become possible to visualize with US progressive sulcal development. In the developing brain, the first sulci appear as straight lines during the fifth month of gestation. The calloso-marginal sulcus complex develops during the sixth month. At this time the sylvian fissure operculates. By the middle of the seventh month, all primary sulci should be present. Secondary sulci develop during the eighth and ninth months (Fig. 4.6). This late and complex development implies that no definite diagnosis of fetal lissencephaly can be ascertained before the seventh month (WORTHEN et al. 1986). Similarly, the development of the cerebellum may be followed;

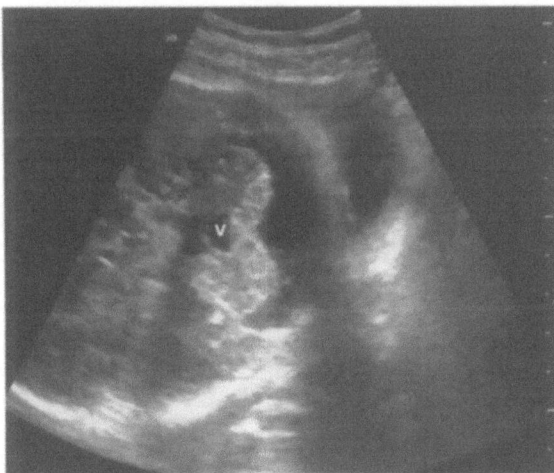

Fig. 4.5. Cerebellum. Third trimester. The sulci are now visible at the surface of the cerebellum. *v* fourth ventricle

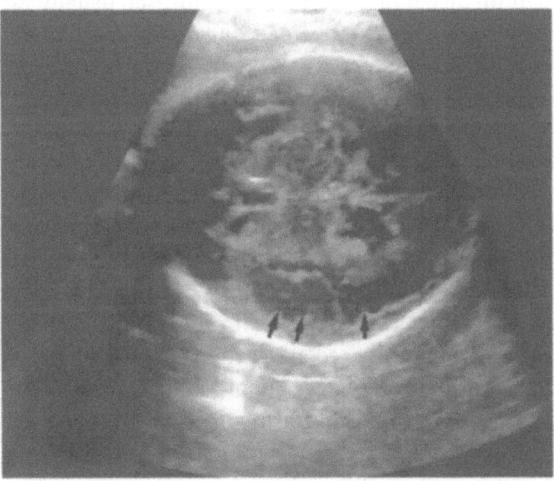

Fig. 4.6. Sulci. Late third trimester. Sulci (*arrows*) are visible indenting the cerebral surface

normal measurements, visualization of the hyper-echoic vermis and the development of sulci help to ascertain normal evolution (MALINGER et al. 2001).

The development of the fetal spine takes even longer and its ossification is not completed until after birth. Ossification of the spine develops in a caudal direction. The three ossification centers of L5 are ossified by week 13. An additional level becomes ossified every 2 weeks from L5 through S5. By week 22, S2 should be ossified. The ossification of the laminae is somewhat delayed in comparison with the vertebral body. During the third trimester, the conus medullaris is clearly defined and its location can be determined normally around L2 (BUDORICK et al. 1991, 1995, WOLF et al. 1992) (see Chap. 9).

> Analysis of the CNS normal anatomy must be meticulous and detailed; knowledge of the stages of brain development is mandatory in order to verify normal echoanatomy.

4.1.2
MR Imaging of the Fetal Brain: Technique and Normal Anatomy

MR imaging must be considered as a complementary method to US for the evaluation of anomalies of the fetal brain. It should be performed only after a complete evaluation has been performed by an experienced sonologist. MR imaging should be performed only if there are doubts about a specific diagnosis or extent of a disease. MR imaging can also be performed when there is a familial risk for the recurrence of a specific disease. To date there are no contraindications to performing the examination other than the usual MR contraindications. Yet, usually no examinations are performed during the fist trimester of the pregnancy (RESTA et al. 1994, SONIGO et al. 1998, BEKKER and VAN VUGT 2001).

The examination can be performed in high and low field magnets. T2- and T1-weighted sequences are mandatory. Rapid Haste T2-weighted sequences are usually sufficient in order to image the fetal morphology. They obviate the need for maternal sedation. T1-weighted sequences are useful for the evaluation of the degree of myelinization after 28 weeks. Body or phased array coils are well suited to the examination. Images should be obtained in the axial, coronal and sagittal planes. On T2-weighted images the cerebrospinal fluid (CSF) has a high signal intensity, the cortex and gray matter a low signal intensity. The germinal matrix and migrating neuronal cells have a low signal intensity also

(Figs. 4.7, 4.8). On T1-weighted images, the CSF has a low signal intensity, the cortex and areas of myelinization a relatively high signal intensity (Fig. 4.9) (AMIN et al. 1999).

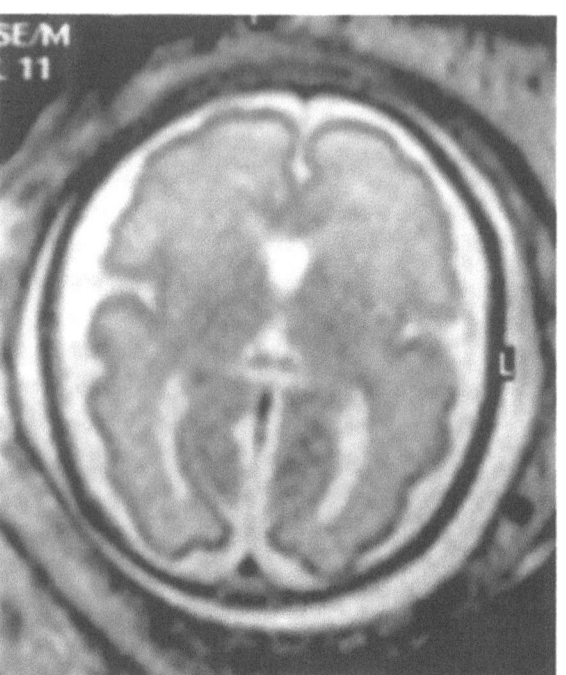

a

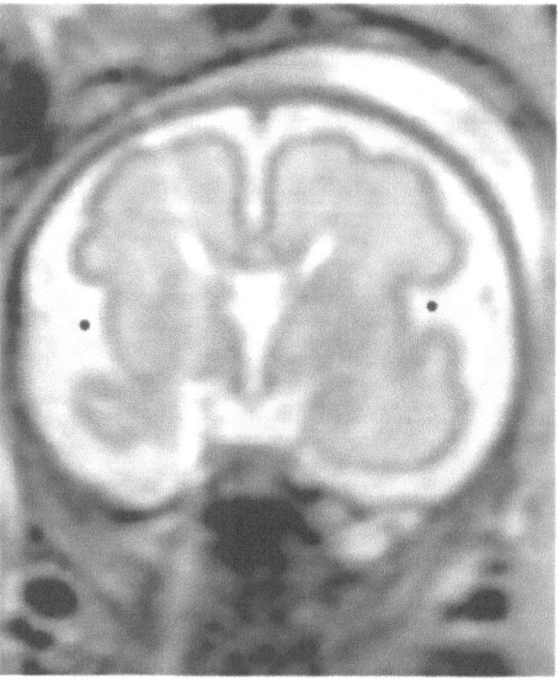

b

Fig. 4.7a, b. MR imaging, T2-weighted sequence: 28 weeks. a Axial view. Few sulci are seen on the surface of the frontal lobes. b Coronal view. Partial operculation of the sylvian fissures (*)

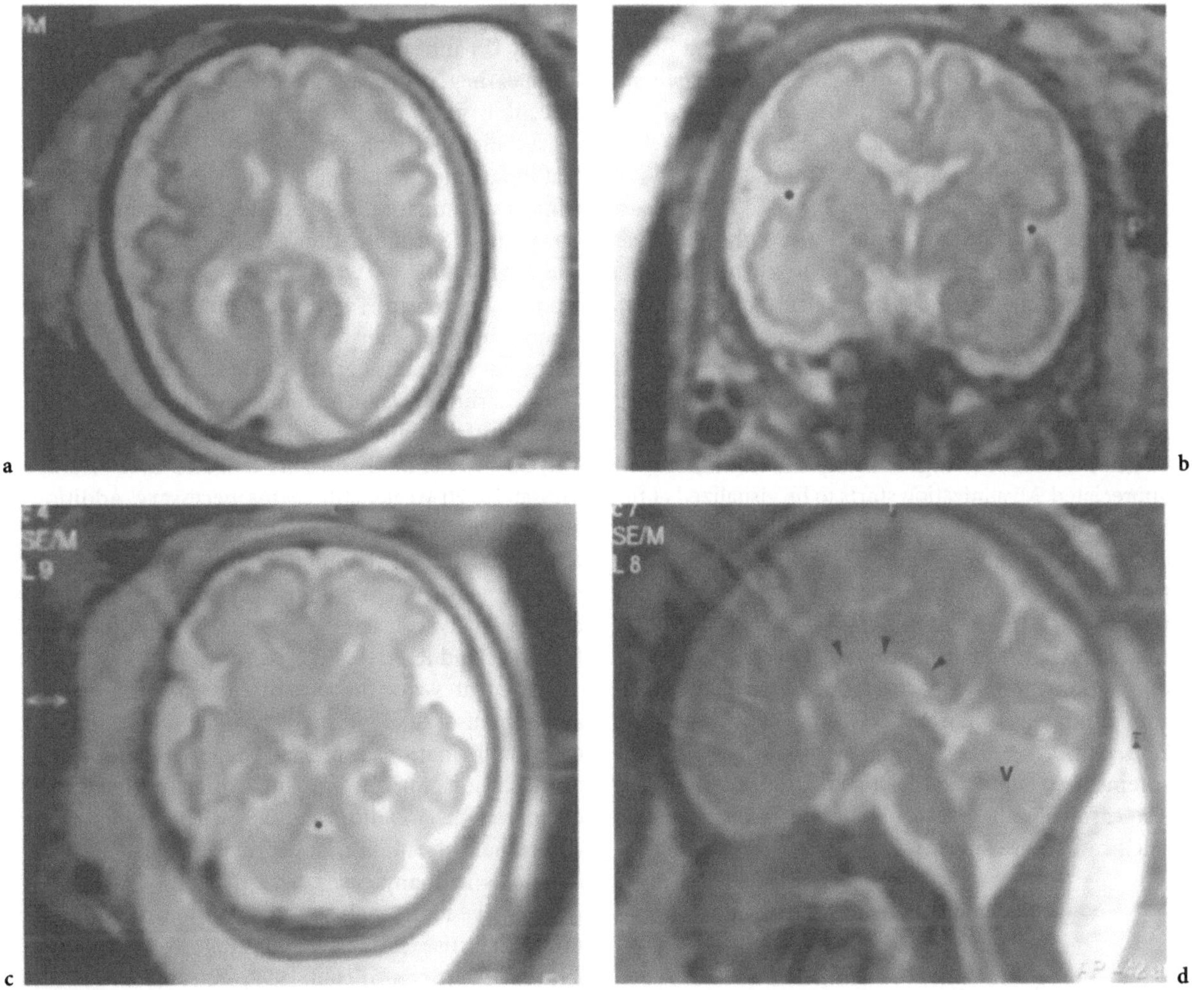

Fig. 4.8a–d. MR imaging, T2-weighted sequence: 32 weeks. **a** Transverse scan. Development of cortical sulci. **b** Coronal view. Progression of operculation (*). **c** Posterior fossa view. Normal cerebellum and fourth ventricle (*). **d** Sagittal view. Normal corpus callosum (*arrowheads*) and vermis (*v*)

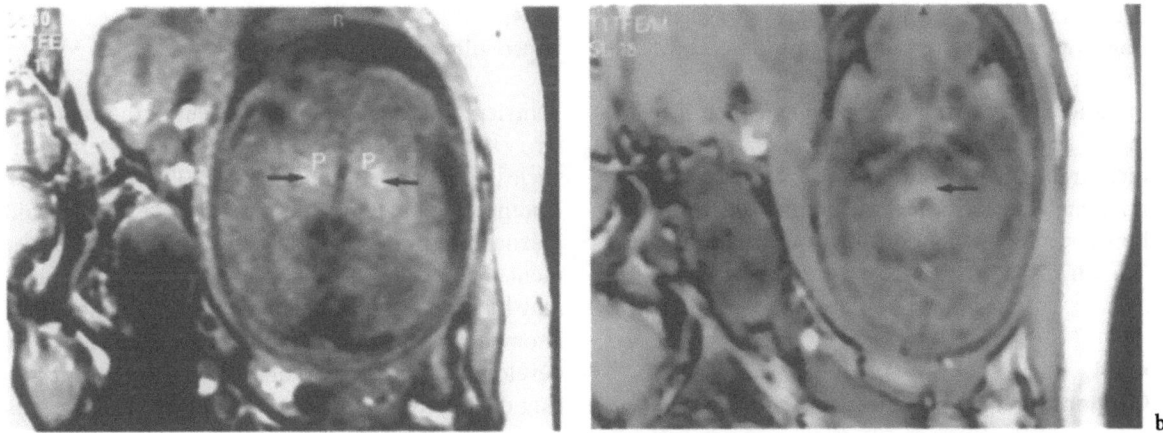

Fig. 4.9a, b. MR imaging, T1-weighted sequence: 34 weeks. **a** Transverse scan through the cerebral peduncles (*p*). Hyperintensity corresponds to myelinization (*arrow*). **b** Posterior fossa and pons. Hyperintensity corresponds to normal myelinization (*arrow*)

Interpretation of images obtained should include measurement of biparietal and fronto-occipital diameters, diameter and surface of the cerebellum. It should also include the evaluation of the cerebral gyri and operculization of the sylvian fissures (Figs. 4.7–4.9). It is noteworthy that between 23 and 28 weeks the normal cerebral cortex appears layered. The deepest layer corresponds to the germinal matrix, the next layer to migrating cells and above that the cortical mantle; with advancing gestation, the matrix and the layers with cells will become thinner. Before 24 weeks very few gyri are seen. They will develop between 24 and 28 weeks. Therefore, MR imaging will become helpful for their evaluation mainly after 28–30 weeks (Figs. 4.7, 4.8). Finally, the degree of myelinization must be appreciated. Myelinization starts to be visualized at the level of the pons, vermis, cerebellar peduncles, internal capsule and central gray nuclei (Fig. 4.9). At the level of the pons, an area of high signal intensity becomes visible around 22 weeks, in the internal capsule around 31 weeks and in the thalami around 28 weeks. The degree of gyration and myelinization is obtained by comparison with tables of normal development (GAREL et al. 2001, GIRARD et al. 1993, YAMASHITA et al. 1997). Measurements of the ventricles (lateral, third, fourth) are also easily obtained. As usual, small cystic lesions and calcifications are poorly visualized on MR imaging.

> Fetal MR imaging provides information about the normal brain anatomy and especially about the development of sulci. Both T1-weighted (for myelinization) and T2-weighted (for morphology) sequences are necessary.

4.1.3
Measurements of Fetal Cerebral Structures

For years, measurements have been part of the routine evaluation of the fetus by obstetrical US (see Chap. 1). Biparietal diameter is the basis of the determination of gestational age. Many other measurements and ratios have been added since. The same measurements and ratios can be obtained by fetal MR imaging. They can be helpful for the evaluation of various pathological states (MONTEAGUDO and TIMOR-TRISCH 1996, SNIJDERS AND NICOLAIDES1994).

4.1.4
Congenital CNS Anomalies

CNS malformations represent a large group (around 3% of births) of congenital malformations detected

in utero (STOLL et al. 1991). The majority are detectable by US and should be visible early in gestation. In Europe, they are usually detected during the routine screening program performed between 17 and 22 weeks. Elevated alpha fetoprotein levels, a previous history of malformation or any abnormality at the clinical examination are supplementary indications for a fetal US examination (PILU et al. 1993, COHEN and HALLER 1994). With the wider use of TVS, the tendency is towards earlier diagnosis of anomalies; several first trimester or early second trimester diagnoses have already been reported. Earlier diagnosis allows earlier decision-making. However, one should be aware of the limitations of the technique; up to now, only 50–60% of anomalies are detected by TVS and a TAS at 18–20 weeks still seems necessary. Additionally, with a scan done early it might be difficult to differentiate between pathology and variants of normal development (BLUMENFELD et al. 1993, BRONSHTEIN et al. 1998b, VAN ZALEN-SPROCK et al. 1995, BONILLO-MUSOLES and RAGA 1994, D'OTTAVIO et al. 1995).

In recent years the use of MR imaging for the assessment of fetal anomalies has increased rapidly; CNS malformations represent the largest proportion of indications for MR imaging, which has been used extensively as an adjunct to US. MR imaging brings additional information and provides more accurate diagnosis in many cases. The US and MR imaging results have to be analyzed together in order to optimize their use (SIMON et al. 2000, HUBBARD and HARTY 1999, SONIGO et al. 1998, WHITBY et al. 2001).

The use of three-dimensional (3D) US and of color Doppler have also gained popularity in several specific indications, but their use remains more limited (MUELLER et al. 1996, JOHNSON et al. 1997, WLADI-MOROFF et al. 1993, HATA et al. 2000).

4.1.4.1
Ventriculomegaly

Ventriculomegaly is an enlargement of the ventricular system, defined as an atrium of the lateral ventricle larger than 12 mm (Fig. 4.10) (FILLY et al. 1991). Another useful sign is the separation of the choroid plexus from the wall of the lateral ventricle. Enlargement may occur early in pregnancy or late, and it may be isolated or associated with CNS or non-CNS anomalies. The malformation may be primary or develop secondary to an acute phenomenon occurring during the course of pregnancy; various events and toxins may interfere with the normal development of the brain. Once ventriculomegaly has been detected the in utero, investigation has to be system-

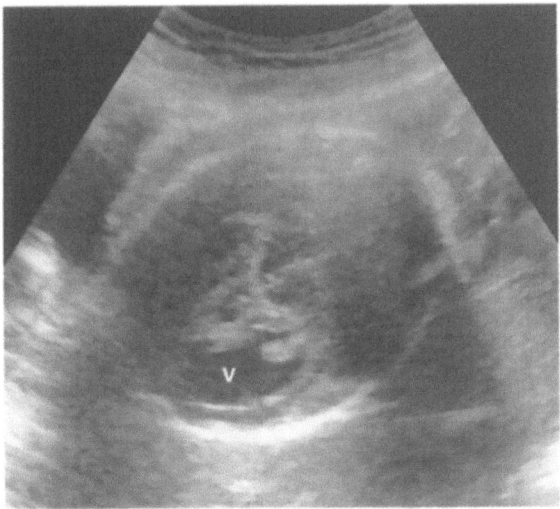

Fig. 4.10. Fetal head in a case of toxoplasmosis. Transverse scan. Moderate ventriculomegaly measured 15 mm at the atrium of the lateral ventricle (*v*)

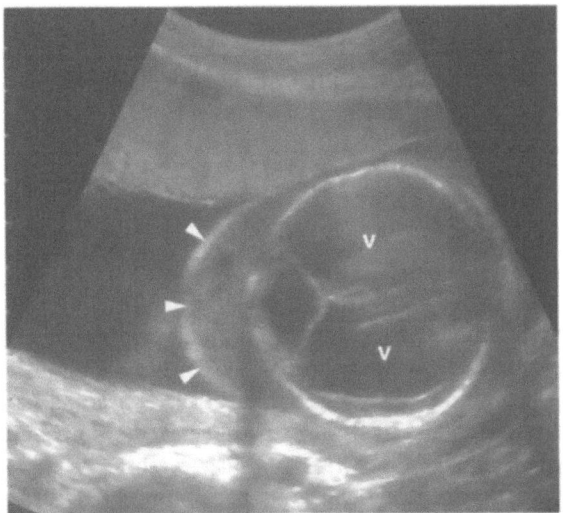

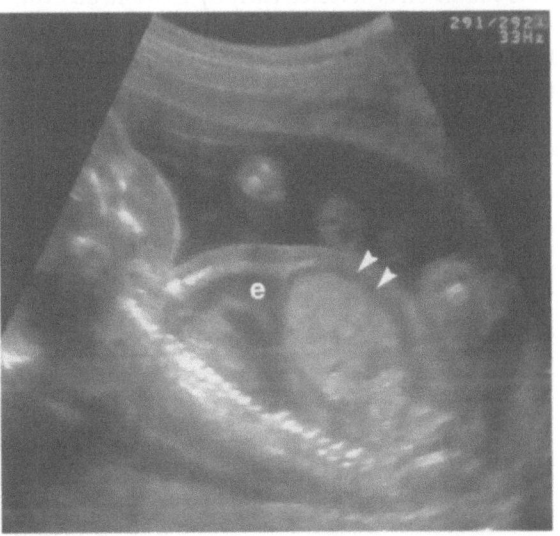

Fig. 4.11a, b. Marked ventriculomegaly and fetal hydrops. **a** Head. Transverse scan. Marked dilatation of the ventricular system (*v*) including the fourth ventricle and thickening of the nuchal soft tissue (*arrowheads*). **b** Trunk. Sagittal scan. Pleural effusion (*e*) and a slight amount of ascites (*arrowheads*)

atic in order to determine the exact diagnosis and prognosis. The degree of dilatation and the level of obstruction must be evaluated carefully. The survey must include careful analysis of other organ systems and chromosome analysis must be performed. In many cases, MR imaging may helpful in order to detect associated anomalies (see below). Isolated uni- or bilateral ventriculomegaly has a much better prognosis than cases with associated malformations (PILU et al. 2000, MONTEAGUDO and TIMOR-TRISCH 1996, DURFEE et al. 2001, KINZLER et al. 2001, KELLY et al. 2001, MERCIER et al. 2001).

Syndromic ventriculomegaly tends to develop earlier and the lateral ventricles present a squared appearance. Acquired dilatation tends to develop later in pregnancy (as a post-infection or post-hemorrhagic phenomenon). Acute and massive dilatations determine a permeation of the septum pellucidum that finally disappears; this phenomenon may render difficult the differential diagnosis with holoprosencephaly. In hydrocephaly, the two thalami remain clearly separated. In the extreme form of hydrocephaly the cerebral mantle is markedly thinned and may even not be visualized (Fig. 4.11) (so-called hydranencephaly).

4.1.4.2
Neural Tube Defects

Neural tube defects (NTD) result from failure of the neural tube to close during primary neurulation. Their incidence is 1.6/1000 births but increases to 5%

if one of the parents is affected and to 10% if two previous siblings were affected. The prevalence at birth has probably diminished since the advent of antenatal diagnosis. NTD are characterized by the presence of a cerebral, spinal or combined cerebro-spinal defect or dysraphism. Most NTD have a polygenic inheritance patterns. Several factors, such as ethnicity, geographical location, nutritional deficiency (folic acid) and medications (valproate) may play a role in their occurrence. It has been hypothesized that NTD are produced by inadequate nutrient supply to the rapidly growing neural folds. A delay in establishing blood flow or abnormal blood supply to the neural tube may interfere with normal closure. The term NTD covers a spectrum of entities, mainly anencephaly, cephalocele and myelomeningocele (HOYME et al. 1981, ROBERTS and MOORE 1995, STEEGERS-THEUNISSEN et al. 1993, STEVENSON et al. 1987).

4.1.4.2.1
Anencephaly

Anencephaly has straightforward US characteristics: no bony structures above the fetal face and relatively scant cerebral tissue (Fig. 4.12). An early diagnosis is achieved in most cases because of a raised alphafetoprotein level. A similar entity is the so-called exencephaly (Fig. 4.13), in which cerebral tissue is present in a larger amount without bony structures. This condition is detected early by TVS and an evolution from ex- to anencephaly has been reported, challenging the classical theories of development of NTD (WILKINS-HAUG and FREEDMAN 1991).

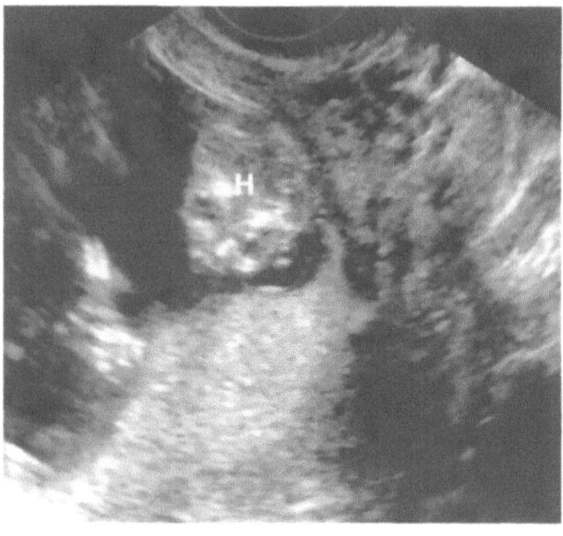

Fig. 4.13. Exencephaly. First trimester. Frontal view of the fetal head (*H*). The brain is visible without a bony skull around it

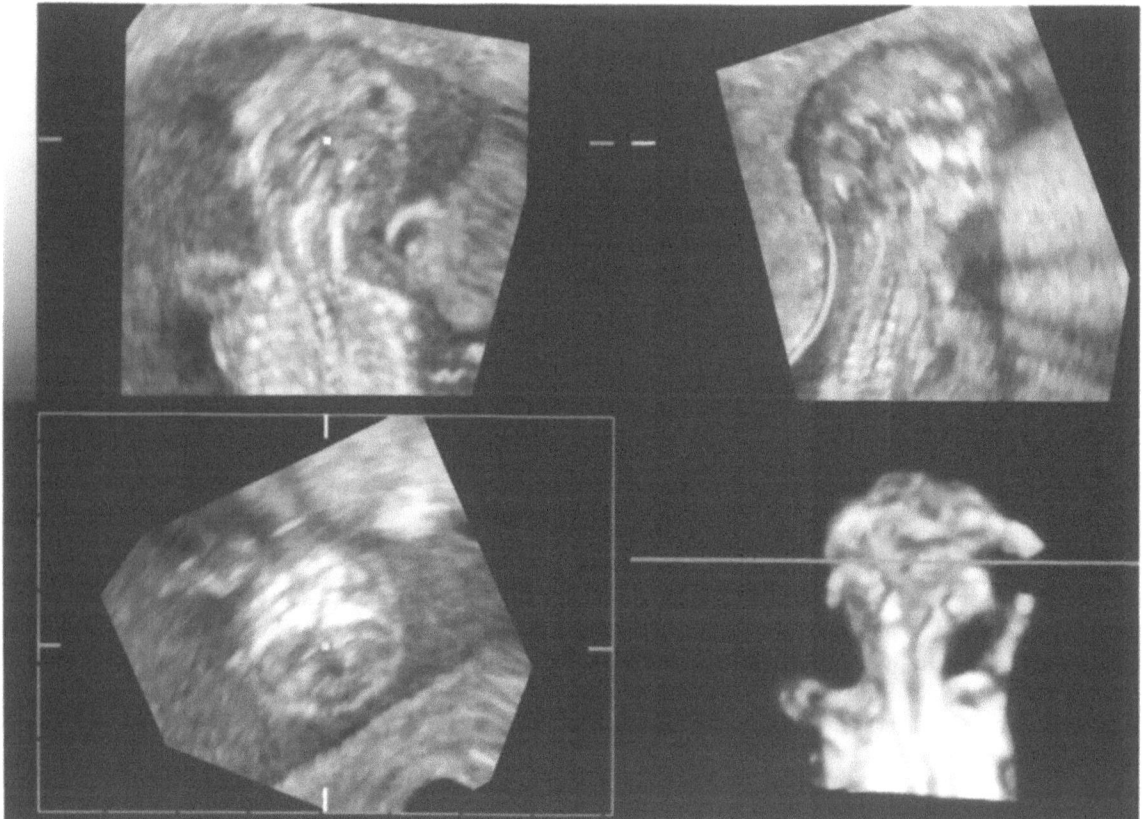

Fig. 4.12. Anencephaly. Second trimester. 2D and 3D visualization of an anencephalic fetus

4.1.4.2.2
Cephalocele

Cephalocele corresponds to the presence of typical cerebral tissue of variable volume outside the cranium (Fig. 4.14). The cerebral tissue extrudes through a bony defect, usually through the occipital bone. The corresponding biparietal diameter is too small. Differential diagnosis includes meningocele (cystic or mixed type mass), cystic hygroma (cystic septated mass outside the skull), hemangioma (highly vascularized extracranial mass and normal brain), teratoma (solid heterogeneous mass) and a scalp cyst (isolated cystic mass in the soft tissues). The amount of herniated cerebral tissue and the size of the ventricles determine the prognosis, which is usually poor. This anomaly may be associated with chromosomal anomalies or is included in polymalformation syndromes that worsen the prognosis (Budorick et al. 1995, Wininger and Donnenfeld 1994).

4.1.4.2.3
Open and Closed Spina Bifida

Open spina bifida occur in 1.25% pregnancies. The anomaly may develop at any level of the spine but predominantly at the lumbosacral spine. The detection by US approximates 100% in the latest series. There are direct and indirect US features. Direct features include the vertebral bony malformation (C-shaped or semilunar-shaped vertebra on a transverse scan), the skin defect and a low back mass (cystic or semicystic) in the case of myelomeningocele (Figs. 4.15–4.17). The mass may be absent in the case of myelocele, or can be more complex and contain echogenic tissue in the case of lipomyelomeningocele. The low insertion of the cord within the mass may be followed in the case of favorable fetal presentation, usually during the late second and third trimesters.

Indirect signs include the lemon sign (Fig. 4.15a; lemon-shaped cranium due to deformity of the frontal bones), the banana sign (Fig. 4.17b; effacement of the cisterna magna and shape of the cerebellum) and ventriculomegaly. Lemon and banana signs are detected during the second trimester whereas ventriculomegaly develops during the third trimester. These features may be difficult to visualize with TAS if there is maternal obesity, breech presentation or oligohydramnios. Additional views with TVS or MR imaging may provide significant diagnostic information (Blumenfeld et al. 1993, Budorick et al. 1995, Goldstein et al. 1989, Van den Hof et al. 1990,

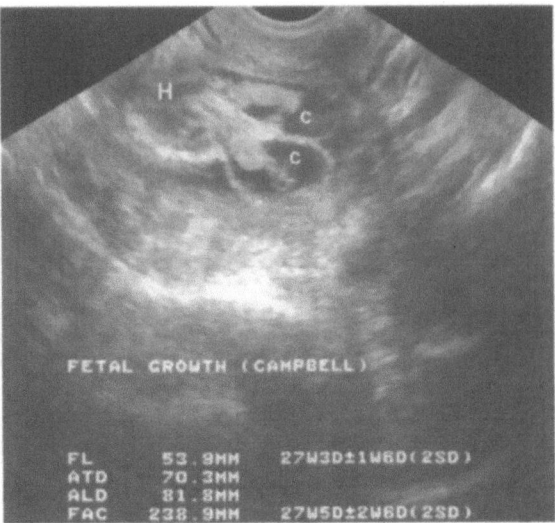

Fig. 4.14. Cephalocele. Early third trimester. Transverse scan of fetal head (H). Bilobed cephalocele (c) extends from the head

Babcook et al. 1994, Hogge et al. 1990, Kollias et al. 1992, Huppert et al. 1999). Closed spina bifida is much more difficult to diagnose, unless a mass is associated with the vertebral anomaly or unless a scoliosis is visualized (Anderson et al. 1994, Chat et al. 2001).

The prognosis depends upon the location of the anomaly, its extent and sensorimotor deficits demonstrated after birth. US analysis can determine with reasonable accuracy the level and extent of the anomaly and helps to predict the motor deficit. However, it is currently impossible to predict the sensory deficits, which are the most important factors for the prognosis. It is important to note that the movements of limbs and bladder function may be normal in utero in patients with NTD, even in the case of anencephaly (Cochrane et al. 1996, Warsof et al. 1988, Seller 1990, Hunt 1990).

4.1.4.3
Microcephaly and Disorders of Neuronal Proliferation

Microcephaly is defined as a fetal head size that falls at least 3 standard deviations below the mean, as measured by the biparietal or (better) the head circumference. This condition is encountered in isolation or may be associated with a variety of conditions including chromosomal anomalies, polymalformation syndromes, gyration disorders or congenital infections (see below). The condition may not be diagnosed until the late second or even third trimester when the

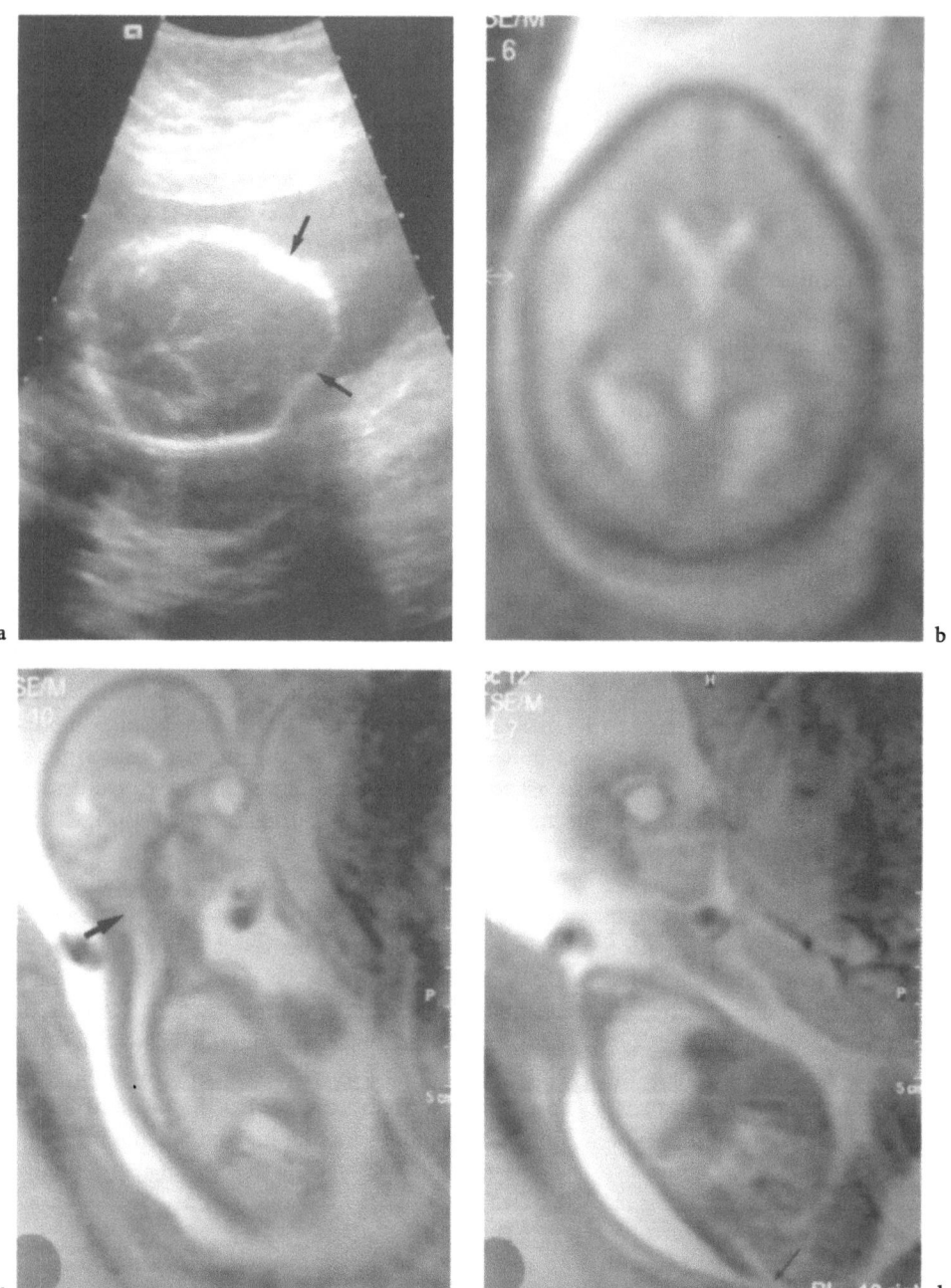

Fig. 4.15a–d. Open spina bifida. 22 week pregnancy. **a** Lemon sign at US. Flattened frontal bones (*arrows*). **b** Lemon sign at MR imaging. There is some associated ventriculomegaly. **c** Chiari malformation. Herniation of the cerebellum is demonstrated (*arrow*) at MR imaging. **d** Open spina bifida at the level of the lower lumbar spine at MRI imaging (*arrow*). The spina bifida was difficult to see on US due to breech presentation and maternal obesity

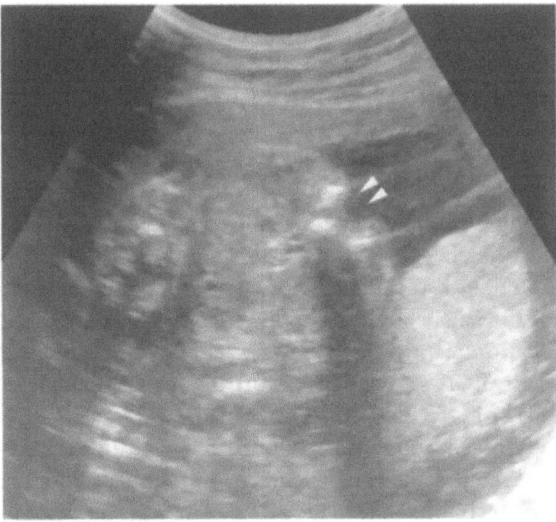

Fig. 4.16. Open spina bifida – bony and skin defect. Transverse scan of the lumbar spine. The open defect is obvious (*arrowheads*)

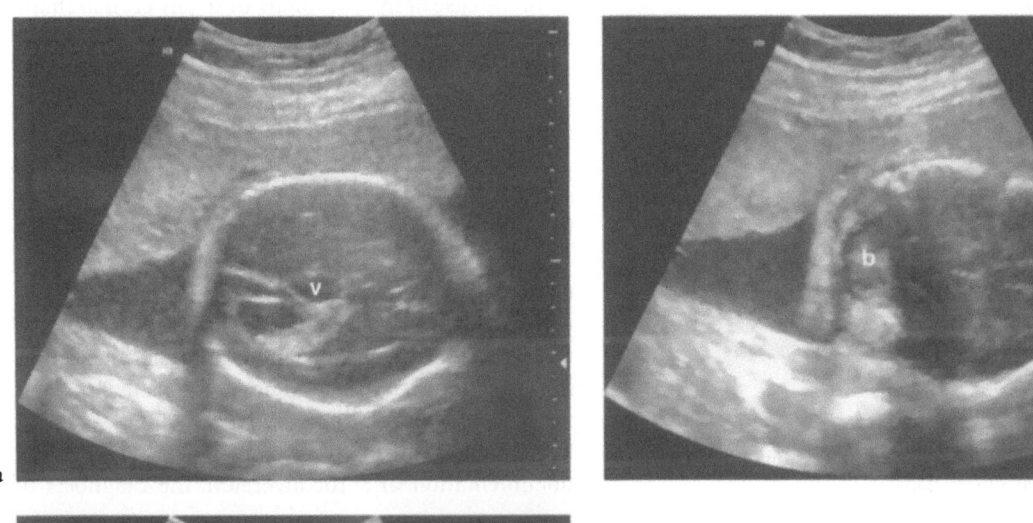

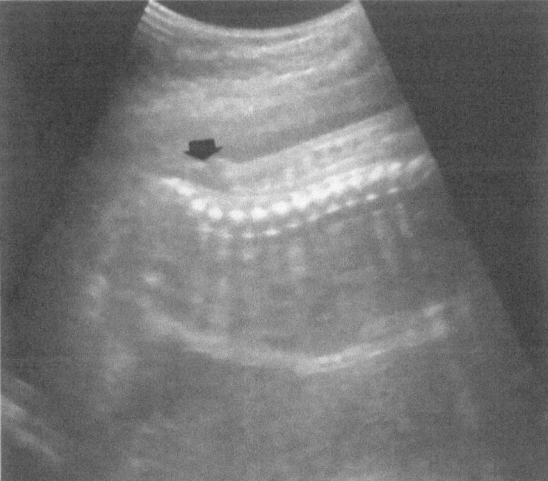

Fig. 4.17a–c. Closed spina bifida. Banana sign. **a** Transverse scan of the head. Ventriculomegaly includes the lateral and third ventricle (*v*). **b** Transverse scan of the posterior fossa. The absence of the cisterna magna and cerebellar herniation determine the banana sign (*b*). **c** Sagittal scan of the sacrum. A small meningocele is visible (*arrow*)

growth of the head slows (Fig. 4.18). It is important to look for associated brain anomalies including midline anomalies, ventriculomegaly, cephalocele or, most important, gyration anomalies and heterotopia. These latter anomalies are difficult to diagnose by US alone. Suggestive signs are a lack of normal development of the sylvian fissures or delay in the appearance of the secondary sulci for gyration anomalies (Figs. 4.19, 4.20). Heterotopia may develop along the ventricular

walls and will determine a nodular pattern. Heterotopia may also develop within the parenchyma or under a band pattern (Fig. 4.21). It is very useful to perform MR imaging in such indications. MR imaging is much more able to demonstrate gyration anomalies or heterotopia, especially band heterotopia (Figs. 4.18–4.21). Using US and MR imaging, one should be able to diagnose lissencephaly or pachygyria, but these diagnoses cannot be ascertained before the seventh month when all the sulci should have developed (WORTHEN et al. 1986, SALZMAN et al. 1991, YUH et al. 1994, HANSEN et al. 1993, GIRARD and RAYBAUD 1992, GRECO et al. 1998, MITCHELL et al. 2000, RYPENS et al. 1996).

Schizencephaly corresponds to a cleft in the cerebral mantle: the ventricle may communicate with the subarachnoid space (Fig. 4.22). This can be demonstrated on US and MR imaging. The condition may be associated with important gyration anomalies.

In the case of microcephaly or in any cranial shape anomalies, the sutures should be verified in order to exclude associated craniosynostosis; this may be easier to demonstrate with 3D US (BENACERAFF et al. 2000).

4.1.4.4
Infections Affecting the CNS

Cytomegalovirus (CMV) and toxoplasmosis are the two most common agents causing infection in the fetus; these infections may induce devastating lesions in the fetal CNS. In pregnancies complicated by CMV, 55% of affected children had permanent sequelae. The diagnosis of primary disease is ascertained by documentation of seroconversion, the diagnosis of

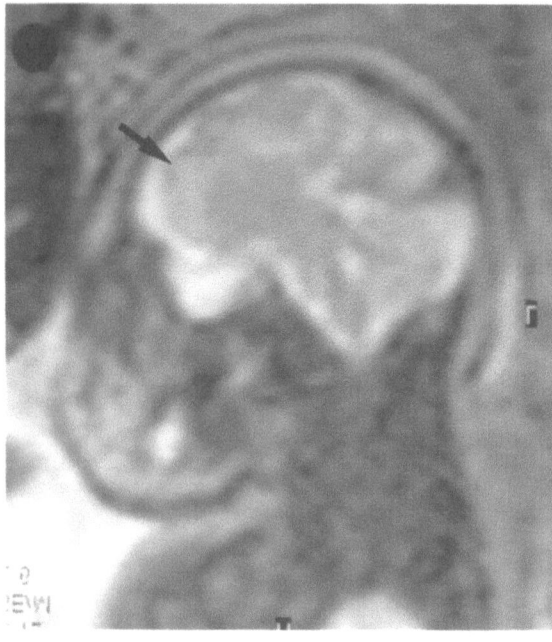

Fig. 4.18. Microcephaly. Third trimester. MR imaging, T2-weighted sequence. Hypoplasia of the frontal lobes (*arrow*). No associated malformations

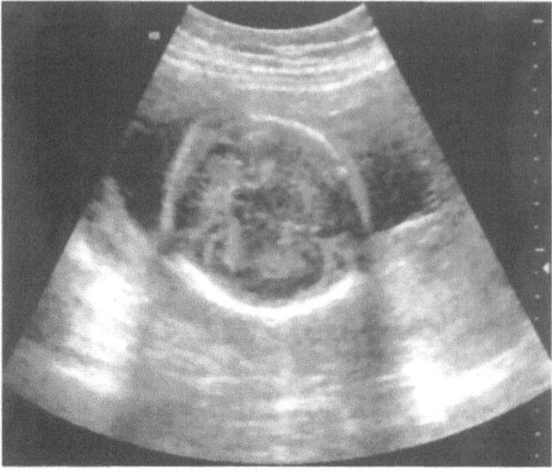
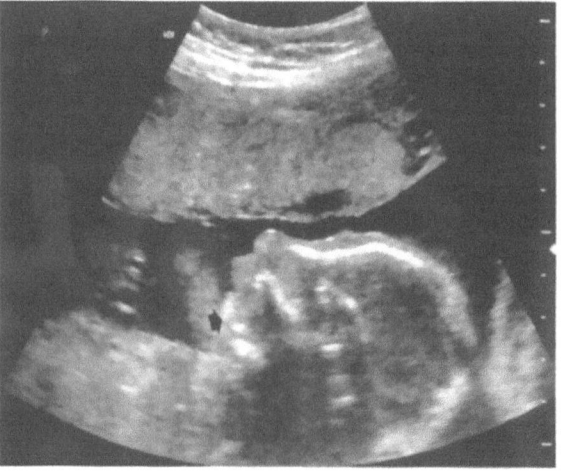

a   b

Fig. 4.19a, b. Abnormal gyration. Second trimester. **a** Transverse scan of the fetal head. No indentation of the sylvian fissure can be seen. **b** Sagittal view of the fetal profile. Micrognathia (*arrow*) as well as frontal hypoplasia

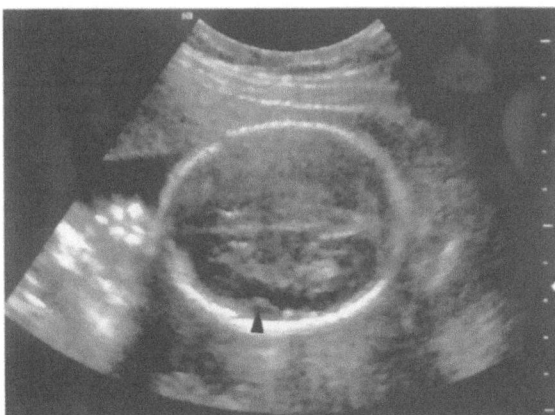

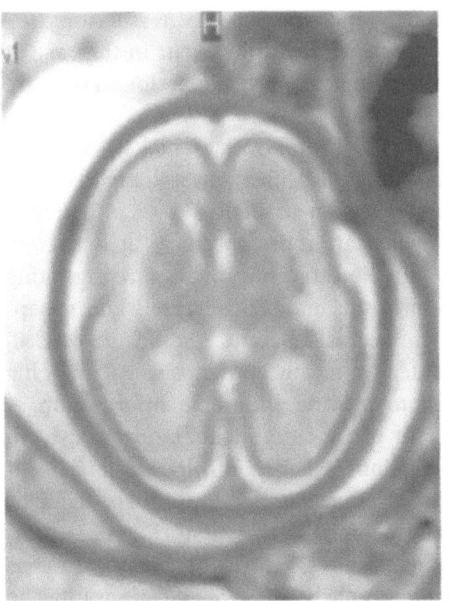

Fig. 4.20a, b. Abnormal gyration (polymalformation syndrome). Second trimester, 25 weeks. **a** US. Poorly indented sylvian fissure (*arrowhead*) on the transverse scan of fetal head. **b** MR imaging confirms abnormal sylvian gyration but no other anomalies are visible

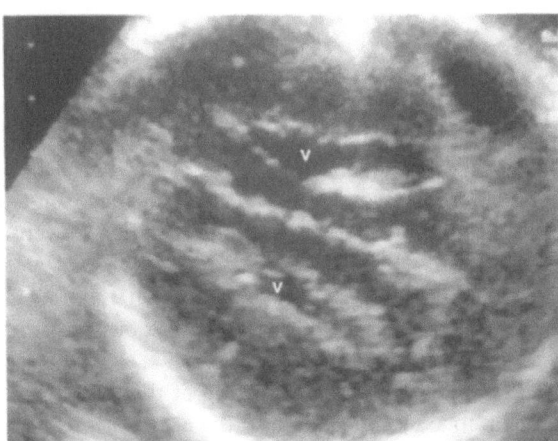

Fig. 4.21a, b. Band heterotopia. Third trimester. **a** US. Transverse scan of the fetal head. Irregular ventricular margins. *V* ventricles. **b** Fetal MR imaging, axial scan T2-weighted sequence. Nodularity of the lateral ventricle walls

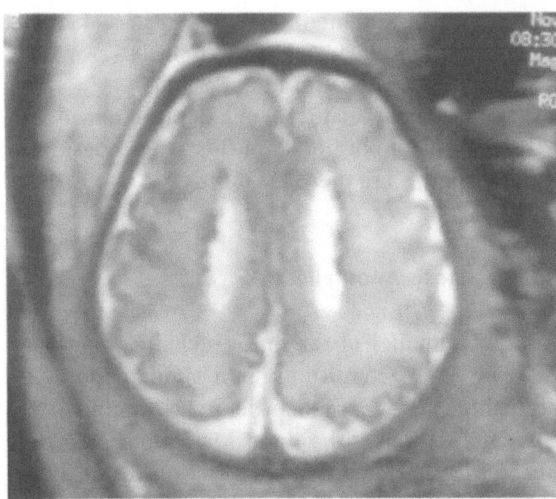

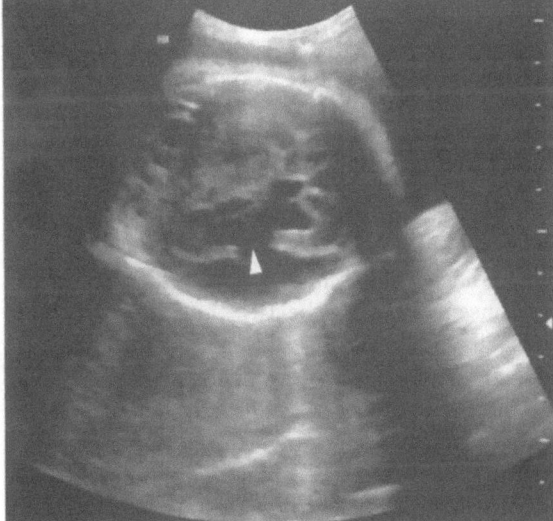

Fig. 4.22. Schizencephaly. Third trimester. Transverse scan. Interruption of the cerebral mantle (*arrowhead*). The ventricle connects with the subarachnoid space

fetal infection by polymerase chain reaction (see Chap. 11). False negative results occur in the case of both CMV and toxoplasmosis; reinfection in the case of CMV does occur.

In the case of CMV, the intracranial US findings include hydrocephalus, calcifications, ischemic destructive lesions and gyration anomalies.

Findings which are more specific, but harder to demonstrate, are linear echogenicities representing mineralization of thalamo-striate vessels and subependymal cystic necrosis. Because the degree of CNS involvement determines the prognosis, MR imaging may be used to provide additional information. A complete survey of the fetus should be performed to look for heart lesions (calcification), liver lesions (ischemia and calcifications) or hydrops. Toxoplasmosis can result in intracranial calcifications (Fig. 4.23), periventricular calcifications, ventriculomegaly with ventriculitis or microcephaly. These calcifications must be differentiated from the hyperechoic tubers observed in tuberous sclerosis (see below) (TASSIN et al. 1991, DROSE et al. 1991, ESTROFF et al. 1992, RADEMAKER et al. 1993, SEIDMAN et al. 1996, AHMAD et al. 2001, ENDERS et al. 2001) (see Chap. 11).

4.1.4.5
Intracranial Hemorrhage and Ischemia

With the use of obstetric US, it has been demonstrated that ischemic or hemorrhagic insults may occur any time during pregnancy and affect any organ of the developing embryo or fetus. The consequences depend on the gestational age of the fetus at the time of insult, and the duration and degree of the insult. Various factors have been shown to increase the risk of an ischemic or hemorrhagic event. Risk factors include twin pregnancies, maternal or fetal trauma, abruptio placentae, maternal shock or hypotension, maternal use of cocaine and maternal diabetes. Hemorrhagic and ischemic insults have devastating consequences on the CNS and the prognosis is usually poor. Early gestation ischemic or hemorrhagic lesions are rarely demonstrated as such but their consequences are usually detected; early insults probably determine schizencephaly, partial corpus callosum agenesis or perisylvian syndrome (KLINGENSMITH and CIOFFI 1986, KUSNIECKY and ANDERMANN 1994, VOLPE 1992). During the third trimester, the US features of in utero ischemia or hemorrhage are similar to those observed in the neonate or premature infant. Ischemic lesions appear as periventricular hyperechogenicity whereas hemorrhagic lesions may appear as echogenic

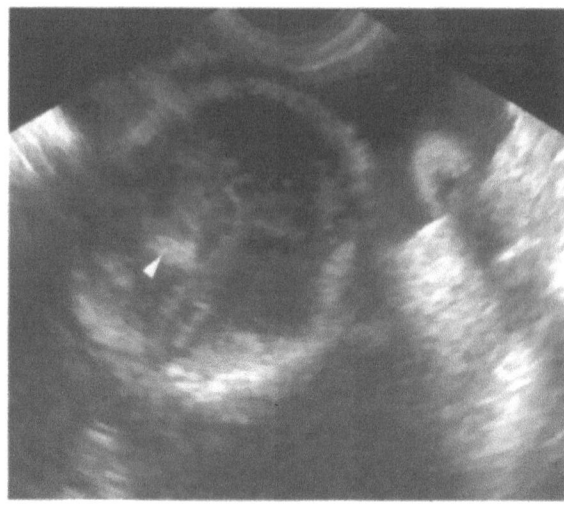

Fig. 4.23. Toxoplasmosis. Transverse scan of the head towards the vertex demonstrating a focus of calcification (*arrow*)

parenchymal foci or intraventricular echogenic debris; an indirect sign of intraventricular hemorrhage is the demonstration of ependymal periventricular hyperechogenicity (Figs. 4.24–4.27). The end result can range from extensive brain destruction to the development of porencephalic cavities or ventriculomegaly (KUSNIECKY and ANDERMANN 1994, ANDERSON et al. 1994, RORKE and ZIMMERMAN 1992, ACHIRON et al. 1993, VOLPE 1992, BARKOVICH et al. 1995, SCHER et al. 1991, KNUPPEL et al. 1994, DEVRIES et al. 1998). MR imaging of the fetal brain can help to assess the extent of the acute lesions and of the sequelae: hemorrhagic foci will appear hyperintense on T1-weighted images (Figs. 4.24, 4.27) (CANAPICCHI et al. 1998, FUKUI et al. 2001, REISS et al. 1996, DE LAVEAUCOUPET et al. 2001).

It is noteworthy that ischemic damage may occur at the level of the brain stem; this type of lesion is rarely recognized in utero (MAMELAK et al. 1994).

4.1.4.6
Organogenesis Anomalies

Midline anomalies of the brain include a heterogeneous group of conditions with similar etiologies and pathogenesis. Each disorder may be found alone or in combination with others. Meticulous scanning is necessary to document each case. Chromosomal analysis is always performed and MR imaging is usually performed to provide complementary information.

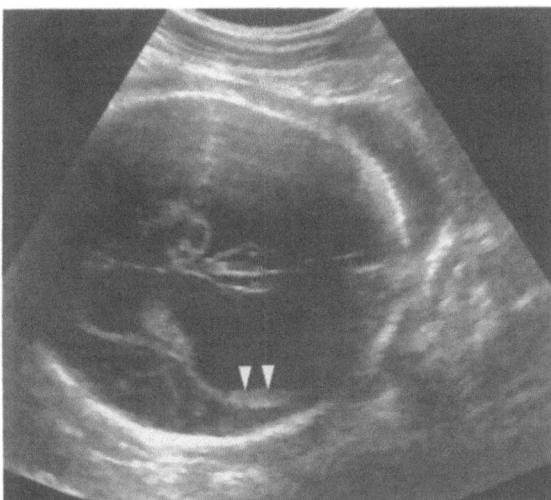

a

Fig. 4.24a–c. Intraventricular hemorrhage. Third trimester. **a** US in utero. Transverse scan. Ventriculomegaly and echogenic deposit (*arrowheads*) in the most dependent part of the ventricle. **b** US at birth. Coronal view. Ventriculomegaly with hyperechoic ependyma (ventricular margins). **c** MR imaging at birth. Coronal view. Right intraventricular hyperintense clot (*arrow*)

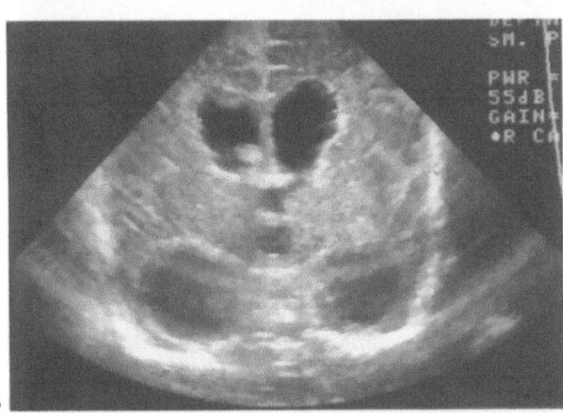

b

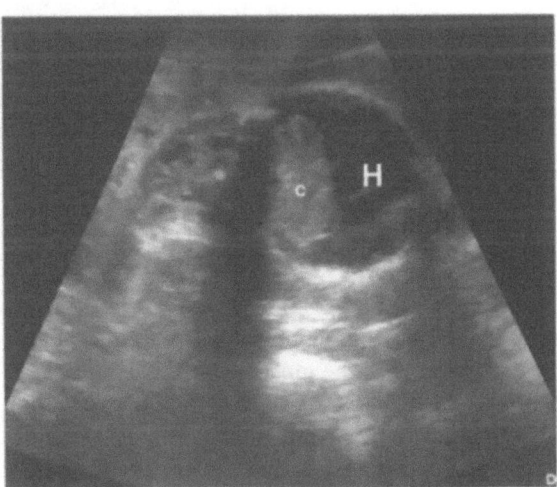

Fig. 4.25. Subependymal hemorrhage. Second trimester. Transverse scan. Hyperechoic "mass" in the subependymal area (*arrowhead*)

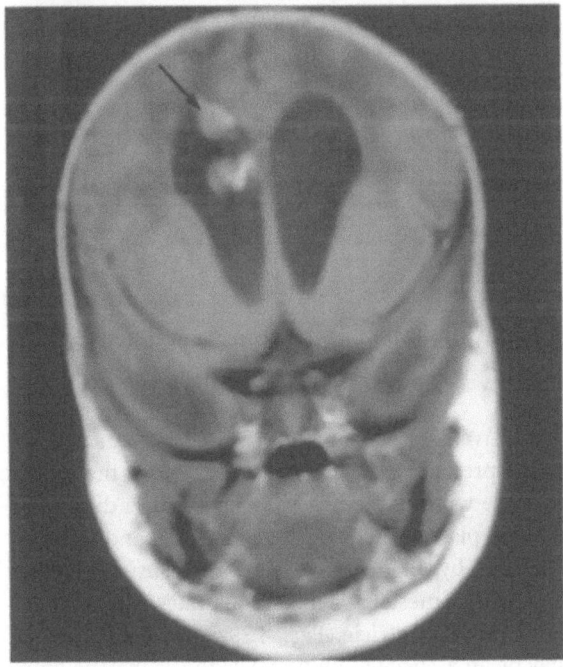

c

Fig. 4.26. Cerebellar hemorrhage (eclamptic mother). Second trimester. Transverse scan. Diffuse hyperechogenicity of the cerebellum (*c*). *H* head

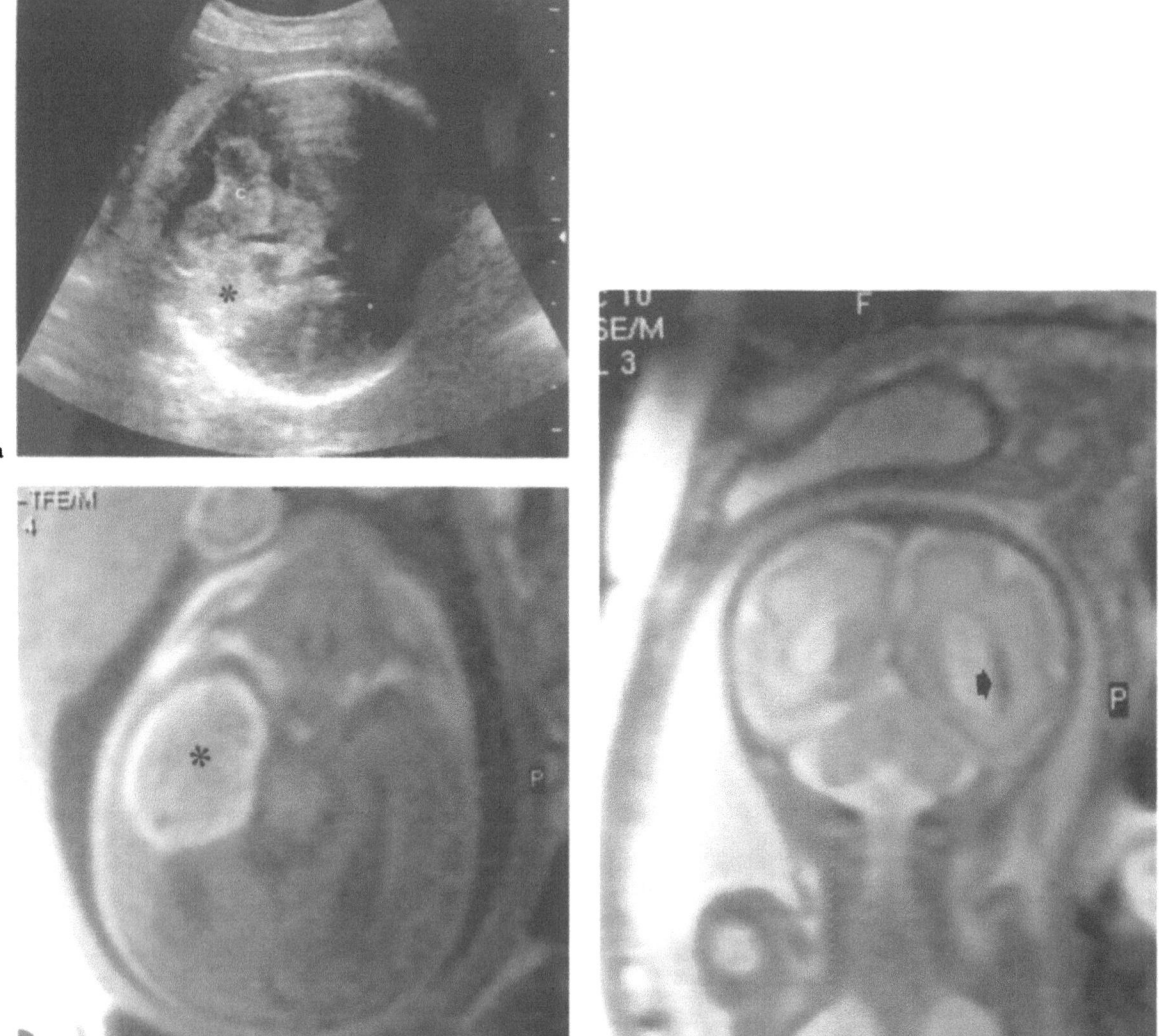

Fig. 4.27a–c. Intraventricular and parenchymal hemorrhage. Third trimester. **a** US. Transverse scan. Hyperechoic focus in temporal and sylvian area (*). *c* cerebellum. **b** Fetal MR imaging. T1-weighted sequence. Temporal hyperintense area of hemorrhage (*). **c** Fetal MR imaging. T2-weighted sequence. Ventriculomegaly and fluid-fluid level (*arrow*) corresponding to blood

4.1.4.6.1
Holoprosencephaly

Among the types of holoprosencephaly, alobar holoprosencephaly has the most typical US appearance: a single ventricle and fused thalami. First trimester or early second trimester diagnosis is possible. The semi-lobar and lobar subtypes are less easily diagnosed and may resemble hydrocephalus. This malformation is important to detect as early as possible since the prognosis is poor with associated malformations (face++), and chromosomal anomalies are very common (trisomy 13 and 18) (Fig. 4.28) (GEMBRUCH et al. 1995) (see Chap. 12).

4.1.4.6.2
Dandy-Walker Malformation and Dandy-Walker Variant

Dandy-Walker malformation (DWM) is characterized by the presence of a marked dilatation of the fourth ventricle with marked vermian hypoplasia displacing the hypoplastic cerebellar lobes laterally and forward. Diagnosis by US is easy in typical cases, usually during the third trimester, as it demonstrates the enlarged cystic fourth ventricle (Figs. 4.29–4.31). Fetal hydrops may be an associated finding. Diagnosis may be more difficult with Dandy-Walker variant (DWV), in which the degree of vermian hypoplasia varies (Fig. 4.32).

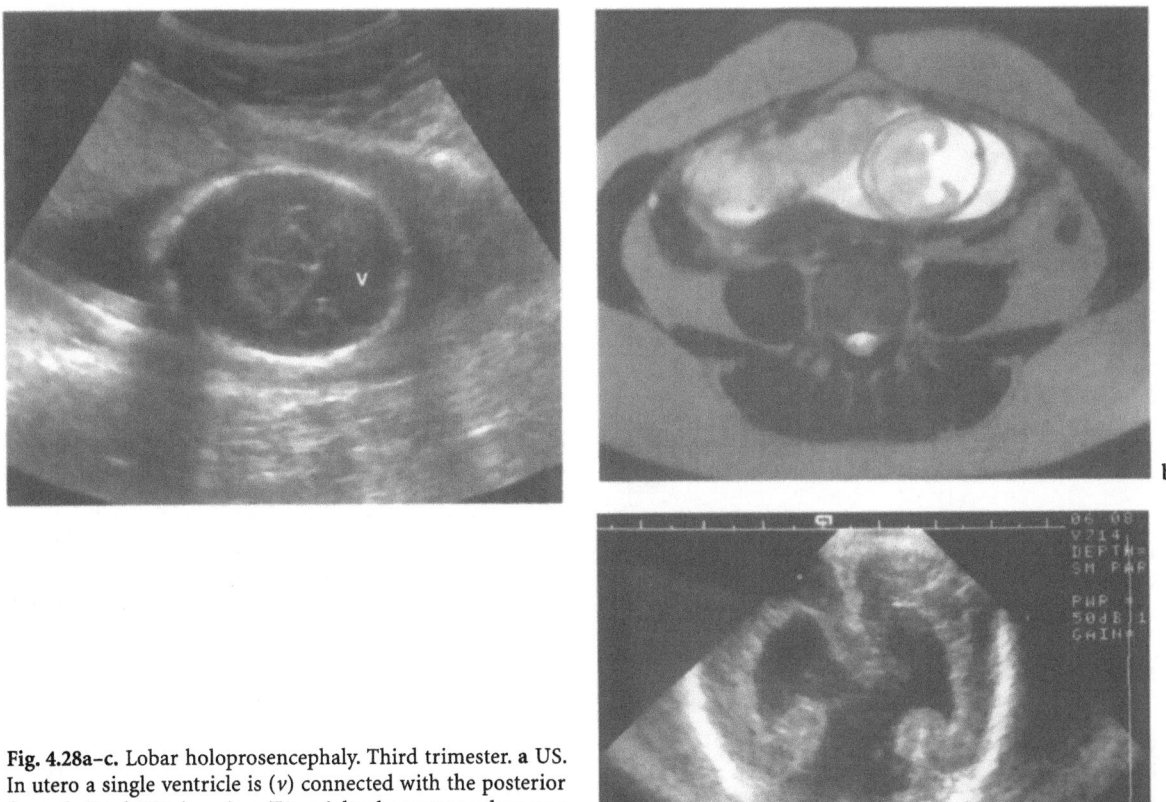

Fig. 4.28a–c. Lobar holoprosencephaly. Third trimester. a US. In utero a single ventricle is (*v*) connected with the posterior fossa. b Fetal MR imaging. T2-weighted sequence does not show additional information. c US. Stillbirth examination, confirming the anomaly

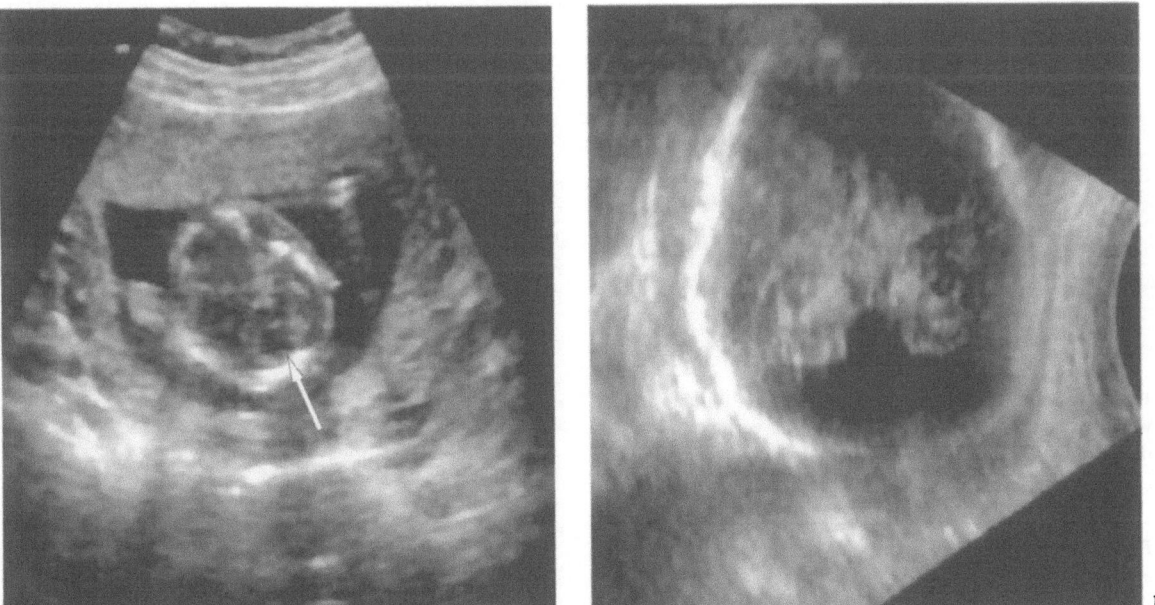

Fig. 4.29a, b. Dandy-Walker malformation: evolution of the cystic dilatation. a Second trimester. Limited cystic dilatation of the fourth ventricle (*arrow*). b Third trimester (same patient). Marked increased dilatation of the fourth ventricle

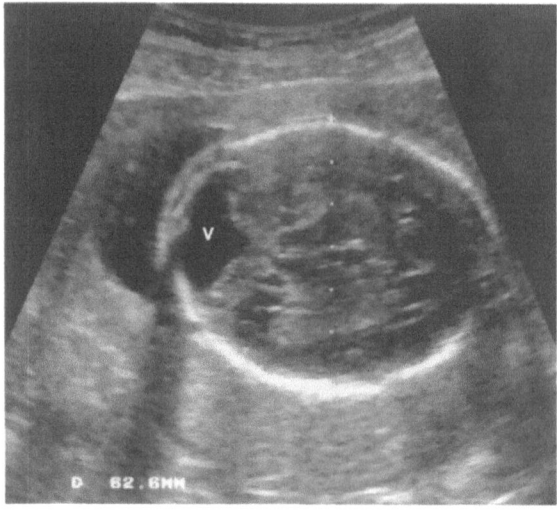

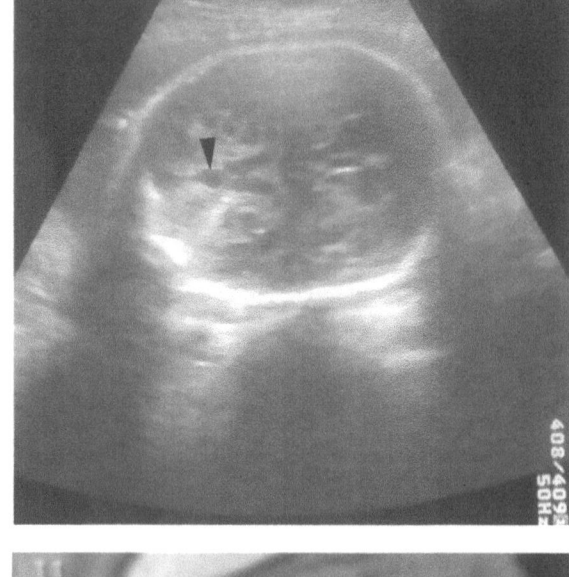

Fig. 4.30. Dandy-Walker malformation. Third trimester. Cystic distension of the fourth ventricle (*v*)

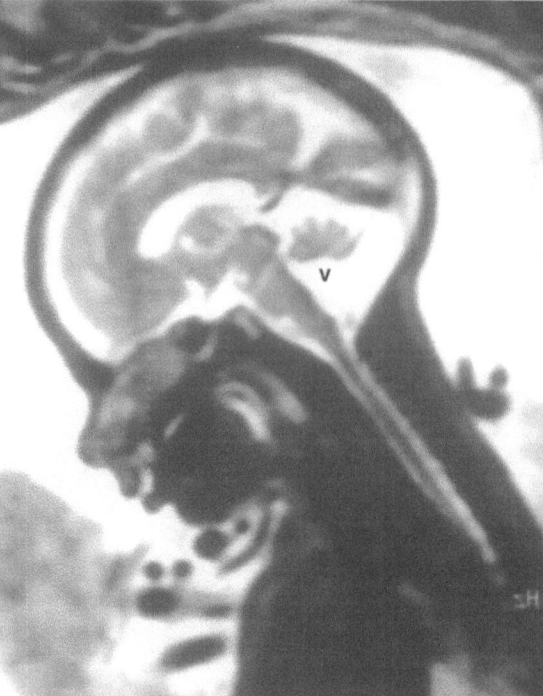

Fig. 4.31. Dandy-Walker malformation. Fetal MR imaging. T2-weighted sagittal scan. Hypoplasia of the vermis and cystic dilatation of the fourth ventricle (*v*)

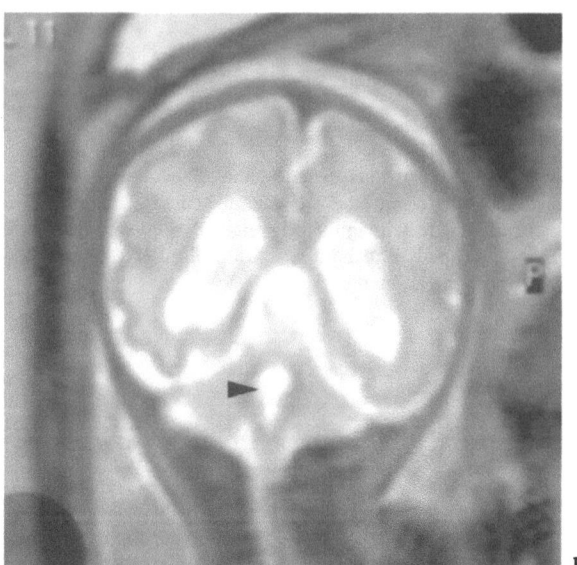

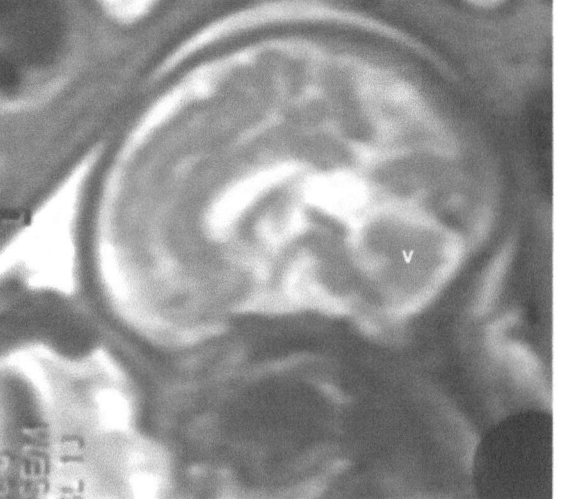

Fig. 4.32a–c. Dandy-Walker variant. Ventriculomegaly and cerebellar sulci hypoplasia. **a** US transverse view. Globular fourth ventricle (*arrowhead*). **b** Fetal MR imaging. Coronal view confirming the ventriculomegaly and cystic dilatation of the fourth ventricle (*arrowhead*). **c** Fetal MR imaging. Sagittal view demonstrating too few sulci at the surface of the vermis (*v*)

Furthermore, as mentioned above, stages of the normal cerebellar development may mimic malformations. The interpretation should be cautious and, MR imaging is helpful in ascertaining the anomaly. Important contributory features by MR imaging would be the demonstration of the shape and size of the vermis (small, abnormal sulci), and the shape and size of the fourth ventricle (round or oval is suggestive of an anomaly). Complete agenesis of the vermis can be part of Joubert syndrome. The prognosis of DWM is unknown but presumed grim, especially with associated malformations (heart ++) (GEMBRUCH 1995, ACHIRON et al. 1993, KEOGAN et al. 1994, BABCOOK 1996a, BROMLEY et al. 1994, CHANG et al. 1994).

4.1.4.6.3
Agenesis of the Corpus Callosum and Related Anomalies

The corpus callosum (CC) is the largest cerebral commissure connecting neocortical areas. It develops late compared with the other cerebral structures. The rostral part develops first around 12 weeks. Development of the CC is completed around 18–20 weeks. At that time, the CC should be visualized with US best on midsagittal views. TVS may give better delineation of the CC in some cases. The presence of a cavum of the septum pellucidum is an indirect sign of the presence of the CC (Figs. 4.2–4.4). The demonstration of pericallosal and anterior cerebral arteries is also a good evidence of the normal development of the CC.

Partial or complete agenesis of the CC is a challenging condition for antenatal US, as regards both diagnosis and management. US diagnosis of complete agenesis of the CC is based on direct and indirect signs (Figs. 4.33–4.35). Direct evidence of absence is nonvisualization of the CC after 20 weeks gestation. Indirect signs include parallel positioning of the lateral ventricles with pointed frontal horns, peculiar globular dilatation of the occipital horns (colpocephaly), ascension of the third ventricle (with the so-called bull horns appearance; Fig. 4.33), and usually widening of the interhemispheric fissure but sometimes interdigitation of the interhemispheric sulci. In cases of complete agenesis, the pericallosal sulci will radiate, perpendicular to the supposed location of the CC. Color Doppler may demonstrate the absence of a normal pericallosal artery. Partial agenesis (dysgenesis) may involve the posterior segment (corresponding to arrested development) or the other segments (resulting from an insult later in pregnancy). This diagnosis is less easily made since the US signs may be partial or mild. MR imaging is very helpful in such

cases in order to verify the extent of the anomaly and to look for associated anomalies. Chromosomal analysis is mandatory too (MALINGER and ZAKU 1993, RUBINSTEIN et al. 1994, PILU et al. 1993).

Pericallosal lipoma may be a rare associated finding. The lipoma appears as a nodular or a tubular echogenic mass paralleling the CC when it is present, or replacing it when the CC is partially or completely absent. The lipoma may extend into the choroid fissures or into the frontal lobes. The condition may be isolated or associated with chromosomal anomalies and syndromes (Goldenhar syndrome) (ICKOWICZ et al. 2001).

Counseling parents of a fetus with an anomaly of the CC is very difficult. An isolated anomaly has apparently a better prognosis than cases with associated malformations. MR imaging may help counseling (GIRARD et al. 1993, GUPTA and ILFORD 1995, VERGANI et al. 1994).

4.1.4.7
CNS Tumors and Vascular Malformations

A choroid plexus cyst is very common finding and is not abnormal when isolated. Otherwise, in cases of cystic-appearing masses, arachnoid cyst must be differentiated from vascular malformations. Arachnoid cysts may develop in any subarachnoid space, more commonly in the midline (suprasellar region or posterior fossa) (Figs. 4.36–4.38). Vascular malforma-

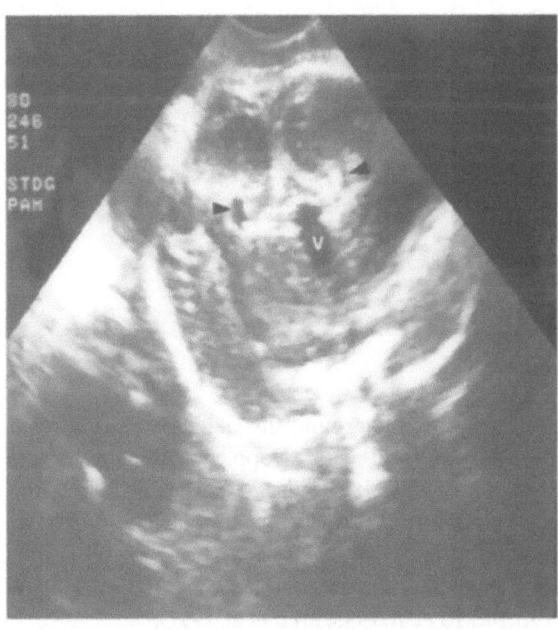

Fig. 4.33. Agenesis of the corpus callosum. Third trimester. Endovaginal US. Coronal view. Typical "bull horns" appearance. *v* third ventricle, *arrowheads* lateral ventricles

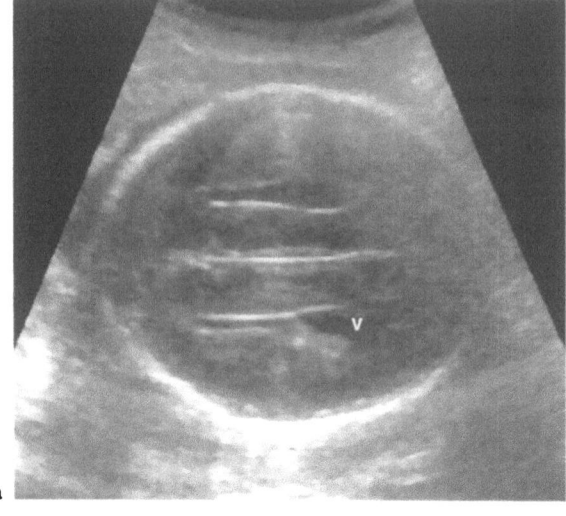

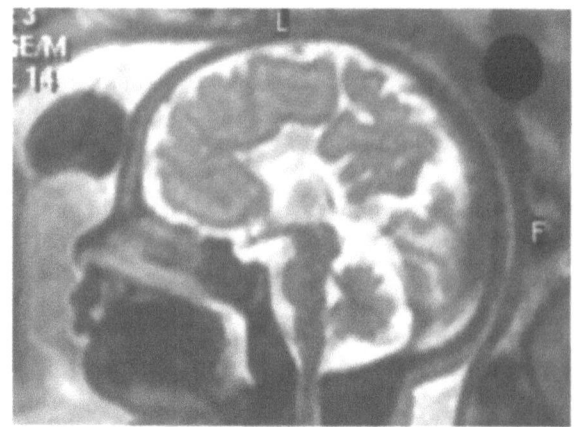

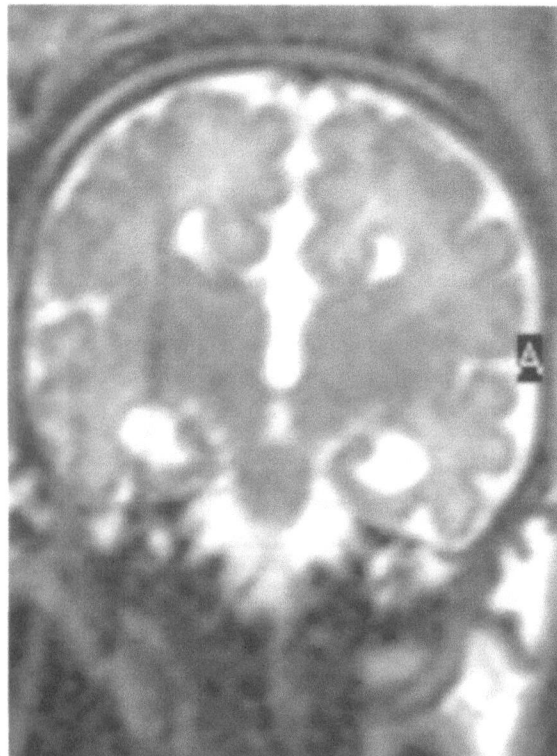

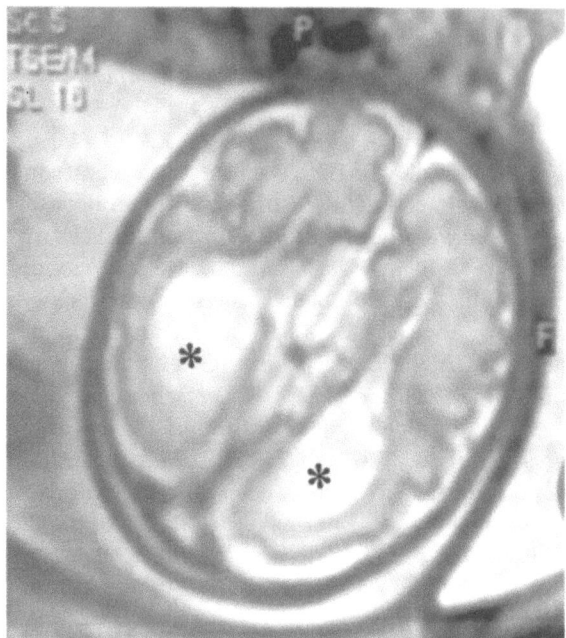

Fig. 4.34a–d. Agenesis of the corpus callosum (ACC). **a** US. Third trimester. The lateral ventricles are too parallel to the falx. Occipital ventriculomegaly (colpocephaly) (*v*). **b** Fetal MR imaging. T2-weighted sagittal view confirming a complete ACC. **c** Fetal MR imaging. T2-weighted coronal view confirming complete ACC. **d** Fetal MR imaging. T2-weighted transverse view confirming the colpocephaly

tion occur mainly around the Galen vein. Aneurysm may develop and color Doppler will demonstrate the hypervascularized enlarged vessel. MR imaging is useful in order to map the vascular anomaly (Fig. 4.39) (see Chap. 13) (COMSTOCK and KIRK 1991, DAN et al. 1992, BANNISTER et al. 1999, BARJOT et al. 1999, D'ADDARIO et al. 1998, PILU et al. 1997).

True CNS tumors are very rare. Intracranial teratoma and glioma have been reported. They appear as large, solid, heterogeneous and hypervascular-ized masses. Differential diagnosis should include pericallosal lipoma (on the midline) (ICKOWICZ et al. 2001) and parenchymal hemorrhage (nonvascu-larized areas) (see Chap. 13).

MR imaging is particularly efficient for the evaluation of patients at risk of developing tuberous sclerosis (either because of the discovery of a car-diac rhabdomyoma or because of a family history). Visualization of cerebral involvement is very difficult on US. On MR imaging, tubers appear hyperintense

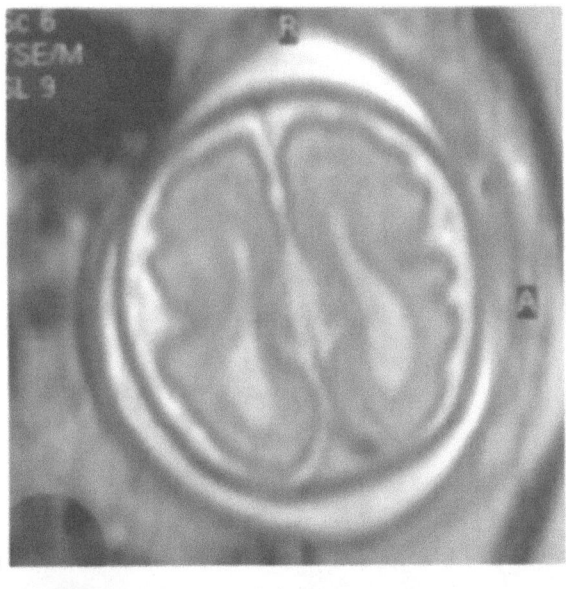

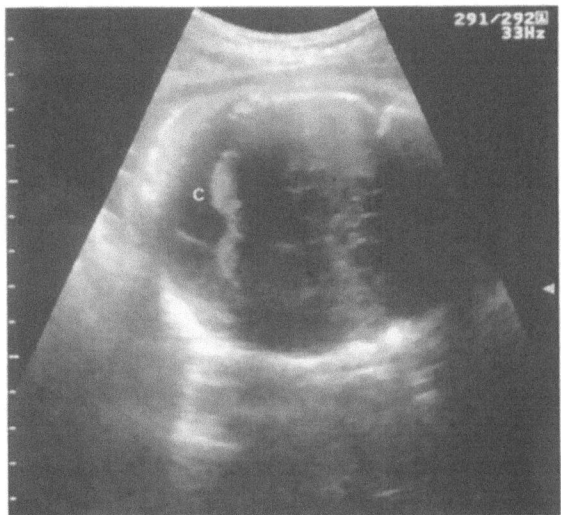

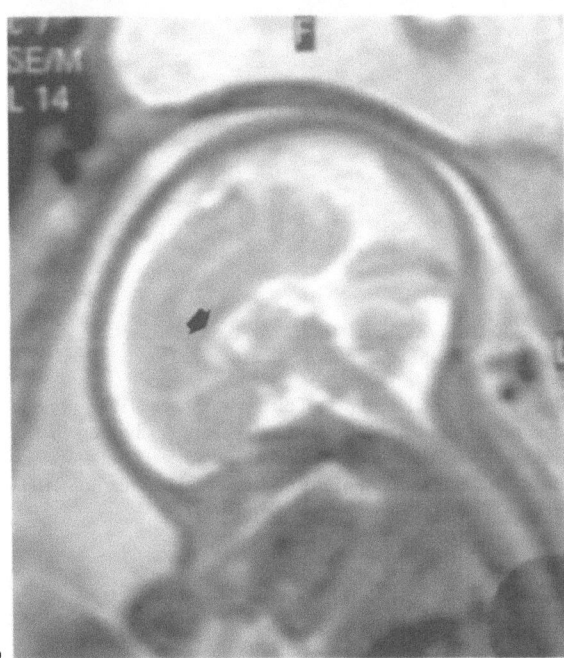

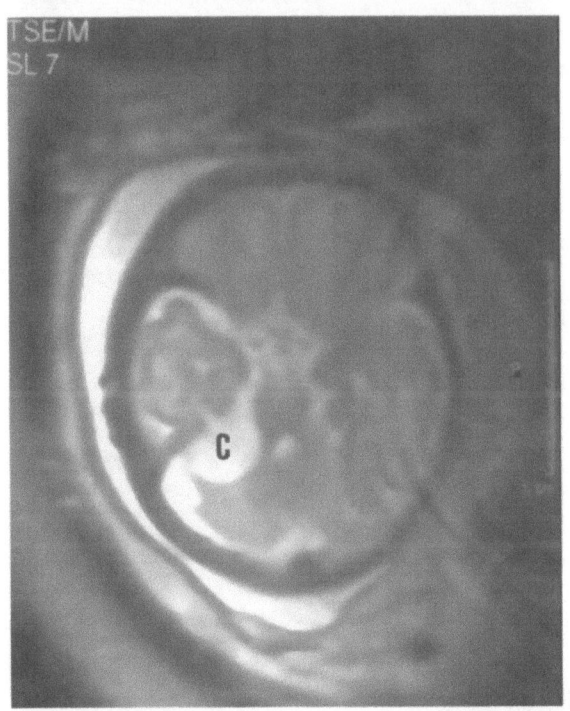

Fig. 4.35a, b. Partial agenesis of the corpus callosum. a Fetal MR imaging. Transverse scan demonstrating mild colpocephaly (and parallel frontal norms). b Fetal MR imaging. Sagittal scan. The anterior part of the corpus callosum is present (*arrow*)

Fig. 4.36a, b. Posterior fossa cyst (*c*) displacing the subarachnoid folds. a US. Third trimester transverse scan. b MR imaging. T2-weighted sequence allows a better delineation of the anomaly

on T1-weighted and hypointense on T2-weighted sequences (LEVINE et al. 2000).

The spectrum of anomalies that can affect the CNS is very wide. Developmental anomalies occur in every structure of the brain. Acquired anomalies may also impair normal brain development.

4.2
Face

Examining the fetal face is an important part of obstetrical US of the developing fetus. On the one hand it symbolizes to the parents their baby-to-be and gives them a closer link with it. On the other hand anomalies of the face may signal more complex

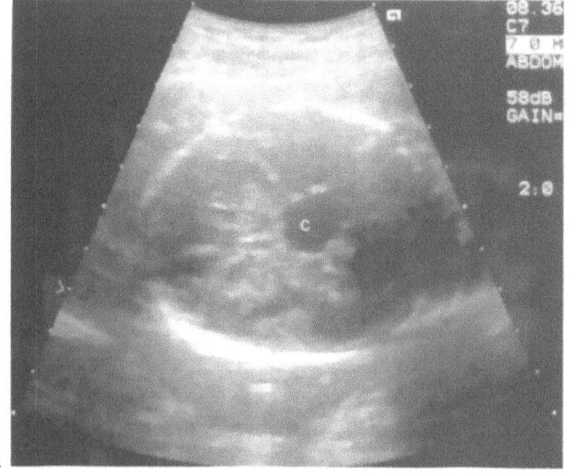

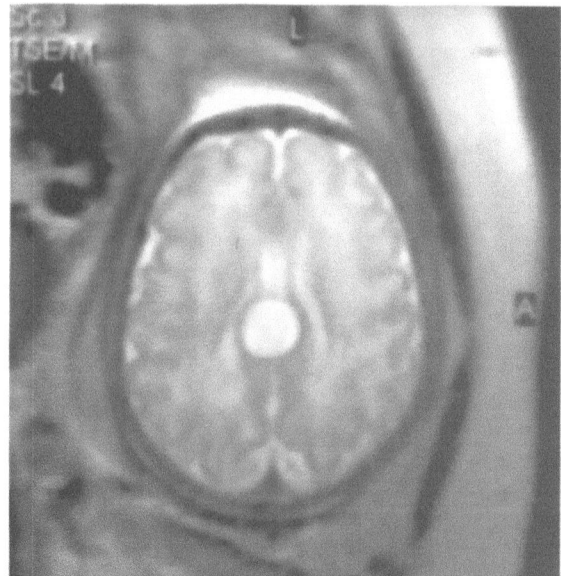

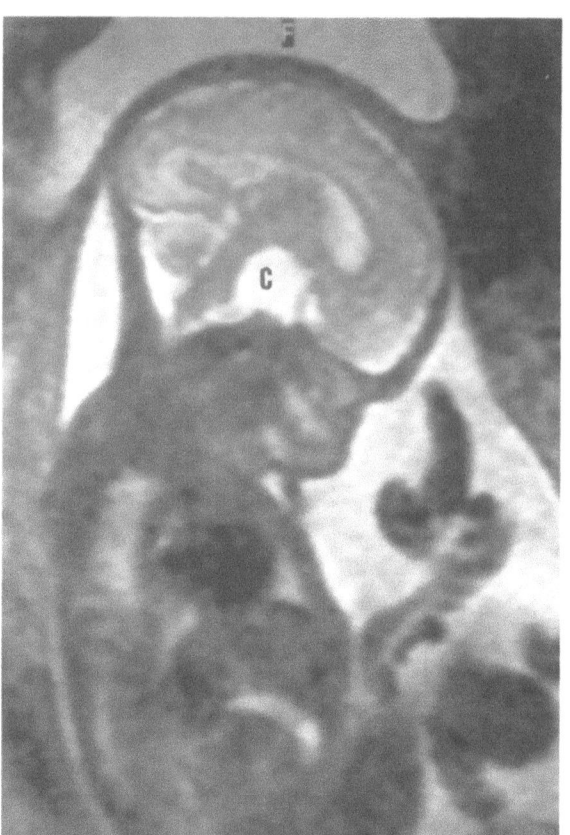

Fig. 4.37a-c. Arachnoid cyst. Third trimester. **a** US. Transverse scan of the fetal head. A cystic structure (*c*) is seen in the middle of the falx. **b** Fetal MR imaging. T2-weghted sequence confirming the location of the cyst. **c** Fetal MR imaging. Sagittal view. The cyst (*c*) indents the pons

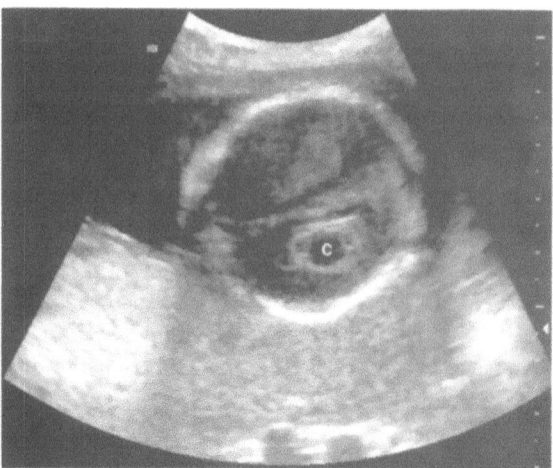

Fig. 4.38. Choroid plexus cyst. Second trimester. Transverse scan demonstrates a choroid plexus cyst (*c*)

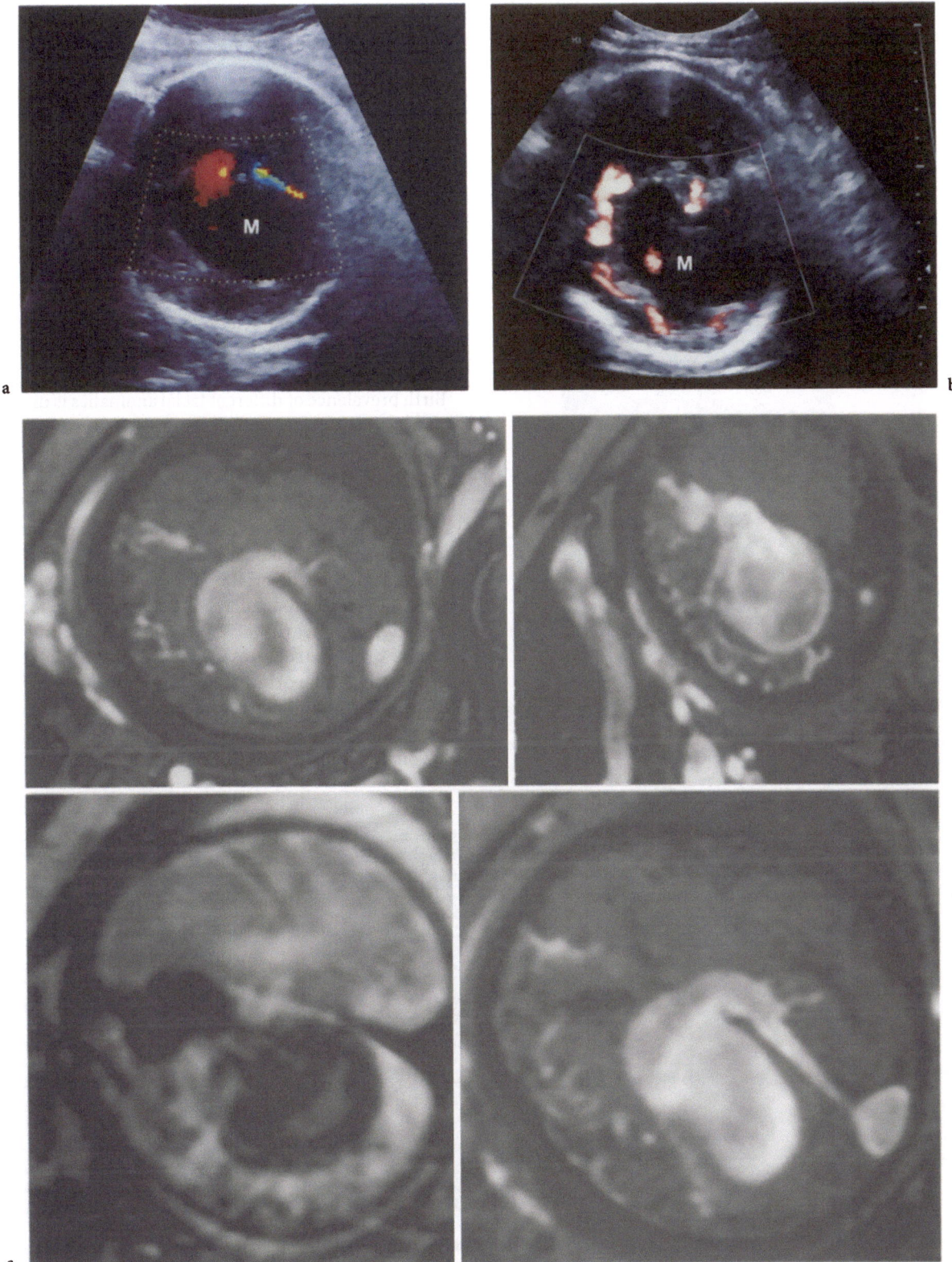

Fig. 4.39a–c. Vascular malformation. Third trimester. **a** US color Doppler. Vascularization around but not within the mass (*M*). **b** US Doppler energy. Abnormal vascular channels around the mass (*M*). **c** MR imaging. Various T1- and T2-weighted sequences confirming the vascular nature of the malformation and the collaterals

malformations. 3D US is modifying our approach to facial anomalies and helps a better understanding of their extent (Fig. 4.40).

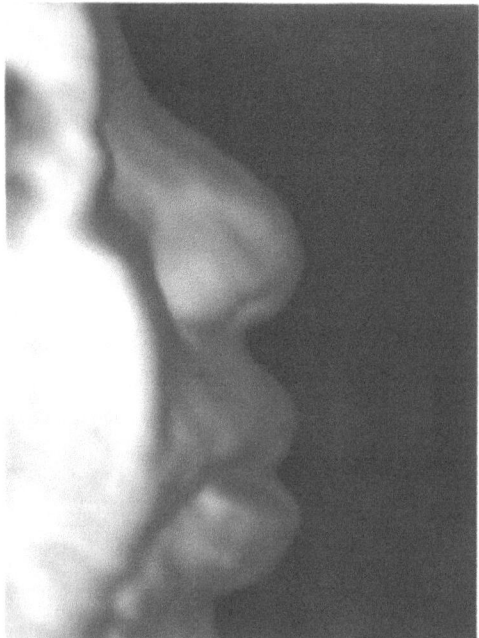

a

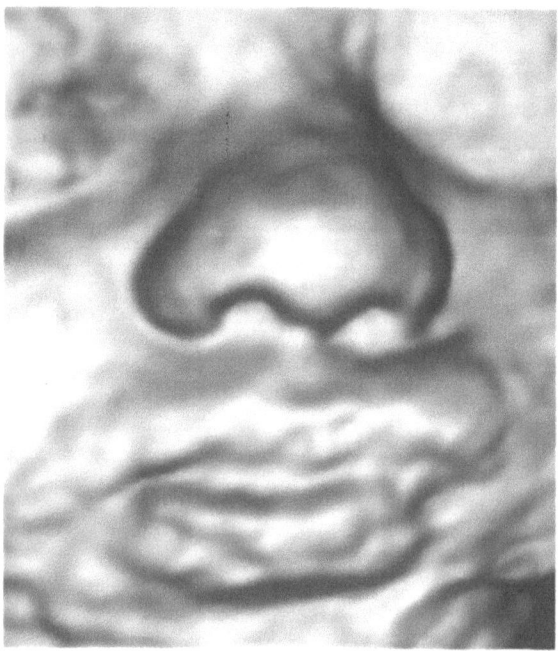

b

Fig. 4.40a, b. 3D display of the nose and mouth. **a** Nose in profile. **b** Nose and mouth, frontal view

4.2.1
Normal Facial Anatomy

Analysis of the normal anatomy should include the lips and maxillae, the nose, the eyes and the fetal profile. There must be an evaluation of the appearance in relation to the gestational age (Figs. 4.40–4.48). Several structures can be measured whenever an anomaly is suspected.

The fetal face is an area of considerable information and should be included in every scan dedicated to the early detection of fetal abnormalities. The early detection of facial defect should initiate a thorough survey for other structural malformations in the fetus, as well as a cytogenetic analysis.

Birth prevalence of different facial anomalies is difficult to estimate correctly because the true prevalence of many specific malformations is either unknown or extremely rare.

The normal facial anatomy should be studied systematically in three planes: sagittal, axial and coronal. The sagittal plane is useful for observing the fetal profile: forehead, nasal bridge, upper and lower lips, and jaw. The coronal plane is the most useful for identifying the integrity of the facial anatomy: lips, nose and orbital structures. The axial plane is best used to evaluate the orbital region, and the anatomy of the maxilla and mandible.

The classification of facial malformations is easy, based on their location: forehead, nose, lips, chin, etc.

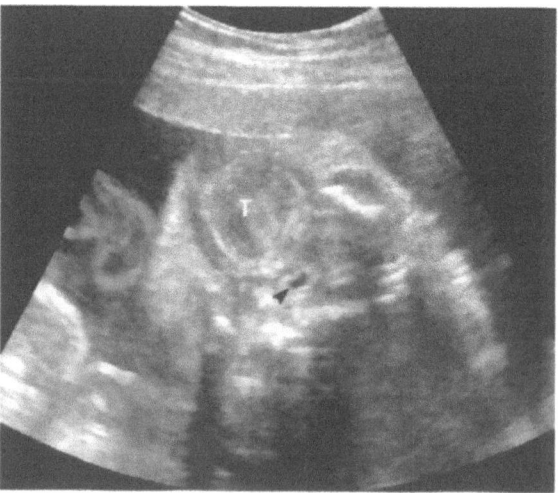

Fig. 4.41. Tongue (*T*). Transverse view. Third trimester. The *arrowhead* points to the larynx

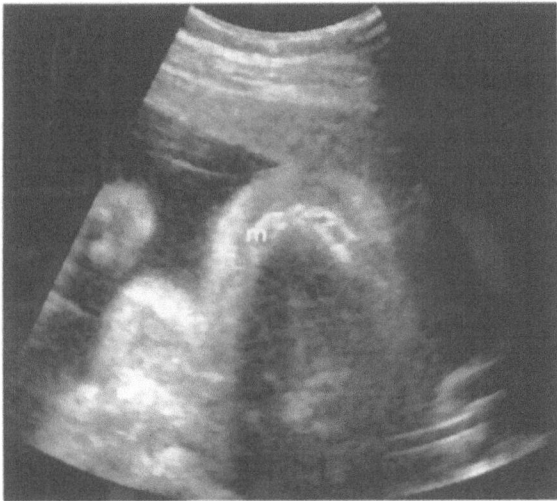

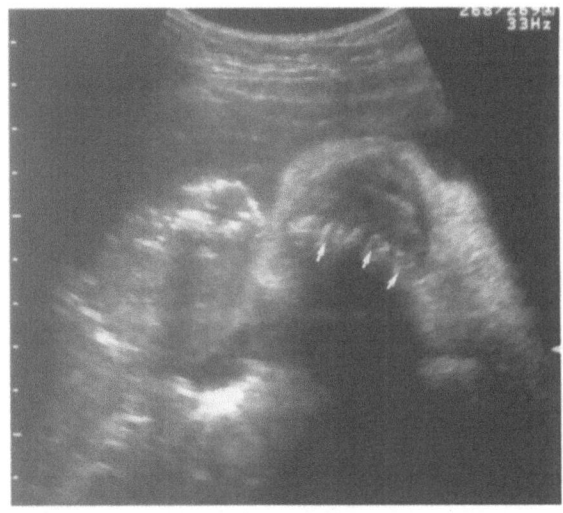

Fig. 4.42. Upper maxilla. Transverse view. The bony maxilla appears hyperechoic (*m*) and correctly positioned

Fig. 4.43. Tooth germs, lower maxilla. Multiple germs are visible (*arrows*)

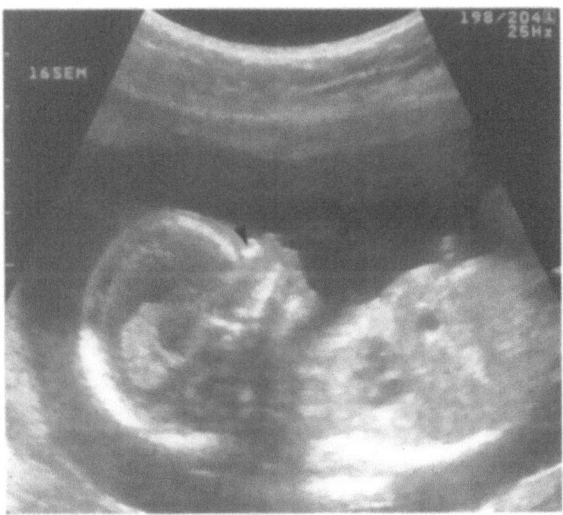

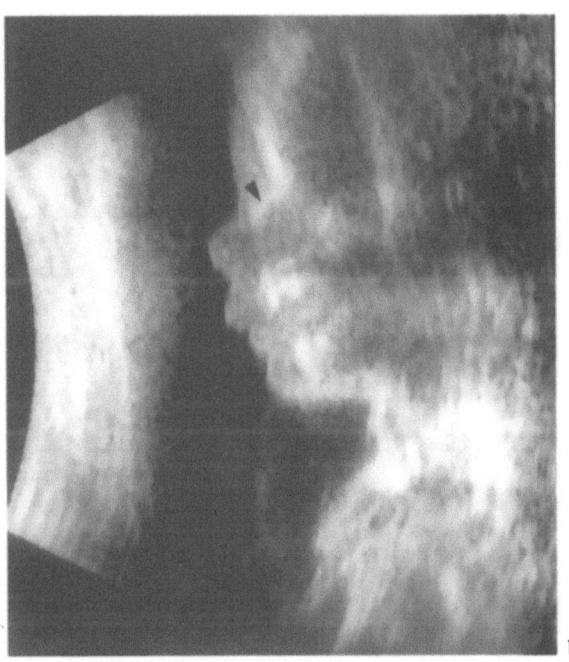

Fig. 4.44a, b. Nose and nasal bone (*arrowhead*). Profile view of the fetal head. **a** Second trimester. **b** Third trimester

The impressive advances in sonographic imaging of the fetus over the last decade have made possible the detailed evaluation of the fetal face in the majority of cases.

4.2.1.1
Lips and Maxillae

The lips must be assessed in a frontal view of the fetal head (Fig. 4.40). The upper and lower lips must be evaluated completely in order to exclude a cleft. The relatively hypoechoic lip is bordered by a hyperechoic margin. The normal anatomy is easier to assess with an open mouth. Another view that allows visualization of the lips is the transverse thoracic view, especially when the head is slightly inclined. The examination should include an evaluation of the mouth and tongue (Fig. 4.41), of the upper and lower maxillae; the bones and tooth germs appear as hyperechoic structures disposed in an arcuate regular shape

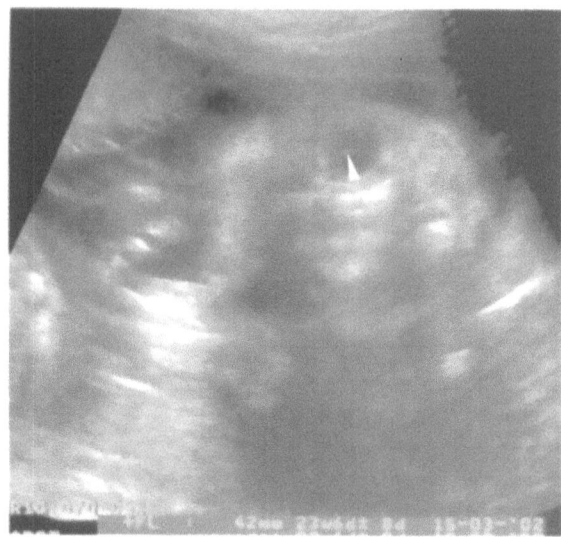
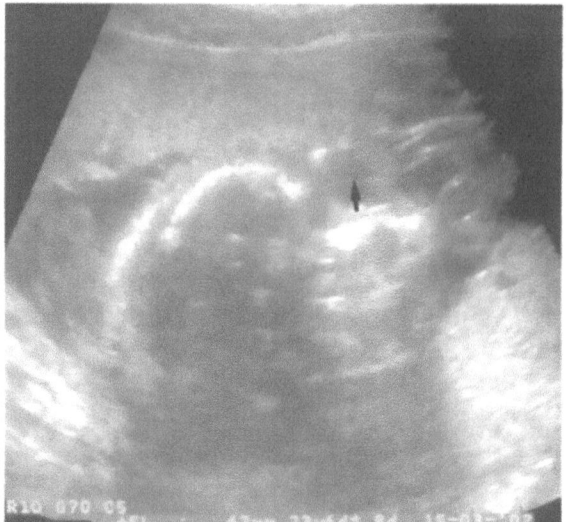

Fig. 4.45a, b. Eye. Transverse view. Second trimester. Normal appearance. **a** Rounded lens (*arrowhead*) is visible within the eyeball. **b** Hyaloid artery (*arrow*)

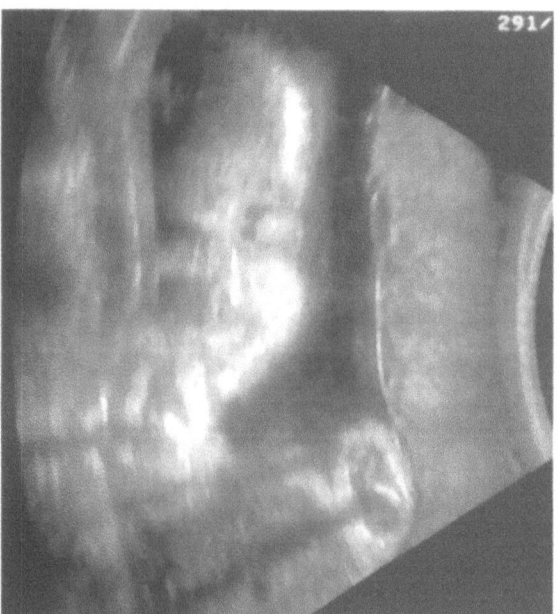
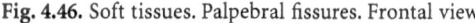

Fig. 4.46. Soft tissues. Palpebral fissures. Frontal view

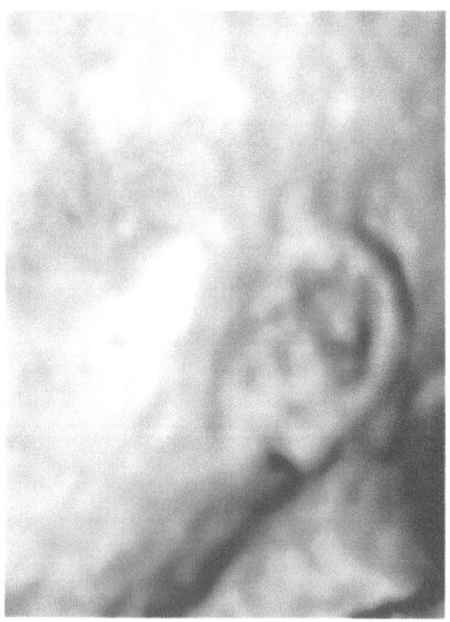

Fig. 4.47. Ear. 3D display. Third trimester

(Figs. 4.42, 4.43) (Babcook et al. 1996b, Cockell and Lees 2000, Ulm et al. 1995).

4.2.1.2
Nose

The nasal bone is best demonstrated and measured on a sagittal view (fetal profile) (Figs. 4.40, 4.44). The nostrils and soft tissues of the nose are best assessed on a

transverse view (fetal profile) where the nasal width can be measured (Ben Ami et al. 1998, Guis et al. 1995).

4.2.1.3
Eyes

Fetal eyes appear as symmetric cystic structures. The lens is identified thanks to its posterior hyperechoic convex limit. During normal development the hyaline

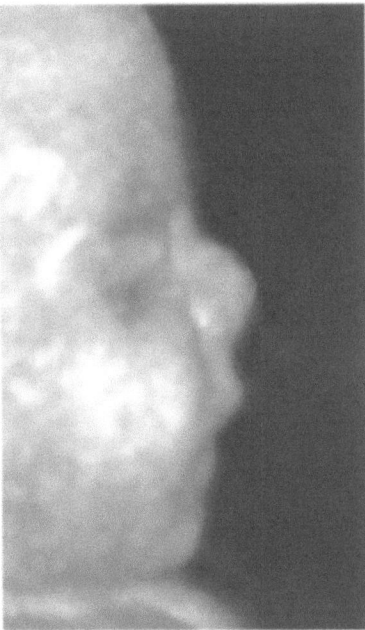

Fig. 4.48. Fetal profile. 3D display

artery is identified best between the 16th and 20th weeks. It involutes progressively and should not be visualized any longer after the 27th week (Fig. 4.45). The eyeballs, and the inter- and intraorbital distances can be measured. Also important are the eye movements (followed thanks to the movements of the lens), which are part of the assessment of fetal well-being (ACHIRON et al. 1995, 2000, HORIMOTO et al. 1993, ROTH et al. 1999, BIRNHOLZ and FARRELL 1988).

4.2.1.4
Ears

In ultrasonographic measurements of the fetal ear the aim is to establish nomograms of fetal ear measurements Abnormalities of auricular configuration are mentioned in as many as 100 syndromes, but in most conditions, ear anomalies are nonspecific. A dysplastic ear is found in 60% of fetuses with T21 (images). The palpebral fissures and soft tissues are best evaluated on a frontal view of the face (Fig. 4.46).

4.2.1.5
Fetal Profile

Fetal profile is interesting to evaluate whenever a polymalformation syndrome is suspected, especially bone dysplasia. Care should be taken in order to obtain a correct midsagittal scan that includes the real profile (Fig. 4.48).

Assessment of the fetal face is of utmost importance since many syndromes and malformations include facial anomalies. 3D imaging greatly facilitates the evaluation of the normal facial structures.

4.2.2
Facial Anomalies

4.2.2.1
Cleft Lip and Palate

Cleft lip is one of the commonest anomalies and occurs in 3.6% of births. The cleft may be uni- or bilateral, and may be associated with cleft palate; the latter can also occur in isolation, without cleft lip. Facial cleft may be part of a polymalformation syndrome. US demonstrates an interruption in the normal curvature of the lip that is, in most circumstances, easy to demonstrate on the mid-trimester US using the facial coronal view or the thoracic transverse scan (Figs. 4.49–4.51). It can be demonstrated even earlier, around 15–16 weeks. Color Doppler may demonstrate flow of amniotic fluid through the cleft. Some fetal presentations may render this visualization more difficult, and TVS or 3D US (Fig. 4.50) may provide a better depiction of the anomaly. Isolated cleft palate is difficult to demonstrate; malpositioning of the tooth germs may be a helpful sign.

Whenever a facial cleft is demonstrated, a complete survey of the fetus and especially of the CNS must be performed in order to look for associated anomalies. Chromosomal analysis is rarely abnormal when the facial cleft is isolated; it becomes frequently abnormal when associated anomalies are detected (CLEMENTI et al. 2000, COCKELL and FARRELL 2000, HATA et al. 1998, JOHNSON et al. 2000, MERNAGH et al. 1999, MONNI et al. 1995, SHERE et al. 1993).

4.2.2.2
Macroglossia

Macroglossia is an unusual finding that may be observed during the third trimester on the scan intended to visualize the fetal profile; in cases of macroglossia the tongue protrudes outside the mouth permanently. The differential diagnosis of such a finding includes real macroglossia, in relation to Beckwith-Wiedemann syndrome (Fig. 4.52), trisomy 21 or hypothyroidism, and oral tumors (gingival epulis, lymphangioma or teratoma) (WEISSMAN et al. 1995, MERNAGH et al. 1999).

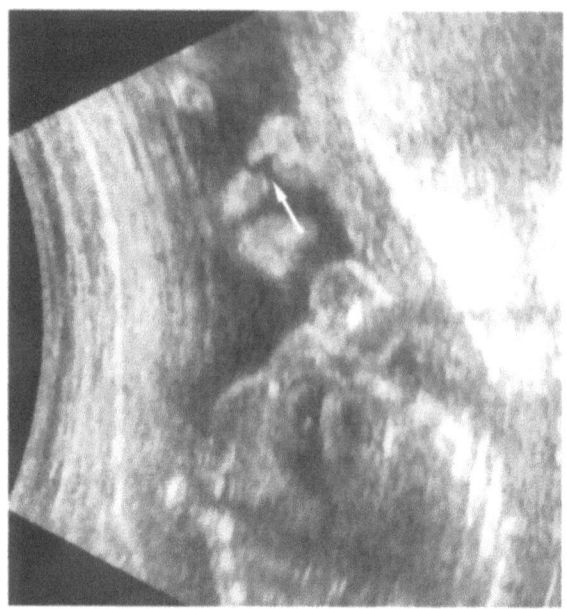

Fig. 4.49. Unilateral cleft lip. Frontal view. Interrupted upper lip (*arrow*) and enlarged nostril

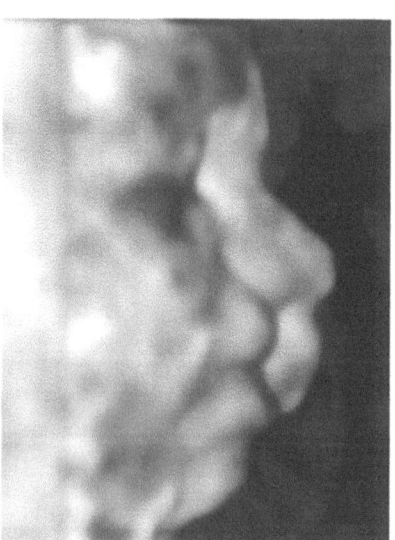

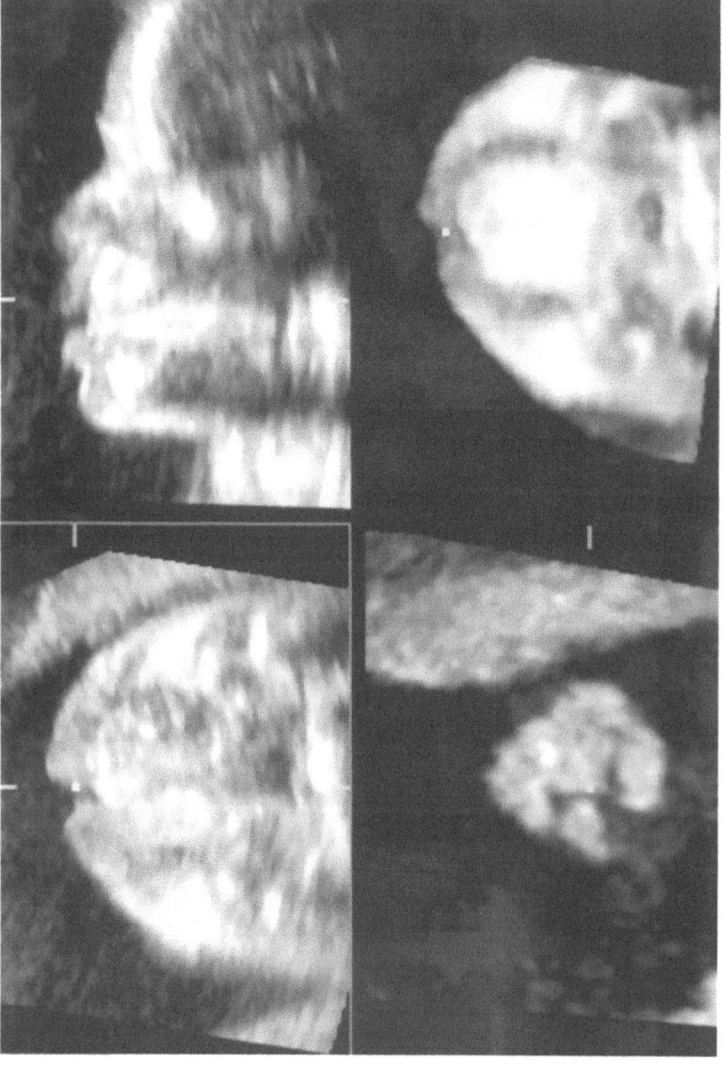

Fig. 4.50a, b. Unilateral cleft lip. 3D display. **a** 2D automated evaluation. **b** 3D rendering

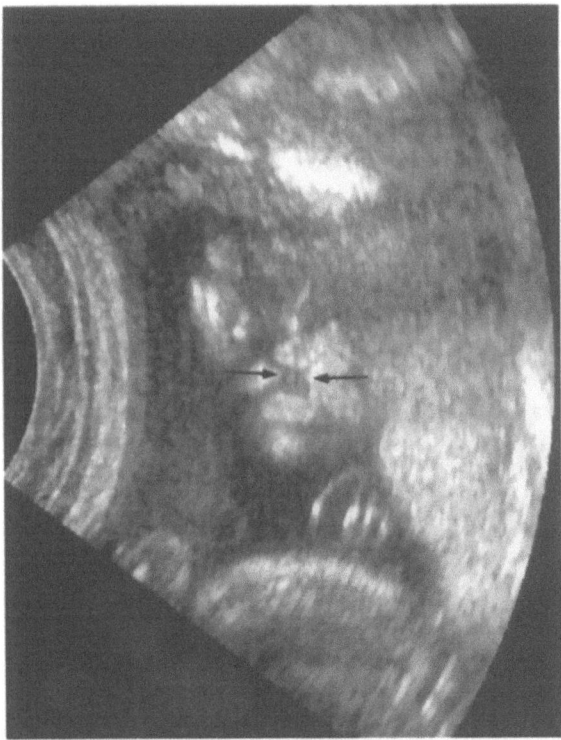

Fig. 4.51. Complex bilateral cleft lip. Frontal view. The upper lip and nose are completely malformed (*arrows*)

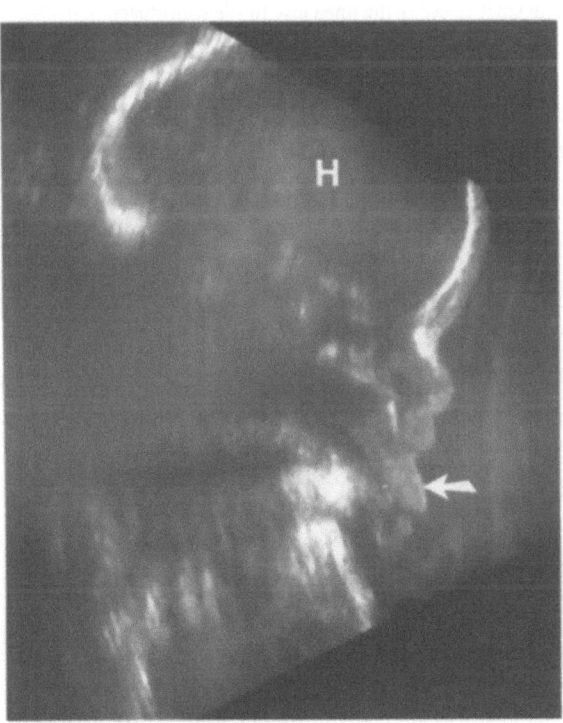

Fig. 4.52. Macroglossia. Case of Beckwith-Wiedemann syndrome. The enlarged tongue protrudes (*arrow*) out of the mouth. *H* fetal head

4.2.2.3
Nasal Malformation

Nasal bone hypoplasia may be an associated finding of the trisomy 21 syndrome. Malformation of the central segment part of the face is an important part of malformation syndromes that include holoprosencephaly. In such anomalies, the nose and the eyes are malformed and replaced by an abnormal structure resembling a proboscis (Fig. 4.53); associated orofacial clefts are also present (MERNAGH et al. 1999, BRONSHTEIN et al. 1998a).

4.2.2.4
Eye Anomalies

Measurement of the interorbital distance may help to assess hypo- or hypertelorism in cases of malformation syndromes (Fig. 4.53b). Anomalies of the eye itself are unusual. Microphthalmy is rarely diagnosed (Fig. 4.54). Cystic masses at the inner part of the eye usually correspond to dacryocystocele (Fig. 4.55) (BRONSHTEIN et al. 1991, MERNAGH et al. 1999).

4.2.2.5
Micrognathia

Micrognathia is frequently seen with morphological and chromosomal anomalies. It is best visualized on a sagittal view of the face. The Pierre Robin sequence is the most common cause (Fig. 4.56) (MERNAGH et al. 1999).

> Cleft lips are common malformations that are best assessed by 3D US. Several other malformations orient towards specific chromosomal anomalies.

4.3
Fetal Neck

Under normal conditions, the evaluation of the fetal neck is limited to the measurement of the thickness of the nuchal soft tissues. Before 13 weeks, this is achieved on a mid-sagittal scan of the fetus, obtained during TVS. During the second trimester examination, the measurement is obtained on a transverse scan of the fetal head at the level of the posterior fossa. The thickness should not measure more than 5 mm. The rest of the survey of fetal neck anatomy may include analysis of the vessels, the cervical spine and the thyroid area (BROMLEY et al. 1992, MERNAGH et al. 1999).

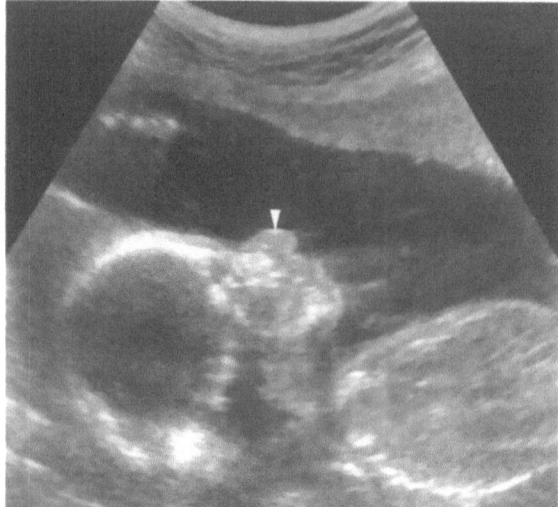

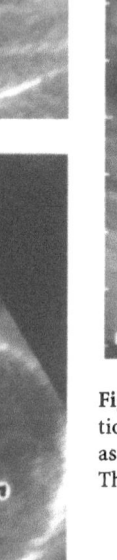

Fig. 4.53a–c. Nasal malformation. Case of trisomy 13. a Profile view. Elongated tribular nasal appendix (*arrowhead*). b Transverse view of the fore head. Marked hypotelorism (*arrowheads* point to the orbit). c Transverse view of the brain. Associated lobar holoprosencephaly with fused thalami (*T*)

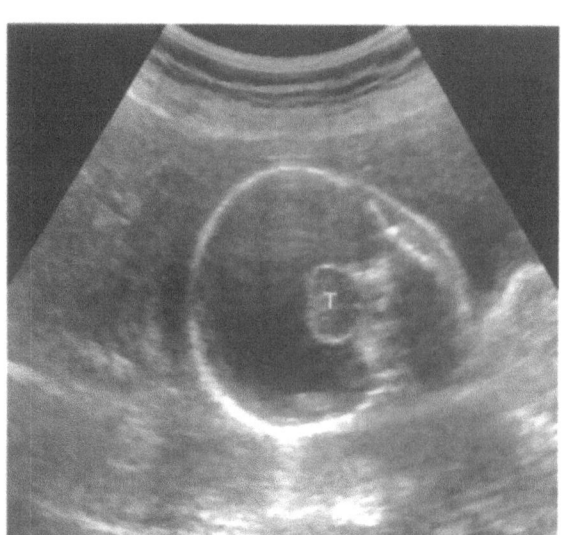

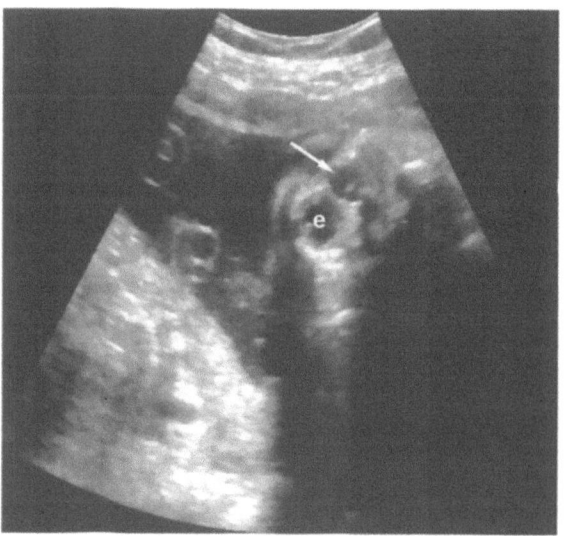

Fig. 4.54. Microphthalmy. Case of chromosome 9 translocation. Asymmetric size of the orbits (*H*). (Microphthalmy was associated with ambiguous genitalia and ventriculomegaly.) The smaller eye is the one close to the transducer

Fig. 4.55. Dacryocystocele. Second trimester. A small cyst (*arrow*) is seen internal to the eye (*e*)

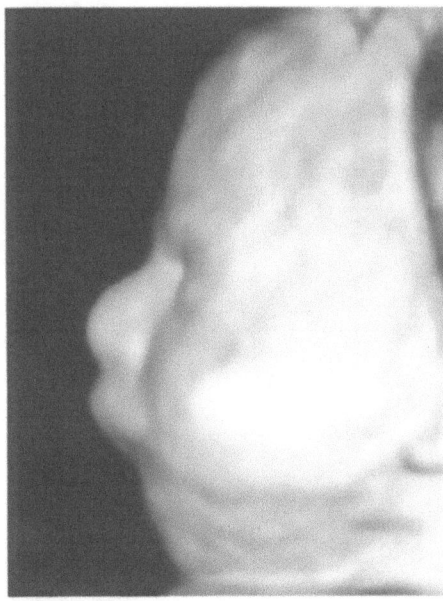

Fig. 4.56. Micrognathia. 3D display

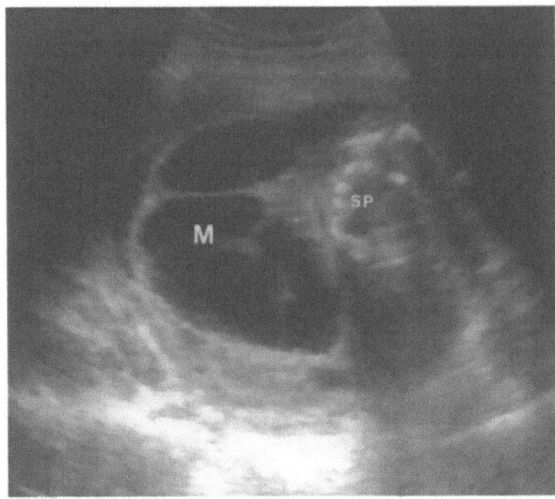

Fig. 4.57. Cystic hygroma. Case of Turner syndrome. Second trimester. Transverse scan of fetal head. A large cystic septated mass (*M*) is seen behind the spine (*sp*)

Anomalies of the neck include posterior, lateral and anterior masses.

4.3.1
Posterior Masses

4.3.1.1
Cystic Hygroma

Cystic hygroma probably results from a lack of connections between developing lymphatics. It may be septated or not. The presence of posterior cystic hygroma should initiate the search for associated anomalies, chromosomal or structural defects (mainly heart defects) (Fig. 4.57). It may be a sign of Turner (XO) or Noonan syndrome. It may also be an isolated finding. The anomaly may resolve spontaneously (MACHEN et al. 1989, BOYD et al. 1996, MERNAGH et al. 1999).

4.3.1.2
Meningo-cephalocele

Meningocele may develop in the cervical area and its US characteristics are similar to those described in the lumbar region. Cephalocele that develops in the nuchal area originates from an occipital bone defect. In such circumstances, there will be associated CNS anomalies such as microcephaly and/or hydrocephalus (REMPEN and FEIGE 1985).

4.3.1.3
Fetal Scalp Cyst

Fetal scalp cyst is an important benign differential diagnosis of posterior masses. It is usually a cystic mass, well limited within the posterior soft tissue and without connection with the brain (Fig. 4.58) (OGLE and JAUNIAUX 1999, LAU et al. 2001).

4.3.2
Lateral Masses

The differential diagnosis of lateral neck masses includes mainly (hemo-)lymphangioma, teratoma and branchial cleft cysts. Lymphangioma tends to be a cystic septated mass (Fig. 4.59), whereas teratoma is more commonly solid and calcified, and branchial cleft cysts are rarely septated. Color Doppler may reveal the type of vascularization of the mass. Fetal MR imaging may be helpful in order to determine the extent of the mass (Fig. 4.59b, c) (SUCHET 1995).

4.3.3
Anterior Masses

Teratoma and lymphangioma may extend towards the anterior part of the neck. An important differential diagnosis is enlargement of the fetal thyroid

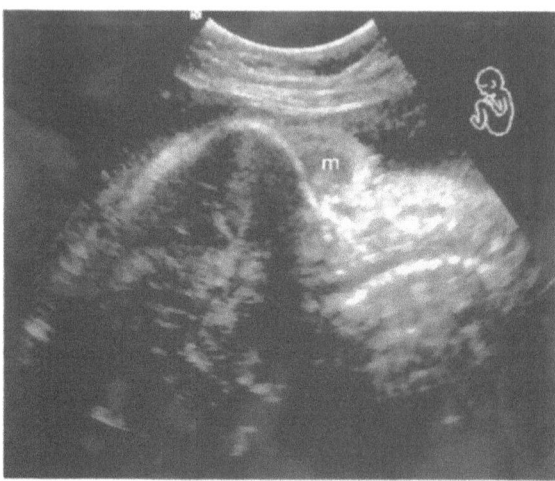

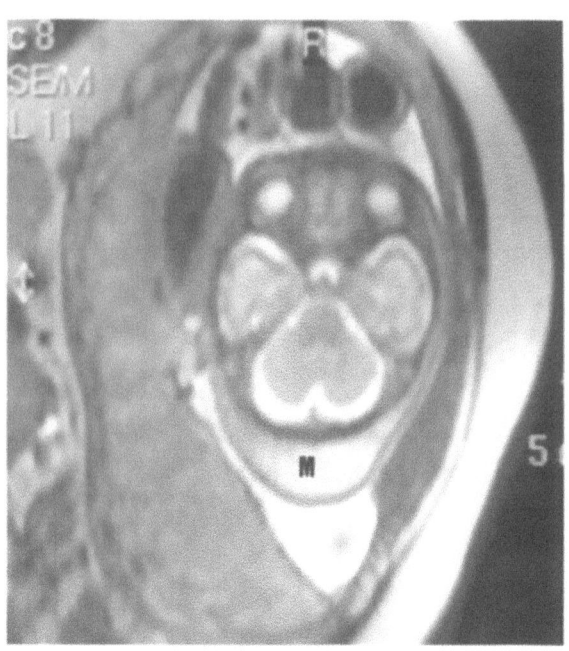

Fig. 4.58a, b. Fetal scalp cyst. **a** US. Third trimester. A cystic posterior mass (*M*) is visible within the soft tissue of the neck. H head. **b** Fetal MR imaging demonstrating the poorly delineated cystic mass (*m*) and absence of any connection with the posterior fossa

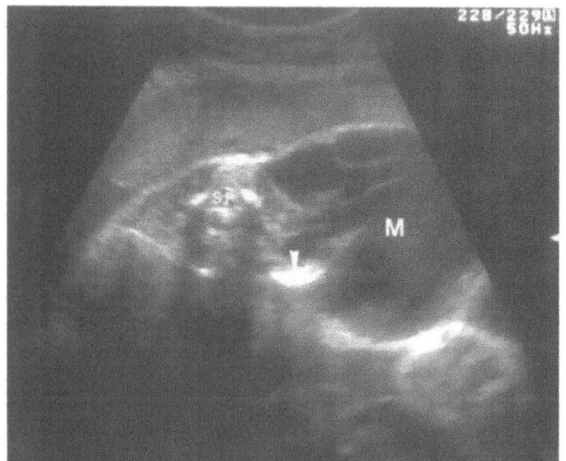

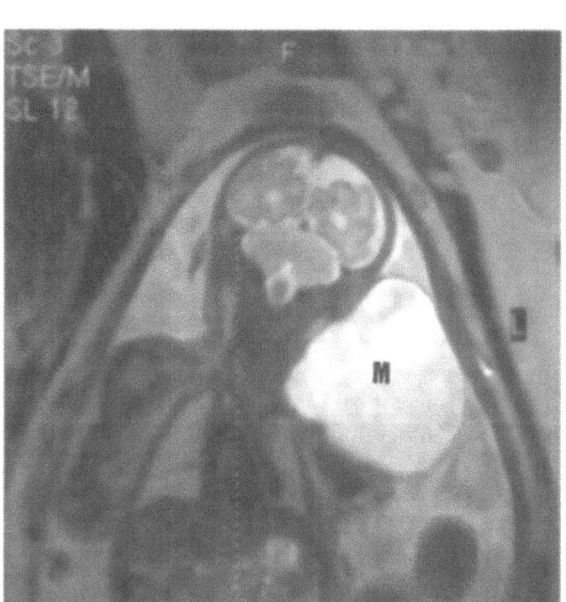

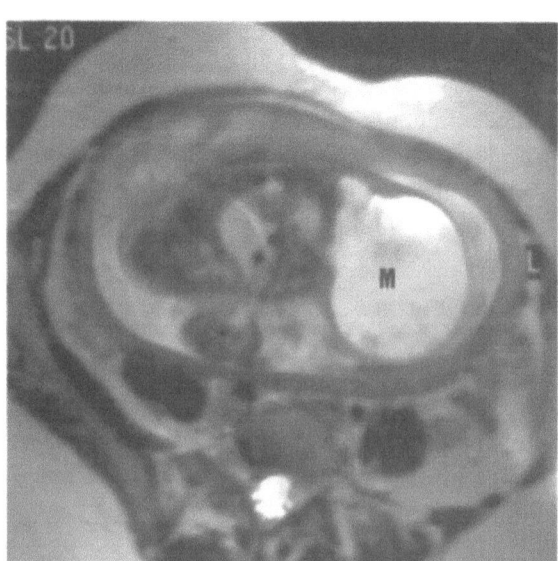

Fig. 4.59a–c. Lateral neck lymphangioma. Third trimester. **a** US. Transverse scan. A cystic septated mass (*M*) is located lateral to the cervical spine (*sp*) and behind the clavicula (*arrowhead*). **b** Fetal MR imaging. T2-weighted sequence. Frontal view. *M* mass. **c** Fetal MR imaging. Axial view. *M* mass. Good delineation of the tumoral extension

gland. In utero goiter will appear as a symmetric anterior mass around the tracheal lumen (Fig. 4.60) (sagittal measurement exceeds 10 mm). The fetal neck may be in hyperextension. Swallowing may be disturbed and induce polyhydramnios. Maternal thyroid disease is a helpful feature in order to diagnose the condition. Other associated findings are IUGR, cardiac rhythm anomalies and delayed ossification of the epiphyses of the long bones (SUCHET 1995, AVNI et al. 1992, MERNAGH et al. 1999, YANCEY et al. 1993, PRADEEP et al. 1991, BROMLEY et al. 1992, RANZINI et al. 2001, VOLUMENIE et al. 2000).

> Lymphangioma is the commonest mass of the neck; fetal MR imaging may provide complementary information on the tumoral extent.

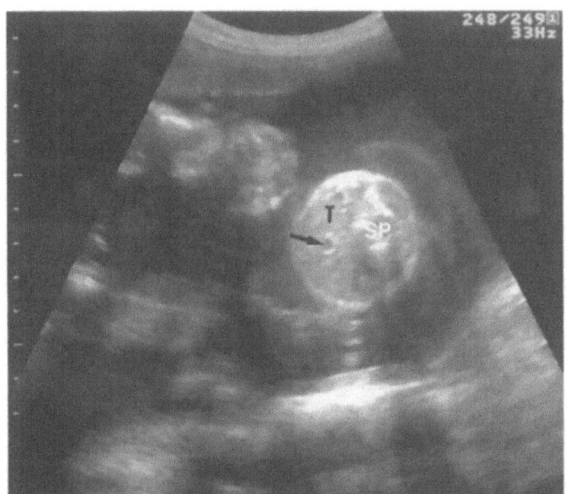

a

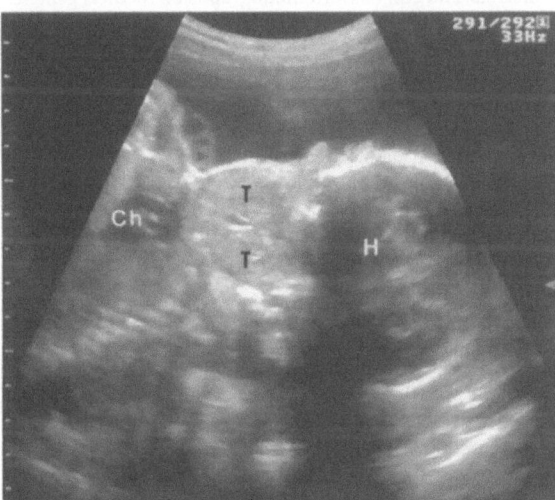

b

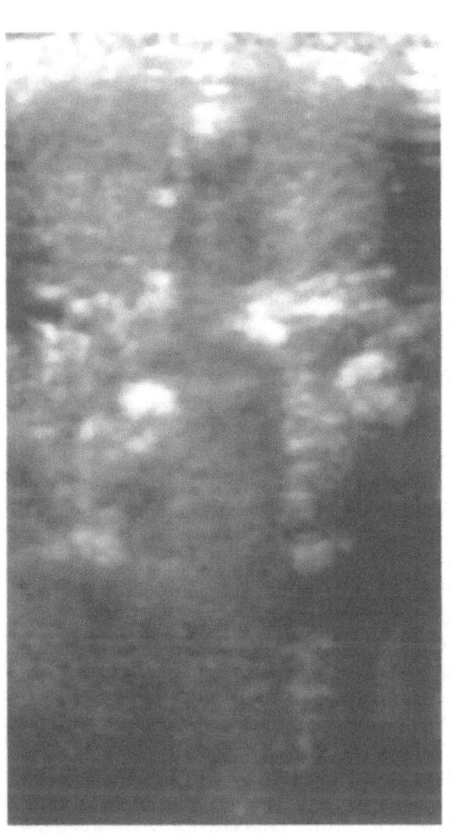

c

Fig. 4.60a–c. Fetal goiter. **a** US. In utero, third trimester. Transverse scan of the neck. Sp spine, T thyroid, arrow trachea. **b** US. In utero. Coronal view. H fetal head, T enlarged thyroid, Ch chest. **c** US. At birth. Persistently enlarged thyroid (T) lobe. (It resolved spontaneously in subsequent examination)

References

Aase JM, Wilson AC, Smith WD (1973) Small ears Down's syndrome: a helpful diagnostic aid. Brief clinical and laboratory observations. J Pediatr 82:845–847

Achiron R, Achiron A, Yagel S (1993) First trimester TVS diagnosis of DWM. J Clin Ultrasound 21:62–64

Achiron R, Hamiel PO, Reuchman B, et al (1993) Fetal intracranial hemorrhage. Br J Obstet Gynaecol 100:995–999

Achiron R, Kreiser D, Achiron A, et al (2000) Axial growth of the fetal eye and evaluation of the hyaloid artery. Prenat Diagn 20:894–899

Achiron R, Gotlieb Z, Yaron Y, et al (1995) The development of the eye: in utero US measurements. Prenat Diagn 15:155–160

Ahmad ZA, Vial Y, Fawer CL, et al (2001) Prenatal diagnosis of CMV, Obstet Gynecol ;7:443–408

Anderson MW, McGahan JP (1994) US detection of an in utero intracranial hemorrhage in the second trimester. J Ultrasound Med 13:315–318

Amin RS, Nikolaidis P, Kawashima A, et al (1999) Normal anatomy of the fetus at MR imaging. Radiographics 19:S201-S214

Anderson NG, Jordan S, MacFailane S, et al (1994) Diastematomyelia: diagnosis by prenatal US. AJR Am J Roentgenol 163:911–914

Avni F, Rodesch F, Vandemerckt C, Vermeylen D (1992) Detection and evaluation of fetal goiter by US, Br J Radiol 65:302–305

Babcook CJ, Goldstein RB, Barth RA, et al (1994) Prevalence of ventriculomegaly in association with myelomeningocele. Radiology 190:703–707

Babcook CJ, Chong BW, Salamt S, et al (1996) US anatomy of the developing cerebellum: normal embryology can resemble pathology. AJR Am J Roentgenol 166:427–423

Babcook CJ, McGahan JP, Chong BW (1996) Evaluation of fetal midface anatomy related to facial clefts: use of US. Radiology 201:113–118

Bannister CM, Russel SA, Rimmer S, Mowle DH (1999). Fetal arachnoid cysts. Eur J Pediatr Surg 9:27–28

Barjot P, Von Theobald P, Refahi N (1999) Diagnosis of arachnoid cysts on prenatal US. Fetal Diagn Ther 14:306–309

Barkowich AJ, Rowley H, Bollen A (1995) Correlation of prenatal events with the development of polymicrogyria. AJNR Am J Neuroradiol 16:822–827

Baumeister LA, Herzberg BS, McNally PJ, et al (1994) Fetal 4th ventricle: US appearance and frequency of depiction. Radiology 192:333–336

Bekker MN, van Vugt JMG (2001) The role of MR imaging in prenatal diagnosis of fetal anomalies. Eur J Obstet Gynaecol Reprod Biol 965:173–176

Benaceraff BR, Spiro R, Mitchell AG (2000) Using 3D US to detect craniosynostosis in a fetus with Pfeiffer syndrome. Ultrasound Obstet Gynecol 16:391–394

Benaceraff BA (1987). Asymptomatic cysts of the fetal choroid plexus. J Ultrasound Med 6:475–478

Ben Ami M, Weiner E, Perlitz Y, Shalev E (1998) US evaluation of the width of the fetal nose. Prenat Diagn 18:1010–1013

Birnholz JC, Farrell TA (1988) Fetal hyaloid artery. Radiology 166:781–783

Boyd PA, Anthony MY, Manning N, et al (1996) Antenatal diagnosis of cystic hygroma or nuchal pad. Arch Dis Child 74: F38-F42

Blaas HG, Eik-Neis SH, Kiserud T, et al (1995) Early development of the hindbrain: a longitudinal US study from 7–12 weeks of gestation. Ultrasound Obstet Gynecol 5:151–160

Blumenfeld Z, Siegler E, Bronshtein M (1993) The early diagnosis of NTD. Prenat Diagn 13:863–871

Bonilla-Musoles FM, Raga F Ballester MJ, Sezra P (1994) Early detection of embryonic malformation by transvaginal and color Doppler US. J Ultrasound Med 13:347–355

Bromley B, Nader AS, Pauker S, Estroff J (1994) Closure of the cerebellar vermis: evaluation with second trimester US. Radiology 193:761–763

Bromley B, Frigoletto FD, Cramer D, et al. (1992) The fetal thyroid: normal and abnormal US measurements. J Ultrasound Med 11:25–28

Bronshtein M, Zimmer E, Gershoni-Baruch R, et al (1991) First and second trimester diagnosis of fetal ocular defects. Obstet Gynecol 77:443–449

Bronshtein M, Blumenfeld I, Zimmer EZ, et al (1998) Prenatal US diagnosis of nasal malformations. Prenat Diagn 18:447–454

Bronshtein M, Zimmer EZ, Blazer S (1998) Isolated large 4th ventricle in early pregnancy: a possible benign transient phenomenon. Prenat Diagn 18:997–1000

Budorick NE, Pretorius DH, Grafe MR, et al (1991) Ossification of the fetal spine. Radiology 181:561–565

Budorick NE, Pretorius DH, Nelson TR (1995) US of the fetal spine: technique, imaging findings and clinical implications. AJR Am J Roentgenol 164:421–428

Budorick NE, Pretorius DH, McGahan JP, et al (1995) Cephalocele detection in utero: US and clinical features. Ultrasound Obstet Gynecol 5:77–85

Canapicchi R, Cioni G, Strigini F, et al (1998) Prenatal diagnosis of periventricular hemorrhage by fetal brain magnetic resonance imaging. Childs Nerv Syst 14:689–692

Chang MC, Russell SA, Callen PW (1994) US detection of inferior vermian agenesis in DWM. Radiology 193:765–770

Chat L, Sonigo P, Simon I, et al (2001). Sémiologie anténatale des diasténatomyélies. J Radiol 82:661–663

Clementi M, Tenconi R, Bianchi F, et al (2000) Evaluation of prenatal diagnosis of cleft lip by US. Prenat Diagn 20:870–875

Cockell a Lees M (2000) Prenatal diagnosis and management of orofacial clefts. Prenat Diagn 20:149–151

Cochrane DD, Wilson RD, Steinbock P, et al (1996) Prenatal spinal evaluation and functional outcome of patients born with myelo-meningocele. Fetal Diagn Ther 11:159–168

Cohen HL, Haller JO (1994) Advances in perinatal neurosonography. AJR Am J Roentgenol 163:801–810

Cohen Michael M Jr (1997) The child with multiple birth defects, 2nd edn (Oxford monographs on medical genetics 31). Oxford University Press,, Oxford, pp 62–90

Comstock CH, Kirk JS (1991). Arteriovenous malformations: locations and evolution in the fetal brain. J Ultrasound Med 10:361–365

Cyr DR, Mack LA, Nyberg DA, et al (1988) Fetal rhombencephalon: normal US findings. Radiology 166:691–692

D'Addario V, Pinto V, Moo F, Resta M (1998) The specificity of US in fetal intracranial tumors. Perinat Med 26:480–485

Dan U, Shalev E, Greif M, Weiner E (1992). Prenatal diagnosis of fetal brain A-V malformations. J Clin Ultrasound 20: 149–151

D'Ottavio G, Meir YJ, Rustico MA, et al (1995) Pilot screening for fetal malformations: possibilities and limits of TVS, J Ultrasound Med 14:575–580

De Elejade MM, de Elejade BR (1985) Visualization of the fetal spine: a proposal of a standard system to increase reliability. Am J Med Genet 21:445–456

De Laveaucoupet J, Audibert F, Guis F, et al (2001) Fetal MR imaging of ischemic brain damage. Prenat Diagn 21:729–736

DeVries LS, Groenendaal F, Rademaker KJ, et al (1998) Antenatal onset of hemorrhage and ischemia in preterm infants Arch Dis Child 78:F51-F56

Drose JA, Dennis MA, Thickman D (1991) Infection in utero: US findings in 19 cases. Radiology 12:117–122

Durfee SM, Kim FM, Benson CM (2001) Postnatal outcome of fetuses with the prenatal diagnosis of asymmetric hydrocephalus. J Ultrasound Med 20:263–268

Ecker J, Schipp TD, Bromley B, et al (2000) The US diagnosis of DWM and DWV. Prenat Diagn 20:328–332

Enders G, Bäder U, Linderman L, et al (2001) Prenatal diagnosis of CMV in 189 pregnancies with known outcome. Prenat Diagn 21:362–377

Estroff JA, Parad RB, Teele RL (1992) Echogenic vessels in the fetal thalami and basal ganglia associated with CMV infection. J Ultrasound Med 11:686–688

Filly RA, Cardoza RD, Goldstein RB, Barkovitch J (1989) Detection of fetal CNS anomalies: a practical level of effort for a routine sonogram. Radiology 172:403–408

Filly RA, Golddstein R, Callen PW (1991) Fetal ventricle: importance in routine obstetric US. Radiology 181:1–7

Fukui K, Morioka T, Nishio S, et al (2001) Fetal germinal matrix and intraventricular hemorrhage diagnosed by MRI. Neuroradiology 43:68–72

Garel C, Chantrel E, Brisse H, et al (2001) Fetal cerebral cortex: normal gestational landmarks. AJNR Am J Neuroradiol 22:184–189

Gembruch U, Baschat AA, Reusch E, et al (1995) First trimester diagnosis of holoprosencephaly with a DWM by TVS, J Ultrasound Med 14:619–622

Girard NJ, Raybaud CA (1992) In vivo MRI of fetal brain cellular migration. J Comput Assist Tomogr 16:265–267

Girard N, Raybaud C, Dercole C, Boubli L, Chau C, Cahen S, Potier A, Gamerre M (1993) In vivo MRI of the fetal brain. Neuroradiology 35:431–436

Goldstein RB, Podrasky AE, Filly RA, Callen PW (1989) Effacement of the cisterna magna in association with myelomeningocele. Radiology 172:409–413

Greco P, Resta M, Vimercati A, et al (1998) Antenatal diagnosis of isolated lissencephaly by US and MR imaging. Ultrasound Obstet Gynecol 12:276–279

Guis F, Ville Y, Vincent Y, et al (1995) US evaluation of the length of the fetal nasal bones throughout gestation. Ultrasound Obstet Gynecol 5:304–307

Gupta JK, Lilford RJ (1995) Assessment and management of fetal agenesis of the CC. Prenat Diagn 15:301–312

Hansen PE, Ballesteros MC, Soila K, et al (1993) MRI of the developing human brain. Radiographics 13:21–36

Hata T, Yonehara T, Aoki S, et al (1998) 3D US visualization of the fetal face. AJR Am J Roentgenol 170:481–483

Hata T, Yanagihara T, Matsumoto M, et al (2000) 3D US features of fetal CNS anomaly. Acta Obstet Gynecol Scand 79:635–639

Hogge WA, Dungan JS, Brooks MP, et al (1990) Diagnosis and management of prenatally detected myelomeningocele. Am J Obstet Gynecol 163:1061–1065

Horimoto N, Hepper PG, Shahidullah S, et al (1993) Fetal eye movements. Ultrasound Obstet Gynecol 3:362–369

Hoyme HE, Higginbottom MC, Jones KL (1981) Vascular etiology of disruptive structural defects in monozygotic twins. Pediatrics 67:288–291

Hubbard AM, Harty P (1999) Prenatal MR imaging of fetal anomalies. Semin Roentgenol 34:41–47

Hunt GM (1990) Open spina bifida: outcome for a complete cohort treated unselectively and followed into adulthood. Dev Med Child Neurol 32:108–118

Ickowicz V, Eurin D, Rypen F, et al (2001) Prenatal diagnosis and postnatal follow-up of pericallosal lipoma. AJNR Am J Neuroradiol 22:767–772

Johnson DD, Pretorius DH, Budorick NE, et al (2000) Fetal lip and primary palate: 3D vs 2D US. Radiology 217:236–239

Johnson DD, Pretorius DH, Riccabona M, et al (1997) 3D US of the fetal spine. Obstet Gynecol 89:434–438

Huppert BJ, Brandt KR, Ramin KD, et al (1999) SSFSE MR imaging of the fetus. Radiographics 19:S215-S217

Keogan MT, DeAtkine AB, Hertzberg BS (1994) Cerebellar vermian defects: antenatal US appearance and clinical significance. J Ultrasound Med 13:607–611

Kelly EN, Allen VM, Seaward G, et al (2001) Mild ventriculomegaly in the fetus: a literature review. Prenat Diagn 21:697–700

Kinzler WL, Smulian JC, McLean DA, et al (2001) Outcome of prenatally diagnosed mild unilateral cerebral ventriculomegaly. J Ultrasound Med 20:257–262

Klingensmith WC, Cioffi DT (1986) Schizencephaly: diagnosis and progression in utero. Radiology 159:617–618

Knuppel RA, Salvatore DD, Agarwal R, Leiman S, Sikka A (1994) Documented fetal brain damage resulting from a motor vehicle accident. J Ultrasound med 13:402–404

Knutzon RK, McGahan JP, Salamat S, et al (1991) Fetal cisterna magna septa: a normal anatomic finding. Radiology 180: 799–801

Kölble N, Wisser J, Kurmanavicius J, et al (2000) DWM: prenatal diagnosis and outcome. Prenat Diagn 20:318–327

Kollias SS, Goldstein RB, Cogen PH, Filly RA (1992) Prenatally detected myelomeningoceles: US accuracy. Radiology 185:109–112

Kushnir U, Shalev U, Bronstein M, et al (1989) Fetal intracranial anatomy in the first trimester of pregnancy: TVS evaluation. Neuroradiology 31:222–225

Kuzniecky R, Andermann F (1994) The congenital bilateral perisylvian syndrome. AJNR Am J Neuroradiol 15:139–144

Lau TK, Leung BTY, Pang M, et al (2001) Fetal scalp cysts. J Ultrasound Med 20:175–177

Lee W, Kirk JS, Shaheen KW, et al (2000) Fetal cleft lip and palate detection by 3D US. Ultrasound Obstet Gynecol 16:314–320

Levine D, Barnes P, Korf B, et al (2000) Tuberous sclerosis in the fetus: second trimester diagnosis of tubers with ultrafast MR imaging. AJR Am J Roentgenol 175:1067–1069

Macken MB, Grantmyre EB, Vincer MJ (1989) Regression of nuchal cystic hygroma in utero. J Ultrasound Med 8:101–103

Malinger G, Zaku H (1993) The corpus callosum: normal fetal development as shown by TVS. AJR 161:1041–1043

Malinger G, Ginath S, Lerman-Sagie T, et al (2001) The fetal cerebellar vermis: normal development as shown by TVS. Prenat Diagn 21:687–692

Mamelak AN, Cogen PH, Barkovich AJ (1994) The filum intermedium sign: focal in utero spinal cord infarct. J Neurosurg 81:941–946

Mercier A, Eurin D, Mercier PY, et al (2001) Isolated mild fetal cerebral ventriculomegaly. Prenat Diagn 21:589–595

Mernagh JR, Mohide PT, Lappalainen RE, et al (1999) US assessment of the fetal head and neck. Radiographics 19:S229-S241

Mirlesse V, Wener H, Jacquemard F, et al (1992) Magnetic resonance imaging in antenatal diagnosis of tuberous sclerosis. Lancet 340:1163

Mitchell LA, Simon EM, Filly RA, et al (2000) Antenatal diagnosis of subependymal heterotopia. AJNR Am J Neuroradiol 21:296–300

Monni G, Ibba RM, Olla G, et al (1995) Color Doppler US and prenatal diagnosis of cleft palate. J Clin Ultrasound 23:189–191

Monteagudo A (1996) Haratz-Rubinstein Timor-Trisch biometry of the fetal brain> In: Timor-Trisch IE (ed) US of the fetal and neonatal brain. Appleton and Lange, Stanford, pp 89–146

Monteagudo A, Timor-Trisch IE (1996) Fetal neurosonography of congenital brain malformation. In: Timor-Trisch IE (ed) US of the fetal and neonatal brain. Appleton and Lange, Stanford, pp 147–220

Mueller GM, Weiner CP, Yankowitz J (1996) 3D US in the evaluation of fetal head and spine. Obstet Gynecol 88:372–378

Ogle RF, Jauniaux E (1999) Fetal scalp cysts: dilemmas in diagnosis. Prenat Diagn 19:1157–1159

Pilu G, Sandri A, Perolo A, et al (1993) US of fetal agenesis of the CC. Ultrasound Obstet Gynecol 3:318–329

Pilu G, Falco P, Perolo A (2000) US evaluation of the fetal neural axis. In: Callen's US in obstetrics and gynecology, 4th edn. WB Saunders, Philadelphia, pp 277–306

Pilu G, Falco P, Perolo A, et al (1997) Differential diagnosis and outcome of fetal intracranial hypoechoic lesions. Ultrasound Obstet Gynecol 9:229–236

Pooh RK, Aono T (1996) TVS power Doppler angiography of the fetal brain. Ultrasound Obstet Gynecol 8:417–421

Pradeep VM, Ramachandran K, Sasidharan K, et al (1991) Fetal goiter: a case detected by US. J Clin Ultrasound 19:571–574

Rademacker KJ, De Vries LS, Barth PG (1993) Subependymal pseudocysts: US diagnosis and findings at follow-up. Acta Paediatr 82:394–399

Ranzini AC, Ananth CV, Smulian JC, et al (2001) US of the fetal thyroid. J Ultrasound Med 20:613–617

Reiss I, Gortner L, Möller J, et al (1996) Fetal intracerebral hemorrhage in the second trimester. Ultrasound Obstet Gynecol 7:49–51

Rempen A, Feige A (1985) Differential diagnosis of US detected tumors in the fetal cervical region. Eur J Obstet Gynecol 20:89–105

Resta M, Greco P, D'Addario V, Florio C, Dardes N, Caruso G, Spagnolo P, Clemente R, Vimercati A, Selvaggi L (1994) Magnetic resonance imaging in pregnancy: study of fetal cerebral malformations. Ultrasound Obstet Gynecol 4:7–20

Roberts HE, Moore CA, Cragan JD, et al (1995) Impact of prenatal diagnosis on the birth prevalence of NTD. Pediatrics 96:880–883

Rorke LB, Zimmerman RA (1992) Prematurity, postmaturity and destructive lesions in utero. AJNR Am J Neuroradiol 13:517–536

Roth PH, Roth A, Clerc-Berin F, et al (1999) Mesures échographiques anténatales de l'œil et de la distance interorbitaire. J Gynecol Obstet Biol Reprod 28:343–351

Rubinstein D, Youngman V, Hise JH, et al (1994) Partial development of the CC. AJNR Am J Neuroradiol 15:869–875

Rypens F, Sonigo P, Avni F (1996) Diagnostic anténatal des anomalies du corps calleux. Radiologie J CEPUR 16:33–37

Rypens F, Sonigo P, Aubry MC, Delezoide AL, Brunelle F (1996) Prenatal MR diagnosis of cerebral abnormal gyration and neuronal heterotopia in a fetus presenting with a thick corpus callosum. AJNR Am J Neuroradiol 17:1918–1920

Salzman DH, Kraus CM, Goldman JM, et al (1991) Prenatal diagnosis of lissencephaly. Prenat Diagn 11:139–143

Scher MS, Belfar H, Martin J, et al (1991) Destructive lesions of presumed fetal onset: antepartum causes of cerebral palsy. Pediatrics 88:898–906

Seidman DS, Nass D, Mendelson E, et al (1996) Prenatal US diagnosis of fetal hydrocephalus due to infection with parainfluenza virus type 3. Ultrasound Obstet Gynecol 7:52–54

Seller MJ (1990) Is antenatal selection for spina bifida possible? BMJ 301:251–252

Sherer DM, Abramowicz JS, Jaffe R, et al (1993) Cleft palate: confirmation of prenatal diagnosis by color Doppler US. Prenat Diagn 13:953–956

Simon EM, Goldstein RB, Coakley FV, et al (2000) Fast MR imaging of fetal CNS anomalies in utero. AJNR Am J Neuroradiol 21:1688–1698

Snijders RJM, Nicoilaides KH (1994) Fetal biometry at 14–40 weeks gestation. Ultrasound Obstet Gynecol 4:34–48

Sonigo P, Rypens FF, Carteret M, et al (1998) MR imaging of fetal cerebral anomalies. Pediatr Radiol 28:212–222

Sonigo P, Elmaleh A, Fermont L, et al (1996) Prenatal MRI diagnosis of fetal cerebral tuberous sclerosis. Pediatr Radiol 26:1–4

Sonigo P, Rypens F, Carteret M, et al (1998) MR imaging of fetal cerebral anomalies. Pediatr Radiol 28:212–222

Steegers-Theunissen RPM, Smithelis RW, Eskes TKAB (1993) Update of new risk factors and prevention of NTD. Obstet Gynecol Surv 48:287–293

Stevenson RE, Kelly JC, Arylswoth AS, et al (1987) Vascular basis of NTD: a hypothesis. Pediatrics 80:102–106

Stoll C, Dott B, Alembik Y, et al (1991) Malformations congénitales observés dans une série de 131,760 naissances consécutives pendant 10 ans. Arch Fr Pediatr 48:549–554

Suchet IB (1995) US of the fetal neck in the second and third trimester. Can Assoc Radiol J 46:426–433

Tassin GB, Maklad NF, Stewart RR, Bell ME (1991) CMV infection: intrauterine US diagnosis using findings involving the brain. AJNR Am J Neuroradiol 12:117–122

Timor-Trisch IE, Monteguado A, Warren B (1991) TVS definition of the CNS in the first and early second trimester. Am J Obstet Gynecol 164:497–504

Timor-Trisch IE, Monteguado A (1996) Normal neurosonography of the prenatal brain. In: Timor-Trisch IE (ed) US of the prenatal and neonatal brain. Appleton and Lange, Stanford, pp 11–87

Timor-Trisch IE, Monteguado A (1996) Transvaginal fetal neurosonography: standardization of the planes and sections by anatomic landmarks. Ultrasound Obstet Gynecol 8:42–47

Toma P, Lucigrai G, Ravegnani M, Cariati M, Mugnano G, Lituania M (1990) Hydrocephalus and porencephaly: prenatal diagnosis by ultrasonography and MR imaging. J Comput Assist Tomogr 14:843–845

Ulm MR, Chalubinski K, Ulm C, et al (1995) US depiction of fetal tooth germs. Prenat Diagn 15:368–372

Van den Hof MC, Nicolaides KH, Campbell J, et al (1990) Evaluation of the lemon and banana signs in 130 fetuses with open spina bifida. Am J Obstet Gynecol 162:322–327

VanZalen-Sprock RM, vanVugt JM, van Geijn HP (1995) First and early second trimester diagnosis of anomalies of the fetal CNS. J Ultrasound Med 14:603–610

Vergani P, Ghildini A, Strobelt N, et al (1994) Prognostic indicators in the prenatal diagnosis of agenesis of the CC. Am J Obstet Gynecol 170:753–758

Volpe JJ (1992) Effect of cocaine use on the fetus. N Engl J Med 327:399–401

Volumenie JL, Polak M, Guibourdenche J, et al (2000) Management of fetal thyroid goiters. Prenat Diagn 20:799–806

Warsof SL, Abramowicz JS, Sayegh SK, et al (1988) Lower limb movements and urologic function in fetuses with NTD and other CNS defects. Fetal Ther 3:129–133

Weissman A, Maschiach S, Achiron R (1995) Macroglossia: prenatal US diagnosis. Prenat Diagn 15:66–69

Wenstrom KD, Williamson RA, Weiner CP, et al (1991) Magnetic resonance imaging of fetuses with intracranial defects. Obstet Gynecol 77:529–532

Werner H, Mirlesse V, Jacquemard F, et al (1994) Prenatal diagnosis of tuberous sclerosis: use of magnetic resonance imaging and its implications for prognosis. Prenat Diagn 14:1151–1154

Whitby E, Paley MN, Davies N, et al (2001) Ultrafast MR imaging of CNS abnormalities in utero. Br J Obstet Gynecol 108:519–526

Wilkins-Haug L, Freedman W (1991) Progression of exencephaly to anencephaly in the human fetus. Prenat Diagn 11:227–233

Wininger SJ, Donnenfeld AE (1994). Syndromes identified in fetuses with prenatally diagnosed cephaloceles. Prenat Diagn 14:839–843

Wladomoroff JW, Heydanus R, Stewart PA (1993) Doppler color flow mapping of fetal intracerebral arteries in the presence of CNS anomalies. Ultrasound Med Biol 19:355–357

Wolf S, Schreibe S, Tröger J (1992) The conus medullaris; time of ascendance to the normal level. Pediatr Radiol 22:590–592

Worthen NJ, Gilbertson V, Lau C (1986) Cortical sulcal development seen on sonography. J Ultrasound Med 5:153–156

Yamashita Y, Namimoto T, Abe Y, Takahashi M, Iwamasa J, Miyazaki K, Okamura H (1997) MR imaging of the fetus by a HASTE sequence. AJR Am J Roentgenol 168:513–519.

Yancey MK, Lasley D, Richards DS (1993) An unusual mass in a fetus with Klippel Trenaunay syndrome. J Ultrasound Med 12:779–782

Yuh WTC, Nguyen HD, Fischer DJ, et al (1994) MRI of fetal CNS abnormalities. AJNR Am J Neuroradiol 15:459–464

5   The Fetal Chest

FRANÇOISE RYPENS, ANDRÉE GRIGNON, FRED E. AVNI

CONTENTS

5.1   Introduction 77
5.2   Fetal Lung Development 78
5.3   Normal Appearance of Fetal Thora
         on US and MRI 79
5.3.1   Normal US Appearance 79
5.3.2   Normal MR Appearance 80
5.4   General Considerations 81
5.5   Specific Fetal Lung Malformations 82
5.5.1   Ultrasound Characteristics 82
5.5.2   Congenital Cystic Adenomatoid Malformation 83
5.5.2.1 In Utero Appearance 83
5.5.2.2 Management 83
5.5.2.3 Differential Diagnosis 86
5.5.3   Sequestration 86
5.5.3.1 Management and Prognosis 86
5.5.3.2 Differential Diagnosis 88
5.5.4   Bronchogenic Cyst 88
5.5.5   Tracheal, Laryngeal and Bronchial Atresia 90
5.5.6   Congenital Lobar Emphysema 91
5.5.7   Mucous Plug 91
5.5.8   Postnatal Presentation 91
5.6   Diaphragmatic Herniation 91
5.6.1   Left Diaphragmatic Hernia 92
5.6.2   Right Diaphragmatic Hernia 93
5.6.3   Bilateral Diaphragmatic Hernia 94
5.6.4   Management and Prognosis 94
5.6.5   Diaphragmatic Hypoplasia 94
5.6.6   Parasternal Morgagni Herniation 95
5.7   Pleural Effusion 95
5.8   Pulmonary Hypoplasia 97
5.9   Mediastinal Anomalies 97
5.9.1   Neurenteric Cyst 97
5.9.2   Pericardial Teratoma 98
5.9.3   Thymic Lesion 98
5.10   Thoracic Parietal Malformations 98
         References 98

FRANÇOISE RYPENS, MD; ANDREE GRIGNON, MD
Department of Medical Imaging, Sainte Justine Hospital, 3175
Côte-Sainte-Catherine, Montréal, Québec H3T 1C5, Canada
FRED E. AVNI, MD, PhD
Department of Pediatric Imaging, University Children's
Hospital, Queen Fabiola, Avenue J. J. Crocg 15, 1020 Brussels,
Belgium

5.1
Introduction

The study of the fetal chest is an important component of the standard fetal US examination. Congenital thoracic malformations may be responsible for fetal or neonatal death due to mediastinal compression or respiratory distress (HUBBARD and CROMBLE-HOLME 1998a). The discovery of a fetal thoracic malformation modifies the perinatal management and implies a transfer to a specialized neonatal department. The discovery of a fetal thoracic anomaly may also lead to the diagnosis of a polymalformation syndrome or to a chromosomal anomaly (GOLDSTEIN 2000).

Systematic US screening during pregnancy has led to the diagnosis of more thoracic fetal malformations and to better knowledge of their natural history (BROMLEY et al. 1995, ADZICK et al. 1998, BUNDUKI et al. 2000). The prognosis of some pulmonary malformations, such as sequestration or cystic adenomatoid malformation, appears much better than had been supposed from clinical series usually based on symptomatic cases detected postnatally (HEIJ et al. 1990, THORPE-BEESTON and NICOLAIDES 1994, KHAKOO et al. 1993). Improvement of prenatal US screening, better knowledge of the natural history of fetal malformations, and the development of fetal MRI, led some teams to perform fetal surgery in some specific and selected circumstances (HUBBARD et al. 1998b, ADZICK et al. 1998).

Yet, in spite of these improvements, prenatal diagnosis still has significant limitations. We are still unable to predict the individual prognosis for a fetus with diaphragmatic herniation, or the precise severity of an associated pulmonary hypoplasia (CANNON et al. 1996, DOMMERGUES et al. 1996).

In this chapter, we will first describe the embryological development of the fetal lungs and the corresponding normal US appearance of the fetal chest. We will then describe in turn the in utero appearance and management of parenchymal lung malformations, diaphragmatic herniation, pleural effusions and mediastinal anomalies. Heart anomalies will be discussed in Chap. 6.

5.2
Fetal Lung Development

The laryngotracheal diverticulum evaginates from the ventral wall of the primitive pharynx during the middle of the 4th week of embryological development. The endodermal lining of this bud gives rise to the inferior respiratory epithelium and to the tracheobronchial glands. The surrounding mesenchyme will produce the conjunctival tissue, cartilage, muscles, blood and lymphatic vessels. Numerous interactions occur between the mesenchyme and the mesoderm. Until the 30th day of embryological development, blood flow to the fetal lungs originates only from systemic vessels. These vessels, branches of the aorta, involute progressively while the pulmonary arteries develop (MOORE and PERSAUD 1993).

The primary lung bud divides itself into two bronchial buds during the beginning of the 5th week of embryological development. These endodermal buds grow laterally into the pericardioperitoneal canals, which are the primordia of the pleural cavities. Each bronchial bud enlarges, forming a primary bronchus, and divides into two secondary bronchi and then into segmentary bronchi. By 24 weeks of development, about 17 successive divisions have taken place and respiratory bronchioles exist. Seven new successive divisions occur after birth. Surrounding mesenchyme forms cartilaginous plates, bronchial smooth vasculature and pulmonary connective tissue as the bronchi develop. The visceral pleura originates from the splanchnic mesenchyme and the parietal pleura is derived from the somatic mesoderm.

Lung development can be arbitrarily divided into four stages. During the pseudoglandular period (6–16 weeks of development), the main airways not involved in gaseous exchange are formed. From the 16th to the 25th–28 weeks of development (canalicular stage), the lumen of the bronchi and bronchioles enlarges. Respiratory bronchioles and alveolar ducts appear. The parenchyma is highly vascular. Breathing becomes possible at the end of this period. During the saccular period, from 25–28 weeks of development until birth, alveolar ducts give rise to the terminal sacs forming the primitive alveoli. Their epithelium is initially cuboid and gets thinner at about 26 weeks. Capillary network and lymphatic vessels develop. Type 2 pneumocytes produce surfactant, starting at the 20th

week. This production increases at the end of the pregnancy. The alveolar period begins at 32 weeks gestation and lasts until late childhood. Type 1 pneumocytes get thinner and capillary vessels bulge inside the terminal sacs. The alveolocapillary membrane is sufficiently thin to allow gas exchange and respiration. After birth, the primitive alveoli enlarge. Most growth in the size of the lungs results from an increase in the number of respiratory bronchioles and primitive alveoli. Most mature alveoli appear after birth. At birth, about 50 million alveoli are present in a full-term neonate. This represents one sixth of the adult number (LANGSTON et al. 1984, LARSEN 1997, LAUDY and WLADIMIROFF 2000).

The diaphragm develops from four embryonic structures: the septum transversum, the pleuroperitoneal membranes, the paraxial mesoderm of the body wall, and the esophageal mesenchyme (LARSEN 1997). Breathing movements are observed already in utero (LAUDY and WLADIMIROFF 2000). They allow exchange between the intrapulmonary fluid and the amniotic fluid (NOBUHARA and WILSON 1996).

Conditions necessary for the normal development of the lung include: (a) normal thoracic shape and size, (b) adequate amniotic and intrapulmonary fluid volume, (c) breathing movements, (d) functioning fetal kidneys, and (e) a functional hypothalamo-hypophyseal axis (BALLARD 1980, KITTERMAN 1988, LAUDY and WLADIMIROFF 2000). Any condition interfering with one of these factors may lead to insufficient lung development and to its ultimate complications: lung hypoplasia and neonatal death (NOBUHARA and WILSON 1996). The degree of lung hypoplasia depends on the timing and the severity of the alteration.

The diversity of lung malformations is better understood in the light of embryogenesis. Persistence of systemic vessels as pulmonary vascularization, other than bronchial arteries, is the proposed mechanism for the development of pulmonary sequestrations. The numerous interactions occurring between the mesenchyme and the endoderm explain the association of anomalies sometimes observed in fetuses with thoracic malformations (i.e., sequestration and cystic adenomatoid malformation, diaphragmatic herniation and sequestration or cystic adenomatoid malformation, cardiac malformations, etc.). The complexity of the development also explains the existence of a continuous spectrum of malformations, from normal lung parenchyma supplied by abnormal vessels (sequestration) to abnormal parenchyma supplied by normal vessels (lobar emphysema) (SADE et al. 1974, HEITZMAN 1984, CLEMENTS and WARNER 1987).

5.3
Normal Appearance of Fetal Thorax on US and MRI

5.3.1
Normal US Appearance

On an axial scan, the fetal thorax appears round or oval; in sagittal and coronal planes, the transition between the fetal thorax and the abdomen is smooth. The fetal lungs are homogeneously echogenic throughout gestation. Their echogenicity relative to the liver increases with time (Figs. 5.1, 5.2). Trachea and main bronchi may be observed as hypoechoic tubular structures limited by hyperechoic borders. The pleural space is normally not discernible with any imaging techniques.

The heart is the main mediastinal structure, occupying 25–30% of the chest volume (Fig. 5.3) (PALADINI 1990). Using color and power Doppler it is possible to follow the aorta and pulmonary arterial branches (Fig. 5.4). Inferior and superior vena cava are visible in frontal and sagittal scans (Fig. 5.5).

The normal thymus is visible as early as the end of the second trimester of gestation in most fetuses (FELKER et al. 1989, HATA and DETER 1992). It has a homogeneous hypoechoic appearance compared with the adjacent lungs (Figs. 5.3, 5.6). Its absence during a third trimester US examination must induce the search for associated cardiac malformations and DiGeorge syndrome.

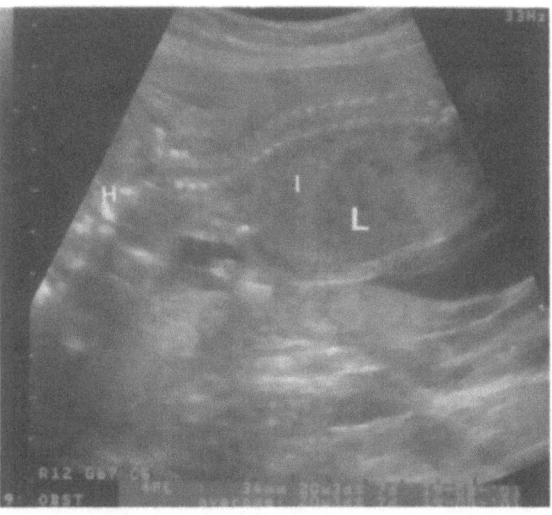

Fig. 5.2. Chest sagittal scan. Second trimester. The lungs (*l*) are clearly demarcated from the liver (*L*). *H* head

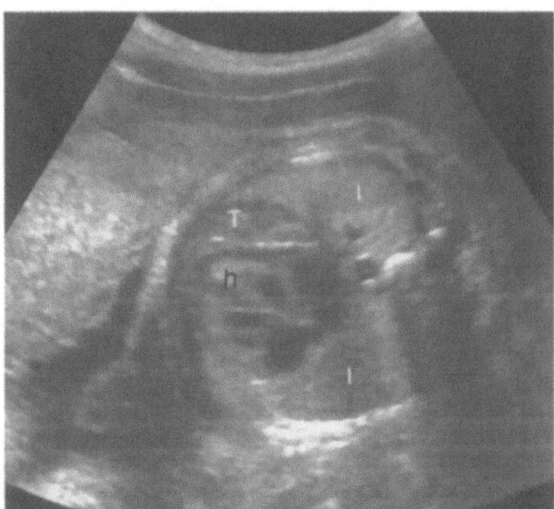

Fig. 5.3. Chest. Four-chamber view. Third trimester. Transverse scan demonstrates the heart (*h*), the lungs (*l*) and the thymus (*T*)

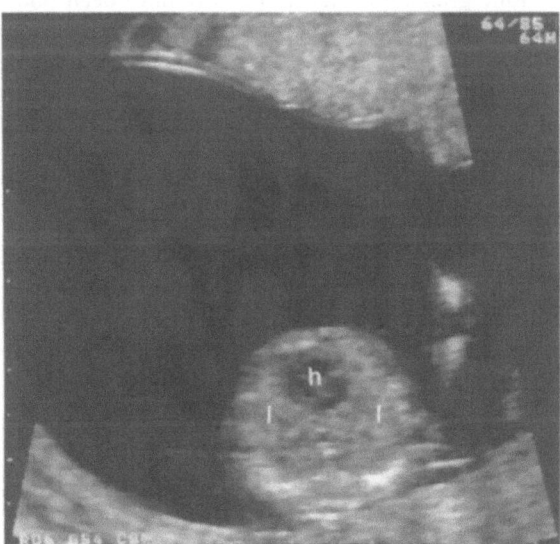

Fig. 5.1. Chest. Transverse scan. Early second trimester. The lungs (l) appear as diffusely echogenic areas on both sides of the heart (*h*)

The normal esophagus is visible inside the mediastinum as a hyperechoic, thick tubular structure. Its appearance changes during pregnancy. During the end of the first trimester it appears as a hyperechoic single-layer tubular structure (COOPER et al. 1985). By the end of the second trimester its wall has thickened and at least two layers are seen. Progression of swallowed amniotic fluid inside its lumen may also be followed during the US examinations.

The diaphragm is visible as a thin hypoechoic membrane between the liver or the spleen and the

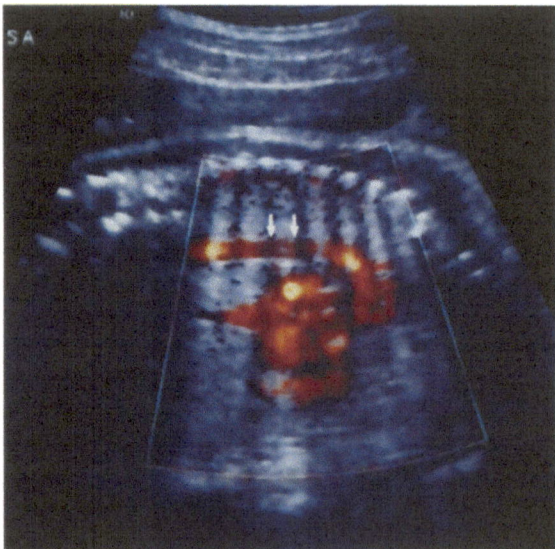

Fig. 5.4. Aortic cross (*arrows*). Sagittal view with power Doppler

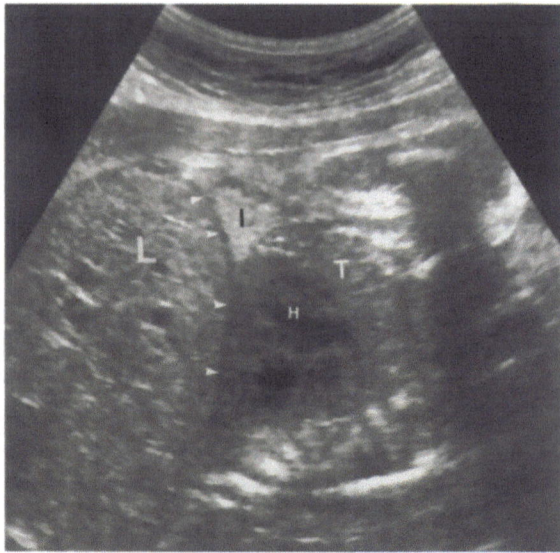

Fig. 5.6. Diaphragm. Third trimester. Sagittal scan. The diaphragm appears as a hypoechoic line (*arrowheads*) separating chest from abdomen. *L* liver, *h* heart, *T* thymus, *l* lung

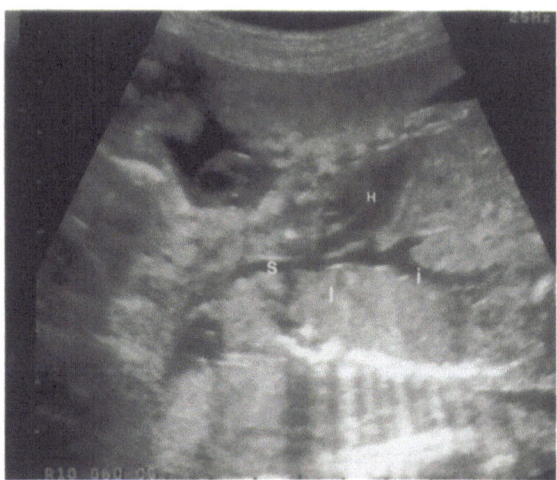

Fig. 5.5. Superior (*s*) and inferior (*i*) vena cava view. Sagittal scan. Third trimester. *H* head, *l* lung

ture. Clavicles and scapula are easily identified on axial and parasagittal scans. The sternal ossification centers appear first in the manubrium and then in the sternal body. They are hyperechoic inside the hypoechoic sternal cartilage (McCormick and Nichols 1981, Odita et al. 1985, Zalel et al. 1999).

Normal breathing motion is visible as early as the end of the second trimester, as well as normal episodes of hiccup.

Nomograms for fetal thorax size have been published (Chitkara 1987, Merz 1995).

5.3.2
Normal MR Appearance

T2-weighted sequences are the most informative due to the natural high contrast between the hyperintense lungs, and the mediastinum and thoracic wall (including the diaphragm), which appear hypointense. These sequences are also rapidly obtained (Yamashita et al. 1997, Huppert et al. 1999, Rypens 2001). Gradient echo T1-weighted sequences, necessitating a longer acquisition time, are useful in selected circumstances, particularly for the precise determination of the nature of a structure (for example the content of a diaphragmatic herniation).

On T2-weighted scans, fetal lungs appear homogeneous and hyperintense (Fig. 5.7). The boundaries with the mediastinum, the parietal wall and the dia-

lung. It presents with an inferior concavity (Figs. 5.2, 5.6). Flattening or inversion of the normal curvature of the diaphragm suggests the presence of a thoracic mass. Conversely, in cases of abdominal distension, the diaphragm may be displaced upwards, which decreases the intrathoracic volume and interferes with fetal lung growth.

The bony chest wall is clearly visible as early as 14 weeks of gestation. The ribs are regularly and symmetrically positioned with a smooth regular curva-

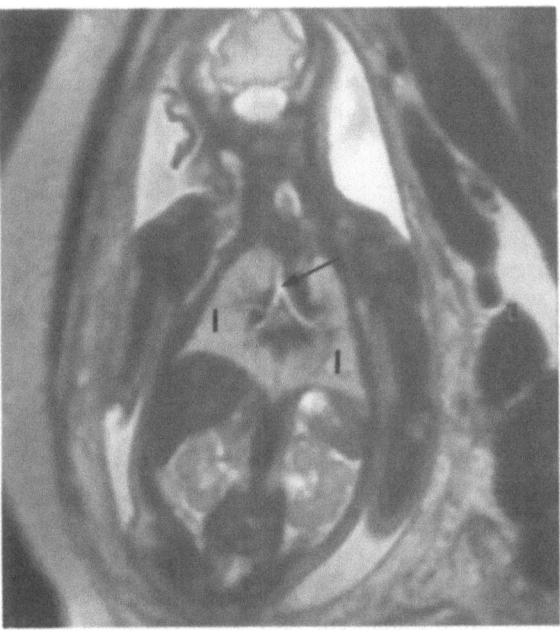

Fig. 5.7. Normal MR appearance of the lungs (*l*) and of the trachea (*arrow*). T2-weighted sequence

phragm are clearly seen. On T1-weighted sequences, the lungs, hypointense and homogeneous, have a less intense signal than the liver or the spleen. The fetal airways are easily demonstrated by fetal MRI, which is now able to display these structures up to the lobar bronchi. On T2-weighted scans, the liquid inside the trachea and main bronchi is hyperintense, and seems to have the same intensity as the amniotic fluid. The wall of the airways appears hypointense and is not precisely demarcated from the adjacent vessel walls (Fig. 5.7). On T1-weighted gradient-echo sequences, the motion of the fluid inside the airways is clearly detected, allowing perfect delineation of the piriform sinuses, the glottis, trachea and bronchi. This could be useful in cases of large mediastinal or cervicothoracic masses capable of displacing or compressing the fetal airways at birth. This sequence is also sensitive to the blood circulation, allowing demonstration of the four cardiac chambers and of the main mediastinal vessels more clearly than with T2-weighted sequences. The heart cavities and the large mediastinal vessels are hypointense on T2-weighted scans. The myocardium is more intense than the blood on this type of sequence. However, US and Doppler US remain the modalities of choice to study the vascular structures in a fetus.

The inferior part of the thoracic esophagus is usually visible on T2-weighted axial and coronal scans. The normal thymus has a higher signal intensity than the heart and main mediastinal vessels on T2-weighted scans. The thyroid gland is easily detected on T1-weighted sequences as a result of its high signal intensity.

The diaphragm may be seen on T2-weighted scans. It has a hypointense signal, and separates the lungs from the infradiaphragmatic organs.

Thanks to the natural high contrast that exists between the lungs and their boundaries on T2-weighted sequences, it is possible to measure the fetal lung volume by MRI using planimetry or semi-automatic volumetric measurements (BAKER et al. 1994, DUNCAN 1999a, COAKLEY et al. 2000, RYPENS et al. 2001). In contrast to US studies, volumetric measurements with MRI are possible in normal and abnormal circumstances such as diaphragmatic herniation and oligohydramnios. Fetal lung volume normally increases with gestational age. There is a constant relation between the left and right lung volumes, the right lung being slightly larger than the left (RYPENS 2001). The utility of this measurement in fetuses at risk for lung hypoplasia is currently under study.

Other teams have also used MRI to perform spectrometry in order to study the properties of the fetal lung and the degree of maturation of the fetal lungs (FENTON et al. 1998, 2000, DUNCAN et al. 1999b). These studies are promising.

5.4
General Considerations

Prenatal diagnosis of thoracic anomalies is mainly based on US and Doppler findings. Most thoracic malformations are discovered fortuitously during the second trimester US examination. Rarely, abnormal clinical examination (abnormal uterine size, suspicion of hydramnios, abnormal fetal monitoring, etc.) will lead to the discovery of a large malformation during the third trimester of gestation.

The natural history and the prognosis are very different depending on the origin of the malformation. Pulmonary malformations (the more frequent being cystic adenomatoid malformation and sequestration) have a globally favorable prognosis. In contrast, nonparenchymal malformations such as diaphragmatic hernia or large pleural effusions have a worse prognosis. The anomaly may be primarily thoracic or may be the consequence of another malformation (e.g., pleural effusion in the case of hydrops). The prognosis and the management will depend on the primary disease. Finally, the thoracic malformation may be isolated (e.g., cystic adenomatoid malformation) or associated with other malformations (e.g., diaphragmatic herniation in Fryns syndrome, rib anomalies associated with various skeletal disease). In all those circumstances, the prognosis, the management and the investigations required will be very different. A complete US survey is thus always mandatory in order to detect possible associated malformations and the possible repercussions for the developing fetus.

All significant thoracic malformations are likely to produce a mass effect on the adjacent lung, the mediastinum or the diaphragm, and to affect the normal physiology and development of the fetus. It is still impossible to quantify individually and precisely the degree of lung hypoplasia associated with a large thoracic malformation, yet this is the most crucial criterion for postnatal adaptation. Usually, the prognosis of a large malformation can not be evaluated at first examination and US follow-up will be necessary (BROMLEY et al. 1995). In the case of diaphragmatic herniation, and large thoracic masses, a complementary detailed fetal cardiac examination must be performed and, if necessary, repeated. Karyotype analysis is systematically indicated in cases of diaphragmatic hernia. The presence of hydrops detected early during pregnancy carries a poor prognosis.

In most circumstances, US and Doppler US will be enough to propose a presumptive diagnosis based on the anatomical location of the malformation. In some difficult circumstances, MRI may be proposed as a complementary examination (DUNCAN et al. 1997, HUBBARD 1999a). Thanks to its three-dimensional imaging capabilities, and accurate depiction of fetal airways, MRI may be useful when the malformation is particularly large with possible compression of the fetal airways and when the perinatal team considers an ex utero intrapartum treatment (EXIT procedure) (HUBBARD 1998b). MRI may also determine the exact anatomical extent of a large malformation, particularly when it encroaches upon the neck, the abdomen or the spine as is sometimes the case with large cystic lymphangioma or teratoma. MRI is also particularly useful in cases of diaphragmatic herniation in order to assess the content of the malformation (which is essential in cases of fetal surgery), the extent of the diaphragmatic defect and the volume of the fetal lung (HUBBARD et al. 1997, 1999b, RYPENS et al. 2001).

In each case, the obstetrician, the pediatrician, the neonatologist and the pediatric surgeon must be informed. The mode of delivery is usually not affected by the presence of a thoracic malformation unless it is responsible for maternofetal disproportion. How-

ever, birth must take place in a tertiary level hospital because respiratory distress is always possible even if the malformation seems to have involuted spontaneously (OLUTOYE et al. 2000).

5.5
Specific Fetal Lung Malformations

5.5.1
US Characteristics

The US appearances of the various parenchymal lung malformations are not specific and are in general the same: a hyperechoic mass, either homogeneous or containing cysts of various sizes (McCULLAGH et al. 1994, SAKALA et al. 1994). The cystic part may predominate. The malformation may produce a mass effect on the adjacent lung parenchyma that will appear hyperechoic itself and may be confused with part of the malformation. Two distinct pathological entities may coexist in the same malformation (e.g., cystic adenomatoid malformation and sequestration) (MORIN et al. 1989, CASS et al. 1997). These mixed lesions are more frequent than previously reported: the association of cystic adenomatoid malformation type II and extralobar sequestration has been found in up to 50% of the American Forces Institute of Pathology material (CONRAN and STOCKER 1999). The lack of specificity of US for an accurate diagnosis must be taken into account but in most circumstances will not modify the obstetrical management. Nevertheless, some US criteria still help in the differential diagnosis: most solid echogenic masses are cystic adenomatoid malformation or sequestration. Most malformations are unilateral. In cases of bilateral malformation, congenital high airway obstructions (CHAOS) must be suspected.

On the whole, the prognosis of a parenchymal malformation is favorable. More than 50% of cystic adenomatoid malformations and sequestrations become smaller during pregnancy (BROMLEY et al. 1995, MILLER et al. 1996, ADZICK et al. 1998, DE SANTIS et al. 2000). Smaller masses and absence of mediastinal shift or hydrops are usually associated with a better outcome as well. Larger malformations rarely enlarge enough to compress the mediastinum and to induce hydramnios, cardiac failure, hydrops, fetal death or significant lung hypoplasia and neonatal respiratory distress or death. Hydramnios may result from two different mechanisms: increased secretion of lung fluid by the malformation, and compression of the fetal esophagus.

5.5.2
Congenital Cystic Adenomatoid Malformation

Cystic adenomatoid malformation (CAM) is the most common pulmonary malformation detected in utero (ROSADO-DE-CHRISTENSON and STOCKER 1991, BROMLEY et al. 1995). This hamartomatous lesion is characterized by abnormal growth of the terminal bronchioles without alveolar differentiation. It results probably from a vascular insult leading to bronchial atresia, cessation of the distal bronchiolar development and dilatation of the immature parenchyma distal to the atresia. The malformation is linked with the airways by abnormal channels, which explains the progressive aeration of the malformed area after birth. The discovery of this sporadic anomaly is usually fortuitous during the second trimester US examination.

5.5.2.1
In Utero Appearance

The malformation is typically unilateral and can involve any lobe or segment. It is limited to one lobe or segment in more than 95% of cases. Bilateral involvement is rare (less than 2%). In cases of bilateral involvement, the anomaly must be differentiated from tracheal atresia, which may have the same appearance. (In tracheal atresia, both lungs are enlarged and appear hyperechoic, reversing the diaphragm.) CAM is usually avascular on Doppler US. Abnormal systemic vessels may be observed when it is associated with an intralobar sequestration.

Stocker's histological classification distinguishes three types of CAM (STOCKER et al. 1977). Type 1 lesions (more than 50% of cases) contain multiple cysts larger than 2 cm. One cyst usually predominates (Fig. 5.8). On US, the lesion has a multicystic appearance, one or a few large cysts being associated with smaller ones. Type 2 (30–40% of cases) includes lesions with 0.5–2 cm cysts. The US appearance is mixed, consisting of numerous small cysts and associated echogenic tissue (Fig. 5.9). Type 3 (less than 10% of cases) contains microcysts giving a solid hyperechoic appearance (Figs. 5.10, 5.11). ADZICK and coworkers have proposed another simplified classification, based on the US appearance of the malformation (ADZICK et al. 1985). They distinguish macrocystic malformation, including cysts of more than 5 mm, and microcystic lesions. If these classifications illustrate the various US appearances of CAM, they do not have a practical clinical consequence, unless a therapeutic approach is planned

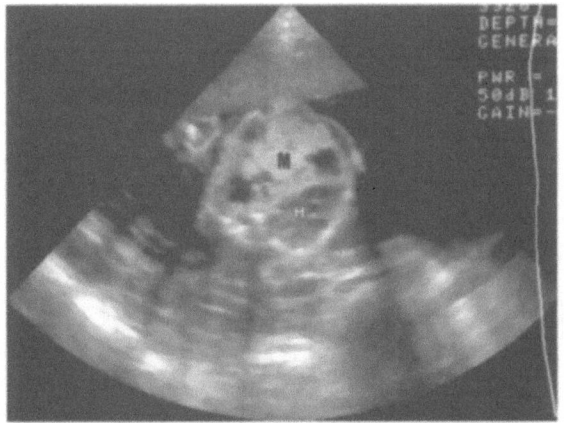

a

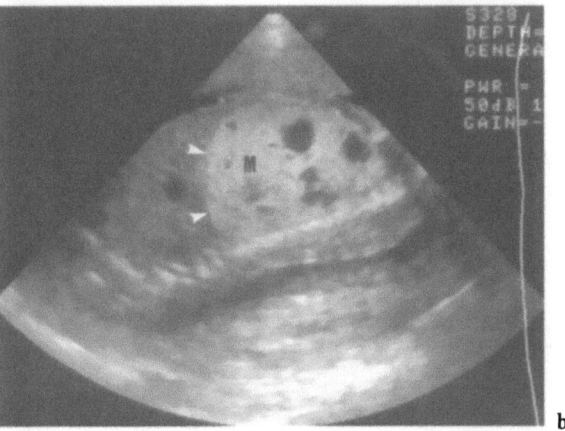

b

Fig. 5.8a, b. CAM type I. a Axial fetal chest US scan in a 20-week-old fetus. Right thoracic echogenic mass (*M*) with macrocysts displacing the heart (*H*) towards the left side of the chest. b Parasagittal US scan of the same fetus illustrates the mass (*M*) effect on the diaphragm, which bulges downwards (*arrowheads*)

(i.e., intrauterine drainage in the case of large type 1 malformation or fetal surgery in the case of type 3 malformation associated with hydrops before 32 weeks of gestation).

5.5.2.2
Management

In utero, CAM generally exists in isolation. However, it is wise to search for possible associated malformations (urinary, cardiac and digestive). Previous retrospective studies have suggested the association of systemic malformations or karyotypic anomalies with type 2 CAM (BROMLEY et al. 1995). These associations are not confirmed by the most recent prospective fetal series. Karyotype analysis was historically

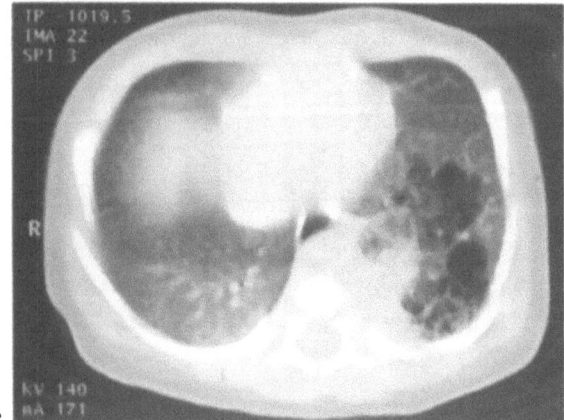

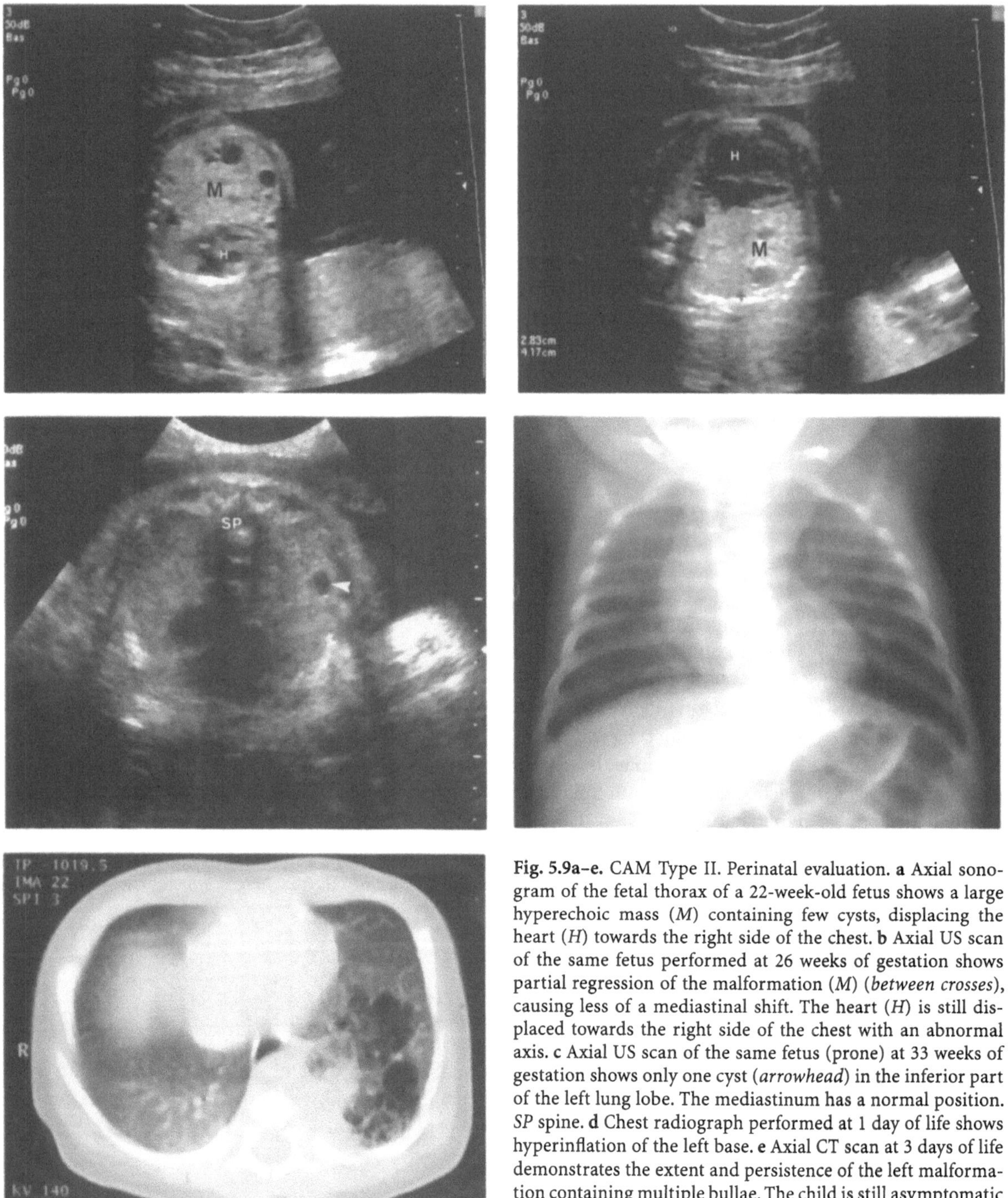

Fig. 5.9a–e. CAM Type II. Perinatal evaluation. a Axial sonogram of the fetal thorax of a 22-week-old fetus shows a large hyperechoic mass (*M*) containing few cysts, displacing the heart (*H*) towards the right side of the chest. b Axial US scan of the same fetus performed at 26 weeks of gestation shows partial regression of the malformation (*M*) (*between crosses*), causing less of a mediastinal shift. The heart (*H*) is still displaced towards the right side of the chest with an abnormal axis. c Axial US scan of the same fetus (prone) at 33 weeks of gestation shows only one cyst (*arrowhead*) in the inferior part of the left lung lobe. The mediastinum has a normal position. *SP* spine. d Chest radiograph performed at 1 day of life shows hyperinflation of the left base. e Axial CT scan at 3 days of life demonstrates the extent and persistence of the left malformation containing multiple bullae. The child is still asymptomatic after 3 years of follow-up

strongly recommended in cases of type 2 malformation but is now debatable when the malformation is isolated (SAKALA et al. 1994, HUBBARD 1998a). The prognosis depends on the size of the mass and on the impairment of lung development and fetal hemodynamics. If the mass is big enough to compress the mediastinum, hydramnios or hydrops may supervene. However, only hydrops seems to represent a negative predictor of outcome in the most recent series (DE SANTIS et al. 2000). In such rare circumstances, cystic drainage or surgical intervention are proposed by some teams. In the absence of hydrops, conservative management is mandatory. A US follow-up of the malformation is necessary in order to appreciate the evolution of the mass and its possible effects. CAM can grow during pregnancy, but also

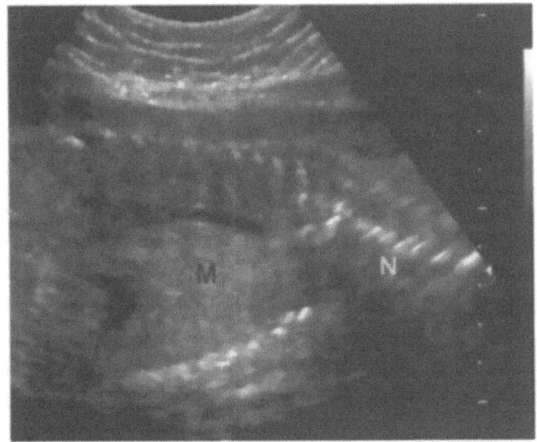

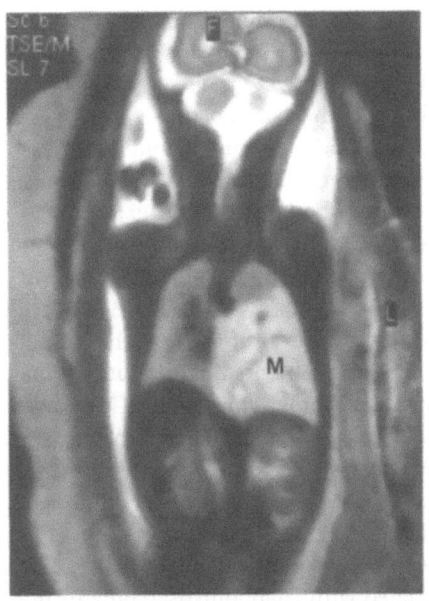

Fig. 5.10a, b. CAM type III. Third trimester. **a** Sagittal US. scan showing a homogeneous mass (*M*) (3.5 cm; *N* neck, between the crosses). **b** Fetal MRI was performed at 28 weeks of gestation and shows the extent of the mass (*M*) that occupies most of the left chest and appears hyperintense on this T2-weighted sequence

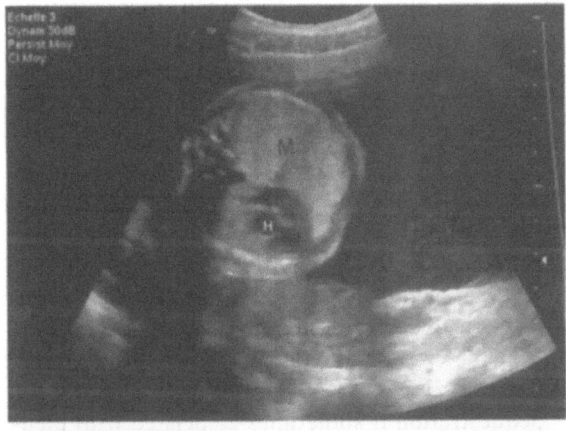

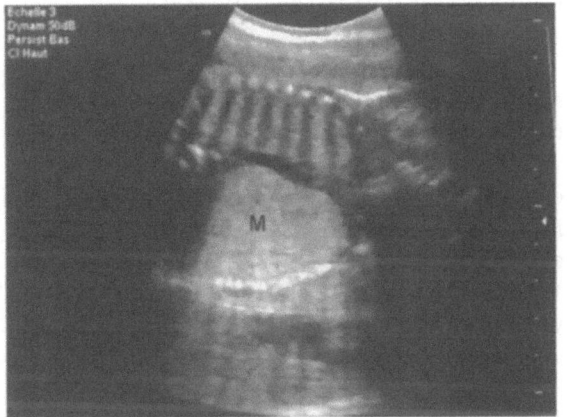

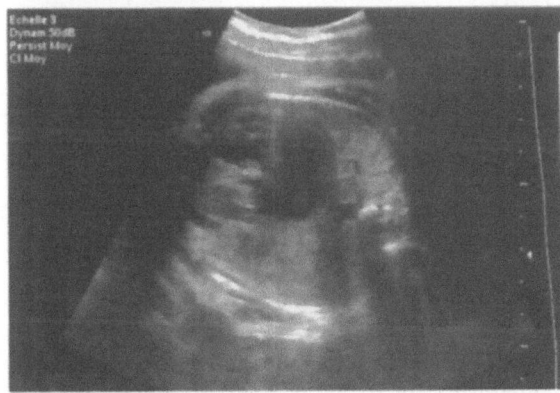

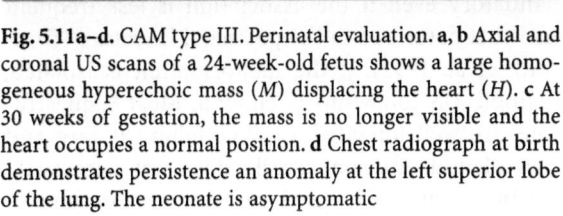

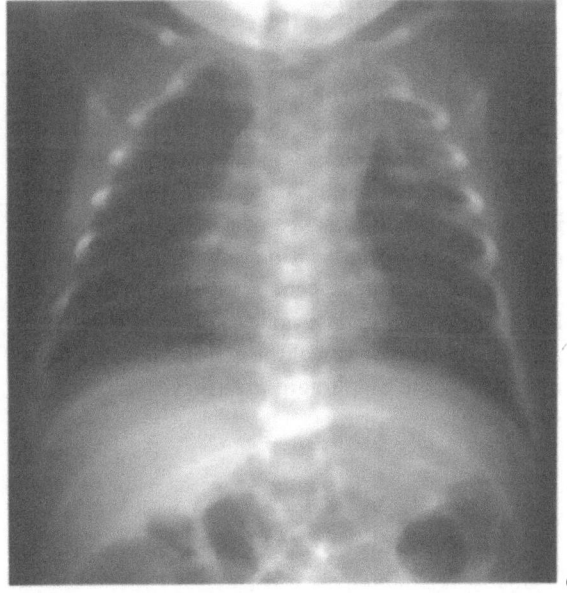

Fig. 5.11a–d. CAM type III. Perinatal evaluation. **a, b** Axial and coronal US scans of a 24-week-old fetus shows a large homogeneous hyperechoic mass (*M*) displacing the heart (*H*). **c** At 30 weeks of gestation, the mass is no longer visible and the heart occupies a normal position. **d** Chest radiograph at birth demonstrates persistence an anomaly at the left superior lobe of the lung. The neonate is asymptomatic

slowly regress and even disappear on US (this evolution has been observed in up to 30% of cases) (BARRET et al. 1995) (Figs. 5.9, 5.11).

After birth, in each case, postnatal imaging is necessary (Figs. 5.9, 5.11). Thoracic and abdominal radiographs, US, thoracic CT scan or MRI will be necessary to determine the location and extent of the mass (MATA et al. 1990, WINTERS et al. 1997). CT and MRI show more precisely the residual lesion (WINTERS et al. 1997, VAN LEEUWEN et al. 1999). This assessment is necessary even if the mass has apparently disappeared on US before birth, because it may still be present and become symptomatic (MEAGHER et al. 1993). This is why birth must occur in a tertiary center with an experienced team.

After birth, CAM may remain asymptomatic, become infected, or grow progressively due to a valve-like phenomenon (HEIJ et al. 1990). Rare cases of CAM associated with rhabdomyosarcoma or pulmonary blastoma have been described in children (MURPHY et al. 1992, D'AGOSTINO et al. 1997, GRANATA et al. 1998).

Treatment is still debated, some teams proposing surgical resection in each case and others preferring to reserve surgery for symptomatic cases and conservative management for the other patients (KHAKOO et al. 1993, THORPE-BEESTON and NICOLAIDES 1994, MORIN et al. 1994, BROMLEY et al. 1995, ADZICK et al. 1998, BAGOLAN et al. 1999, VAN LEEUWEN et al. 1999, DE SANTIS et al. 2000). However, there is still no well-performed prospective study to suggest the best approach.

5.5.2.3
Differential Diagnosis

In the case of a unilocular cystic appearance of the malformation, bronchogenic cyst and mediastinal cystic malformations are the main differential diagnoses. When the lesion appears solid and hyperechoic, sequestration or rarely bronchial atresia have to be discussed. The presence of a systemic vessel and an inferior thoracic location suggest sequestration. In the case of a heterogeneous cystic mass, the differential diagnosis must include diaphragmatic herniation. Demonstration of the abdominal viscera and integrity of the diaphragm are clues to the diagnosis.

5.5.3
Sequestration

Bronchopulmonary sequestration contains nonfunctional lung tissue without normal connection with the airways and with a systemic arterial blood supply (usually from the thoracic descending aorta or abdominal aorta). Intralobar sequestration has the same pleural wrapping and venous drainage as the adjacent lung. Extralobar sequestration has its own pleural envelope and an abnormal venous drainage towards the vena cava, the azygos system or the portal system. Although it represents only 25% of sequestrations, the extralobar form is the most frequently observed before birth (most intralobar sequestrations diagnosed after birth are in fact acquired lesions associated with chronic infection) (STOCKER 1986, ROSADO-DE-CHRISTENSON et al. 1993). Usually, the sequestration appears as a hyperechoic mass located in the posteroinferior part of the thorax between the inferior lung lobe and the diaphragm, more often on the left side (Fig. 5.12). It can sometimes be in a paramedian juxtamediastinal location or even below the diaphragm (MARIONA et al. 1986, WHITE et al. 1994, CURTIS et al. 1997, HERNANZ-SCHULMAN et al. 1997) (Fig. 5.13). The appearance can be the same as any type of CAM. The diagnosis will depend on the demonstration of an abnormal systemic vessel with color or power Doppler US (LOPOO et al. 1999, BECMEUR et al. 1998) (Fig. 5.12b). US and Doppler US are not always able to detect the abnormal systemic vascularization, the vessels being discovered during arteriography, surgery or at pathological examination.

Sequestration is sometimes associated with pleural effusion (suggesting a torsion of the sequestration) or with diaphragmatic hernia (HERNANZ-SCHULMAN et al. 1991). Rarely, it communicates with the digestive tract; an esophago-bronchopulmonary malformation is fully diagnosed after birth (SRIKANTH et al. 1992).

5.5.3.1
Management and Prognosis

In utero, a search for associated malformations is mandatory even if the association is less frequent than that described in the postnatal literature (DOLKART et al. 1992). If the malformation is isolated, a simple US follow-up is enough. Most sequestrations are well tolerated. Cardiac failure is rare and even pleural effusion usually does not necessitate any interventional procedure. Spontaneous involu-

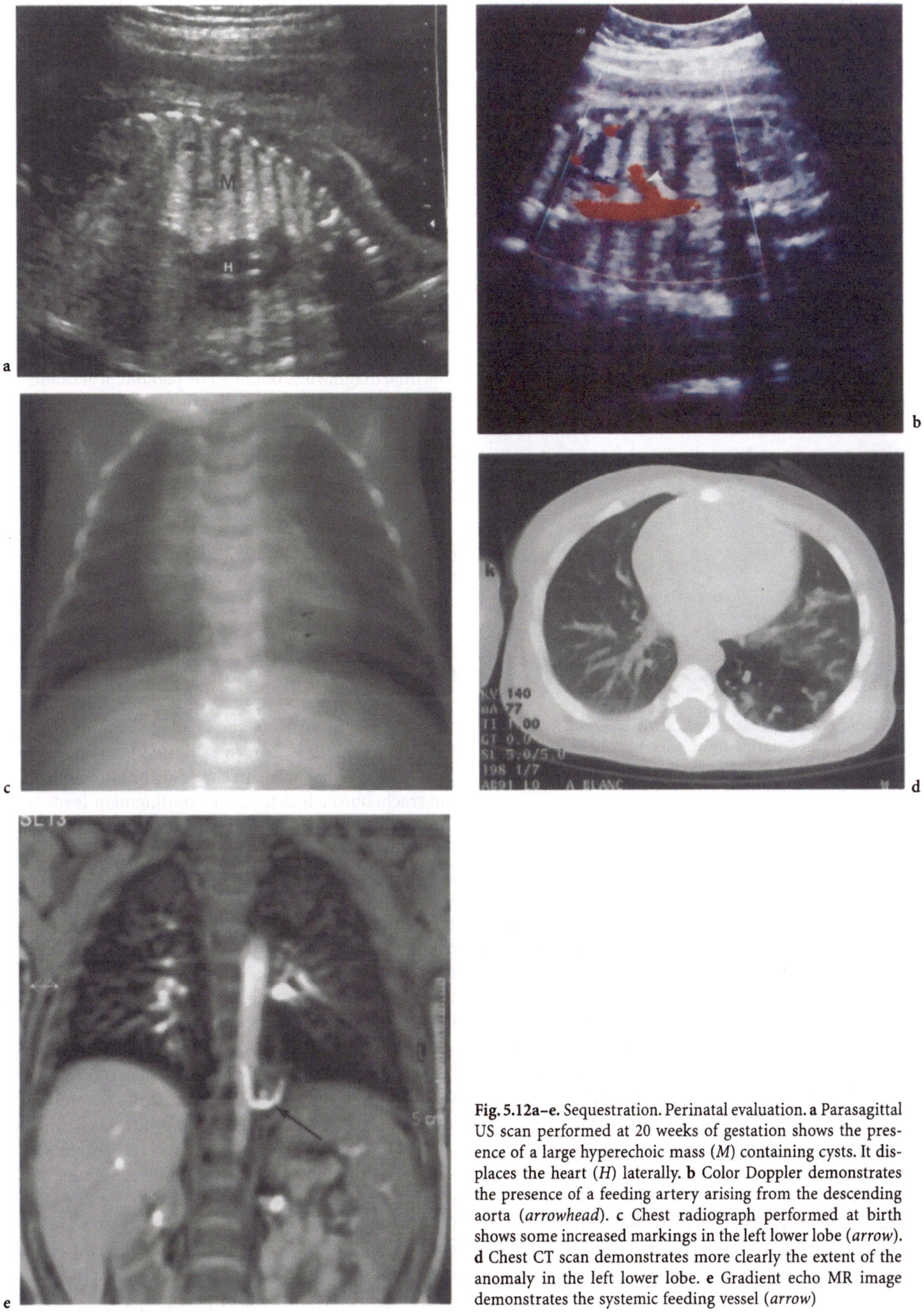

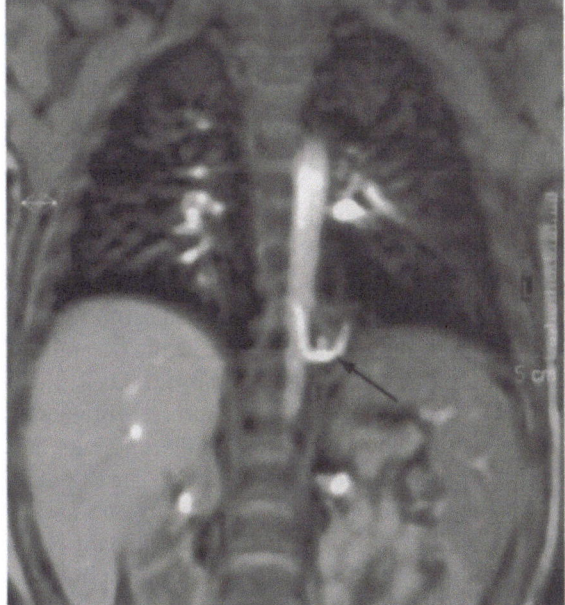

Fig. 5.12a–e. Sequestration. Perinatal evaluation. **a** Parasagittal US scan performed at 20 weeks of gestation shows the presence of a large hyperechoic mass (*M*) containing cysts. It displaces the heart (*H*) laterally. **b** Color Doppler demonstrates the presence of a feeding artery arising from the descending aorta (*arrowhead*). **c** Chest radiograph performed at birth shows some increased markings in the left lower lobe (*arrow*). **d** Chest CT scan demonstrates more clearly the extent of the anomaly in the left lower lobe. **e** Gradient echo MR image demonstrates the systemic feeding vessel (*arrow*)

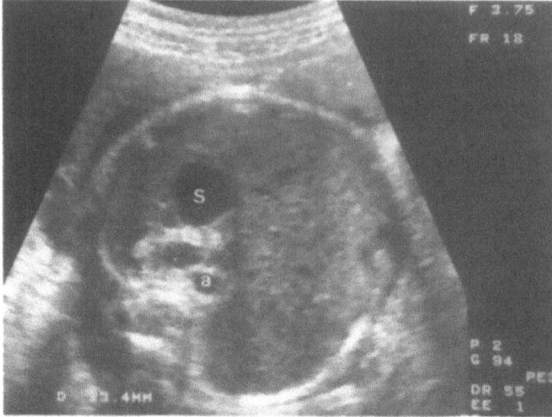

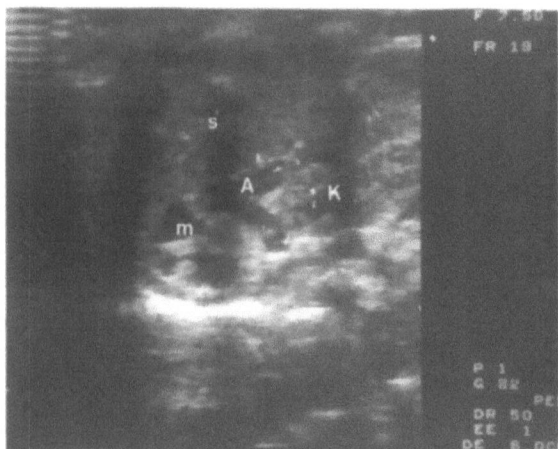

Fig. 5.13a, b. Infradiaphragmatic sequestration. **a** Axial sonogram performed during third trimester shows a heterogeneous hyperechoic mass (between *crosses*) containing a cystic part and located behind the stomach (*S*). *a* aorta. **b** Sagittal US scan performed at birth demonstrates the mass (*m*) distinct from the adrenal (*A*) and kidney (*k*). *s* spleen

tion during pregnancy is possible and observed more often than with CAM (LANGER et al. 1995, HUBBARD 1998a).

At birth, most sequestrations are asymptomatic. A thoracic radiograph, US and CT scan or MRI are performed after birth in order to delineate precisely the anatomical location and extent of the malformation as well as the importance of the systemic vessels (Fig. 5.12) (WEST et al. 1989, FELKER and TONKIN 1990). Some of these vessels are not visualized even on a good CT scan examination or angiography and are finally discovered during surgical resection. Treatment is also controversial: conservative observation, resection or embolization have been proposed, depending on the clinical situation and

the local expertise (BROMLEY et al. 1995, ADZICK et al. 1998, DANEMAN et al. 1997, PARK et al. 1998, LOPOO et al. 1999, BECMEUR et al. 1998, BRATU et al. 2001). Conservative management in cases of regressing sequestration is a clear trend in the recent literature.

5.5.3.2
Differential Diagnosis

The same differential diagnosis as for CAM can be discussed. Depending on the appearance and location, CAM, bronchial atresia, mucous plug, bronchogenic foregut malformation (Fig. 5.14), duplication and bronchogenic cyst can be included in the discussion. The final diagnosis is obtained by pathological examination and is not significant for the discussion of fetal prognosis. In the case of a juxtamediastinal or infradiaphragmatic location (Fig. 5.13), neuroblastoma must be included in the differential diagnosis. Neuroblastoma is usually diagnosed during the third trimester of gestation and does not have a preferential left-sided location (CURTIS et al. 1997). An abnormal systemic feeding artery helps to suggest sequestration.

5.5.4
Bronchogenic Cyst

A bronchogenic cyst is rarely diagnosed in utero (MAYDEN et al. 1984, YOUNG et al. 1989). It originates from an abnormal bronchial budding or branching of the tracheobronchial tree. Bud confinement leads to the formation of a cyst containing mucus. The cyst wall may contain cartilage and muscle. The malformation is typically located along the tracheobronchial tree, most often within the mediastinum. The cyst may be located in the hilum, or inside the lung parenchyma (25% of cases) (Fig. 5.15). Usually, the cyst does not communicate with the tracheobronchial tree; rare communications have been observed in the intraparenchymal form (Fig. 5.15b).

At US, a bronchogenic cyst appears as a unilocular hypoechoic intraparenchymal or mediastinal structure. Atypical content may complicate the US appearance: internal septa may give an appearance similar to CAM. The cyst can also compress a bronchus, increasing the echogenicity of the adjacent lung: this gives the appearance of a typical CAM. The differential diagnosis is obtained at pathological examination only. When located in the mediastinum, the differential diagnosis must include esophageal duplication, neurenteric cyst, teratoma or pericardial cyst.

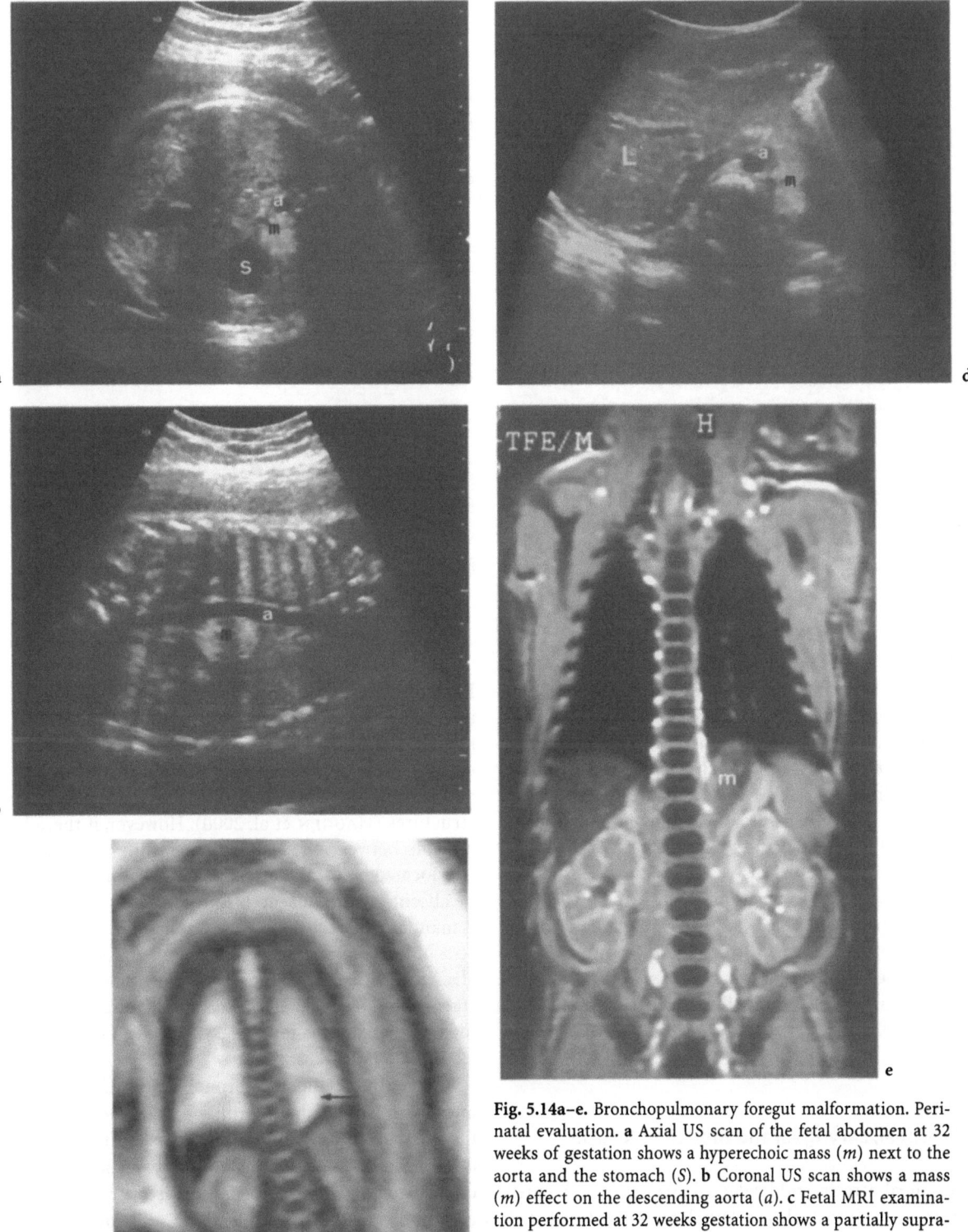

Fig. 5.14a–e. Bronchopulmonary foregut malformation. Perinatal evaluation. **a** Axial US scan of the fetal abdomen at 32 weeks of gestation shows a hyperechoic mass (*m*) next to the aorta and the stomach (*S*). **b** Coronal US scan shows a mass (*m*) effect on the descending aorta (*a*). **c** Fetal MRI examination performed at 32 weeks gestation shows a partially supradiaphragmatic mass with a cystic component (*arrow*). **d** Axial US scan performed at birth shows the persistence of the mass (*m*) against the diaphragm. *a* aorta, *L* liver. **e** Coronal TFE. T1-weighted sequence performed when the baby was 3 months old shows the persistence of a hypointense peridiaphragmatic mass (*m*), separated from the adrenal. At the follow-up performed 3 months later, the mass was no longer visible

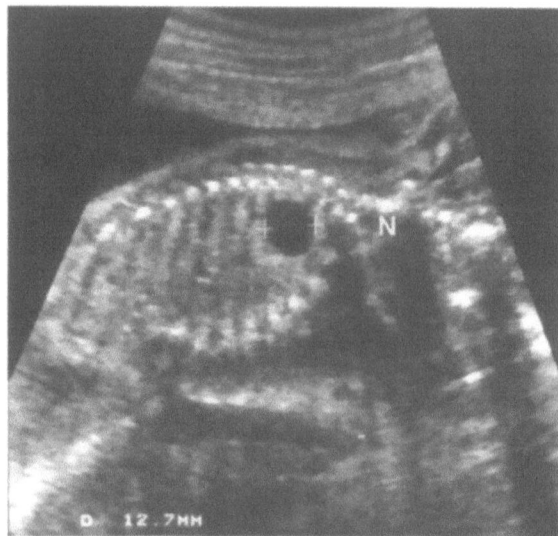

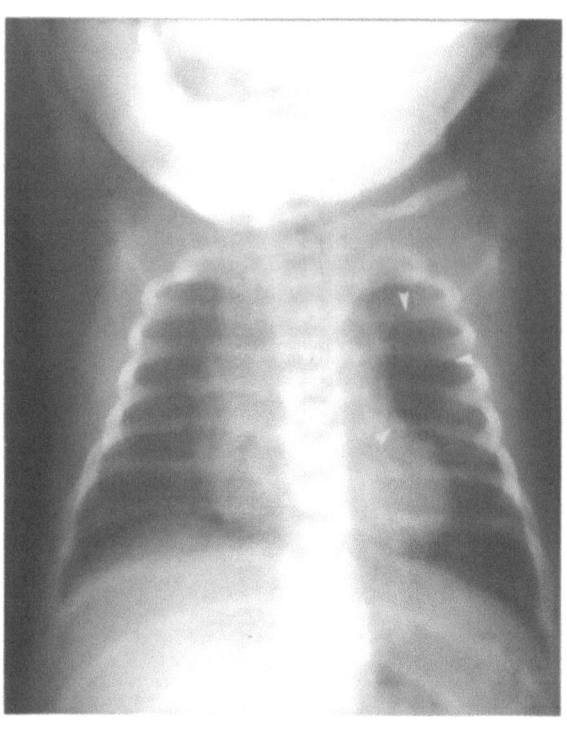

Fig. 5.15a, b. Bronchogenic cyst. **a** Parasagittal US scan performed at 30 weeks of gestation shows a cyst (between *crosses*) inside the left lung parenchyma. *N* fetal neck. **b** Radiograph at 2 days of life shows a bulla (*arrowheads*) in the left upper lung corresponding to a bronchogenic cyst

Most bronchogenic cysts are isolated. They are usually well tolerated in utero. Hydramnios and hydrops are only observed when the malformation is large and compresses the fetal esophagus or displaces the mediastinum. Most cysts remain asymptomatic after birth. Nevertheless some will enlarge and compress adjacent structures (esophagus or bronchi) leading to respiratory distress in infancy (Hernanz-Schulman 1993). Infection may also contribute to symptoms when the cyst communicates with the tracheobronchial tree (Bolton and Shahian 1992). Spontaneous pneumothorax has also been described in association with bronchogenic cyst (Matzinger et al. 1992).

5.5.5
Tracheal, Laryngeal and Bronchial Atresia

Tracheal atresia and laryngeal atresia are extremely rare and almost always lethal malformations. Left untreated, these congenital high airway obstructions (CHAOS) lead to death within minutes after birth from respiratory obstruction. The anomaly (atresia, stenosis or web) affects the larynx or the upper part of the trachea. In the typical US presentation, both lungs appear highly hyperechoic and enlarged (De

Hullu et al. 1995). The diaphragm is flattened or inverted and fetal ascites, polyhydramnios or oligohydramnios, and signs of hydrops, may be present. In some circumstances, the fluid-filled bronchi and trachea may be detected as tubular hypoechoic structures (Haugen et al. 2000). However, if there is a fistula between the esophagus and the respiratory tree located below the atresia, these US findings may be absent. A careful search for associated anomalies is mandatory because they are observed in more than 50% of fetuses with laryngeal obstruction. Laryngeal atresia may be part of Fraser's syndrome combining tracheal or laryngeal atresia, uropathy, oligohydramnios, ocular anomalies and syndactyly (Taybi and Lachman 1996).

If the atresia affects a bronchus, the US appearance is indistinguishable from a large type III CAM: the obstructed fluid-filled lung distal to the atresia appears on US as a homogeneous hyperechoic parenchymal mass. This malformation is observed most commonly in the left upper lobe and more rarely involves the lower lobes, in contrast to pulmonary sequestrations or diaphragmatic herniations. The location of the malformation, respecting anatomical boundaries, is a useful diagnostic criterion which may be used in order to suggest the diagnosis when observed with fetal MRI.

5.5.6
Congenital Lobar Emphysema

Congenital lobar emphysema (CLE) is rarely diagnosed in utero (RICHARDS et al. 1992, OLUTOYE et al. 2000). It is secondary to focal abnormal bronchial cartilage that may be associated with intrinsic or extrinsic bronchial compression. CLE appears in utero as a homogeneous hyperechoic mass usually located in the upper or middle lobe. Its appearance is similar to those of type 3 CAM or sequestration. Spontaneous involution has been described in utero (RICHARDS et al. 1992, OLUTOYE et al. 2000). Symptoms may be observed after birth even after spontaneous in utero resolution because the malformation is still present and may enlarge after birth due to a valve mechanism (OLUTOYE et al. 2000). This congenital malformation is more often detected during the first year of life when the infant suffers from respiratory symptoms due to lobar hyperinflation. In some cases, the malformation may appear opaque soon after birth, due to the persistence of fluid inside the involved lobe.

5.5.7
Mucous Plug

Spontaneous involution of intraluminal mucous plugs has also been suggested as the origin of the resolution of some intraparenchymal hyperechoic masses when no bronchial malformation is detected. The appearance is then similar to the solid type of CAM (MEIZNER and ROSENAK 1995, ACHIRON 1995a).

5.5.8
Postnatal Presentation of Congenital Lung Malformations

Congenital lung malformations may become symptomatic after birth by three mechanisms: air trapping, infection, and cardiac failure (ALFORD et al. 1993). Communications with the tracheobronchial tree lead to the progressive ventilation of the malformation and to its possible distension by a valve mechanism. This may lead to respiratory distress soon after birth. A solid intraparenchymal mass which progressively aerates with time is usually a CAM or rarely a CLE or a bronchogenic cyst. Infection may also lead to the discovery of congenital malformations. Abnormal airways connections may be responsible for abnormal ventilation and repeated pulmonary infections. Repeated infections in the same anatomical location in a child must induce the search for an associated congenital malformation or an inhaled foreign body. Thoracic CT scans and endoscopy are then the clues for the diagnosis of CAM, sequestration or bronchogenic cyst. Rarely, sequestration may manifest as cardiac failure due to its hemodynamic effect.

Finally, congenital pulmonary malformations may be fortuitously discovered when performing a thoracic radiograph in a child or adult.

5.6
Diaphragmatic Herniation

Diaphragmatic herniation corresponds to the intrathoracic presence of abdominal viscera within the chest. It results from an anomaly of the partitioning of the celomic cavity. The malformation may be due to a primitive defect of the diaphragm (anomalous closing of the pericardioperitoneal canal by the septum transversum or anomalous muscularization). Other possible pathogenic mechanisms have also been proposed: excessively early intra-abdominal reintegration of the primitive bowel or primitive anomalous lung development. The most frequent diaphragmatic anomaly is the Bochdalek hernia, occurring in 90% of cases and characterized by a posterolateral diaphragmatic defect. The defect is most frequently unilateral and left-sided (80%), more rarely right-sided (15%) or bilateral (5%). Diaphragmatic hypoplasia (eventration), parasternal Morgagni hernia and hiatal hernia are other diaphragmatic malformations rarely diagnosed in the fetus.

Diaphragmatic herniation is relatively frequent and observed in 1/2,200 to 1/5,000 live births. It is usually isolated and sporadic, more rarely familial or associated with antiepileptic medications (GIBBS et al. 1997, ENNS et al. 1998). It may also be part of a polymalformation syndrome (Fryns syndrome, Cornelia de Lange syndrome, Beckwith-Wiedemann syndrome, etc.) or be associated with chromosomal anomalies (MANNI et al. 1994, ENNS et al. 1998).

The rate of US diagnosis of diaphragmatic hernia is variable, depending on the content and the size of the hernia. Furthermore the herniation may occur late during pregnancy, or even after birth.

5.6.1
Left Diaphragmatic Hernia

Diagnosis of a left diaphragmatic hernia relies upon the discovery of intra-abdominal viscera inside the left hemithorax and their absence in the fetal abdomen (Figs. 5.16, 5.17). The diaphragmatic defect itself is usually more difficult to demonstrate. The herniated viscera displace the mediastinum to the right and may compress the heart (KASALES et al. 1998). The fetal stomach appear as a left paracardiac cystic structure. The spleen often follows

the stomach and appears as a hypoechoic homogeneous structure, sometimes located behind the heart. Its appearance must be differentiated from lung sequestration or CAM, which can be associated with diaphragmatic hernia (sequestration and CAM appear more echogenic than the splenic

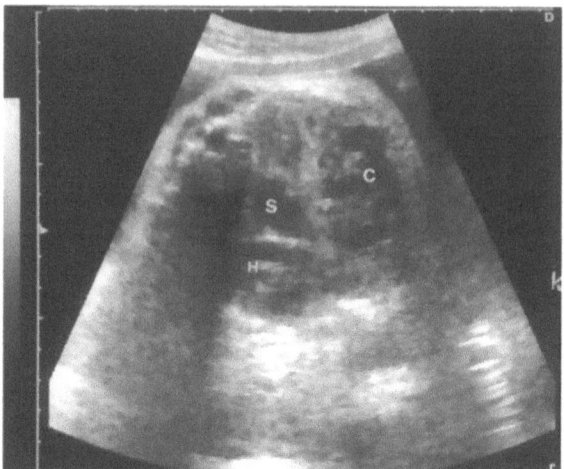

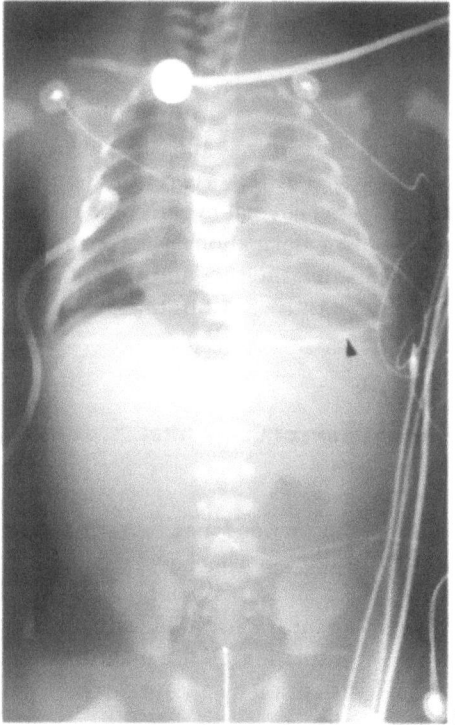

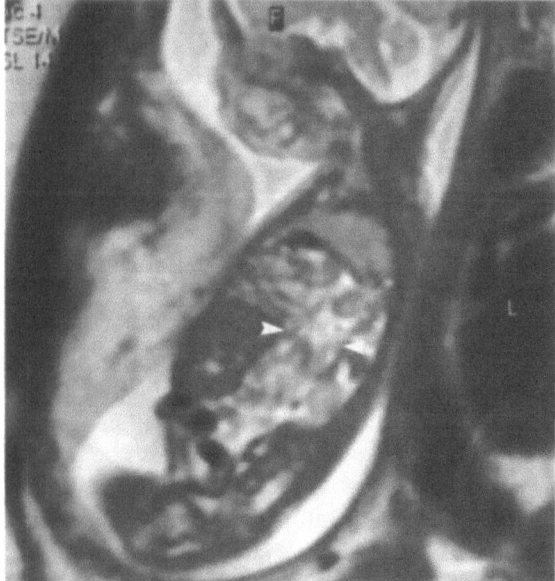

Fig. 5.16a, b. Left diaphragmatic hernia. Second trimester. a Axial US scan of the chest in a 22-week-old fetus (the fetus is prone). Displacement of the mediastinum by a hyperechoic mass corresponding to small bowel (b). h heart. b Parasagittal T2-weighted MR scan at 22 weeks shows the extent of the diaphragmatic defect (arrowheads), and the herniated small bowel

Fig. 5.17a, b. Left diaphragmatic hernia. Third trimester. a Axial chest US scan performed in a 30-week-old fetus. The heart (H) is displaced and compressed by the stomach (S), the small bowel, and the colon (C) herniated inside the chest. b Chest and abdominal radiograph of the neonate. Mediastinal shift and partial aeration of the left herniated intestines. Note the location of the gastric tube (arrowhead)

tissue) (Fig. 5.18). Small bowel loops and sometimes the colon may also be herniated. The intrathoracic location of the left hepatic lobe is detected by the displacement of the umbilical and hepatic veins. The diaphragmatic herniation may be associated with pleural effusion and hydramnios.

5.6.2
Right Diaphragmatic Hernia

Right diaphragmatic hernia is more difficult to diagnose due to the similar echogenicity of the liver and the lung. The liver is herniated inside the thorax and displaces the heart towards the left. The liver and the gallbladder are located high in the chest and the hepatic vascular network appears disorganized (BOTASH and SPIRT 1993) (Fig. 5.19). The intra-abdominal stomach has a more midline and

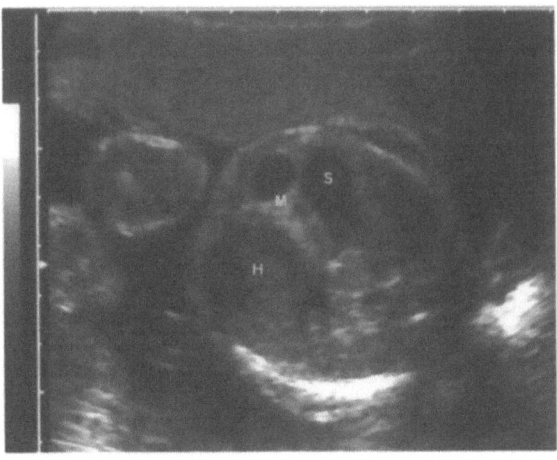

Fig. 5.18. Association between diaphragmatic herniation and CAM. Axial US scan of a 24-week-old fetus shows the intrathoracic presence of the stomach (*S*) close to an echogenic mass (*M*) with a cystic component as well as the mediastinal shift. *H* heart

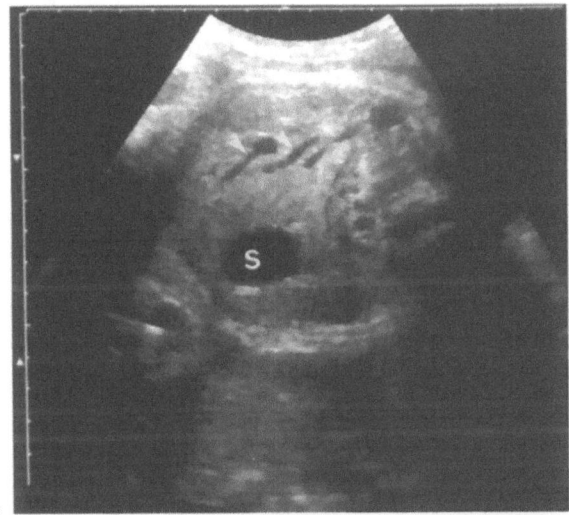

a

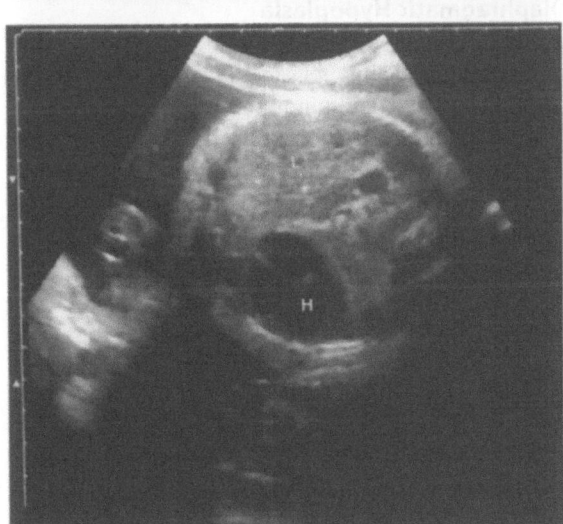

c

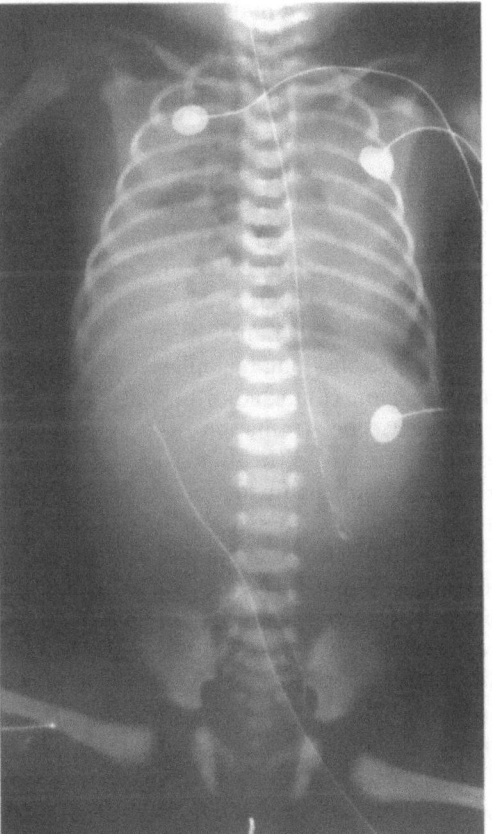

b

Fig. 5.19a–c. Right diaphragmatic hernia. Third trimester. **a** Axial US scan performed in a 32-week-old fetus shows displacement of the heart (*H*) inside the left hemithorax by the herniated liver (*L*). **b** Transverse scan of the abdomen. The liver vessels converge towards the diaphragmatic defect (*arrowheads*). *S* stomach. **c** Radiograph performed after birth shows the right thoracic opacity with left mediastinal shift

horizontal location. The appearance of the herniated lobe, associated with collapsed bowel loops, must be differentiated from a solid type of CAM. Rarely, this diagnosis is not achieved with US alone and complementary prenatal MRI may be proposed (HUBBARD 1999a, b).

5.6.3
Bilateral Diaphragmatic Hernia

Bilateral diaphragmatic hernia can be overlooked because there may be no mediastinal shift.

5.6.4
Management and Prognosis

A complete and careful US fetal survey, especially a cardiac examination, are necessary and are usefully repeated. Associated malformations are found in 25–75% of cases. They can affect every system. Karyotype analysis is mandatory because chromosomal abnormality is present in 10–20% of cases (KATZ et al. 1998, GEARY 1998, GOLDSTEIN 2000).

The consequences of the malformation for fetal well-being must also be assessed, including an evaluation on the degree of mediastinal shift, cardiac hemodynamic consequences and lung volume. The mortality of diaphragmatic hernia diagnosed in utero remains higher than 50% due to the associated malformations, lung hypoplasia and pulmonary hypertension (BERESFORD and SHAW 2000). However, precise determination of prognosis for the individual fetus is difficult. Associated cardiac malformations, polymalformation syndrome and karyotype anomalies worsen the prognosis, and in these circumstances pregnancy termination may be proposed. In isolated forms, indicators of a poor prognosis are a large mediastinal shift, heart compression with asymmetrical size of ventricles (left heart hypoplasia discovered before 24 weeks of gestation seems to be correlated with a 100% mortality rate) and/or cardiac failure (CRAWFORD et al. 1989, THÉBAUD et al. 1997). Prognosis is also poor when the lung volume is reduced: a contralateral lung surface area less than one hemithorax is also a poor prognostic indicator (GUIBAUD et al. 1996). Lung-to-head ratio also seems useful to help predict neonatal outcome (LIPSHUTZ et al. 1997). Intrathoracic location of the fetal stomach, or of the liver, presence of hydramnios and early diagnosis of the malformation (before 24 weeks of gestation)

are more controversial factors. In fact, no US criteria allow the precise determination of the degree of lung hypoplasia and the prediction of the postnatal survival rate (CANNON et al. 1996, DOMMERGUES et al. 1996). Birth must occur in a specialized tertiary center with an experienced team. The postnatal management of a neonate with a diaphragmatic hernia remains difficult and problematic (DAVIS and SABHARWAL 1998, BERESFORD and SHAW 2000). Even after successful surgery, the morbidity remains high due to chronic lung disease, persistent feeding problems (including digestive dysmotility and gastroesophageal reflux) and delay in neurological development (BERNBAUM et al. 1995, IJS-SELSTIJN et al. 1997, DAVIS and SABHARWAL 1998). No agreement exists on the postnatal management (extracorporeal membrane oxygenation or not). The experience in fetal surgery remains limited to a few teams. If fetal surgery is planned, MRI seems to be a useful complementary examination, providing more precise information on the content of the hernia (the fetal liver, the spleen and the intestinal structures are more easily detected and differentiated using T1- and T2-weighted sequences) but also on the extent of the diaphragmatic hernia and on the lung volume (HUBBARD et al. 1997, HARRISON 1998, WALSH et al. 2000, PAEK et al. 2001). This information is also important for the neonatologists and pediatric surgeons who will take care of the neonate.

The search for better prognostic factors and therapeutic management in diaphragmatic herniation is still relevant.

5.6.5
Diaphragmatic Hypoplasia

In diaphragmatic hypoplasia, the diaphragm is present but the muscular component is partially or totally lacking and replaced by fibrous tissue. An upper bulging of the abdominal content is detected before or more often after birth. When the anomaly reaches the entire dome, the US appearance is similar to that of a true diaphragmatic hernia. The prognosis depends on the extent of the anomaly: in the case of large hypoplasia, the management and prognostic criteria of a true diaphragmatic hernia are used. This information is more easily provided by fetal MRI (Fig. 5.20).

Diaphragmatic eventration may also be acquired during the delivery or after surgical lesion of the phrenic nerve (DE VRIES et al. 1998).

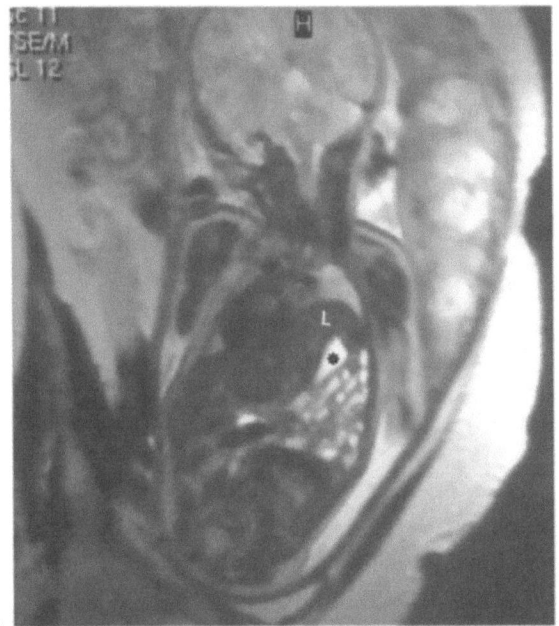

a

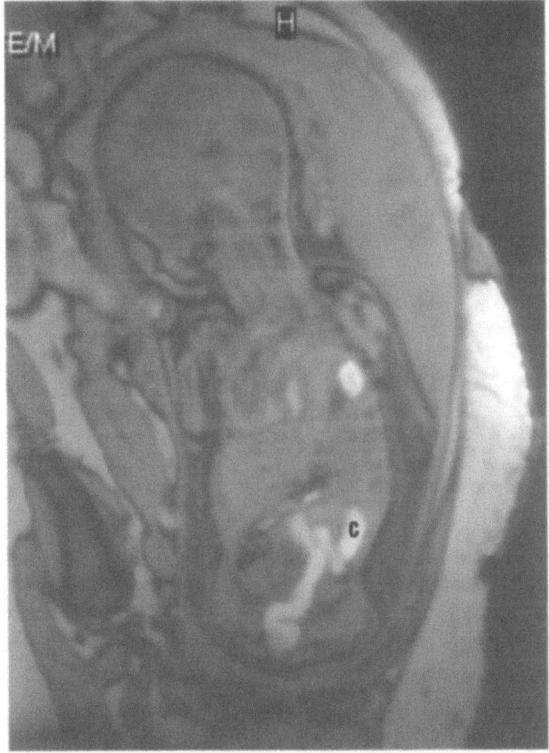

b

Fig. 5.20a, b. Diaphragmatic eventration. Discovery of a "left diaphragmatic hernia" during the third sonographic examination performed at 31 weeks gestation in a twin pregnancy. **a** Coronal T2-weighted MR scan shows high positioning of the left liver lobe, of the stomach and of the small bowel. The boundary between the left lung and the "herniated viscera" appears complete and smooth, suggesting diaphragmatic eventration, confirmed after birth at surgery. *L* liver, *asterisk* stomach. **b** Coronal gradient echo T1-weighted MR scan confirms the intra-abdominal location of the stomach and colon (*c*)

5.6.6
Parasternal Morgagni Herniation

The parasternal Morgagni type of anterior herniation is very rarely diagnosed in utero. The liver or a colonic loop may be herniated. The diagnosis must be considered in the case of a precardiac mass. The herniation may even enter the pericardium. Pericardial and pleural effusion may be associated findings.

5.7
Pleural Effusion

Pleural effusion in a fetus is always abnormal. It is easily detected as an anechoic fluid accumulation between the thoracic wall and the hyperechoic lung (Figs. 5.21, 5.22). The effusion may be unilateral or bilateral, primary (1/12,000 live births) or more frequently secondary (1/1,500 live births).

The prognosis depends on the uni- or bilaterality of the disease, the presence or absence of associated anomalies, the presence or absence of hydrops and the evolution of the effusion.

A complete US survey is mandatory to search for associated malformations. Other sites for fluid accumulations (pericardium, peritoneal cavity, subcutaneous tissue) must be looked for, because pleural effusion can be the first sign of hydrops. Detailed cardiac US, amniocentesis or cordocentesis (for viral studies and karyotype analysis) are essential components of management. Chromosomal anomalies are found in up to 5% of the cases in some series (ACHIRON et al. 1995b).

The discrimination between primary and secondary forms of hydrothorax is not always easy. Unilateral and isolated effusions responsible for mediastinal shift are more probably primary. If the pleural effusion is isolated, chylothorax or idiopathic effusion is the probable diagnosis and US survey alone is proposed. (Chylothorax can be isolated or associated with diffuse lymphangiomatosis, congenital lymphedema, pulmonary lymphangiectasias, anomalies of the thoracic duct or a sequestration). Secondary effusions are more often bilateral, cause less mediastinal shift, and are associated with other abnormalities.

The natural history of pleural effusion is variable: spontaneous resolution may occur in utero (in 10–20% of cases) or after birth (LONGAKER et al. 1989, WEBER and PHILIPSON 1992, AUBARD et al. 1998) (Figs. 5.21, 5.22). Unilateral and limited effusion usually has a good prognosis. In contrast, in cases of

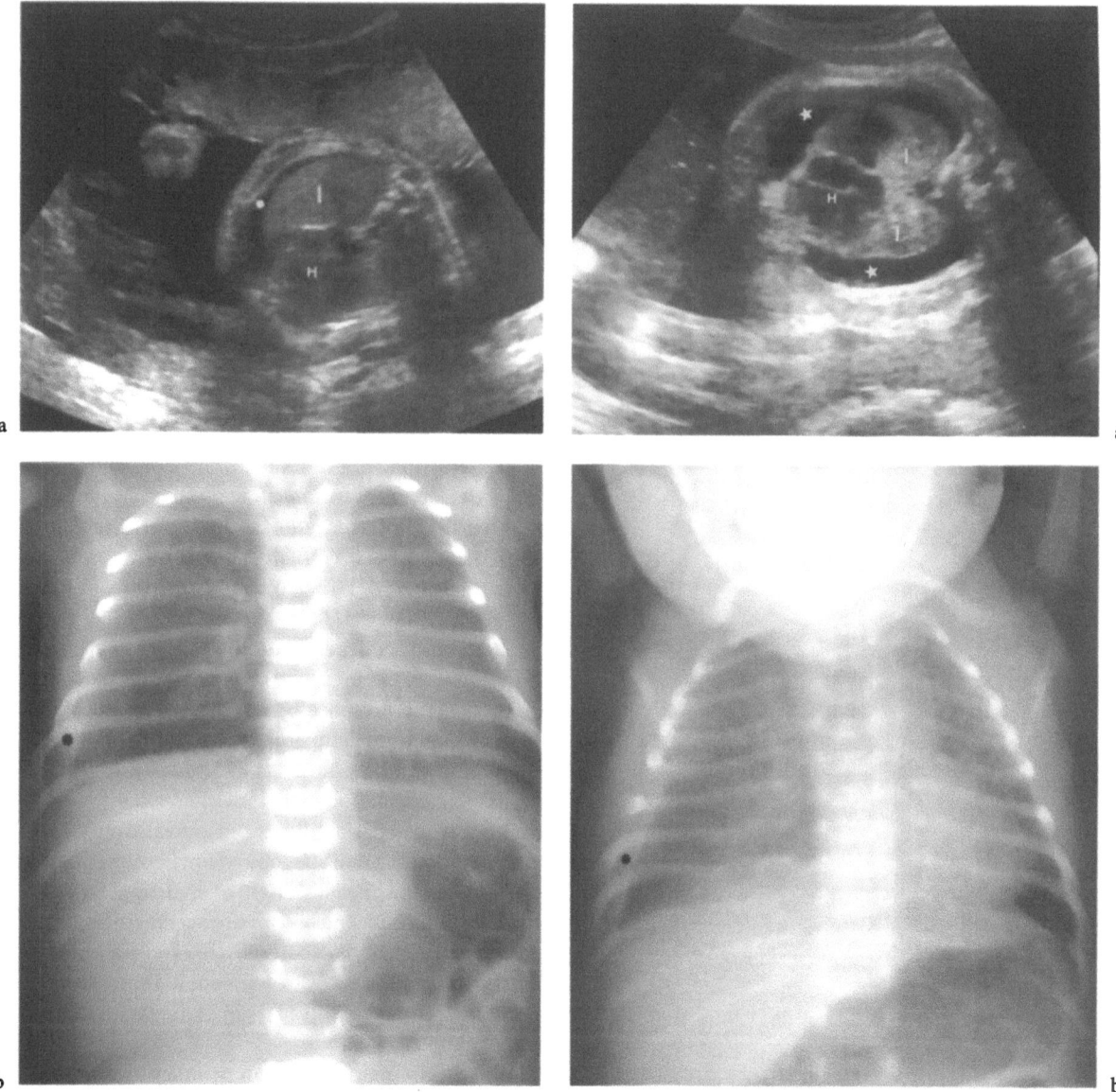

Fig. 5.21a, b. Unilateral pleural effusion. **a** Axial US performed at 21 weeks of gestation shows a small unilateral pleural effusion (*asterisk*). *l* lung, *H* heart. **b** Chest radiograph at birth. Persisting effusion (*asterisk*) (it resolved spontaneously on follow-up)

Fig. 5.22a, b. Bilateral effusion. Third trimester. **a** Axial US scan shows bilateral pleural effusions (*star*). *H* heart, *l* lungs. **b** Radiograph of the same baby performed at 3 days of life shows persistence of a right pleural effusion (*asterisk*) with increased interstitial markings. It corresponded to a chylothorax

pleural effusion with hydrops, the mortality rate rises above 90% if other malformations are found. If the effusion is limited and isolated or regresses spontaneously, a simple US survey is sufficient. If the pleural effusion increases and compresses the mediastinum or the lungs, pleural centesis or thoracoamniotic shunting can be considered in utero depending on the gestational age and the evolution of the condition. In cases of chylothorax, analysis of the clear pleural fluid usually reveals lymphocytosis higher than 70–80%, but this sign is neither specific nor sensitive. The possible failures and risks of shunt placement (migration and clogging of the catheter, fetal death) must be considered in the management discussion (BERNASCHEK et al. 1994).

Presence of a pleural effusion usually does not modify the type of delivery but birth must ideally take place in a tertiary center. Respiratory care and parenteral nutrition may be necessary after birth (MUSSAT et al. 1995).

5.8
Pulmonary Hypoplasia

Unilateral lung agenesis has rarely been detected in utero (YANCEY and RICHARDS 1993, KALACHE et al. 1997, BROMLEY and BENACERRAF 1997). It is due to an arrest in development. Agenesis can affect a single lobe, an entire lung or rarely be bilateral (KRAVITZ 1994). In cases of entire unilateral agenesis, the prenatal landmark is mediastinal shift in the absence of evidence of diaphragmatic hernia (KALACHE et al. 1997, BROMLEY and BENACERRAF 1997). Color Doppler may show the absence of pulmonary vessels. After birth, the chest initially has a normal shape, but as the patient ages, asymmetry develops (KRAVITZ 1994).

Right lung hypoplasia has also been detected in utero, usually associated with mediastinal shift and heart anomaly. It may be associated with scimitar syndrome (ABDULLAH et al. 2000).

Bilateral lung hypoplasia occurs more frequently. It is usually secondary to a persistent oligohydramnios (due to premature membrane rupture, renal abnormalities or intrauterine growth retardation) or to an intrathoracic mass (i.e., diaphragmatic herniation, massive hydrothorax). Lethal bone dysplasia and absence of fetal motion (fetal akinesia sequence) are rarer causes of lung hypoplasia (see Chap. 9). The pulmonary hypoplasia is worse if the associated malformation occurs early in development and persists during pregnancy.

Lung hypoplasia is characterized by insufficient development of pulmonary airways, alveoli, and vessels (KALOUSEK et al. 1990). In the fetus, the size of the lungs is normally correlated with the fetal weight (CHAPMAN et al. 1990). The fetal weight is not directly and precisely determinable in utero. Study of the pulmonary vasculature in utero is based on Doppler US but results of published studies are contradictory (RASANEN et al. 1996, LAUDY et al. 1996, CYNOBER et al. 1997, ROTH et al. 1998). Prenatal diagnosis of lung hypoplasia thus relies upon the diagnosis of a small lung. This diagnosis is difficult and remains an unsolved problem. Usually, the size of the lungs is correlated with the size of the thorax. Reference US measurements are available for the fetal thoracic circumference, for various ratios and also for fetal lung areas and volumes (CHITKARA et al. 1987, VINTZILEOS et al. 1989, D'ALTON et al. 1992, HARSTADT et al. 1993, D'ARCY et al. 1996, LEE et al. 1996, YOSHIMURA et al. 1996). Measurements of thoracic circumference are of no interest in cases of diaphragmatic herniation

or pleural effusion. Furthermore, in cases of severe oligohydramnios, these US measurements are difficult to obtain due to technical limitations. MRI shows interesting potential in evaluating the fetal lung volume, being able to measure the fetal lung volume in these circumstances (COAKLEY et al. 2000, RYPENS et al. 2001, PAEK et al. 2001). Studies are still at the investigative stage.

5.9
Mediastinal Anomalies

Except for cardiac and pericardiac anomalies, mediastinal malformations are rare. They can produce a mass effect on the adjacent structures and, if sufficiently large, be responsible for fetal hydrops. These malformations are usually discovered after birth due to mediastinal compression. They may remain asymptomatic for years and be discovered fortuitously on a radiograph or CT scan performed for other reasons. Bronchogenic cyst, lymphangioma, esophageal duplication, neurenteric cyst, pericardial and thymic cyst are the possible entities to discuss in the case of an abnormal mediastinal cystic structure (JACQUEMARD et al. 1991, RAHMANI et al. 1995, MARKERT et al. 1996). Bronchogenic cyst, neurenteric cyst and esophageal duplication have the same US appearance and, most often, the diagnosis is achieved following pathological investigation. Their discovery in utero implies a complete US examination. The location of the mass helps for the differential diagnosis (i.e., intrathymic or pericardial location). Lymphangiomas are usually not limited to a mediastinal location and can be found throughout the neck, the axillary or the retroperitoneal regions. In the case of a large malformation, fetal MRI can be used to determine the extent of the lesion and its relation with the fetal airways. After birth, thoracic radiograph, CT scan or MRI, and digestive tract opacification are necessary (HADDON and BOWEN 1991). (see Chap. 13).

5.9.1
Neurenteric Cyst

Neurenteric cyst results from notochordal defects and is a part of the split notochord syndrome. In the complete form, a stalk connects the skin of the back to the digestive lumen, throughout the intraspinal space; this communication is usually not found in utero. The malformation can be in connection with the small intestine through the diaphragm. Vertebral defects, including abnormalities of segmentation (hemivertebrae, fused vertebrae, cleft vertebrae) or diastematomyelia, can be also observed. The cyst is usually located inside the posterior mediastinum. As for bronchogenic cyst or esophageal duplication, this malformation is usually diagnosed after birth and may be responsible for respiratory distress (MACAULAY et al. 1997).

5.9.2
Pericardial Teratoma

Pericardial teratoma is rare and has a complex heterogeneous US appearance. It is usually associated with pericardial effusion. It can be differentiated from cardiac tumors by its pericardial location and its heterogeneous appearance (rhabdomyomas and myxomas usually have a more homogeneous solid appearance). Hydrops is a poor prognostic indicator (TODROS 1991).

5.9.3
Thymic Lesion

Thymic cysts are remnants of the third branchial pouch. They are usually isolated. They have rarely been discovered in utero. The differential diagnosis must include CAM, sequestration, bronchogenic cyst and other rarer cystic mediastinal lesions. They may be completely asymptomatic (DE MIGUEL CAMPOS et al. 1997).

5.10
Thoracic Parietal Malformations

Thoracic parietal malformations are rarely isolated. Simple and isolated rib malformations (i.e., bifid or hypoplastic rib) are rarely diagnosed in utero. They are usually found incidentally after birth on a chest radiograph performed for another reason or because of a thoracic deformity. Abnormal rib morphology must induce the search for associated vertebral malformations (i.e., hemivertebra, segmental anomalies) or skeletal dysplasia (see Chap. 9). Diffuse abnormal rib morphology must induce the search for an associated osseous disease (i.e., osteogenesis imperfecta and the multiple syndromes associated with short ribs and polydactyly). An abnormal small chest can

interfere with the normal development of the lung and can be a cause of pulmonary hypoplasia.

Pentalogy of Cantrell is a rare malformation characterized by ectopia cordis, omphalocele, defect of the inferior sternum, defect of the anterior diaphragm and of the diaphragmatic pericardium. Cardiac anomalies are usually associated, as well as craniofacial ones. Trisomy 13 and 18 have been reported with this anomaly. A karyotype is systematically indicated as well as a cardiac US examination and a specific search for associated anomalies. The ectopia cordis may be manifest by a simple bulging of the anterior thoracic wall through an inferior sternal defect, to a true herniation of the heart. Anterior parietal defect is also one of the malformations observed in limb body wall defect.

References

Abdullah MM, Lacro RV, Smallhorn J, et al (2000) Fetal cardiac dextroposition in the absence of an intrathoracic mass: sign of significant right lung hypoplasia. J Ultrasound Med 19:669–676

Achiron R, Strauss S, Seidman DS, Lipitz S, Mashiach S, Goldman B (1995a) Fetal lung hyperechogenicity: prenatal ultrasonographic diagnosis, natural history and neonatal outcome. Ultrasound Obstet Gynecol 6:40–42

Achiron R, Weissman A, Lipitz S, Mashiach S, Goldman B (1995b) Fetal pleural effusion: the risk of fetal trisomy. Gynecol Obstet Invest 39:153–156

Adzick NS, Harrison MR, Glick PL, et al (1985) Fetal cystic adenomatoid malformation: prenatal diagnosis and natural history. J Pediatr Surg 20:483–488

Adzick NS, Harrison MR, Crombleholme TM, Flake AW, Howell LJ (1998) Fetal lung lesions: management and outcome. Am J Obstet Gynecol 179:884–889

Alford BA, McIlhenny J, Jones JE, et al (1993) Asymmetric radiographic findings in the pediatric chest: approach to early diagnosis. Radiographics 13:77–93

Aubard Y, Derouineau I, Aubard V, Chalifour V, Preux PM (1998) Primary fetal hydrothorax: a literature review and proposed antenatal clinical strategy. Fetal Diagn Ther 13:325–333

Bagolan P, Nahom A, Giorlandino C, et al (1999) Cystic adenomatoid malformation of the lung: clinical evolution and management. Eur J Pediatr 158:879–882

Baker PN, Johnson IR, Gowland PA, Freeman A, Adams V, Mansfield P (1994) Estimation of fetal lung volume using echo-planar magnetic resonance imaging. Obstet Gynecol 83:951–954

Ballard PL (1980) Hormonal influences during fetal lung development. Ciba Found Symp 78:251–274

Barret J, Chitayat D, Sermer M, et al (1995) The prognostic factors in the prenatal diagnosis of the echogenic fetal lung. Prenat Diagn 15:849–853

Becmeur F, Horta-Geraud P, Donato L, Sauvage P (1998) Pulmonary sequestrations: prenatal ultrasound diagnosis, treatment, and outcome. J Pediatr Surg 33:492–496

Beresford MW, Shaw NJ (2000) Outcome of congenital diaphragmatic hernia. Pediatr Pulmonol 30:249–256

Bernaschek G, Deutinger J, Hansmann M, Bald R, Holzgreve W, Bollmann R (1994) Feto-amniotic shunting: report of the experience of four European centres. Prenat Diagn 14: 821–833

Bernbaum J, Schwartz IP, Gerdes M, D'Agostino JA, Coburn CE, Polin RA (1995) Survivors of extracorporeal membrane oxygenation at 1 year of age: the relationship of primary diagnosis with health and neurodevelopmental sequelae. Pediatrics 96:907–913

Bolton JW, Shahian DM (1992) Asymptomatic bronchogenic cysts: what is the best management? Ann Thorac Surg 53:1134–1137

Botash RJ, Spirt BA (1993) Color Doppler imaging aids in the prenatal diagnosis of congenital diaphragmatic hernia. J Ultrasound Med 12:359–361

Bratu I, Flageole H, Chen MF, Di Lorenzo M, Yazbeck S, Laberge JM (2001) The multiple facets of pulmonary sequestration. J Pediatr Surg 36:784–790

Bromley B, Parad R, Estroff JA, Benacerraf BR (1995) Fetal lung masses: prenatal course and outcome. J Ultrasound Med 14:927–936

Bromley B, Benacerraf BR (1997) Unilateral lung hypoplasia: report of three cases. J Ultrasound Med 16:599–601

Bunduki V, Ruano R, da Silva MM, et al (2000) Prognostic factors associated with congenital cystic adenomatoid malformation of the lung. Prenat Diagn 20:459–464

Cannon C, Dildy GA, Ward R, Vaner MW, Dudley DJ (1996) A population-based study of congenital diaphragmatic hernia in Utah: 1988–1994. Obstet Gynecol 87:959–963

Cass DL, Crombleholme TM, Howell LJ, Stafford PW, Ruchelli ED, Adzick NS (1997) Cystic lung lesions with systemic arterial blood supply: a hybrid of congenital cystic adenomatoid malformation and bronchopulmonary sequestration. J Pediatr Surg 32:986–990

Chapman B, O'Callaghan C, Coxon R, et al (1990) Estimation of lung volume in infants by echoplanar imaging and total body plethysmography. Arch Dis Child 65:168–170

Chitkara U, Rosenberg J, Chervenak FA, et al (1987) Prenatal sonographic assessment of the fetal thorax: normal values. Am J Obstet Gynecol 156:1069–1074

Clements BS, Warner JO (1987) Pulmonary sequestration and related congenital bronchopulmonary-vascular malformations: nomenclature and classification based on anatomical and embryological considerations. Thorax 42:401–408

Coakley FV, Lopoo JB, Lu Y, et al (2000) Normal and hypoplastic fetal lungs: volumetric assessment with prenatal single-shot rapid acquisition with relaxation enhancement MR imaging. Radiology 216:107–111

Conran RM, Stocker JT (1999) Extralobar sequestration with frequently associated congenital cystic adenomatoid malformation, type 2: report of 50 cases. Pediatr Dev Pathol 2:454–463

Cooper C, Mahony BS, Bowie JD, Albright TO, Callen PW (1985) Ultrasound evaluation of the normal fetal upper airway and esophagus. J Ultrasound Med 4:343–346

Crawford DC, Wright VM, Drake DP, Allan LD (1989) Fetal diaphragmatic hernia: the value of fetal echocardiography in the prediction of postnatal outcome. Br J Obstet Gynaecol 96:705–710

Curtis MR, Mooney DP, Vaccaro TJ, et al (1997) Prenatal ultrasound characterization of the suprarenal mass: distinction between neuroblastoma and subdiaphragmatic extralobar pulmonary sequestration. J Ultrasound Med 16:75–83

Cynober E, Cabrol D, Haddad B, et al (1997) Fetal pulmonary artery Doppler waveform: a preliminary report. Fetal Diagn Ther 12:226–231

D'Agostino S, Bonoldi E, Dante S, Meli S, Cappellari F, Musi L (1997) Embryonal rhabdomyosarcoma of the lung arising in cystic adenomatoid malformation: case report and review of the literature. J Pediatr Surg 32:1381–1383

D'Alton M, Mercer B, Riddick E, Dudley D (1992) Serial thoracic versus abdominal circumference ratios for the prediction of pulmonary hypoplasia in premature rupture of the membranes remote from term. Am J Obstet Gynecol 166:658–663

Daneman A, Baunin C, Lobo E, et al (1997) Disappearing suprarenal masses in fetuses and infants. Pediatr Radiol 27:675–681

D'Arcy TJ, Hughes SW, Chiu WSC, et al (1996) Estimation of fetal lung volume using enhanced 3-dimensional ultrasound: a new method and first result. Br J Obstet Gynaecol 103:1015–1020

Davis CF, Sabharwal AJ (1998) Management of congenital diaphragmatic hernia. Arch Dis Child Fetal Neonatal Ed 79:F1–F3

de Hullu JA, Kornman LH, Beekhuis JR, Nikkels PG (1995) The hyperechogenic lungs of laryngotracheal obstruction. Ultrasound Obstet Gynecol 5:271–274

de Miguel Campos E, Casanova A, Urbano J, Delgado Carrasco J (1997) Congenital thymic cyst: prenatal sonographic and postnatal magnetic resonance findings. J Ultrasound Med 16:365–367

De Santis M, Masini L, Noia G, Cavaliere AF, Oliva N, Caruso A (2000) Congenital cystic adenomatoid malformation of the lung: antenatal ultrasound findings and fetal-neonatal outcome. Fifteen years of experience. Fetal Diagn Ther 15:246–250

de Vries TS, Koens BL, Vos A (1998) Surgical treatment of diaphragmatic eventration caused by phrenic nerve injury in the newborn. J Pediatr Surg 33:602–605

Dolkart LA, Reimers FT, Helmuth WV, Porte MA, Eisinger G (1992) Antenatal diagnosis of pulmonary sequestration: a review. Obstet Gynecol Surv 47:515–520

Dommergues M, Louis-Sylvestre C, Mandelbrot L, et al (1996) Congenital diaphragmatic hernia: can prenatal ultrasonography predict outcome? Am J Obstet Gynecol 174:1377–1381

Duncan K, Baker P, Johnson I (1997) The complementary role of echoplanar magnetic resonance imaging and three-dimensional ultrasonography in fetal lung assessment. Am J Obstet Gynecol 177:244–245

Duncan KR, Gowland PA, Moore RJ, Baker PN, Johnson IR (1999a) Assessment of fetal lung growth in utero with echoplanar MR imaging. Radiology 210:197–200

Duncan KR, Gowland PA, Freeman A, Moore R, Baker PN, Johnson IR (1999b) The changes in magnetic resonance properties of the fetal lungs: a first result and a potential tool for the non-invasive in utero demonstration of fetal lung maturation. Br J Obstet Gynaecol 106:122–125

Enns GM, Cox VA, Goldstein RB, Gibbs DL, Harrison MR, Golabi M (1998) Congenital diaphragmatic defects and associated syndromes, malformations, and chromosome anomalies: a retrospective study of 60 patients and literature review. Am J Med Genet 79:215–225

Felker RE, Cartier MS, Emerson DS, Brown DL (1989) Ultrasound of the fetal thymus. J Ultrasound Med 8:669–673

Felker RE, Tonkin IL (1990) Imaging of pulmonary sequestration. AJR Am J Roentgenol 154:241–249

Fenton BW, Lin CS, Seydel F, Macedonia C (1998) Lecithin can be detected by volume-selected proton MR spectroscopy using a 1.5 T whole body scanner: a potentially non-invasive method for the prenatal assessment of fetal lung maturity. Prenat Diagn 18:1263–1266

Fenton BW, Lin CS, Ascher S, Macedonia C (2000) Magnetic resonance spectroscopy to detect lecithin in amniotic fluid and fetal lung. Obstet Gynecol 95:457–460

Geary M (1998) Management of congenital diaphragmatic hernia diagnosed prenatally: an update. Prenat Diagn 18:1155–1158

Gibbs DL, Rice HE, Farrell JA, Adzick NS, Harrison MR (1997) Familial diaphragmatic agenesis: an autosomal-recessive syndrome with a poor prognosis. J Pediatr Surg 32:366–368

Goldstein RB (2000) Ultrasound evaluation of the fetal thorax. In: Callen PW (ed) Ultrasonography in obstetrics and gynecology, 4th edn. WB Saunders, Philadelphia, pp 426–455

Granata C, Gambini C, Balducci T, et al (1998) Bronchioloalveolar carcinoma arising in congenital adenomatoid malformation in a child: a case report and review on malignancies originating in congenital cystic adenomatoid malformation. Pediatr Pulmonol 25:62–66

Guibaud L, Filiatrault D, Garel L, et al (1996) Fetal congenital diaphragmatic hernia: accuracy of sonography in the diagnosis and prediction of the outcome after birth. AJR Am J Roentgenol 166:1195–1202

Haddon MJ, Bowen A (1991) Bronchopulmonary and neurenteric forms of foregut anomalies. Imaging for diagnosis and management. Radiol Clin North Am 29:241–254

Harrison MR, Mychaliska GB, Albanese CT, et al (1998) Correction of congenital diaphragmatic hernia in utero. IX. Fetuses with poor prognosis (liver herniation and low lung-to-head ratio) can be saved by fetoscopic temporary tracheal occlusion. J Pediatr Surg 33:1017–1022

Harstad TW, Twickler DM, Leveno KJ, Brown CE (1993) Antenatal prediction of pulmonary hypoplasia: an elusive goal? Am J Perinatol 10:8–11

Hata T, Deter RL (1992) A review of fetal organ measurements obtained with ultrasound: normal growth. J Clin Ultrasound 20:155–174

Haugen G, Jenum PA, Scheie D, Sund S, Stray-Pedersen B (2000) Prenatal diagnosis of tracheal obstruction: possible association with maternal pertussis infection. Ultrasound Obstet Gynecol 15:69–73

Heij HA, Ekkelkamp S, Vos A (1990) Diagnosis of congenital cystic adenomatoid malformation of the lung in newborn infants and children. Thorax 45:122–125

Heitzman ER (1984) The lung, radiologic-pathologic correlations, 2nd edn. Mosby, St Louis

Hernanz-Schulman M, Stein SM, Neblett WW, et al (1991) Pulmonary sequestration: diagnosis with color Doppler sonography and a new theory of associated hydrothorax. Radiology 180:817–821

Hernanz-Schulman M (1993) Cysts and cystlike lesions of the lung. Radiol Clin North Am 31:631–649

Hernanz-Schulman M, Johnson JE, Holcomb GW 3rd, Neblett WW 3rd, Heller RM, Ambrosino MM (1997) Retroperitoneal pulmonary sequestration: imaging findings, histopathologic correlation, and relationship to cystic adenomatoid malformation. AJR Am J Roentgenol 168:1277–1281

Hubbard AM, Adzick NS, Crombleholme TM, Haselgrove JC (1997) Left-sided congenital diaphragmatic hernia: value of prenatal MR imaging in preparation for fetal surgery. Radiology 203:636–640

Hubbard AM, Crombleholme TM (1998a) Anomalies and malformations affecting the fetal/neonatal chest. Semin Roentgenol 33:117–125

Hubbard AM, Crombleholme TM, Adzick NS (1998b) Prenatal MRI evaluation of giant neck masses in preparation for the fetal exit procedure. Am J Perinatol 15:253–257

Hubbard AM, Adzick NS, Crombleholme TM, et al (1999a) Congenital chest lesions: diagnosis and characterization with prenatal MR imaging. Radiology 212:43–48

Hubbard AM, Crombleholme TM, Adzick NS, et al (1999b) Prenatal MRI evaluation of congenital diaphragmatic hernia. Am J Perinatol 16:407–413

Huppert BJ, Brandt KR, Ramin KD, King BF (1999) Single-shot fast spin-echo MR imaging of the fetus: a pictorial essay. Radiographics 19:S215–S227

Ijsselstijn H, Tibboel D, Hop WJ, Molenaar JC, de Jongste JC (1997) Long-term pulmonary sequelae in children with congenital diaphragmatic hernia. Am J Respir Crit Care Med 155:174–180

Jacquemard F, Palavric JC, Cousin C, d'Herve D, Conan H, Giraud JR (1991) Aspect échographique anténatal d'une duplication oesophagienne. A propos d'un cas. J Gynecol Obstet Biol Reprod 20:963–967

Kalache KD, Chaoui R, Paris S, Bollmann R (1997) Prenatal diagnosis of right lung agenesis using color doppler and magnetic resonance imaging. Fetal Diagn Ther 12:360–362

Kalousek DK, Fitch N, Paradice BA (1990) Respiratory tract defects. In: Pathology of the human embryo and previable fetus: an atlas. Springer, Berlin Heidelberg New York, pp 116–119

Kasales CJ, Coulson CC, Meilstrup JW, Ambrose A, Botti JJ, Holley GP (1998) Diagnosis and differentiation of congenital diaphragmatic hernia from other noncardiac thoracic fetal masses. Am J Perinatol 15:623–628

Katz AL, Wiswell TE, Baumgart S (1998) Contemporary controversies in the management of congenital diaphragmatic hernia. Clin Perinatol 25:219–248

Khakoo GA, Jawad MH, Bush A, Warner JO, Shirley IS, Buchdahl RM (1993) Conservative management of foetal lung lesions. Early Hum Dev 35:55–62

Kitterman JA (1988) Physiological factors in fetal lung growth. Can J Physiol Pharmacol 66:1122–1128

Kravitz RM (1994) Congenital malformations of the lung. Pediatr Clin North Am 41:453–472

Langer B, Donato L, Riethmuller C, et al (1995) Spontaneous regression of fetal pulmonary sequestration. Ultrasound Obstet Gynecol 6:33–39

Langston C (1983) Normal and abnormal structural development of the human lung. Prog Clin Biol Res 140:75–91

Langston C, Kida K, Reed M, Thurlbeck WM (1984) Human lung growth in late gestation and in the neonate. Am Rev Respir Dis 129:607–613

Larsen WJ (1997) Embryonic folding. In: Larsen WJ (ed) Human embryology, 2nd edn. Churchill Livingstone, New York, pp 127–149

Laudy JA, Gaillard JL, vd Anker JN, Tibboel D, Wladimiroff JW (1996) Doppler ultrasound imaging: a new technique to detect lung hypoplasia before birth? Ultrasound Obstet Gynecol 7:189–192

Laudy JA, Wladimiroff JW (2000) The fetal lung. 1. Developmental aspects. Ultrasound Obstet Gynecol 16:284–290

Lee A, Kratochwil A, Stumpflen I, Deutinger J, Bernaschek G (1996) Fetal lung volume determination by three-dimensional ultrasonography. Am J Obstet Gynecol 175:588–592

Lipshutz GS, Albanese CT, Feldstein VA, et al (1997) Prospective analysis of lung-to-head ratio predicts survival for patients with prenatally diagnosed congenital diaphragmatic hernia. J Pediatr Surg 32:1634–1636

Longaker MT, Laberge JM, Dansereau J, et al (1989) Primary fetal hydrothorax: natural history and management. J Pediatr Surg 24:573–576

Lopoo JB, Goldstein RB, Lipshutz GS, Goldberg JD, Harrison MR, Albanese CT (1999) Fetal pulmonary sequestration: a favorable congenital lung lesion. Obstet Gynecol 94:567–571

Macaulay KE, Winter TC 3rd, Shields LE (1997) Neuroenteric cyst shown by prenatal sonography. AJR Am J Roentgenol 169:563–565

Manni M, Heydanus R, Den Hollander NS, Stewart PA, De Vogelaere C, Wladimiroff JW (1994) Prenatal diagnosis of congenital diaphragmatic hernia: a retrospective analysis of 28 cases. Prenat Diagn 14:187–190

Mariona F, McAlpin G, Zador I, Philippart A, Jafri SZ (1986) Sonographic detection of fetal extrathoracic pulmonary sequestration. J Ultrasound Med 5:283–285

Markert DJ, Grumbach K, Haney PJ (1996) Thoracoabdominal duplication cyst: prenatal and postnatal imaging. J Ultrasound Med 15:333–336

Mata JM, Caceres J, Lucaya J, Garcia-Conesa JA (1990) CT of congenital malformations of the lung. Radiographics 10:651–674

Matzinger MA, Matzinger FR, Sachs HJ (1992) Intrapulmonary bronchogenic cyst: spontaneous pneumothorax as the presenting symptom. AJR Am J Roentgenol 158:987–988

Mayden KL, Tortora M, Chervenak FA, Hobbins JC (1984) The antenatal sonographic detection of lung masses. Am J Obstet Gynecol 148:349–351

McCormick WF, Nichols MM (1981) Formation and maturation of the human sternum. Am J Forensic Med Pathol 2:323–328

McCullagh M, MacConnachie I, Garvie D, Dykes E (1994) Accuracy of prenatal diagnosis of congenital cystic adenomatoid malformation. Arch Dis Child 71:F111–F113

Meagher SE, Fisk NM, Harvey JG, Watson GF, Boogert A (1993). Disappearing lung echogenicity in fetal bronchopulmonary malformations: a reassuring sign? Prenat Diagn 13:495–501

Meizner I, Rosenak D (1995) The vanishing fetal intrathoracic mass: consider an obstructing mucous plug. Ultrasound Obstet Gynecol 5:275–277

Merz E, Wellek S, Bahlmann F, Weber G (1995) Normal ultrasound curves of the fetal osseous thorax and fetal lung. Geburtshilfe Frauenheilkd 55:77–82

Miller JA, Corteville JE, Langer JC (1996) Congenital cystic adenomatoid malformation in the fetus: natural history and predictors of outcome. J Pediatr Surg 31:805–808

Moore KL, Persaud TVN (1993) The respiratory system. In: Moore KL, Persaud TVN (eds) The developing human: clinically oriented embryology, 5th edn. WB Saunders, Philadelphia, pp 226–236

Morin C, Filiatrault D, Russo P (1989) Pulmonary sequestration with histological changes of cystic adenomatoid malformation. Pediatr Radiol 19:130–132

Morin L, Crombleholme T M, D'Alton ME (1994) Prenatal diagnosis and management of fetal thoracic lesions. Semin Perinatol 18:228–253

Murphy JJ, Blair GK, Fraser GC, et al (1992) Rhabdomyosarcoma arising within congenital pulmonary cysts: report of three cases. J Pediatr Surg 27:1364–1367

Mussat P, Dommergues M, Parat S, et al (1995) Congenital chylothorax with hydrops: postnatal care and outcome following antenatal diagnosis. Acta Paediatr 84:749–755

Nobuhara KK, Wilson JM (1996) The effect of mechanical forces on in utero lung growth in congenital diaphragmatic hernia. Clin Perinatol 23:741–751

Odita JC, Okolo AA, Omene JA (1985) Sternal ossification in normal newborn infants. Pediatr Radiol 15:165–167

Olutoye OO, Coleman BG, Hubbard AM, Adzick NS (2000) Prenatal diagnosis and management of congenital lobar emphysema. J Pediatr Surg 35:792–795

Paek BW, Coakley FV, Lu Y, et al. (2001) Congenital diaphragmatic hernia: prenatal evaluation with MR lung volumetry – preliminary experience. Radiology 220:63–67

Paladini D, Chita SK, Allan LD (1990) Prenatal measurement of cardiothoracic ratio in evaluation of heart disease. Arch Dis Child 65:20–23

Park ST, Yoon CH, Sung KB, et al. (1998) Pulmonary sequestration in a newborn infant: treatment with arterial embolization. J Vasc Interv Radiol 9:648–650

Rahmani MR, Filler RM, Shuckett B (1995) Bronchogenic cyst occurring in the antenatal period. J Ultrasound Med 14:971–973

Rasanen J, Huhta JC, Weiner S, Wood DC, Ludomirski A (1996) Fetal branch pulmonary arterial vascular impedance during the second half of pregnancy. Am J Obstet Gynecol 174:1441–1449

Richards DS, Langham MR Jr, Dolson LH (1992) Antenatal presentation of a child with congenital lobar emphysema. J Ultrasound Med 11):165–168

Rosado-de-Christenson ML, Stocker JT (1991) Congenital cystic adenomatoid malformation. Radiographics 11:865–886

Rosado-de-Christenson ML, Frazier AA, Stocker JT, Templeton PA (1993) From the archives of the AFIP. Extralobar sequestration: radiologic-pathologic correlation. Radiographics 13:425–441

Roth P, Agnani G, Arbez-Gindre F, et al (1998) Use of energy color Doppler in visualizing fetal pulmonary vascularization to predict the absence of severe pulmonary hypoplasia. Gynecol Obstet Invest 46:153–157

Rypens F, Metens T, Rocourt N, et al (2001) Fetal lung volume: estimation at MR imaging – initial results. Radiology 219:236–241

Sade R M, Clouse M, Ellis FH (1974) The spectrum of pulmonary sequestration. Ann Thorac Surg 18:644–658

Sakala EP, Perrott WS, Grube GL (1994) Sonographic characteristics of antenatally diagnosed extralobar pulmonary sequestration and congenital cystic adenomatoid malformation. Obstet Gynecol Surv 49:647–655

Srikanth MS, Ford EG, Stanley P, Mahour GH (1992) Communicating bronchopulmonary foregut malformations: classification and embryogenesis. J Pediatr Surg 27:732–736

Stocker JT, Madewell JE, Drake RM (1977) Congenital cystic adenomatoid malformation of the lung. Classification and morphologic spectrum. Hum Pathol 8:155–171

Stocker JT (1986) Sequestrations of the lung. Semin Diagn Pathol 3:106–121

Taybi H, Lachman RS (1996) Radiology of syndromes, metabolic disorders, and skeletal dysplasias, 4th edn. Mosby, St Louis

Thébaud B, Azancot A, de Lagausie P, et al (1997) Congenital diaphragmatic hernia: antenatal prognostic factors. Does cardiac ventricular disproportion in utero predict outcome and pulmonary hypoplasia? Intensive Care Med 23: 1062–1069

Thorpe-Beeston JG, Nicolaides KH (1994) Cystic adenomatoid malformation of the lung: prenatal diagnosis and outcome. Prenat Diagn 14:677–688

Todros T, Gaglioti P, Presbitero P (1991) Management of a fetus with intrapericardial teratoma diagnosed in utero. J Ultrasound Med 10:287–290

van Leeuwen K, Teitelbaum DH, Hirschl RB, et al (1999) Prenatal diagnosis of congenital cystic adenomatoid malformation and its postnatal presentation, surgical indications, and natural history. J Pediatr Surg 34:794–798

Vintzileos AM, Campbell WA, Rodis JF, Nochimson DJ, Pinette MG, Petrikovsky BM (1989). Comparison of six different ultrasonographic methods for predicting lethal fetal pulmonary hypoplasia. Am J Obstet Gynecol 161:606–612

Walsh DS, Hubbard AM, Olutoye OO, et al (2000) Assessment of fetal lung volumes and liver herniation with magnetic resonance imaging in congenital diaphragmatic hernia. Am J Obstet Gynecol 183:1067–1069

Weber AM, Philipson EH (1992) Fetal pleural effusion: a review and meta-analysis for prognostic indicators. Obstet Gynecol 79:281–286

West MS, Donaldson JS, Shkolnik A (1989) Pulmonary sequestration. Diagnosis by ultrasound. J Ultrasound Med 8:125–129

White J, Chan YF, Neuberger S, Wilson T (1994) Prenatal sonographic detection of intra-abdominal extralobar pulmonary sequestration: report of three cases and literature review. Prenat Diagn 14:653–658

Winters WD, Effmann EL, Nghiem HV, Nyberg DA (1997) Disappearing fetal lung masses: importance of postnatal imaging studies. Pediatr Radiol 27:535–539

Yamashita Y, Namimoto T, Abe Y, Takahashi M, Iwamasa J Miyazaki K (1997) MR imaging of the fetus by a HASTE sequence. AJR Am J Roentgenol 168:513–519

Yancey MK, Richards DS (1993) Antenatal sonographic findings associated with unilateral pulmonary agenesis. Obstet Gynecol 81:847–849

Yoshimura S, Masuzaki H, Gotoh H, Fukuda H, Ishimaru T (1996) Ultrasonographic prediction of lethal pulmonary hypoplasia: comparison of eight different ultrasonographic parameters. Am J Obstet Gynecol 175:477–483

Young G, L'Heureux PR, Krueckeberg ST, Swanson DA (1989) Mediastinal bronchogenic cyst: prenatal sonographic diagnosis. AJR Am J Roentgenol 152:125–127

Zalel Y, Lipitz S, Soriano D, Achiron R (1999) The development of the fetal sternum: a cross sectional sonographic study. Ultrasound Obstet Gynecol 13:187–190

6 Heart Disease in the Fetus – Diagnosis and Management

Guy Vaksmann and Yann Robert

CONTENTS

6.1   Diagnosis of Congenital
        Cardiac Malformations   104
6.1.1   When Is a Congenital Cardiac
        Malformation Discovered?   104
6.1.2   How Is a Routine Echocardiography
        Performed?   104
6.1.2.1 B-Mode Echocardiography   104
6.1.2.2 M-Mode Echocardiography   109
6.1.2.3 Doppler Echocardiography   110
6.1.3   How Can a Congenital Cardiac
        Malformation Be Discovered?   110
6.1.3.1 Four-Chamber View:
        Atrioventricular Cavity Abnormality   110
6.1.3.2 Four-Chamber View: Septal Anomalies   113
6.1.3.3 Four-Chamber View:
        Right Ventricular Enlargement   115
6.1.3.4 Four-Chamber View: Cardiomegaly   117
6.1.3.5 Four-Chamber View: Cardiac Tumors   117
6.1.3.6 Great Vessels Views: Conotruncal Lesions   118
6.1.3.7 Great Vessels Views:
        Transposition of the Great Arteries   120
6.2   Arrhythmias   121
6.2.1   Assessment of Fetal Dysrhythmias   121
6.2.2   Mechanism of Fetal Dysrhythmias   121
6.2.2.1 Irregular Heart Rhythm   121
6.2.2.2 Tachycardias   122
6.2.2.3 Bradycardia   123
        References   124

Congenital heart disease (CHD) is the most common cause of congenital malformation with an approximate incidence of about 8–9 in 1000 live births (Hoffman and Christianson 1978), but its real incidence in the fetus is certainly higher since early fetal loss is often the result of complex extracardiac anomalies or chromosomal defects that are often associated with cardiac defects. Approximately half the cases of CHD are minor or easily correctable by surgery or interventional catheterization. Prenatal

Guy Vaksmann, MD
Pediatric Cardiology Service, Hôpital Cardiologique, CHRU
Lille, 2 Avenue Oscar Lambret, Lille 59037, France
Yann Robert, MD
Department of Imaging, Hôpital Jeanne de Flandre, CHRU
Lille, rue E. Avinée, 59037 Lille Cedex, France

diagnosis is important since it allows for better pregnancy counseling and improved neonatal outcome of several severe CHDs (Bonnet et al. 1999, Tworetzky et al. 2001).

Technological advancements as well as increased operator ability to interpret echocardiography provide increasing information about the anatomy of the heart and great vessels, allowing a more frequent depiction of cardiac abnormalities in the fetus. However, despite these improvements, the rate of detection of CHD remains very variable from one institution to another.

The objectives of ultrasound scanning are:

- to detect those CHDs with a poor prognosis, leading to a discussion of medical abortion
- to recognize CHDs commonly associated with chromosomal abnormalities (atrioventricular septal defect, ventricular septal defect, tetralogy of Fallot, truncus arteriosus)
- to initiate and follow transplacental treatment of cardiac dysrhythmias
- to identify CHDs (transposition of the great arteries, aortic arch hypoplasia/atresia, pulmonary artery atresia) which will require immediate postnatal management.

Conversely, observation of normal fetal cardiac anatomy is reassuring for parents in the case of a maternal history of cardiac disease, or may help for counseling when other malformations have been found.

The optimal period for fetal cardiac scanning is the second trimester, usually between 18 and 22 weeks gestational age, but standards differ from one country to another and are related to local practice, the maternal echogenicity and medical gestational interruption laws. The transvaginal approach allows an earlier cardiac evaluation (10–14 weeks of gestation) but one should not forget that cardiac malformation may be small and/or progressive and that in some cases will require a third trimester evaluation, even if the technical conditions are becoming more difficult with the advancement of pregnancy.

6.1
Diagnosis of Congenital Cardiac Malformations

6.1.1
When Is a Congenital Cardiac Malformation Discovered?

CHD can be discovered in four main circumstances:
- *Routine obstetric study.* The main discovery circumstance is the routine fetal cardiac sonographic scan, especially since heart evaluation with a four-chamber-view has become a systematic approach (FERMONT et al. 1986).
- *Abnormal findings related to the heart malformation.* When a nuchal translucency in first trimester has been found and a chromosomal abnormality excluded, CHD, which represents the second major cause, has to be searched for. Fetal cardiac arrhythmia may lead the sonographer to a careful evaluation of cardiac anatomy, particularly when the fetal heart rate is very slow (<80 beats per minute). The association of complete heart block with a CHD has a poorer prognosis. Tachycardia is less frequently associated with a CHD. Although less specific, the presence of pleural, pericardial and/or abdominal fluid and nonimmune fetal hydrops can have a cardiac origin. An oligo- or polyhydramnios is also associated with an increased risk of CHD.
- *An extracardiac abnormal finding in the fetus on a routine obstetric study.* Many malformations must lead to a particular evaluation of the heart and great vessels, particularly malformations of the alimentary tract (esophageal atresia, duodenal atresia, omphalocele, diaphragmatic hernia, situs abnormality) or urinary tract (renal agenesis or dysplasia) and skeletal abnormalities (spine malformation, radial aplasia, hexadactyly, etc.), but also cerebral malformations (holoprosencephaly, Dandy-Walker malformation, encephalocele, corpus callosum agenesis) and facial abnormalities (micrognathism, cleft lip/palate). The malformations may be a part of a syndrome (VACTERL, Holt–Oram, DiGeorge, Cornelia de Lange, Ellis–Van Crefeld, etc.).
- *Family history of cardiac malformation or maternal disease.* Less frequently, ultrasonography may be indicated because of a family history of cardiac malformation, or mendelian syndromes associated with CHD (Holt–Oram, Noonan, DiGeorge, tuberous sclerosis). The rate of recurrence remains low when one child was affected, but is significantly increased when more than one sibling or parent was affected. Fetal cardiac development may also be influenced by maternal disease (diabetes mellitus, phenylketonuria, connective tissue disease), or maternal exposure to drugs or teratogens (lithium, anticonvulsants, alcohol).

6.1.2
How Is a Routine Echocardiography Performed?

For both routine sonographic scanning and scanning dedicated to the heart and great vessels, a systematic evaluation has to be performed, using a real-time probe with B-mode and if necessary M-mode, pulsed and color flow Doppler ultrasound. Whenever possible, the highest frequency probe (5–7 MHz), giving the best resolution, should be used; sometimes a lower-frequency transducer has to be used to allow deeper penetration. The scanning sector has to be at its minimum, providing a higher frame rate. Image magnification facilitates the analysis of cardiac morphology, as well as the cineloop, which allows slower motion reviewing. The best access is usually through the abdomen and anterior chest wall, but a posterior approach through the lung avoiding the spine also gives an accurate view of the fetal heart (BROWN et al. 1993).

6.1.2.1
B-Mode Echocardiography

Step 1: Cardiac Position

After evaluation of the fetus and determination of the right and left, cardiac localization can be performed. The fetal heart orientation is analyzed on a thoracic transverse cross-sectional view. Normally, the heart is located in the left part of the chest, with the cardiac apex pointing to the left side. The angle between the ventricular septum and the median thoracic axis is approximately $45°±20°$, defining the normal levocardia (Fig. 6.1).

Abnormal heart positions are:
- dextrocardia: the heart is located in the right part of the thorax, with the cardiac apex pointing to the right
- dextroposition: the heart is located in the right part of the thorax, with the cardiac apex pointing to the left
- mesocardia: the heart is located on the middle, with the cardiac apex pointing to the front
- extreme levocardia: the septum axis is more than 65°.

In the same way, cardiac orientation has to be compared with the position of the abdominal vis-

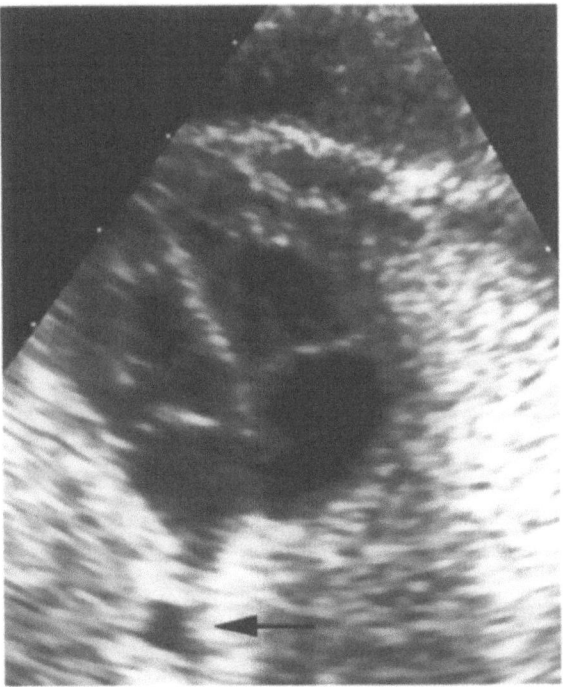

Fig. 6.1. Normal heart dextroposition. Descending aorta (*arrow*) is located on the left of the spine

cera for situs evaluation. The situs is defined by the atrial position: the left atrium receiving the pulmonary veins lies close to the spine. In case of situs solitus (normal localization), the left atrium is in its normal position close to the spine, with the right ventricle close to the chest wall (levocardia); the stomach and liver are located on the left and the right respectively. In the case of situs inversus, the descending aorta and the stomach are on the right and the inferior vena cava and the liver on the left. When the situs is ambiguous, there is either left atrial isomerism or right atrial isomerism. Left isomerism includes bilateral left atria, both lungs with two lobes, left inferior vena cava which is interrupted above the renal veins with lower body venous drainage achieved by the azygos veins, and polysplenia with multiple small accessory spleen, mainly located along the great flexure of the stomach. Right isomerism includes bilateral right atria, both lungs with three lobes, a liver often located on the middle and asplenia. Ambiguous situs is often associated with complex cardiac malformation and right isomerisms usually have a poorer prognosis.

An abnormal position may also be related to the malformation of a structure adjacent to the heart, such as diaphragmatic hernia, lung mass or lung hypoplasia, which have to be excluded (ABDULLAH et al. 2000).

Step 2: The Four-Chamber View

This systematic view of the fetal heart is the easiest to obtain and one of the more informative. It is usually easily obtained with a transverse section of the fetal thorax. There are several points that must be noted in the four-chamber view:

- the fetal heart area is approximately one third that of the thoracic cavity.
- the two atrial chambers are of similar size, with the foraminal flap moving into the left atrium, which lies close to the descending aorta and the spine and receives the pulmonary veins (Fig. 6.2).
- the two ventricular chambers are approximately of equal size, with the right ventricle just behind the sternum. The apex points to the anterior left chest wall. The thickness of the ventricular walls and the septum are about equal, but the apex of the right ventricle is coarse whereas the left ventricle is smooth (Fig. 6.3).
- the atrioventricular valves function properly at every cardiac cycle, with the tricuspid valve located slightly more apically than the mitral valve (Fig. 6.4).
- the junction of the atrioventricular valves with atrial and ventricular septum is intact, imaging the "cross of the heart" during ventricular systole.
- A hyperechoic focus may be seen in the ventricles, most often in the left. This hyperechogenicity of papillary muscle or valve chordae is considered to be a marker of aneuploidy. However, echogenic intracardiac focus may be found in 4–5% of

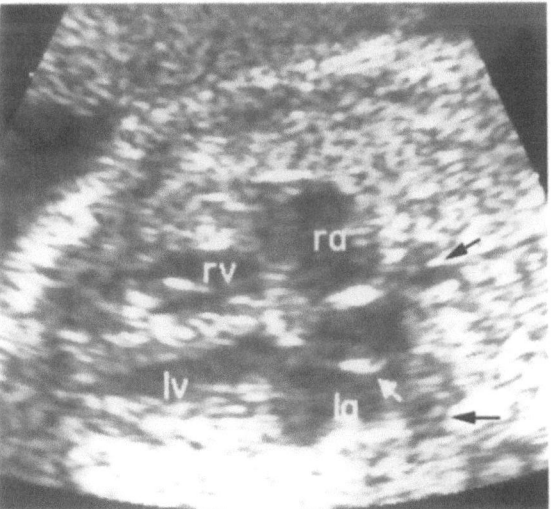

Fig. 6.2. Four-chamber view with the foraminal valve or Vieussen's valve (*white arrow*) moving in the left atrium (*la*), which receives the pulmonary veins (*black arrows*). Left ventricle (*lv*), right ventricle (*rv*) and right atrium (*ra*)

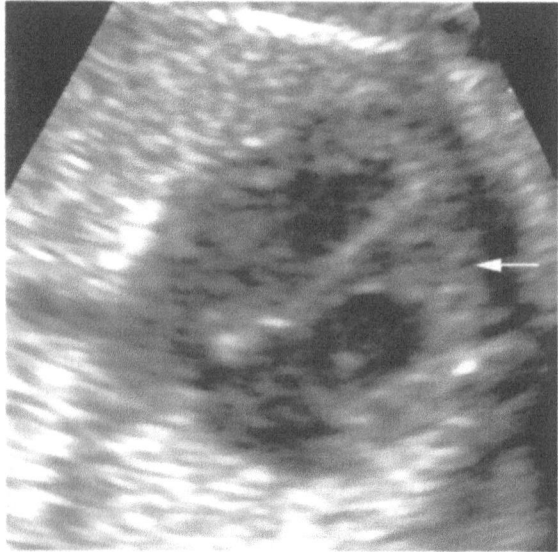

Fig. 6.3. The two ventricular chambers with a coarse appearance of the right apex (*arrow*), close to the sternum

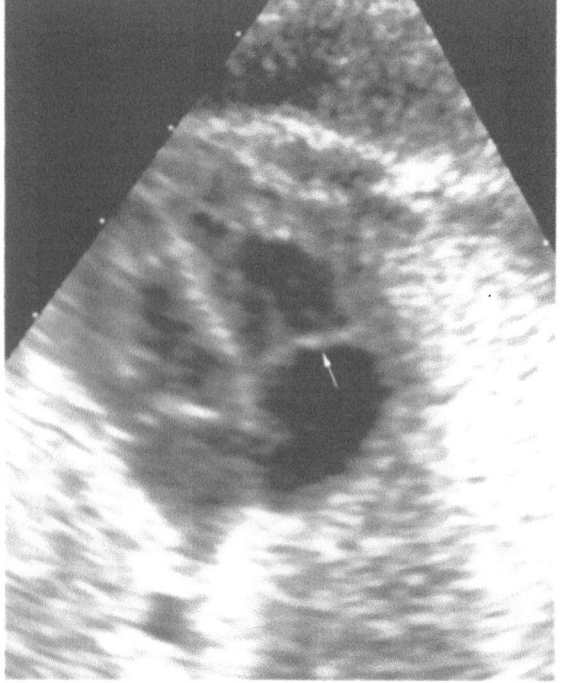

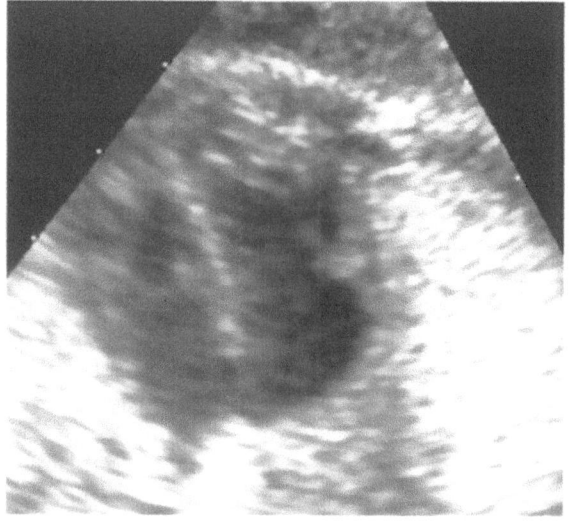

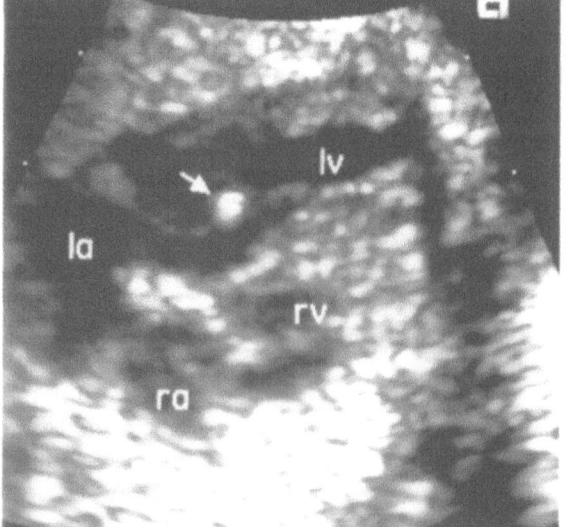

Fig. 6.4. The atrioventricular valves at systole (**a**) and diastole (**b**). Note the more apical position of the right atrioventricular valves. (**c**) Echogenic intracardiac focus located on the mitral valve chordae (*arrow*). Left ventricle (*lv*), right ventricle (*rv*) and right atrium (*ra*)

normal fetuses, so other malformations have to be looked after before deciding to perform genetic amniocentesis (NYBERG and SOUTER 2001).

Although the four-chamber view is very informative, one has to be aware that this cross-sectional image cannot detect many common forms of major defects such as tetralogy of Fallot and transposition of the great arteries (Table 6.1). Thus, heart analysis requires other views for a better analysis of the aorta and pulmonary artery and their connection with the ventricles.

Table 6.1. Congenital cardiac malformations often associated with a normal four-chamber view

Tetralogy of Fallot
Transposition of the great arteries
Small ventricular septal defects
Mild valvular aortic or pulmonary artery stenosis
Mild coarctation

Step 3: The Five-Chamber View

The five-chamber view, also called the long axis view of the aorta, is obtained from the four-chamber view, with an angulation of the transducer in the left ventricular long axes allowing imaging of the origin of the aorta from the left ventricle. With this view, the aortic valves, the flow from the left ventricle to the ascending aorta and the septal continuity with the anterior wall of the aorta can be seen (Fig. 6.5). Most septal defects requiring surgical treatment or associated with complex cardiac malformation are located in the subaortic area. Transposition of the great arteries can be suggested with this when the two great vessels are seen together and parallel.

Step 4: The Transverse Great Vessels View

The transverse great vessels view can be obtained by moving the transducer cranially from the four-chamber view or rotating the transducer 90° from its long axis view. The aorta is centrally located, appearing as a circular structure with the pulmonary artery coursing around it (Figs. 6.6, 6.7). The aortic, pulmonary

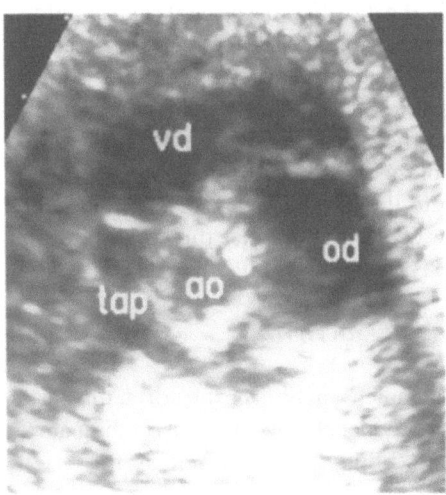

Fig. 6.6. The pulmonary artery trunk (*tap*) is anterior and coming on the left side of the aorta (*ao*). Right ventricle (*vd*) and right atrium (*od*)

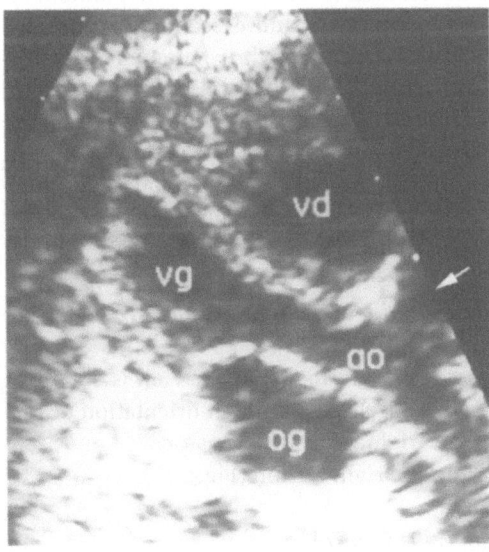

Fig. 6.5. Five-chamber view with the aorta (*ao*) coming from the left ventricle. Left ventricle (*vg*), right ventricle (*vd*), left atrium (*og*), right atrium (*arrow*)

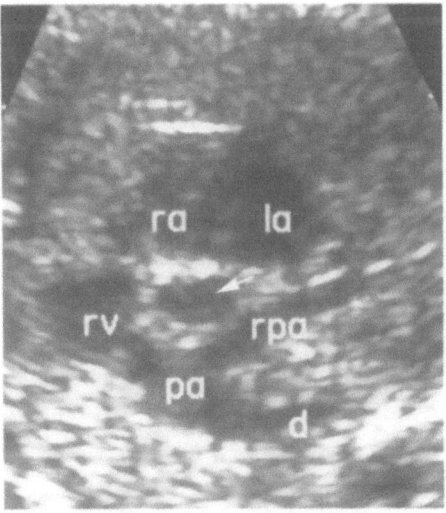

Fig. 6.7. The relationships of the aorta and pulmonary artery can be clearly seen on this view. Aorta (*arrow*), pulmonary artery (*pa*), right pulmonary artery (*rpa*), descending aorta (*d*), right ventricle (*rv*), right atrium (*ra*), left atrium (*la*)

and tricuspid valves are usually well visualized in this view. The pulmonary artery trunk diameter is slightly larger than that of aorta. This short axis view confirms the perpendicular relationship of the great vessels, excluding malformation such as transposition of the great arteries or truncus arteriosus (Yoo et al. 1999a, ALLAN 1997), and allows measurements of the great vessels to look for abnormal discrepancy.

Step 5: Long Axis View of the Pulmonary Artery

The long axis view of the pulmonary artery can be visualized from the five-chamber view by rotating the transducer in the direction of the fetal right shoulder. It allows visualization of the right ventricle ejection chamber and the pulmonary artery origin, coming from the right to the left, the sigmoid valves and the flow through the pulmonary artery trunk (Fig. 6.8). Angulation of the transducer from the long axis view of the aorta to the long axis view of the pulmonary artery is a way of checking that the crossing of the great vessels is normal.

Step 6: The Aortic Arch View

For a more complete analysis of the aorta, the aortic arch view gives a global view of the ascending aorta, arch and descending aorta, as well as the origin

of head and neck vessels (Fig. 6.9). This plane is obtained by a 90° clockwise rotation of the transducer from the longitudinal aorta view, with a slight oblique angulation between the left shoulder and the right chest. This cross-sectional view is required for evaluation of aortic narrowing, particularly coarctation which is located in the isthmus.

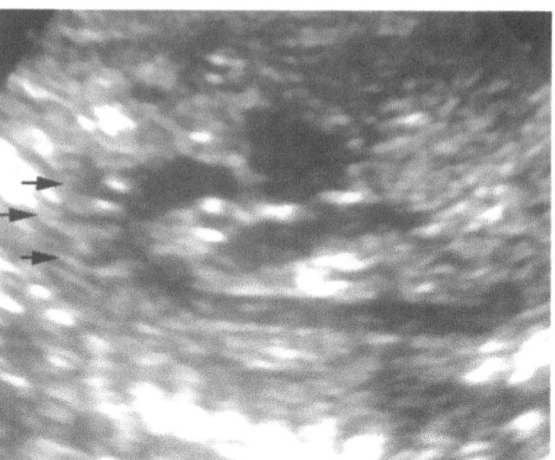

Fig. 6.9. The aortic arch view with the brachiocephalic vessels (*arrows*)

Step 7: The Ductal Arch View

The ductal arch view is obtained by returning to a more anteroposterior axis of the thorax. It can also be obtained from a short axis view of the great vessels. The ductal arch is composed of the pulmonary artery, ductus arteriosus and descending aorta. The appearance of the ductal arch is flatter than that of the aortic arch (Fig. 6.10). No vessels coming out from the arch can be seen. This view allows flow analysis through the ductus arteriosus. The systolic and diastolic velocity increase with gestational age. When the systolic velocity is greater than 1.4 m/s, a restrictive ductus arteriosus has to be suspected.

Step 8: The Superior and Inferior Vena Cava View

The superior and inferior vena cava view is obtained from the aortic arch view with an orientation of the probe to the right. The two venae cavae are seen draining into the right atrium (Fig. 6.11).

Step 9: Checklist Control

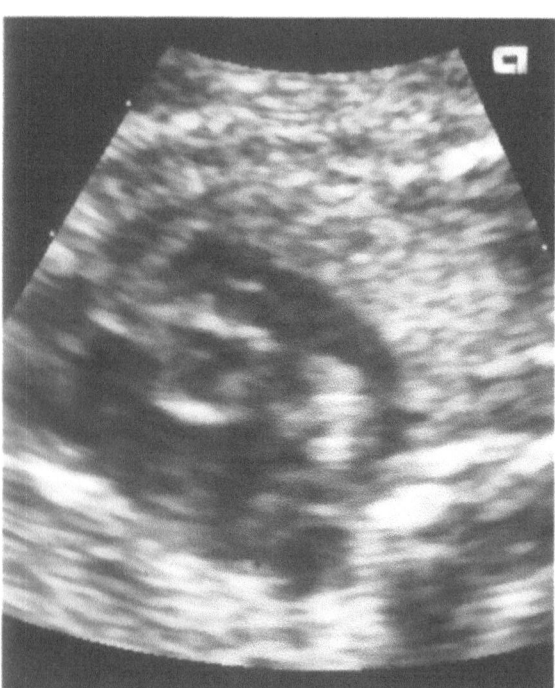

Fig. 6.8. Pulmonary trunk coming from the right ventricle ejection chamber

At the end of the evaluation make sure that all the cardiac structures have been seen (Table 6.2).

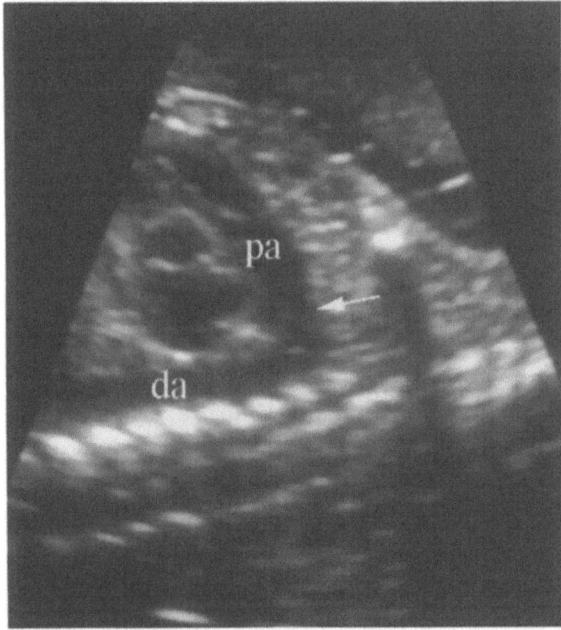

Fig. 6.10. The ductal arch with the pulmonary artery (*pa*), ductus arteriosus (*arrow*) and descending aorta (*da*)

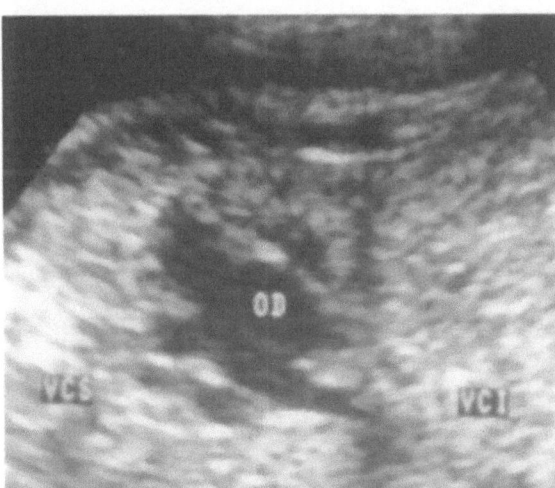

Fig. 6.11. The superior vena cava (*VCS*) and inferior vena cava (*VCI*) are draining into the right atrium (*OD*)

Table 6.2. What should be seen during the routine cardiac examination

---

Heart and stomach are on the same side (left)

Pulmonary veins drain into the left atrium and vena cava in the right atrium

Normal four-chamber view

Normal outflow tracts and great arteries

Normal and regular cardiac frequency

6.1.2.2
M-Mode Echocardiography

M-mode echocardiography is an additional tool to B-mode for the evaluation of wall thickness, ventricular size and ventricular contractility, as well as atrioventricular valve motion and cardiac arrhythmia (BROWN 1997) (Fig. 6.12). The high sample rate allows an accurate analysis of the structural motion, particularly tachycardia. Evaluation of ventricular size and motion requires a transverse view of the ventricles or a four-chamber view, when the septum can be perpendicularly analyzed.

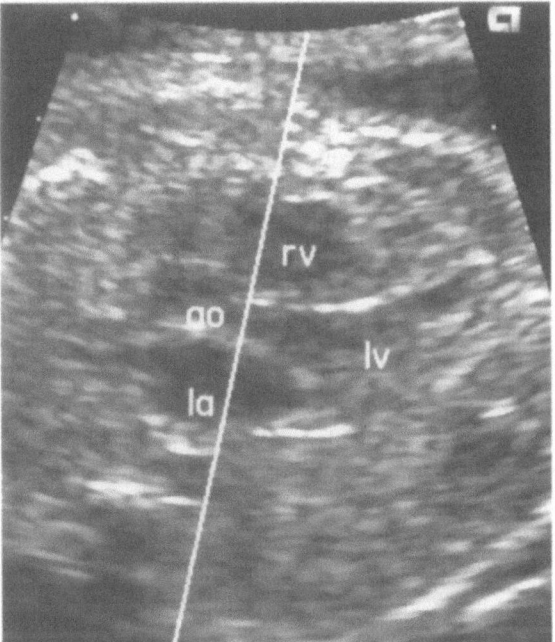

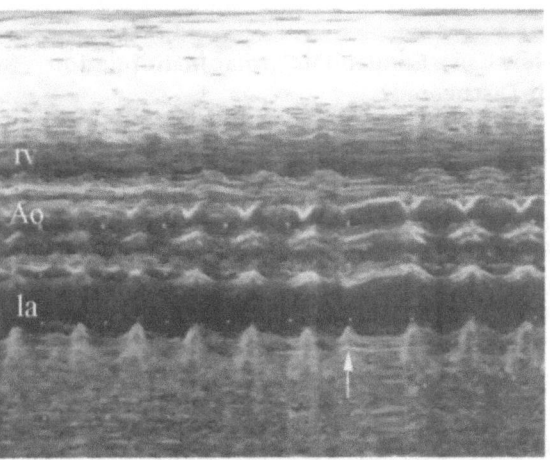

Fig. 6.12. a The drawn *line* illustrates a M-mode recording coming from the right ventricle (*rv*) to the left atrium (*la*) through the aorta. Left ventricle (*lv*) and aorta (*ao*). **b** TM recording in blocked atrial extrasystole (*arrow*)

6.1.2.3
Doppler Echocardiography

Pulsed Doppler Ultrasonography. Pulsed Doppler demonstrates the direction and characteristics of the blood flow through the foramen ovale, the atrioventricular valves and the great vessels, including the ductus arteriosus. Doppler sampling has to be adequate in order to avoid the evaluation of two different but very close structures. A biphasic flow with a low velocity is observed at the foramen ovale level, coming from the right to the left atrium. The flow through the atrioventricular valves is characterized by a biphasic pattern: the first peak is related to the passive ventricular venous filling, followed by a higher second peak as a result of atrial contraction. The flow through the great vessels valves is monophasic. The ductus arteriosus flow has a systolic and a diastolic component, coming from the pulmonary artery to the descending aorta.

Color Doppler Ultrasonography. Color-coded Doppler flow mapping evaluates both the morphology and hemodynamics of the heart and great vessels. When the flow is coming toward the probe the coded color is red, and when the flow is away from the probe the coded color is blue. A quicker assessment of a stenosis, a valvular leak or an abnormal intracardiac communication (Fig. 6.13) can be obtained with color Doppler, as well a rapid visualization of the aortic arch or ventricular outflow chamber, but its use has to be limited to avoid unnecessary exposure to ultrasonic energy above 100 mW/cm^2.

6.1.3
How Can a Congenital Cardiac Malformation Be Discovered?

Throughout the routine and systematic cardiac analysis, abnormal findings may be observed that will either lead to a diagnosis of a congenital cardiac malformation by the sonographer alone, or at the least, to the suspicion of an abnormality which will be further evaluated by a fetal echocardiographic specialist.

6.1.3.1
Four-Chamber View: Atrioventricular Cavity Abnormality

Univentricular Heart. When only one ventricular chamber can be seen, the diagnosis of univentricular malformation can be suggested. Univentricular heart

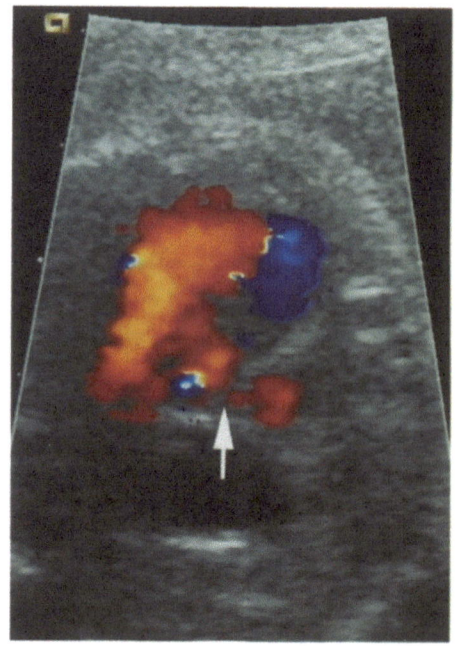

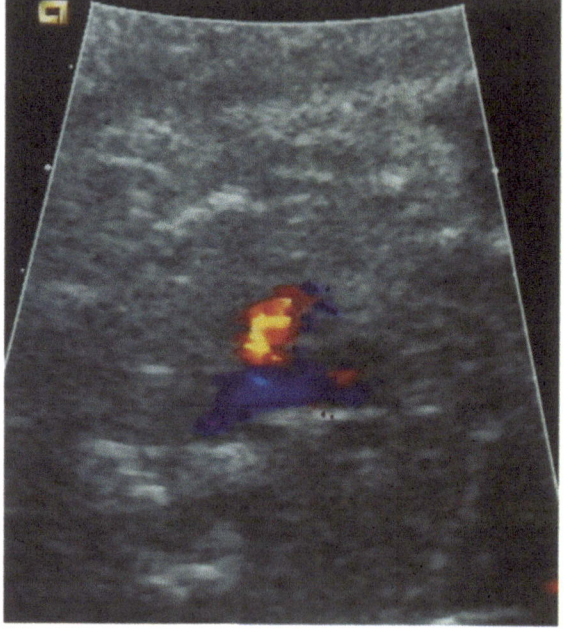

Fig. 6.13. a Hypoplastic left heart syndrome with flow coming through the ventricular septal defect (*arrow*). **b** The aorta, smaller than pulmonary artery, was more clearly depicted with color Doppler; note the reverse flow in comparison with the normal flow in the pulmonary artery

or double inlet ventricle includes a group of defects in which there is primarily a single large ventricle that receives both the mitral and the tricuspid valve (Fig. 6.14) or a common atrioventricular valve. The valve cord should not to be confused with a septum. A small and rudimentary ventricle chamber, with-

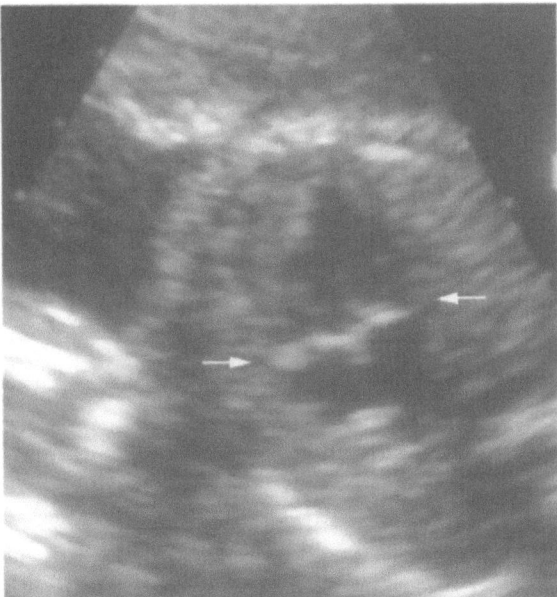

Fig. 6.14. Univentricular heart. A single large ventricle with the both mitral and the tricuspid valves (*arrows*)

out any connection with the atrial cavities, is often observed. The great vessels must be assessed since they frequently display an abnormal position, with the aorta anterior to the pulmonary artery, and pulmonary stenosis or atresia or aortic coarctation are common. In addition, the determination of cardiac situs is mandatory in this malformation, in which abnormalities of cardiac position is not rare.

The first step in postnatal treatment consists of palliative surgery. The strategy is to band the pulmonary artery in patients in whom there is excessive pulmonary blood flow or to create a shunt between systemic and pulmonary circulation when severe pulmonary stenosis is present, thereby maintaining adequate pulmonary perfusion. As in all cardiac malformations in which there is only a single functional ventricle, definitive surgical correction involves the creation of a total cavopulmonary anastomosis. After this operation the single ventricle pumps blood to the systemic circulation whereas pulmonary blood flow is passive and does not directly depend on ventricular contraction. This is a two-stage procedure in which the first operation is a bi-directional Glenn shunting in which the superior vena cava is connected to the right pulmonary artery, directing desaturated blood to right and left pulmonary branches. The second stage of the procedure is a derivation of blood from inferior vena cava to the pulmonary artery with the creation of an intracardiac or extracardiac tunnel.

Early and medium-term surgical results for this operation are encouraging but the long-term outcome is still under evaluation. Driscoll and colleagues (1992) reported a 5-year survival of more than 85% and a 10-year survival above 65%. Cardiac transplantation can be considered after total cavopulmonary connection if there is significant atrioventricular valve regurgitation, ventricular dysfunction or protein losing enteropathy.

Hypoplastic Left Heart Syndrome. Hypoplastic left heart syndrome is one of the most common serious cardiac defects diagnosed prenatally (ALLAN et al. 1994, MONTANA et al. 1996). This evolutive malformation is characterized by a reduced volume of the left heart tract with a small left ventricle also associated with a small aorta and a small left atrium related to the flow decrease (Fig. 6.15 ; see also Fig. 6.13). Experimentally in animal models, the reduction of blood flow between the two atria through the foramen ovale leads to a left heart hypoplasia (HARTH et al. 1973). In the human fetus, a misalignment of the atrial septum could be the cause of this malformation, leading to the blood flow in the vena cava to be preferentially oriented to the right heart tract. The diagnosis is suggested on the four-chamber view by the demonstration of a small left ventricle, which can sometimes be hyperechogenic due to endocardial fibroelastosis, a small motionless mitral valve or poorly moving thickened valves, and a dilated right ventricle which constitutes the cardiac apex. The atrial septum usually bulges into the right atrium, but will be seen bulging to the left in the case of tricuspid regurgitation. Using the other views, the aorta is difficult to depict, whereas the dilated pulmonary artery is clearly seen. With Doppler, the decreased flow can be shown at atrioventricular and aortic levels whereas reversed flow can be observed coming from the ductus arteriosus into the aortic arch.

Newborns with hypoplastic left heart syndrome may be asymptomatic but become severely ill as the ductus closes. Without treatment this defect is almost always rapidly lethal. Current surgical strategy includes staged palliative surgery leading to total cavopulmonary connection or cardiac transplantation (TWORETZKY et al. 2001).

Hypoplastic Right Heart Syndrome. This malformation is related to a flow reduction through the right heart tract, thus impeding its ability to develop properly. It can be the consequence of severe pulmonary stenosis or pulmonary atresia with intact ventricular septum or tricuspid atresia. Thus, when a small right

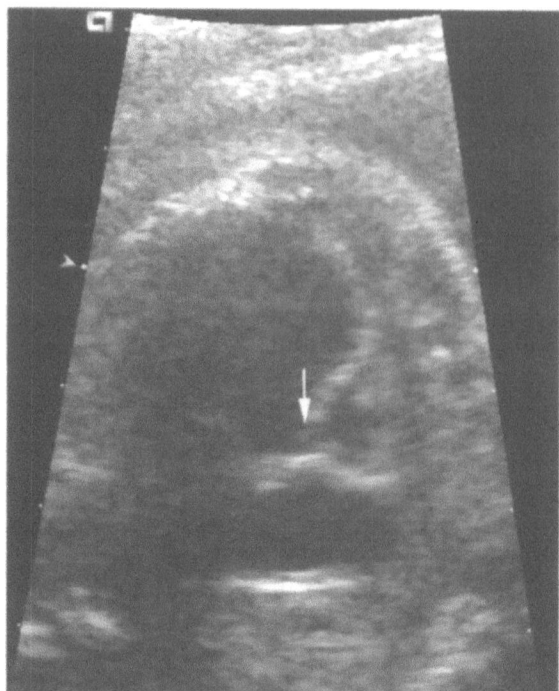

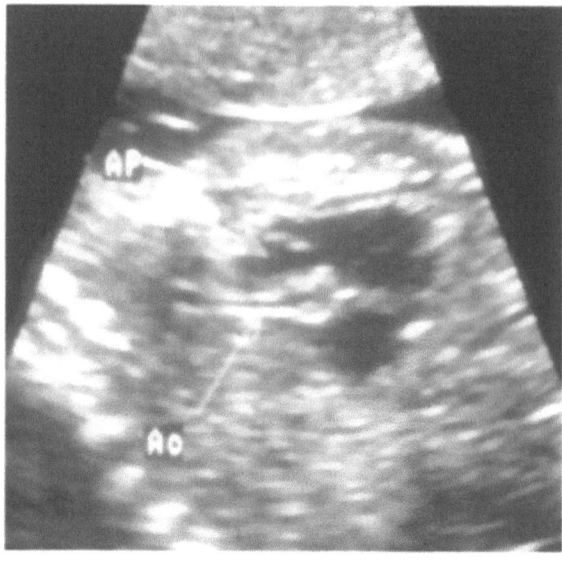

Fig. 6.15. a Hypoplastic left heart syndrome. Hypoplastic left ventricle in comparison with the enlarged right ventricle, communicating through a ventricular septal defect (*arrow*). b In this case the ascending aorta (*Ao*) was very hypoplastic, whereas the pulmonary artery was enlarged (*AP*)

ventricle has been identified, the tricuspid valves and pulmonary artery have to be evaluated to determine the cause. Evaluation of the patency of the tricuspid valves is based on pulsed and color Doppler. In the case of tricuspid atresia, there is a complete agenesis of the tricuspid valve resulting in the absence of communication between right atria and right ventricle (Fig. 6.16). Almost always a ventricular septal defect is present and allows a communication between the enlarged left ventricle and the hypoplastic right ventricle. Transposition of the great arteries is encountered in 20% of cases (ANDERSON et al. 1987). When the relationship between the great vessels is normal, pulmonary stenosis or atresia is often present. Postnatal strategy is the same as in univentricular heart.

In the case of pulmonary atresia with intact ventricular septum, the tricuspid valve may also appear small and hyperechoic but flow can be observed in diastole. In addition, tricuspid regurgitation is often detected. The pulmonary artery is small and atretic with thickened and poorly moving valves. No flow through the pulmonary artery can be recorded with pulsed or color Doppler and reverse flow can be seen from the ductus arteriosus. Both the left ventricle and left atrium are dilated secondary to a volume overload from the right atrium.

Neonates with pulmonary atresia with intact ventricular septum require administration of prostaglandin E_1, to maintain ductal patency until surgery

is performed. If the right ventricle is only moderately hypoplastic, surgical valvulotomy or transcatheter radiofrequency perforation with balloon dilatation of the pulmonary valve can be proposed. In patients in whom the right ventricle is considered unsuitable for biventricular circulation a systemic to pulmonary artery shunt is performed during the neonatal period prior to performing a cavopulmonary shunt.

Enlarged Right Atrium. When the right atrium is enlarged, tricuspid valve abnormality has to be searched for. Two diagnosis have to be searched for: Ebstein anomaly and tricuspid valve dysplasia. *Ebstein anomaly* is a congenital malformation in which the septal and mural leaflets of the tricuspid valve are displaced downward into the inlet portion of the right ventricle. There is usually some dysplasia of the leaflets. Exposure to lithium during pregnancy has been associated with this anomaly. *Tricuspid valve dysplasia* is characterized by abnormal thickened leaflets that have a normal insertion. Both malformations are responsible for tricuspid insufficiency easily recordable by pulsed and color Doppler. The pulmonary trunk is often moderately hypoplastic. Cardiomegaly can be massive and can impair normal development of the lungs. This lesion can also be associated with fetal hydrops or fetal tachycardia.

Some of these babies die in the postnatal life because they cannot be adequately ventilated, but

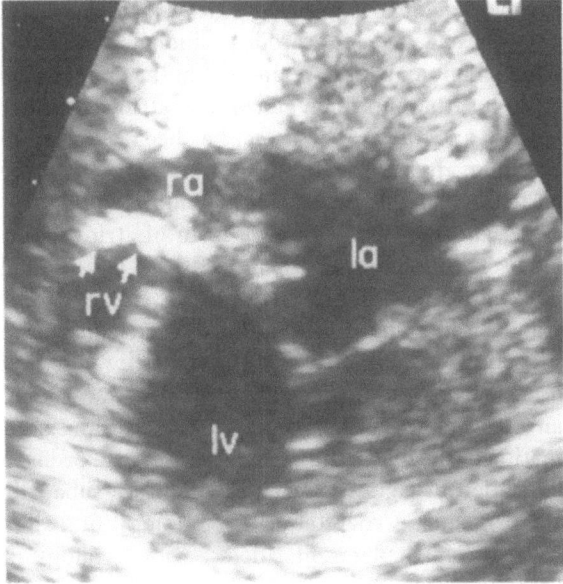

Fig. 6.16. Hypoplastic right ventricle with tricuspid atresia. The right ventricle (*rv*) and atrium (*ra*) are smaller than the left ventricle (*lv*) and left atrium (*la*); the tricuspid valve is thickened and hyperechoic (*arrows*)

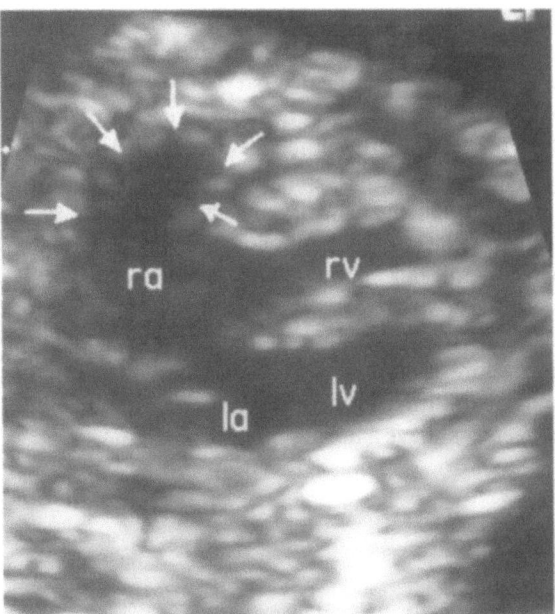

Fig. 6.17. Idiopathic enlargement of the right atrium (*arrows*). Right atrium (*ra*), left atrium (*la*), right ventricle (*rv*), left ventricle (*lv*)

even neonates with massive cardiomegaly, severe cyanosis and congestive heart failure may dramatically improve with the decrease in pulmonary vascular resistance that occurs after birth, and may remain stable for long periods. Isolated enlargement of the right atria without tricuspid malformation suggests the diagnosis of *idiopathic right atrial enlargement*, which has a favorable antenatal and postnatal prognosis (Fig. 6.17).

6.1.3.2
Four-Chamber View: Septal Anomalies

Ventricular Septal Defect. Isolated ventricular septal defect is the commonest congenital heart disease detected in infancy accounting for more than 30% of cases of heart malformations. However, it constitutes less than 10% of sonographically recognized fetal cardiac abnormalities since perimembranous and small muscular defects are rarely seen when isolated (ALLAN et al. 1994). Ventricular septal defect is characterized by a septal discontinuity which is best depicted with the ultrasound beam perpendicular to the interventricular septum (Fig. 6.18). When the beam is parallel to the interventricular septum, dropout can often be seen at the crux of the heart where the septum is thin and membranous. The four-chamber view can miss a subaortic perimembranous defect that is better depicted in the five-cham-

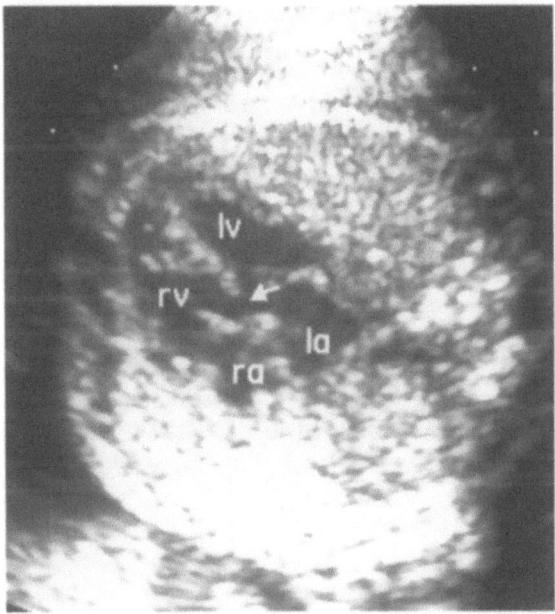

Fig. 6.18. Ventricular septal defect (*arrow*). Right atrium (*ra*), left atrium (*la*), right ventricle (*rv*), left ventricle (*lv*)

ber view. Blood flow identification through the septal defect with color Doppler may be helpful, particularly in cases of small or muscular defects (see Fig. 6.13). When a large ventricular septal defect has been found, a search for other intracardiac or extracardiac anomalies should be made as well as a search for chromosomal anomalies (Fig. 6.19). However, in cases of a small and isolated muscular defect it is not necessary to perform a karyotype. If a significant ventricular septal defect is found in early pregnancy, follow-up must study the sizes of pulmonary artery and aorta.

After birth, the majority of small ventricular septal defects will resolve spontaneously. Large defects may need medical treatment with diuretics. Surgery is necessary when there is pulmonary hypertension, congestive heart failure or failure to thrive. These procedures have an excellent success rate and the vast majority of infants operated on for ventricular septal defects will have a normal life.

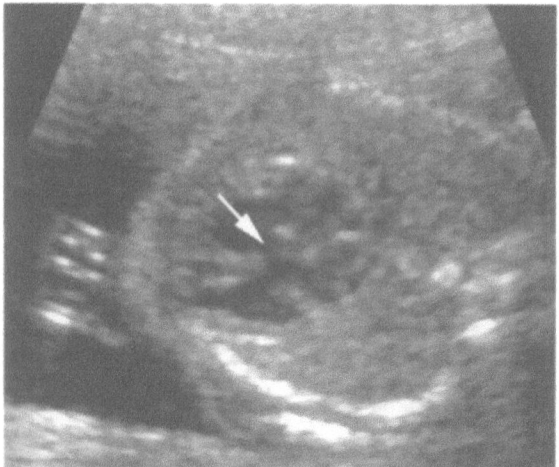

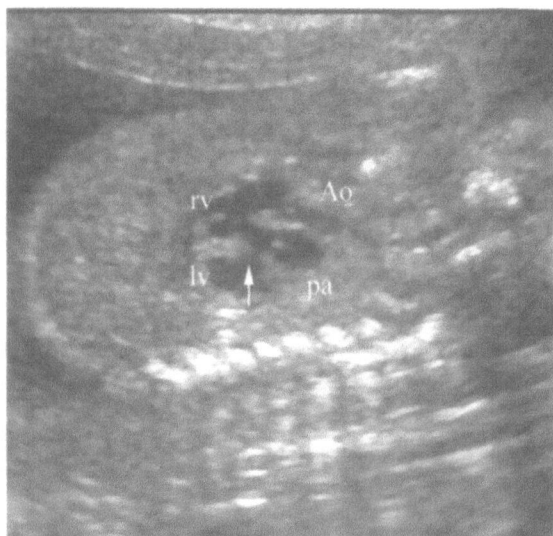

Fig. 6.19a, b. Ventricular septal defect in a complex cardiac malformation. **a** Ventricular septal defect (*arrow*). **b** Further evaluation showed great vessels transposition, with the pulmonary artery (*pa*) over the right ventricle (*rv*) and left ventricle (*lv*). The smaller size of the aorta (*Ao*) was related to a coarctation

Atrioventricular Septal Defect. Atrioventricular septal defect, also called endocardial cushion defect, results from an anomaly of development of the endocardial cushions that normally form the atrioventricular septum and valves. The defect has been reported to occur in approximately 15% of fetuses with CHD and 40% of fetuses with Down syndrome (MACHADO et al. 1998). The complete form of atrioventricular septal defect is characterized by a large septal defect involving both the interatrial and interventricular septa and a common atrioventricular valve that connects both atria and the ventricles. It is best imaged from the four-chamber view (Fig. 6.20). When an atrioventricular septal defect is detected, an examination of the rest of the heart is necessary in order to detect left or right ventricular hypoplasia, subaortic stenosis, aortic coarctation or tetralogy of Fallot. An atrioventricular septal defect with tetralogy of Fallot is frequently associated with Down syndrome (70–75% of cases). Atrioventricular valve regurgitation, easily detectable by color Doppler, can occur and can be responsible for fetal hydrops. In the partial form, two atrioventricular valves are present and the lower portion of the atrial septum (close to the crux of the heart) is absent (Fig. 6.21). The mitral annulus is displaced toward the apex, so that the mitral and tricuspid valves appear to be inserted at the same level.

Surgery for atrioventricular septal defect is indicated earlier in life in the complete form than for the partial form. In the complete form, congestive heart failure usually occurs during infancy, requiring surgery at between 3 and 6 months of age. In the case of unbalanced ventricles or mitral malformation, palliative surgery with pulmonary artery banding may be necessary in order to reduce pulmonary blood flow and heart failure. When possible, primary complete repair is the procedure of choice, with closure of septal defects and reconstruction of the atrioventricular valves. In some patients, significant mitral malformation may require mitral valve replacement. In the partial form, patients are often asymptomatic and surgical repair can be delayed until 3–6 years of age.

Atrial Septal Defect. Absence of the atrial septum, just behind atrioventricular valves which are at the same level, is suggestive of ostium primum atrial septal defect (Fig. 6.22). Ostium secundum atrial septal defect is one of the commonest forms of CHD seen in childhood. Antenatal diagnosis is difficult because of the physiological fetal atrial septal defect that allows blood flow from the right to the left atrium. Atrial

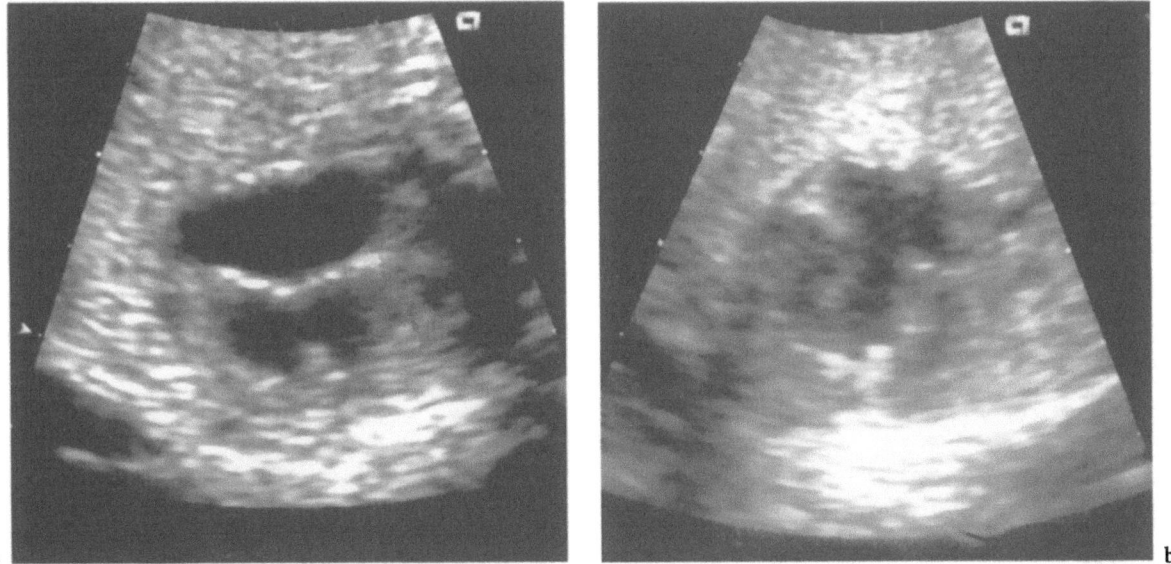

Fig. 6.20a, b. Complete atrioventricular septal defect. **a** Closed and **b** opened atrioventricular valve

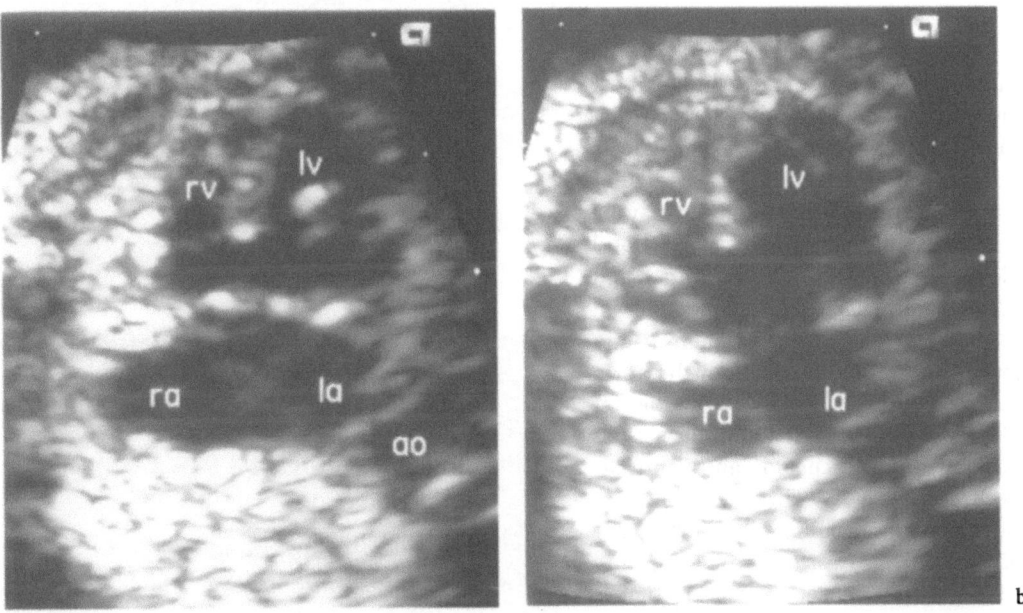

Fig. 6.21a, b. Partial atrioventricular septal defect. **a** Closed and **b** opened atrioventricular valves. Right atrium (*ra*), left atrium (*la*), right ventricle (*rv*), left ventricle (*lv*), aorta (*ao*)

septal defect appears as a larger than expected dropout in the central portion of the septum secundum with a deficient foraminal flap that fails to cover the foramen ovale entirely.

Postnatally, a large number of atrial septal defects close spontaneously during early childhood. The malformation is asymptomatic during childhood but requires closure to avoid pulmonary vascular disease, dysrhythmia or right ventricular failure that

may occur during adulthood. Closure can be done surgically or, in the case of a moderate-sized defect, with percutaneous devices (O'LAUGHLIN 1997).

6.1.3.3
Four-Chamber View: Right Ventricular Enlargement

Coarctation of the Aorta. Coarctation of the aorta is a narrowing of the aortic lumen mainly located at the

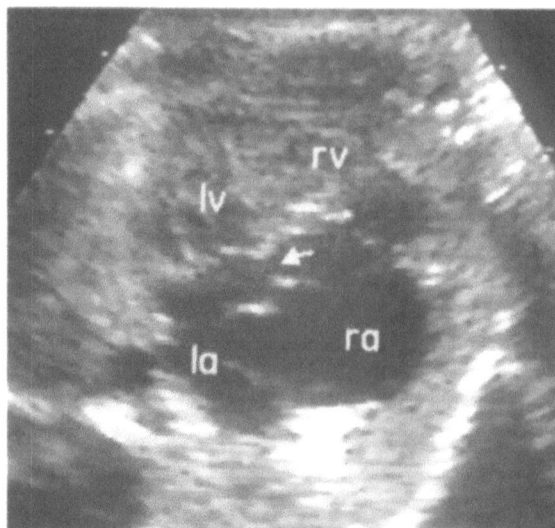

Fig. 6.22. Ostium primum atrial defect (*arrow*). Right atrium (*ra*), left atrium (*la*), right ventricle (*rv*), left ventricle (*lv*)

the body with reduction or abolition of the pulsatility of the femoral pulses. This situation can be tolerated for many years but requires surgery between 1 and 5 years of age, even in the absence of symptoms, to avoid the persistent systemic hypertension that is frequently encountered in patients in whom surgery has been performed after 10 years of age.

Restrictive Ductus Arteriosus. In the normal fetus the ductus arteriosus is widely patent with a flow velocity below 1 m/s. Spontaneously in late pregnancy or

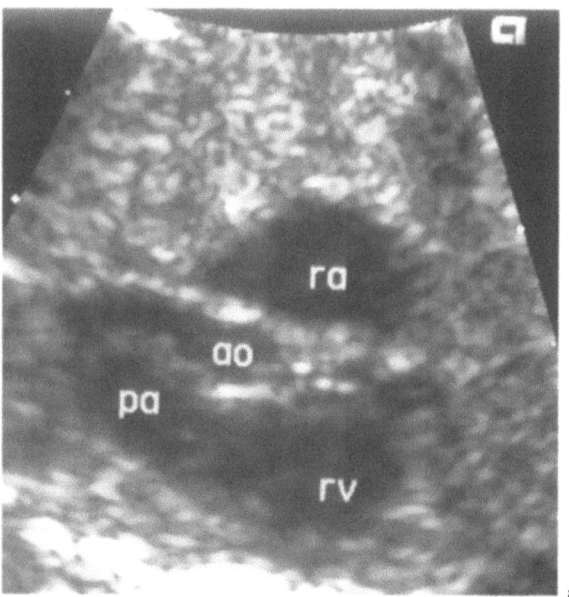

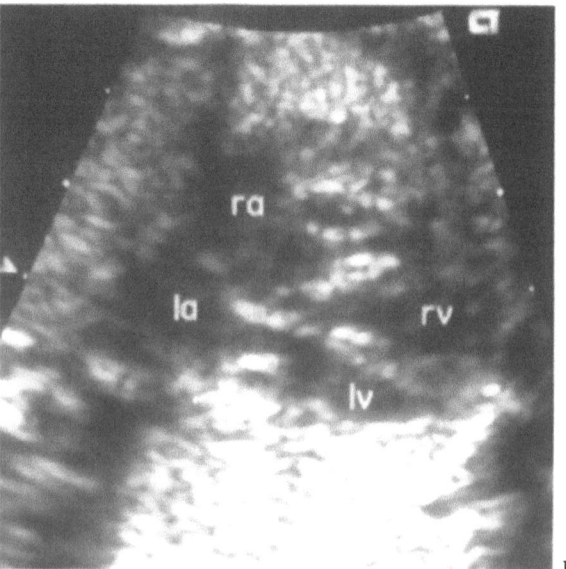

Fig. 6.23a, b. Coarctation of the aorta. **a** The aorta (*ao*) is smaller than the pulmonary artery (*pa*), as well as the left ventricle in comparison with the right ventricle (*rv*). Right atrium (*ra*), left atrium (*la*)

aortic isthmus between the origin of the left subclavian artery and the ductus arteriosus. This narrowing may extend more or less to the aortic arch. The most severe form is interruption of the aortic arch that is almost always associated with intracardiac defects such as ventricular septal defect or aortic valvular stenosis. In utero, diagnosis of coarctation may be very difficult. Some subtle changes may be helpful such as ventricular asymmetry with an enlarged and hypertrophied right ventricle, and a discrepancy in the diameters of the great vessels at their origin with a pulmonary artery 50% larger than the aorta because of the reduction of blood flow in the left heart (Fig. 6.23). Possible associated findings are tricuspid insufficiency, aortic bicuspidy and ventricular septal defect (see Fig. 6.19). Three may be associated chromosomal abnormalities, such as Turner syndrome (45 XO) in the case of coarctation and DiGeorge syndrome (microdeletion 22q.11) that is encountered in 50% of cases of interruption of the aortic arch.

After birth, the clinical manifestations of coarctation of the aorta are very variable. Neonates with severe coarctation or interruption of the aortic arch can develop congestive heart failure and metabolic acidosis that necessitate prostaglandin E_1 infusion prior to surgery to maintain ductus patency and allow perfusion of the lower part of the body. Surgery consists in repairing the aortic arch and associated intracardiac anomalies. Some patients with isolated discrete coarctation of the aorta will present with only systemic hypertension of the upper part of

after maternal administration of anti-inflammatory agents such as indomethacin, aspirin or ibuprofen, the ductus can constrict. Ductal constriction is characterized by an increase in ductal blood flow velocity above 1.4 m/s and is often associated with right ventricular and atrial enlargement with tricuspid insufficiency due to dilation of the right ventricle. Drug-induced ductal constriction is usually reversible within a few days with discontinuation of treatment. Antenatal ductal constriction can be associated postnatally with transient pulmonary hypertension.

6.1.3.4
Four-Chamber View: Cardiomegaly

Cardiomyopathy. A cardiomyopathy is a primary disorder of the cardiac muscle that is not associated with structural anomalies. There are two main presentations in the fetus: dilated and hypertrophic cardiomyopathies.

Dilated cardiomyopathy can be secondary to high-output failure due to severe fetal anemia or volume overload from arteriovenous shunting, or may result from direct myocardial damage encountered in tachycardia-induced cardiomyopathy, fetal infection (DROSE et al. 1991) (parvovirus or TORCH agents) and fetal anoxia. On the four-chamber view there is a cardiomegaly defined by an increase in the cardiac circumference to thoracic circumference ratio (normally approximately 0.5) and by an increase in the cardiac area to thoracic area ratio (normally approximately 0.33). Cardiomegaly can also be assessed by comparison with a published table of M-mode measurements versus gestational age (ALLAN et al. 1992). Impaired ventricular contractility is frequently associated with dilated cardiomyopathy as well as atrio-ventricular regurgitation due to dilatation of the valve annulus and an increased echogenicity of the ventricular wall due to endocardial fibroelastosis.

Hypertrophic cardiomyopathy may be secondary to maternal insulin-dependent diabetes mellitus and is a reversible disorder (WAY et al. 1979). It can also be a primary disorder of the fetal myocardium as seen in Noonan syndrome or glycogen storage disease.

Aortic Valvular Stenosis. The prenatal diagnosis of aortic valvular stenosis can be difficult in moderate forms, in which the left ventricle may appear normal, thickening of aortic valves being a subtle sign in the fetus. Clues to the diagnosis include a post-stenotic dilatation of the proximal aorta and an increased and turbulent aortic flow in the ascending aorta on pulsed or color Doppler. In critical aortic stenosis, the left ventricle is dilated and poorly contracting and often demonstrates endocardial fibroelastosis. Aortic stenosis diagnosed in utero is often severe and usually associated with a high postnatal mortality rate despite successful surgical valvulotomy or percutaneous balloon dilatation (SHARLAND et al. 1991).

6.1.3.5
Four-chamber View: Cardiac Tumors

Cardiac tumors are rare. They include, in decreasing frequency, rhabdomyoma, teratoma, fibroma and hemangioma.

Rhabdomyomas are intramyocardial tumors that tend to be multiple, occurring within the right or left ventricle or within the interventricular septum. Tuberous sclerosis has been reported in up to 80% of patients with multiple rhabdomyoma (Fig. 6.24). Tumors tend to involute postnatally but may sometimes require surgical excision if there is obstruction of blood flow in the outflow tract or in the inlet portion of the ventricles.

Intrapericardial teratomas are usually single, encapsulated, and attached to the base of the heart. They are often associated with pericardial effusion and require surgery in the neonatal period as they cause hemodynamic compromise (Fig. 6.25).

Cardiac fibromas are intracardiac tumors, usually isolated, and often involve the left ventricular free wall or the interventricular septum.

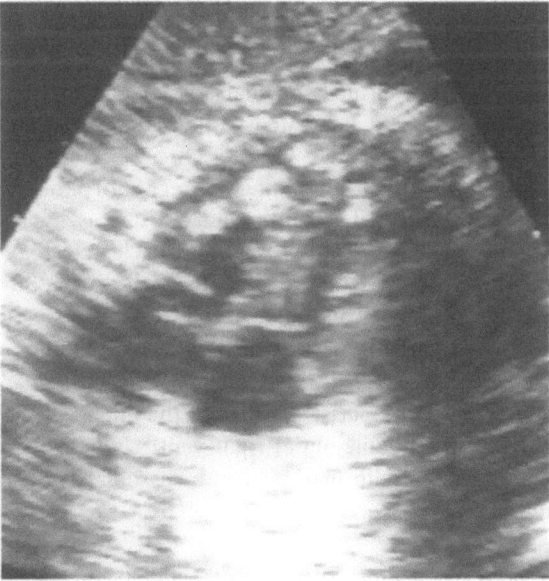

Fig. 6.24. Rhabdomyomas and tuberous sclerosis. Multiple myocardial tumors were found in both ventricles, revealing tuberous sclerosis

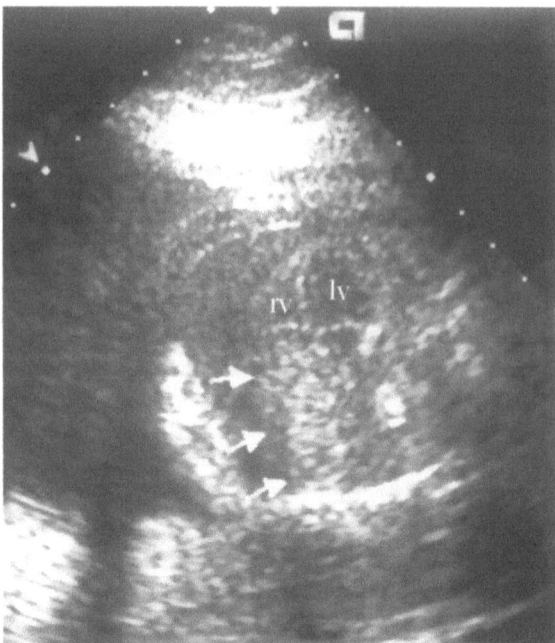

Fig. 6.25. Intrapericardial teratoma

6.1.3.6
Great Vessels Views: Conotruncal Lesions

Conotruncal anomalies are characterized by a defect in the conotruncal septum, and encompass lesions such as tetralogy of Fallot, pulmonary atresia with ventricular septal defect, common arterial trunk and double-outlet right ventricle. These malformations are characterized by a loss of aortic septal continuity in the five-chamber view. In this condition the four-chamber view is usually normal. Loss of aortic septal continuity can be associated with aortic overriding on the interventricular septum. Once aortic over-riding is identified, pulmonary artery morphology must be studied. If the pulmonary artery is hypo-plastic and arising from the right ventricle, tetralogy of Fallot is suggested; if it arises from the aorta, the diagnosis must be common arterial trunk; if it is not connected to the heart, pulmonary atresia with ven-tricular septal defect is likely. Finally, if the two great vessels are seen to arise anterior to the interventric-ular septum, double-outlet right ventricle is proba-ble. All these malformations can be associated with microdeletion 22q.11.

Tetralogy of Fallot. Tetralogy of Fallot is the most common malformation found in children with cya-notic heart disease. It consists of four classic features: subaortic ventricular septal defect, aortic overriding

of the defect, pulmonary stenosis and right ventricu-lar hypertrophy (Yoo et al. 1999b). This last feature may not be present prenatally. In its classic form the pulmonary valves are thickened and their motion is poor, while the pulmonary artery is smaller than the aorta, which can be enlarged by the increased flow (Fig. 6.26). Aneurysmal dilatation of the pulmonary artery associated with significant pulmonary insuffi-ciency on Doppler suggests the diagnosis of tetralogy of Fallot with absence of the pulmonary valves. Post-natal treatment relies on surgery. Infants with favor-able anatomy can undergo primary complete repair soon after the onset of cyanosis. This consists of clos-ing the ventricular septal defect and relieving the right ventricular outflow tract obstruction. Patients with severely hypoplastic pulmonary arteries and multiple ventricular septal defects usually undergo a staged procedure with systemico-pulmonary anasto-mosis prior to complete repair. Patients with absent pulmonary valves and aneurysmal dilatation of the pulmonary artery can present with respiratory dis-tress due to tracheobronchial compression. Surgery consists of complete repair associated with plication of the aneurysmal pulmonary artery branches.

Pulmonary Atresia with Ventricular Septal Defect. The intracardiac anatomy of pulmonary atresia with ventricular septal defect is very similar to that of tetralogy of Fallot but there is no patent communi-

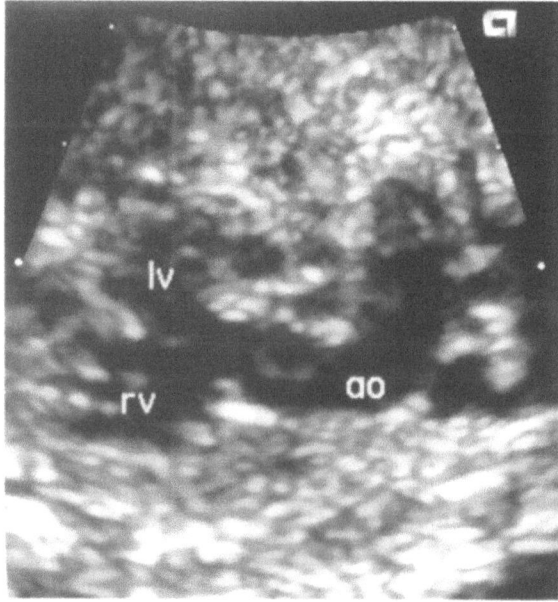

Fig. 6.26. Tetralogy of Fallot. Enlarged aorta (*ao*) overriding the two ventricles (*rv, lv*) communicating by a ventricular septal defect, whereas the pulmonary artery is small with a stenosis at its origin

cation between the right ventricle and pulmonary artery. Pulmonary artery branches are often hypoplastic and may be discontinuous. Echocardiographic features include overriding of a dilated aorta on a ventricular septal defect with no forward flow in the pulmonary artery and reverse flow in the ductus, which has often a more proximal insertion on the aorta than normal.

Common Arterial Trunk. In this malformation, the aorta and pulmonary artery arise from the same common trunk (Fig. 6.27). When the pulmonary

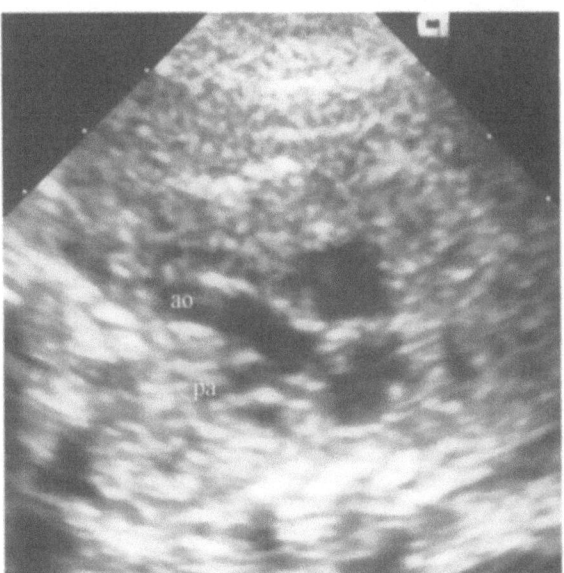

Fig. 6.27. Common arterial trunk. Aorta (*ao*) and pulmonary artery (*pa*) arise from the same common trunk

arteries are seen arising from the posterolateral aspect of the trunk, the diagnosis is straightforward. If the pulmonary arteries are difficult to visualize, the differentiation between this condition and pulmonary artery atresia with ventricular septal defect may be difficult. The truncal valve may exhibit thickening and dysplasia or regurgitation. Postnatally, if pulmonary flow is unrestricted, congestive heart failure rapidly occurs. One-stage correction is usually performed between 1 and 3 months of age and consists of closing the ventricular septal defect and the connecting pulmonary artery with the right ventricle by means of a valved conduit. Truncal valve malformation can necessitate valve repair or replacement.

Double-Outlet Right Ventricle. Double-outlet right ventricle refers to a spectrum of cardiac malforma-

tions in which the two great vessels are seen to arise for more than 50% from the right ventricle. Many different anatomical variants are described according the position of the great vessels relative to the septal defect, the presence of an aortic or pulmonary artery obstruction and the presence of left ventricular hypoplasia. The great vessels are most commonly malpositioned with the aorta right and lateral to the pulmonary artery, but other combinations are possible. Aorta and pulmonary artery may appear parallel at their origin as in transposition of the great arteries (Fig. 6.28). A discontinuity between the mitral valve and either the aortic valve (in normally related great arteries) or the pulmonary valve (in transposition of the great arteries) can be sometimes evidenced prenatally. Echocardiographic evaluation should look for a discrepancy in the great vessels that could suggest associated pulmonary stenosis or coarctation of the aorta. Ventricular septal defect is always present but the spatial relationship between the great vessels and the septal defect may be difficult to determine prenatally. Treatment of double-outlet right ventricle is surgical but the type of surgery will depend on the anatomy and physiology of the malformation as well as the age of the patient.

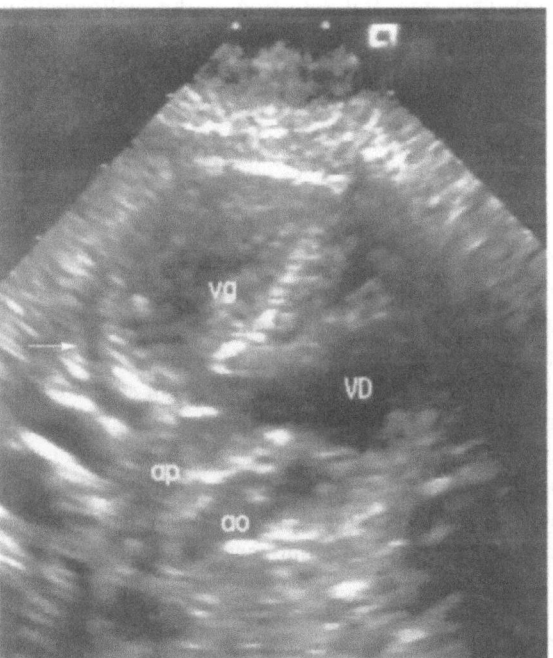

Fig. 6.28. Double-outlet right ventricle. The aorta (*ao*) and pulmonary artery (*ap*) are parallel, coming from the right ventricle (*VD*), displaying a ventricular septal defect. Left ventricle (*vg*)

6.1.3.7
Great Vessels Views: Transposition of the Great Arteries

Isolated Transposition of the Great Arteries (D-transposition). In this malformation, the aorta arises from the right ventricle and the pulmonary artery arises from the left ventricle. Consequently, the pulmonary and systemic circulations function in parallel rather than in series as in normal heart. On echocardiography, the main feature of transposition of the great arteries is the parallel orientation of the great vessels at their origin (Fig. 6.29). Thus, their crossing at the level of the semilunar valves cannot be identified. This can be seen either in the five-chamber view or in the short axis view at the level of the great vessels, where aorta and pulmonary artery appear as circular structures adjacent to each other, instead of having their normal orientation with the right ventricular outflow tract and pulmonary artery coursing around the circular aorta. The four-chamber view is often normal. A ventricular septal defect is present in 20% of cases. Before birth, transposition of the great arteries has little effect on the fetus. Dramatic changes that occur after birth resulting in profound hypoxemia may lead to rapid hemodynamic compromise and death, and require immediate prostaglandin infusion and balloon atrial septostomy (the Rashkind maneuver). Thus, prenatal detection of the malformation may improve neonatal management leading to in utero transfer of fetuses with prenatal diagnosis of transposition of the great arteries to an appropriate unit (BONNET et al. 1999). Surgical repair currently relies on the arterial switch operation, which carries an excellent post-surgical prognosis in most patients.

Corrected Transposition of the Great Arteries (L-transposition). When ventriculo-arterial discordance is associated with atrioventricular discordance, it suggests the diagnosis of corrected transposition of the great arteries. In this cardiopathy, right and left atria remain in their usual location but the morphological right ventricle is on the left and is connected to the left atrium and aorta whereas the anatomical left ventricle is on the right and is connected to the right atrium and the pulmonary artery (Fig. 6.30). On

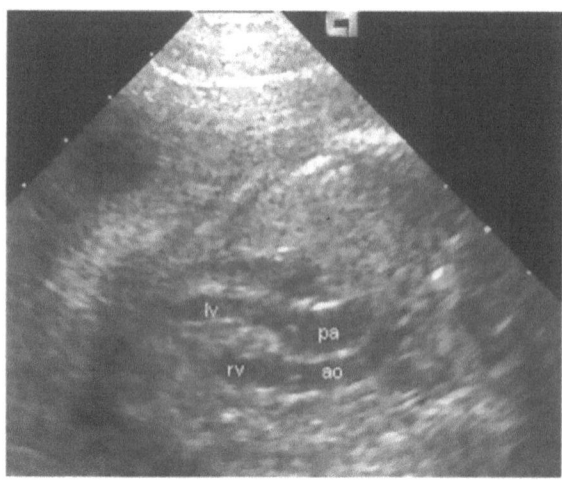

Fig. 6.29. Great arteries transposition. The pulmonary artery (*pa*) and the aorta (*ao*) are parallel and come from the left ventricle (*lv*) and right ventricle (*rv*) respectively

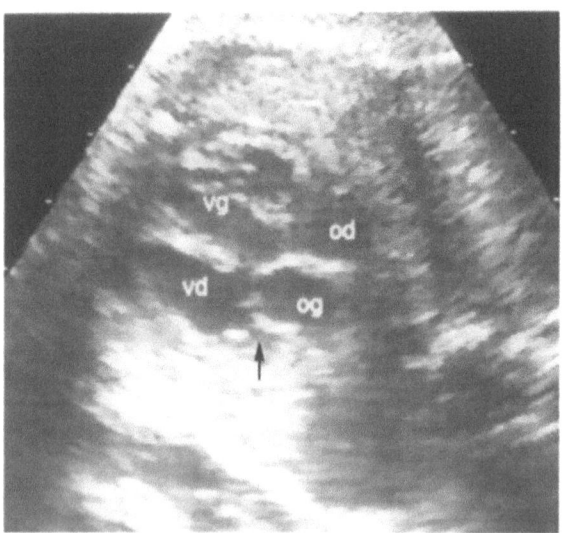

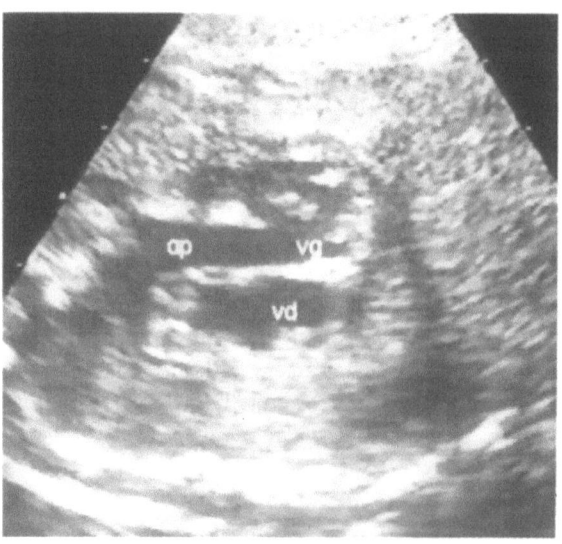

Fig. 6.30a, b. Corrected transposition of the great arteries. **a** Four-chamber view: the "left" atrioventricular valve (*arrow*) is more anterior and so is a tricuspid valve. **b** The pulmonary artery is transposed, coming from the left ventricle. Right ventricle (*vd*), left ventricle (*vg*), pulmonary artery (*ap*), right atrium (*od*), left atrium (*og*)

echocardiography the great vessels are parallel at their origin but, unlike isolated transposition, on the four-chamber view the ventricles are reversed. As a consequence, the left atrioventricular valve, that is the tricuspid valve, is more apically displaced than the right atrioventricular valve, that is the mitral valve. The left atrium is often easily recognizable thanks to the foraminal flap. Associated malformations are frequent, such as ventricular septal defect, pulmonary artery stenosis, Ebstein malformation of the tricuspid valve and atrioventricular block. Corrected transposition of the great arteries does not require surgical repair in itself but surgery may be needed for associated malformations.

6.2
Arrhythmias

Diagnosis of arrhythmias is one area in which prenatal diagnosis has clearly brought practical benefit. Abnormalities of cardiac rhythm can be diagnosed in approximately 1% of fetuses. Normal cardiac rhythm is regular between 100 and 180 beats per minute (bpm). Dysrhythmia is present when the fetal cardiac rhythm is abnormally slow (heart rate below 100 bpm sustained for more than a few minutes), abnormally fast (sustained heart rate of more than 180 bpm) or irregular. Most fetal dysrhythmias are benign and require no treatment. However, some are associated with fetal compromise which may lead to in utero or postnatal death. In such cases transplacental therapy with administration of antiarrhythmic drugs to the mother may be required. For supraventricular tachycardia, the drug of choice is digoxin, since transplacental transfer is as high as 100%. If after a week there is no effect on fetal heart rate, other drugs such as flecainide or sotalol can be added (AZANCOT BENISTY et al. 1997). However, some of these drugs are associated with fetal compromise which may lead to in utero or postnatal death.

6.2.1
Assessment of Fetal Dysrhythmias

The fetal echocardiogram provides information on the atrial rate, ventricular rate and the atrioventricular relationship, and thus allows a precise determination of the type of arrhythmia. Fetal dysrhythmias can be assessed by M-mode and pulsed Doppler tracings (BROWN 1997). Echocardiography also provides a technique to assess the hemodynamic consequences of the arrhythmia. Cardiac failure is evidenced by heart dilatation and hypocontractility, skin edema, fetal ascites, and pleural or pericardial effusion. Finally echocardiography allows detection of associated structural cardiac malformations that can be encountered in up to 15% of fetuses with persistent arrhythmias.

M-mode echocardiographic evaluation of cardiac rhythm involves simultaneous recording of atrial and ventricular contractions. Placement of the M-mode cursor is facilitated after localization of the cardiac structures by two-dimensional echocardiography. Ventricular contractions can also be inferred from the opening of the aortic valves. In pulsed Doppler, the sample volume must be placed in order to record simultaneously the left ventricular inflow and outflow signals. The five-chamber view is the most appropriate for performing the recording. The mitral A wave corresponds to atrial systole whereas left ventricular ejection flow indicates ventricular systole. In the normal heart every ventricular contraction is preceded by atrial contraction.

6.2.2
Mechanism of Fetal Dysrhythmias

6.2.2.1
Irregular Heart Rhythm

Irregular heart rhythm is one of the more common reasons for referral of fetuses for echocardiography. Isolated ectopy is more often of atrial than ventricular origin (see Fig. 6.12b). These premature beats are almost always self-limited and carry a favorable prognosis. It is possible, however, that frequent isolated atrial beats could trigger a re-entrant tachycardia. Occasionally cardiac pauses or sustained bradycardia can be produced by atrial ectopic beats occurring too close to the preceding sinus beat to allow transmission to the ventricle. These are benign arrhythmias that must be distinguished from other forms of bradycardia which carry a different prognosis. In some fetuses atrial ectopic beats can be favored by increased septum primum redundancy in the left atria (Fig. 6.31). Atrial ectopic beats commonly resolve spontaneously during late pregnancy or within the first week of life.

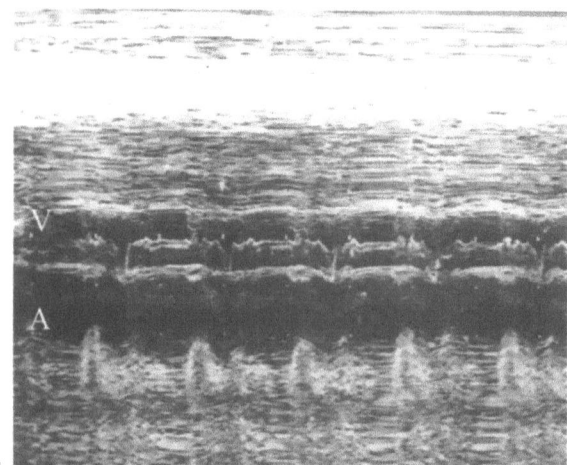

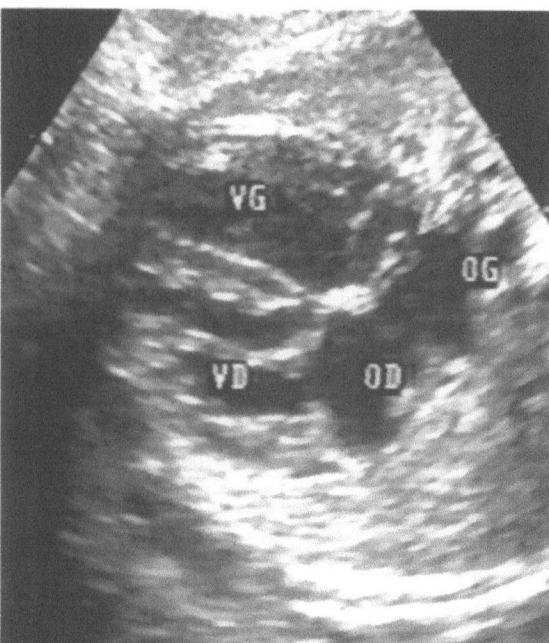

due to a heart rate variability of from 5 to 15 bpm. Sinus tachycardia can be seen in stress situation for the mother or the fetus. *Supraventricular tachycardia* is characterized by a regular tachycardia with a heart rate between 180 and 280 bpm and 1:1 atrioventricular conduction (Fig. 6.32). When intermittent, it is always of sudden onset and offset. The

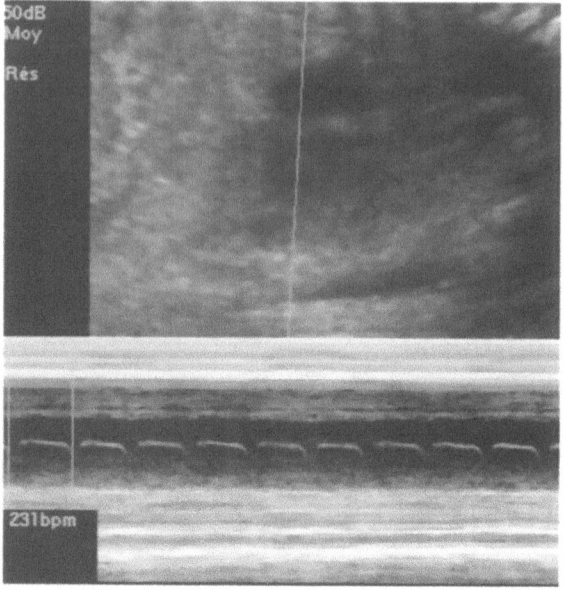

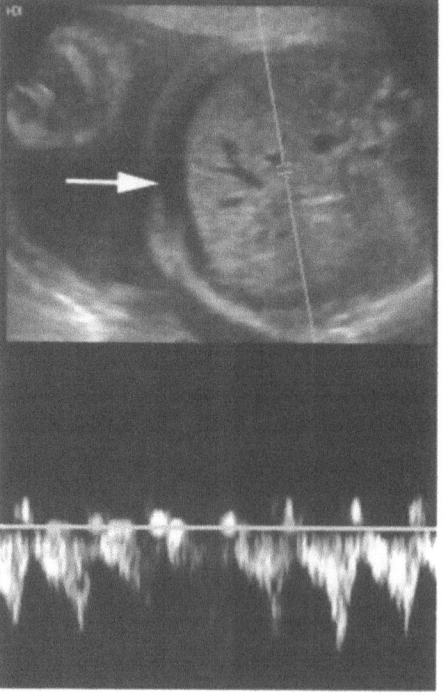

Fig. 6.31. a Atrial dysrhythmia: pseudo-bradycardia related to a blocked atrial bigeminy. **b** Increased septum primum redundancy in the left atria (*arrow*) may be the cause of atrial ectopic beats. Right ventricle (*VD*), left ventricle (*VG*), right atrium (*OD*), left atrium (*OG*)

6.2.2.2
Tachycardias

Tachycardias that have been recognized in utero include sinus tachycardia, supraventricular tachycardia, atrial flutter and ventricular tachycardia. In *sinus tachycardia* heart rate is above 180 bpm with a normal atrioventricular activation sequence. It can be differentiated from supraventricular tachycardia

Fig. 6.32a, b. Supraventricular tachycardia. **a** The heart rate is 230 bpm. **b** With ascites (*arrow*) related to heart failure

examiner should try to determine whether the bradycardia is incessant or intermittent, the latter having less serious hemodynamic effects. The fetus must be examined for signs of heart failure such as cardiac enlargement or hydrops. Supraventricular tachycardia is usually not associated with structural heart defect but such defects must be searched for since hemodynamic effects tend to be worse in fetuses with cardiac defects (Fig. 6.32b). *Atrial flutter* typically has an atrial rate of greater than 300–400 bpm with a varying degree of atrioventricular block, most commonly 2:1 atrioventricular conduction, resulting in a ventricular rate less than the atrial rate (Fig. 6.33). *Ventricular tachycardia* is rare and may be diagnosed when the ventricular rate is higher than the atrial rate with atrioventricular dissociation.

6.2.2.3
Bradycardia

Bradycardia can be of sinus origin or due to complete atrioventricular block. Transient sinus bradycardia is very common and is usually due to factors that increase vagal tone or stimulate baroreceptors, such as uterine compression during the echocardiographic examination. A persistent sinus rate less than 100 bpm is very unusual and can be seen in serious fetal compromise, in long QT syndrome, in sick sinus syndrome or in maternal beta-blocker therapy. Blocked atrial bigeminy must be considered in the differential diagnosis (see Fig. 6.31). Complete atrioventricular block is the most common cause of sinus bradycardia (Fig. 6.34). It manifests as a slow ventricular rate with a faster atrial rate.

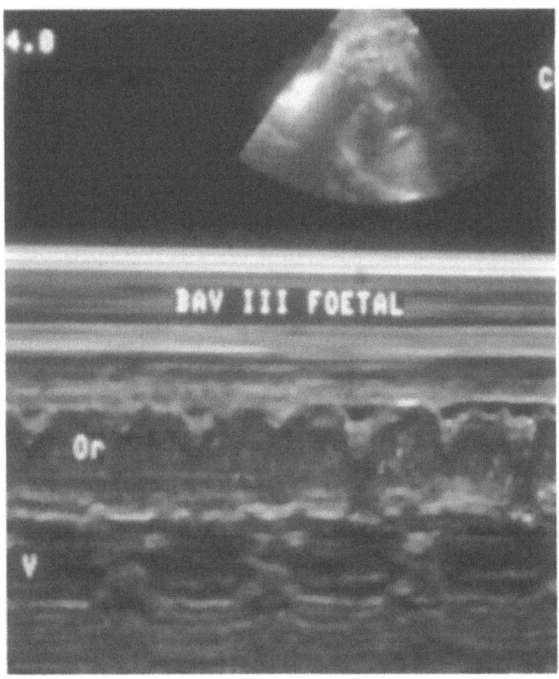

Fig. 6.34. Complete atrioventricular block. Ventricle (*V*), atrium (*Or*)

Complete atrioventricular block can be isolated or associated with structural heart disease such as corrected transposition of the great arteries or atrioventricular septal defect. Isolated complete atrioventricular block is frequently associated with the presence of anti-Ro (SSA) or anti-La (SSB) antibody, either isolated or associated with maternal collagen vascular disease such as Sjögren syndrome, systemic lupus erythematosus or rheumatoid arthritis.

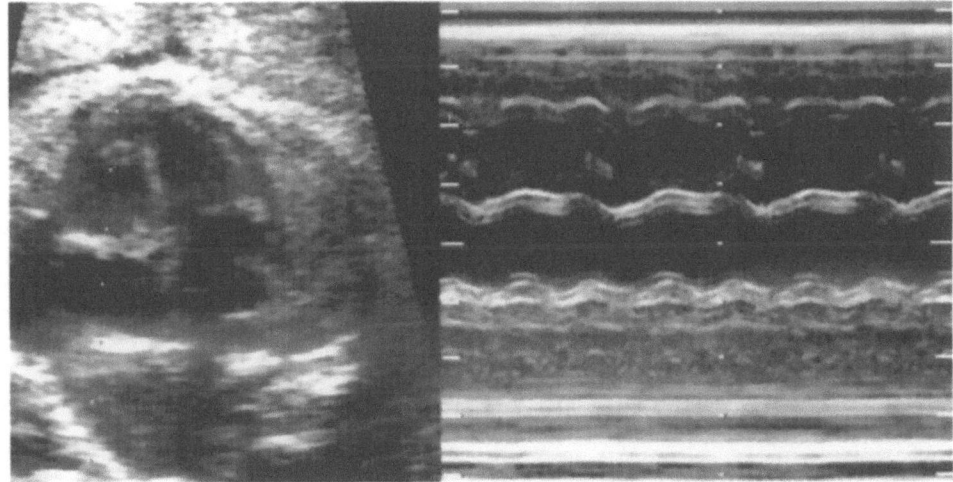

Fig. 6.33. Atrial flutter (commonly 2:1 atrioventricular conduction)

References

Abdullah MM, Lacro RV, Smallhorn J, Chitayat D, Van Der Velde ME, Yoo SJ, Oman-Ganes L, Hornberger LK (2000) Fetal cardiac dextroposition in the absence of an intrathoracic mass: sign of significant right lung hypoplasia. J Ultrasound Med 19:699–676

Allan LD (1997) Sonographic detection of parallel great arteries in the fetus. AJR Am J Roentgenol 168:1283–1286

Allan LD, Joseph MC, Boyd EGCA, et al (1982) M-mode echocardiography in the developing human fetus. Br Heart J 47:573–583

Allan LD, Sharland GK, Milburn A, et al (1994) Prospective diagnosis of 1,006 consecutive cases of congenital heart disease in the fetus. J Am Coll Cardiol 23:1453–1458

Anderson RH, McCartney FJ, Shinebourne EA, Tynan M (eds) (1987) Tricuspid atresia. In: Pediatric cardiology. Churchill Livingstone, Edinburgh, pp 675–697

Azancot Benisty A, Areias JC, Oberhansli I, Schmidt KG, Tulzer G, Viart P (1997) Protocole européen pour la prise en charge des tachycardies supraventriculaires foetales. Arch Mal Coeur 90:735–742

Bonnet D, Coltri A, Gianfranco B, Fermont L, Le Bidois J, Kachaner J, Sidi D (1999) Detection of transposition of the great arteries in the fetus reduces neonatal morbidity and mortality. Circulation 99:916–918

Brown DL (1997) Sonographic assessment of fetal arrhythmias. AJR Am J Roentgenol 169:1029–1033

Brown DL, Disalvo DN, Frates MC, Doubilet PM, Benson CB, Laing, FC, Parness IA (1993) Sonography of the fetal heart: normal variants and pitfalls. AJR Am J Roentgenol 160:1251–1255

Driscoll DJ, Offord KP, Feldt RH, Schaff HV, Puga FJ, Danielson GK (1992) Five to fifteen-year follow-up after Fontan operation. Circulation 85:469–496

Drose JA, Dennis MA, Thickman D (1991) Infection in utero: US findings in 19 cases. Radiology 178:369–374

Fermont L, De Geeter B, Aubry J, et al (1986) A close collaboration between obstetricians and pediatric cardiologists allow detection of severe cardiac malformations by 2D echocardiography. In: Doyle EF, Engle ME, Gersony WM et al (eds) Pediatric cardiology: proceedings of the second world congress. Springer, Berlin Heidelberg New York, pp 34–37

Harth JY, Paul MH, Gallen WJ, et al (1973) Experimental production of hypoplastic left heart syndrome in the chicken embryo. Am J Cardiol 31:51–56

Hoffman JIE, Christianson R (1978) Congenital heart disease in a cohort of 19,502 births with long-term follow-up. Am J Cardiol 42:641–645

Machado MVL, Crawford DC, Anderson RH, et al (1988) Atrioventricular septal defect in the prenatal life. Br Heart J 59:352–355

Montana E, Khoury MJ, Cragan JD, et al (1996) Trends and outcomes after prenatal diagnosis of congenital cardiac malformations by fetal echocardiography in a well defined birth population, Atlanta, Georgia, 1990–1994. J Am Coll Cardiol 28:1805–1809

Nyberg DA, Souter VL (2001) Sonographic markers of fetal trisomies. Second trimester. J Ultrasound Med 20:655–674

O'Laughlin MP (1997) Catheter closure of secundum atrial septal defect. Tex Heart Inst J 24:287–292

Sharland GK, Chita SK, Fagg N, et al (1991) Left ventricular dysfunction in the fetus: relationship to aortic valve anomalies and endocardial fibroelastosis. Br Heart J 66:219–224

Tworetzky W, McElhinney, Reddy M, Brook M, Hanley FL, Silverman N (2001) Improved surgical outcome after diagnosis of hypoplastic left heart syndrome. Circulation 103:1269–1273

Way GI, Wolfe RR, Eshaghpour E, et al (1979) The natural history of hypertrophic cardiomyopathy in infants of diabetic mothers. J Paediatr 95:1025–1029

Yoo SJ, Lee YH, Kim ES, Ryu HM, Kim MY, Yang JH, Chun YK, Hong SR (1999a) Tetralogy of Fallot in the fetus: findings at targeted sonography. Ultrasound Obstet Gynecol 14: 29–37

Yoo SJ, Lee YH, Cho KS (1999b) Abnormal three-vessel view on sonography: a clue to the diagnosis of congenital heart disease in the fetus. AJR Am J Roentgenol 172:825–830

7 Abdomen (Digestive Tract, Wall and Peritoneum)

Josée Dubois and Andrée Grignon

CONTENTS

7.1   Abdominal Wall Defects   125
7.1.1   Introduction   125
7.2   Embryology   126
7.3   Omphaloceles   126
7.3.1   Definition   126
7.3.2   Causes   127
7.3.3   Related Factors   127
7.3.4   US Findings   127
7.3.5   Associated Anomalies   128
7.3.6   Management   129
7.3.7   Prognosis   129
7.4   Pentalogy of Cantrell   130
7.4.1   Definition   130
7.4.2   Cause   130
7.4.3   US Findings   130
7.4.4   Associated Anomalies   130
7.4.5   Prognosis   130
7.4.6   Management   131
7.5   Gastroschisis   131
7.5.1   Definition   131
7.5.2   Cause   131
7.5.3   US Findings   131
7.5.4   Associated Anomalies   132
7.5.5   Management   132
7.5.6   US Follow-up   132
7.5.7   Prognosis   133
7.6   Limb-Body Wall Complex   134
7.6.1   Definition   134
7.6.2   Cause   134
7.6.3   US Findings   134
7.6.4   Associated Anomalies   135
7.6.5   Management   135
7.7   Amniotic Band Syndrome   135
7.7.1   Definition   135
7.7.2   Cause   135
7.7.3   US Findings   135
7.7.4   Associated Anomalies   135
7.7.5   Management   136
7.7.6   Prognosis   136
7.8   Bladder Exstrophy   136
7.8.1   Definition   136
7.8.2   Cause   136
7.8.3   US Findings   136
7.8.4   Associated Anomalies   136
7.8.5   Prognosis   136

7.9   Cloacal Exstrophy   136
7.9.1   Definition and Cause   136
7.9.2   US Findings   136
7.9.3   Associated Anomalies   136
7.9.4   Management   137
7.9.5   Prognosis   137
7.10   Gastrointestinal Tract Anomalies   138
7.10.1 Normal Development, Echoanatomy
        and Physiology   138
7.11   Foregut Pathology   138
7.11.1 Introduction   138
7.11.2 Absence of Visualization of the Stomach   139
7.11.3 Esophageal Atresia   139
7.11.4 Gastric Outlet Obstruction   140
7.11.5 Duodenal Obstruction   140
7.11.6 Duodenal Atresia   141
7.11.7 Small Bowel Pathology   141
7.11.7.1 Echogenic Small Bowel   141
7.11.7.2 Echogenic Dilated Bowel Loops   142
7.11.7.3 Small Bowel Atresia   143
7.11.7.4 Meconium Peritonitis   145
7.11.8 Large Bowel Pathology   146
7.11.8.1 Anorectal Atresia   146
7.11.8.2 Megacystis-Microcolon-Hypoperistalsis
          Syndrome   146
7.11.9 Complementary Studies   146
7.11.10 Postnatal Outcome   146
7.12   Intraperitoneal Masses and Calcifications   146
7.12.1 Abdominal Calcifications   146
7.12.1.1 Meconium Peritonitis and Pseudocyst   147
7.12.1.2 Vascular Calcifications   147
7.12.2 Peritoneal Tumors   147
7.12.2.1 Organomegaly   147
7.12.2.2 Cystic Tumors   147
7.12.2.3 Mixed-Pattern Tumors   147
7.12.2.4 Cystic Lesions   148
          References   149

J. Dubois, MD; A. Grignon, MD
Department of Medical Imaging, Sainte-Justine Hospital, 3175
Côte-Sainte-Catherine, Montréal, Québec H3T 1C5, Canada

7.1
Abdominal Wall Defects

7.1.1
Introduction

The detection and categorization of abdominal wall defects by sonographic examination are challenging problems. A correct diagnosis is mandatory because of its impact on fetal intervention, parental counseling and optimal perinatal management.

This chapter will emphasize key features and practical points that a sonographer has to know concerning the diagnosis of abdominal wall defects. When the diagnosis is made, the pathology, management and outcome must be clearly understood, with particular comprehension of the complications occurring in early infancy. This information allows for more up-to-date and effective counseling of parents of a fetus identified before birth as having such a defect. We will mention only the important aspects of embryology that are vital for diagnosis and we will review the pitfalls.

What to Look for in Abdominal Wall Defects

First Step: To Determine the Location of the Defect and the Relationship of Cord Insertion to the Defect

A. Midline defect:
  1. Cord insertion at the apex of the defect: omphalocele
  2. Defect above the cord insertion: Ectopia cordis, pentalogy of Cantrell.
B. Lateral defect:
  1. Right sided para-umbilical location: Gastroschisis
  2. Large: Limb-body wall complex, amniotic band syndrome.
C. Defect below the cord insertion: Bladder exstrophy, cloacal exstrophy.

Second Step: To Determine Whether the Herniated Content is Covered by a Membrane

A. Covered by a membrane: Omphalocele, pentalogy of Cantrell, ectopia cordis.
B. Not covered: Gastroschisis, amniotic band syndrome, limb-body wall complex.

Third step: To Identify the Eviscerated Organ

Bowel, stomach: Gastroschisis.
Liver: Omphalocele.
Heart: Pentalogy of Cantrell.
Bladder: No visualization = bladder exstrophy.

Fourth step: To Look for Associated Anomalies

Most associated anomalies are related to the gastro-intestinal system, genitourinary system, central nervous system, to the face and skeletal system. But some associated anomalies are more specific:
- Scoliosis: In limb-body wall complex.
- Cleft and cephalocele with gastroschisis: Amniotic band syndrome.
- Heart: Pentalogy of Cantrell.

7.2
Embryology

The most important feature to remember is that by approximately 12 menstrual weeks in a normal fetus, the bowel returns to the abdomen. According to this sequence, anterior abdominal wall defects cannot be reliably diagnosed until 12 menstrual weeks (GRAY et al. 1989). If a defect is suspected at this time, the examination should be repeated at 14 menstrual weeks.

Another embryological concept to keep in mind is the fusion of the amniotic and chorionic membranes. The amniotic cavity continues to expand and eventually obliterates the extraembryonic coelom at about 12 menstrual weeks. Persistence of this space is typical for the limb-body wall complex, but the amnion and chorion can remain separated in a normal fetus, even to term (SPIRT and GORDON 1991).

7.3
Omphaloceles

7.3.1
Definition

Omphaloceles occur in 1 in 4,000 live births (NYBERG and MARK 1990). The prevalence is reported to be similar to that of gastroschisis, at 2.5 in 10,000 births, with a male to female ratio of 1:1. Unlike gastroschisis, omphalocele is reported in older mothers. It is a herniation of the abdominal contents into the base of the umbilical cord (Fig. 7.1). The herniated mass is covered by the parietal peritoneum and the amnion, with Wharton's jelly intervening between the two membrane layers.

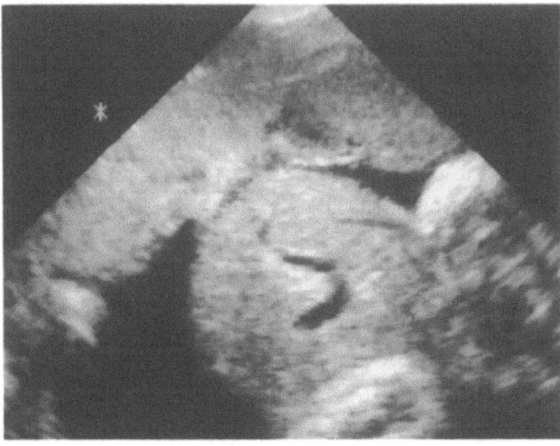

Fig. 7.1. Seventeen weeks of gestation. Transverse scan. Omphalocele with liver herniation

c) Contents:

Typically, omphalocele is represented by a liver herniation (Figs. 7.1, 7.2).

Atypically, omphalocele content is the bowel alone (Fig. 7.3).

Small bowel: more hyperechogenic than the liver. The umbilical vein turns around the eviscerated organ (Fig. 7.4).

Strongly associated with an abnormal karyotype (NYBERG et al. 1989, NICOLAIDES et al. 1992).

d) We divide omphaloceles into giant omphaloceles and ordinary omphaloceles according to the ratio of the transverse diameter of the omphalocele to the transverse diameter of the abdomen.

7.3.2
Causes

- For those containing liver: failure to migrate of the lateral body fold that normally surrounds the abdominal contents at 5–6 weeks (SEASHORE 1978).
- For those containing bowel: persistence of the primitive body stalk with failure of the bowel to return to the abdomen after 12 menstrual weeks (NYBERG and MARK 1990).

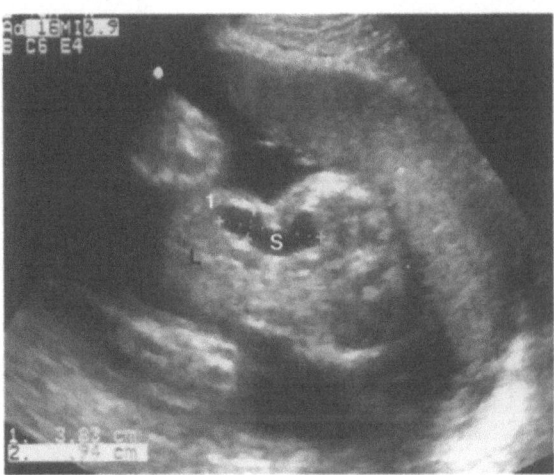

Fig. 7.2. Eighteen weeks of gestation. Transverse scan. Classical omphalocele containing the liver (*L*) and stomach (*S*)

7.3.3
Related Factors

- Higher incidence with increased maternal age (NYBERG et al. 1989).
- Associated chromosomal abnormalities.
- Elevated maternal serum alpha-fetoprotein (AFP).
- Positive acetylcholinesterase (BAIR et al. 1986).

7.3.4
US Findings

a) Position of the umbilical cord: Defect located centrally; cord insertion forms the apex of the defect.

b) Membrane: Eviscerated organs are separated from the surrounding amniotic fluid by a membrane.

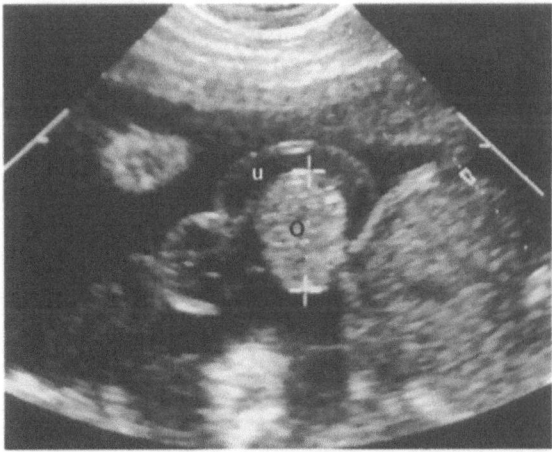

Fig. 7.3. Nineteen weeks of gestation. Transverse section. Small atypical omphalocele (*O*) surrounded by the umbilical cord (*U*)

A giant omphalocele has a ratio over or equal to 0.95 (Fig. 7.4), while an ordinary omphalocele is defined by a ratio that is less than 0.95 (Fig. 7.5).

In the literature, omphaloceles are characterized by the ratio of the herniated mass to the transverse abdominal diameter. When the ratio is less than 60%, the omphalocele is believed to contain only bowel because those that contain liver have a relatively larger defect compared with the abdominal diameter (ROMANO et al. 1988).

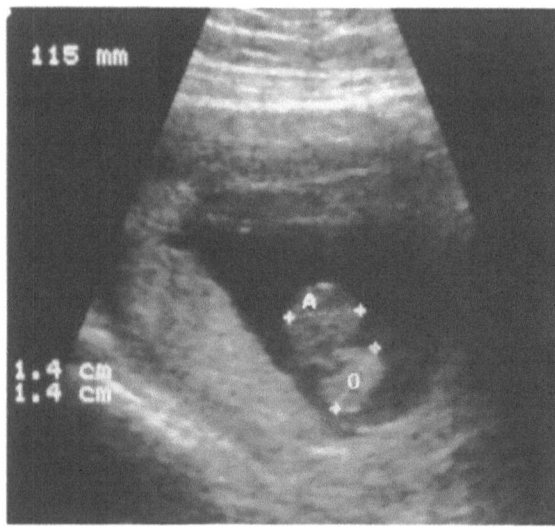

Fig. 7.4. Fifteen weeks of gestation. Giant omphalocele. Abdomen (*A*), omphalocele (*O*)

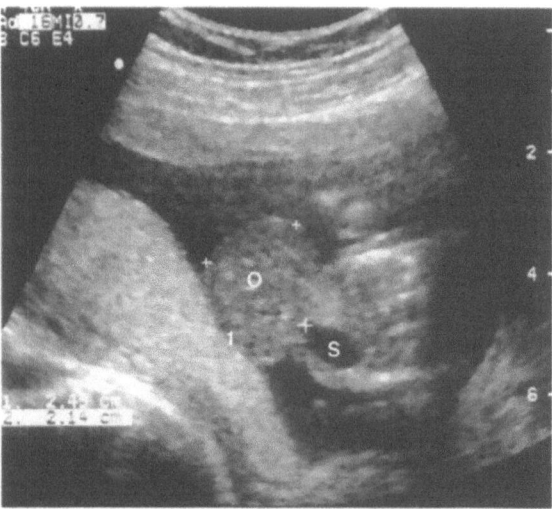

Fig. 7.5. Fifteen weeks of gestation. Transverse abdominal section. Classical giant omphalocele (*O*). Stomach (*S*)

7.3.5
Associated Anomalies

- Can be found in 50–88% of cases (NYBERG and MARK 1990, SEASHORE 1978, NYBERG et al. 1989, MAYER et al. 1980, SCHWAITZBERG et al. 1982, KNIGHT et al. 1981).
- Intestinal atresia.
- Abnormal fixation of the bowel resulting in malrotation.
- Cardiac anomalies (50%) include: ventricular septal defects; atrial septal defects; tetralogy of Fallot; coarctation of the aorta, bicuspid aortic valve; transposition of the great vessels (CRAWFORD et al., 1985, GREENWOOD et al. 1974); association with ectopia cordis and pentalogy of Cantrell.
- Genitourinary: 23% (HUGHES et al. 1989).
- Central nervous system: 27% (HUGHES et al. 1989).
- Gastrointestinal: diaphragmatic hernia; duplication, atresia, ascites; tracheoesophageal fistula; imperforate anus; malrotation.
- Skeletal: 35% (HUGHES et al. 1989).
- Non-gastrointestinal: clubfoot, single umbilical artery, pentalogy of Cantrell, etc.
- Chromosomal abnormalities: 40%–60% (HUGHES et al. 1989, GILBERT and NICOLAIDES 1987):
  - high rate of trisomy 18 (GILBERT and NICOLAIDES 1987);
  - more common if only the small bowel is involved (NYBERG and MARK 1990); most common chromosomal aberrations include trisomy 18 or 13 (NYBERG et al. 1989);
  - also, trisomy 21 with Turner's, Klinefelter's and triploidy syndromes (NYBERG et al. 1989, KNIGHT et al. 1981, GILBERT et al. 1987).
- Beckwith-Wiedemann syndrome: found in 5–10% of infants born with omphalocele (NYBERG et al. 1989).

   Definition: The incidence is 1 in 13,700 live births. It is usually sporadic, but familial occurrence is possible (OSUNA and LINDHAM 1976). Partial duplication of chromosome 11p has been found (WAZIRI et al. 1983). This syndrome consists of the omphalocele, visceromegaly, macroglossia and neonatal hypoglycemia (Fig. 7.6).
   Associated anomalies: Cardiac abnormalities.
   Prognosis: 10% develop malignant tumor in childhood including Wilms' tumor, hepatoblastomas and adrenal tumors (SOTELO-AVILA and GOOCH 1976). Mild to moderate mental deficiency.

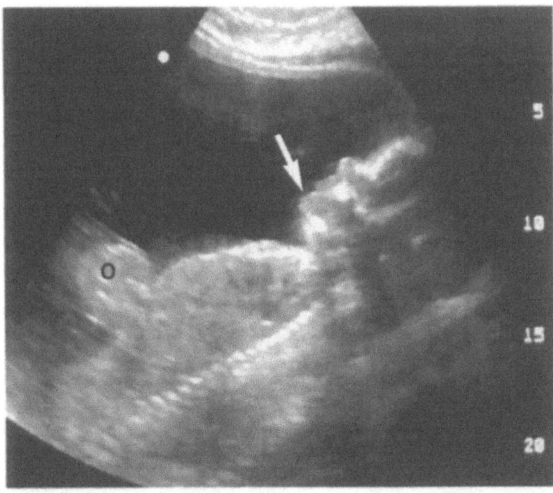

Fig. 7.6. Thirty-eight weeks of gestation. Sagittal section. Omphalocele (*O*) and macroglossia (*arrow*) in a case of Beckwith-Wiedemann syndrome

7.3.6
Management

- Antenatal:
  search for associated anomalies
  echocardiography
  karyotype
  US follow-up
  amniotic fluid: polyhydramnios is noted in
  approximately one-third of fetuses with
  omphalocele (HUGHES et al. 1989, VAN DE
  GEIJN et al. 1991).
- Perinatal:
  delivery in a tertiary care center
  cesarean section is not justified.
- Postnatal: BOYD et al. (1998) reported that 93% of
  born omphaloceles had no long-term problems.

7.3.7
Prognosis

The size of the defect affects the morbidity rate and surgical management but has no direct correlation with the mortality rate. Severe anomalies are responsible for 80–100% of deaths.

The prognosis depends on the presence and severity of the associated anomalies. Death occurs in 10% of cases if there are no other anomalies (MAYER et al. 1980). Mortality increases to 80% for infants with one or more concurrent malformations and to nearly

100% for those with chromosomal or cardiovascular abnormalities (MAYER et al. 1980).

Sepsis and surgical complications occur in 1–10%. There is less than a 1% recurrence risk associated with omphaloceles (MAYER et al. 1980, KNIGHT et al. 1981; HUGHES et al. 1989).

In our series of 73 fetuses with omphalocele diagnosed by second trimester US, we noted 43 ordinary omphaloceles and 30 giant omphaloceles. Sixty-four typical omphaloceles with liver included 34 ordinary and 30 giant omphaloceles compared with nine atypical omphaloceles with bowel alone. Associated anomalies were found in 34 of 43 (80%) ordinary omphaloceles compared with 12 of 30 (40%) giant omphaloceles. Most of the fetuses also had cardiac anomalies and we observed nine cases with Beckwith-Wiedemann syndrome. Chromosomal anomalies were detected in 14% of ordinary omphaloceles and 10% of giant omphaloceles.

It is noteworthy to outline that in cases of atypical omphalocele consisting of bowel alone, five of nine (55%) had chromosomal anomalies.

Regarding the outcome in our series:
- thirty terminations of pregnancy: 13 ordinary omphaloceles and 17 giant omphaloceles.
- three in utero deaths: one ordinary omphalocele and two giant omphaloceles.
- eleven neonatal deaths: seven ordinary omphaloceles and four giant omphaloceles.
- twenty-nine live babies: 22 ordinary omphaloceles and seven giant omphaloceles including the four atypical omphaloceles with normal karyotype.

Why did fetuses die during the neonatal period? In giant omphaloceles, we observed respiratory distress and other pulmonary problems directly related to the volume of the hernia. In seven ordinary omphaloceles, death was related to respiratory distress, cardiopathy, intestinal perforation, renal insufficiency, peritonitis and prematurity with encephalomalacia.

What happened to the survivors? Duration of hospitalization was quite acceptable, with a mean of 13 days for ordinary omphalocele and 34 for giant omphalocele. With new surgical techniques, the number of surgeries per patient was less than before and the hospital stay was decreased. However, we still have to deal with associated anomalies such as Beckwith-Wiedemann syndrome and cardiopathy that are responsible for longer hospitalization in our series.

When we compared our results with the literature, the overall incidence of associated anomalies was lower (38% versus 67%) but the incidence of cardiac abnormalities was similar. Chromosomal aberrations were less frequent than in the literature: 12% versus 30–40%.

Prognostic predictors and corresponding management were the same in our series as in the literature. Ordinary omphalocele is the most frequent. Once chromosomal and associated anomalies have been ruled out, approximately 44% of babies survive without sequelae. Cardiopathy is still the most important associated abnormality. In comparison, giant omphalocele carries high mortality and morbidity in the perinatal period. For atypical omphalocele, once chromosomal anomalies have been excluded, the evolution is favorable.

In conclusion, in the presence of a fetus with an omphalocele, the predictors of a poor prognosis have to be identified, namely chromosomal and associated abnormalities. It must be explained to parents that giant omphalocele is associated with higher mortality and morbidity. New surgical techniques permit less invasive surgery and reduce hospitalization time.

7.4
Pentalogy of Cantrell

7.4.1
Definition

Pentalogy of Cantrell represents a unique association of omphalocele and ectopia cordis (SEASHORE 1978) with diaphragmatic defects, pericardial defects and cardiovascular malformations. The other defects are interposed between the heart and omphalocele: defects of the lower sternum, anterior diaphragm and diaphragmatic pericardium (CRAWFORD et al. 1985, GHIDINI et al. 1988, TOYAMA 1972).

7.4.2
Cause

This defect is secondary to the failure of the lateral body folds to fuse in the thoracic region with variable extension inferiorly that forms at 28–32 menstrual days. The transverse septum that gives rise to the central tendon of the diaphragm does not form and the ventromedial migration of the paired upper abdominal mesodermal folds fails to occur (GHIDINI et al. 1988).

7.4.3
US Findings

Upper abdominal defect (Fig. 7.7):
- Omphalocele is more cephalad than usual.
- Contents: bowel, heart, liver covered by a translucent membrane.
- Ectopia of the heart: simple bulge out of the chest or complete exteriorization.

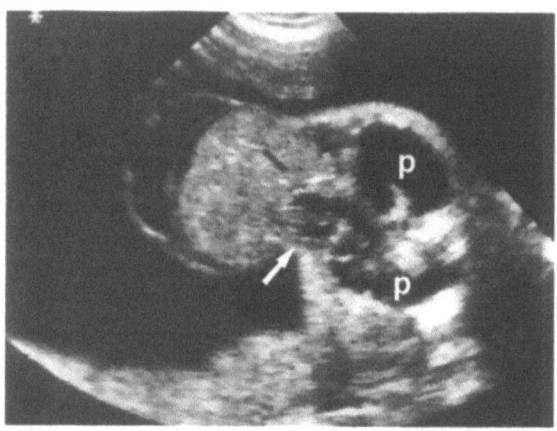

Fig. 7.7. Ectopia cordis. Transverse section. The omphalocele is more cephalad with partial exteriorization of the heart (*arrow*). Pleural effusion (*p*) is present

7.4.4
Associated Anomalies

- Omphalocele.
- Cardiovascular: atrial septal defect (50%), ventricular septal defect (20%), tetralogy of Fallot (10%) (GHIDINI et al. 1988).
- Craniofacial: cleft lip, microphthalmia, low-set ears.
- Others: kyphoscoliosis, vertebral anomalies, clinodactyly, two-vessel cord, ascites.
- Chromosomal abnormalities: usually trisomies 13 and 18 (Fox et al. 1988).

7.4.5
Prognosis

- Mortality: high (BAIR et al. 1986).
- Surgical repair: SILES et al. (1996) reported three cases in which the outcome was favorable despite the occurrence of multiple structural congenital abnormalities in this condition. Prenatal counseling should reflect this fact.

7.4.6
Management

- Antenatal (diagnosis made at mid-second trimester):
  Karyotyping
  Echocardiography
  Search for other anomalies
  In our hospital: therapeutic abortion was performed in all cases except one.
- Postnatal:
  Vaginal delivery or cesarean
  Tertiary center.

7.5
Gastroschisis

7.5.1
Definition

Gastroschisis is a para-umbilical abdominal wall defect with small bowel herniation into the amniotic cavity. The prevalence is 1 in 4,000 live births, the same as for omphalocele (NYBERG and MARK 1990). It is sporadic with no genetic association and no recurrence risk. A few cases of familial occurrence have been reported (MOORE and PERSAUD 1998).

Male predominance is seen (TIBBOEL et al. 1985). Young maternal age, maternal cigarette and cocaine use, and medications with vasoactive properties are associated with an increased risk of gastroschisis.

7.5.2
Cause

Many hypotheses have been proposed. One vascular hypothesis suggests an area of weakness caused by the normal involution of the right umbilical vein (PERRELLA et al. 1991). Disruption of the omphalomesenteric artery produces ischemic damage to the abdominal wall and subsequent herniation (HOYME et al. 1981).

7.5.3
US Findings (Figs. 7.8–7.11)

- Normal umbilical cord insertion.
- Defect almost always on the right.
- No membrane.
- Content: small bowel.
- Occasionally, the stomach or other organs may be herniated.

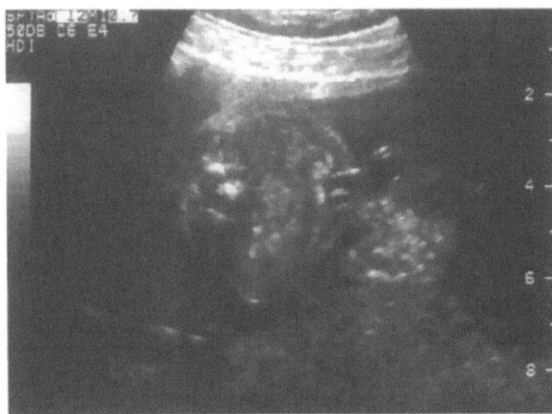

Fig. 7.8. Twenty-four weeks of gestation. Transverse section. Gastroschisis with normal insertion of the cord

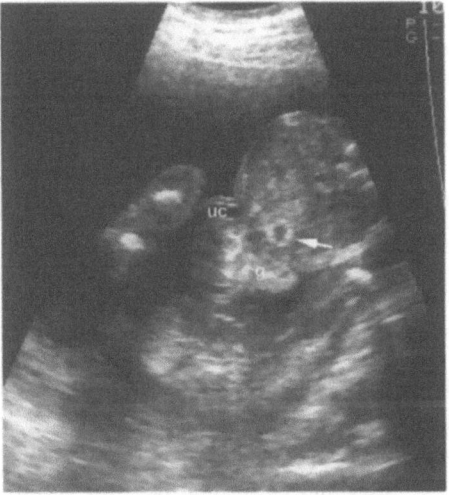

Fig. 7.9. Sixteen weeks of gestation. Atypical gastroschisis (*g*) with normal insertion of umbilical cord (*uc*), complicated by echogenic dilated bowel loops (*arrow*)

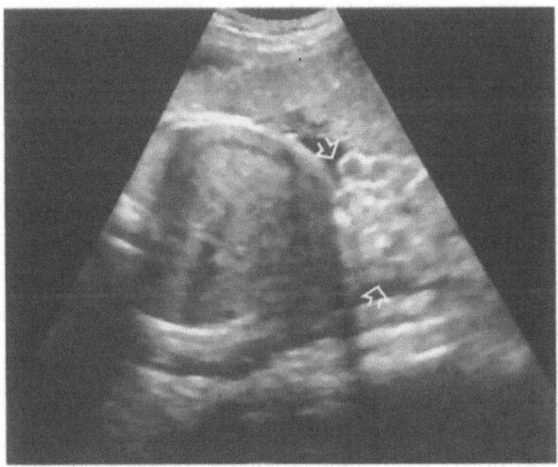

Fig. 7.10. Thirty weeks of gestation. Transverse section. Uncomplicated gastroschisis (*arrows*) with normal intestinal caliber

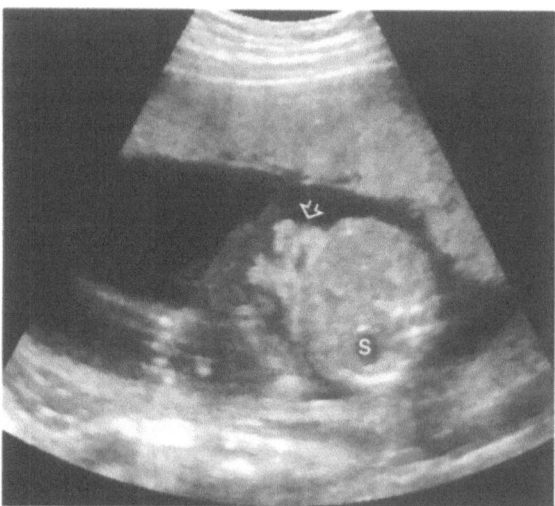

Fig. 7.11. Sixteen weeks of gestation. Transverse section. Classical gastroschisis (*arrow*). Stomach (*s*)

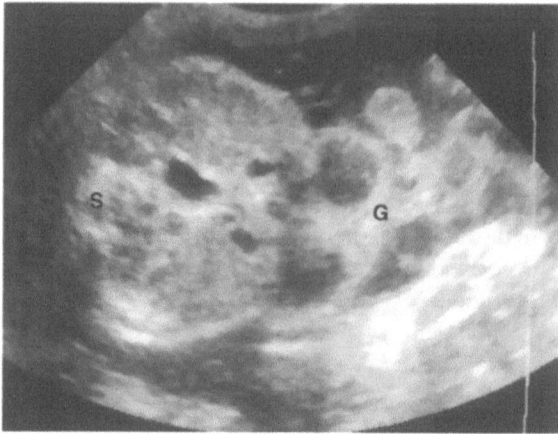

Fig. 7.12. Thirty-five weeks of gestation. Transverse section. Large uncomplicated gastroschisis (*G*). Spine (*S*)

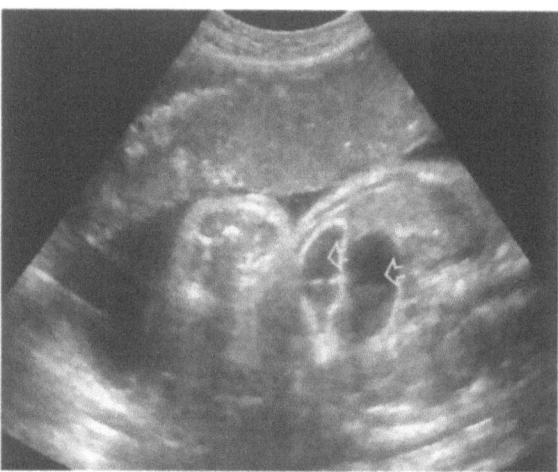

Fig. 7.13. Twenty-eight weeks of gestation. Transverse abdominal scan. Complicated gastroschisis with dilatation of intra-abdominal bowel loops (*arrows*)

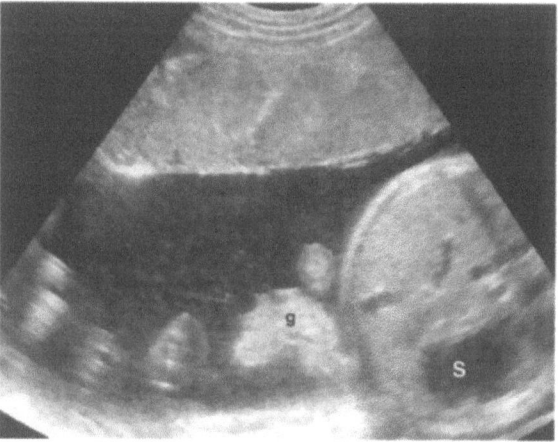

Fig. 7.14. Thirty-four weeks of gestation. Abdominal transverse section. Complicated gastroschisis (*g*) without exteriorized bowel. Stomach (*S*)

7.5.4
Associated Anomalies

Seven to thirty percent (deVries 1980).

- Gastrointestinal abnormalities: related to bowel herniation (20–40%) (Nicolaides et al. 1992, Mayer et al. 1980, Di Lorenzo et al., 1987, Novotny et al. 1993): malrotation or nonrotation; stenosis or atresia secondary to chemical irritation; ischemia; hypoperistalsis.
- Extra-gastrointestinal abnormalities (not significant compared with omphalocele): congenital heart disease, atrial septal defect, ectopia cordis; diaphragmatic hernia; scoliosis; syndactyly; amniotic bands; anencephaly; cleft lip/palate (Redford et al. 1985, Sermer et al. 1987).
- Chromosomal abnormalities: usually not seen.

7.5.5
Management

Antenatal: no karyotyping needed.

7.5.6
US Follow-up (Figs. 7.12–7.15)

- >28 weeks
  a) Bowel dilatation. When the bowel is dilated either >10 mm (small bowel) or >17 mm (colon) in diameter there is a significant risk

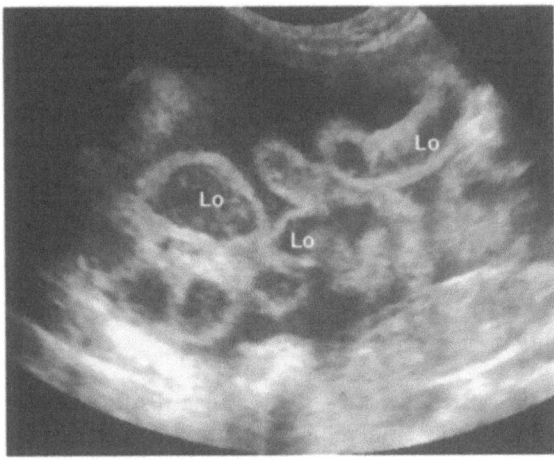

Fig. 7.15. Thirty-six weeks of gestation. Transverse section. Large gastroschisis. Harmonious dilatation of intestinal loops (*Lo*)

f) Screening for intrauterine growth retardation (IUGR). Present in 20–50% with a frequent overestimation due to the small fetal abdomen.

g) Evidence of bowel thickening, as well as other herniated organs, may indicate a less favorable outcome (TIBBOEL et al. 1986).

h) Preterm labor. Occurs in one-third of cases. The bowel develops a fibrous coating which manifests as diffuse thickening when in contact with the amniotic fluid (MAYER et al. 1980, MOLENAAR and TIBBOEL 1993).

i) Polyhydramnios or oligohydramnios (BAIR et al. 1986, CRAWFORD et al. 1992).

j) Sonographic pitfalls. Normal colon may be prominent in diameter. Normal mesentery may create the appearance of a thickened bowel. Also, the intestinal dilatation is frequently transient, as shown by the variable dilatation of the bowel in cases of gastroschisis followed sonographically at 8-h intervals (unpublished data).

for neonatal complications, including delayed enteral feeding, prolonged hospital stay and surgical complications (PRYDE et al. 1994).
Other authors conversely comment on the poor interobserver correlation of abnormal bowel findings, and even disagree with the prognostic predictive value of bowel dilatation (BABCOOK et al. 1994, ALSULYMAN et al. 1996).

b) Asymmetric bowel dilatation. Intra-abdominal dilatation associated with normal extra-abdominal bowel and regression of bowel dilatation during the third trimester carry a high morbidity. In our series of 76 cases of fetal gastroschisis, the pattern of intra-abdominal bowel dilatation and normal extra-abdominal bowel was predictive of short bowel syndrome (80%) (Fig. 7.12).

c) Size of wall defect: No associated morbidity is seen (BOND et al. 1988).

d) Ischemic intestine. Sonographic indicators:
   - thickening of the herniated bowel loops over 3 mm: BOND et al.(1988) found higher postnatal morbidity in these cases
   - polyhydramnios
   - abdominal calcifications
   - meconium cysts: sign of abdominal perforation.

e) Doppler. The pulsatility index of the superior mesenteric artery has been evaluated and reported as being without predictive value for normal outcome or complications (ABUHAMAD et al. 1997).

- Perinatal management:
   - Mode of delivery is controversial (FITZSIMMONS et al. 1988, LENKE and HATCH 1986, GRUNDY et al. 1988)
   - Some authors favor cesarean section (FITZSIMMONS et al. 1988, LENKE and HATCH 1986)
   - Delivery should take place in a tertiary care center.

7.5.7
Prognosis

The survival rate is 80–90%. If no complications occur, the survival rate even approaches 100%. In our series of 76 fetal gastroschises, no chromosomal anomalies were detected. All children were born alive with a mean birth weight of 2,450 g. Five patients died: three from short bowel syndrome, one from respiratory distress and one from intestinal necrosis. Thirty-seven (49%) patients had postnatal complications with a mean hospital stay of 102 days. The complications were ileus (n=37), bowel atresia (n=12) and short bowel (n=5). The overall mortality rate was five of 76 (6%), and the morbidity rate was 37 of 76 (49%). Our morbidity rate (49%) is higher than that reported in the literature (7%).

In accordance with the literature, because of better management and nutrition, especially with infants weighing >2,500 g, the mortality rate has been reduced to less than 10%.

Premature delivery is a more critical factor in determining overall complications. Sepsis and bowel ischemia are the most important complications and the cause of neonatal death. Mean hospital stay has been reported to be 20 days (FITZSIMMONS et al. 1988).

BOYD et al. (1998) reported that 15% of gastroschisis babies had major problems up to the age of 2 years and 12% had long-term developmental problems. The major problems reported are hydrocephalus of postnatal origin, ileostomy performed for ileal atresia, hiatus hernia, dysmorphism and slow development. Eight-eight percent had no long-term problems (BOYD et al. 1998).

7.6
Limb-Body Wall Complex

7.6.1
Definition

Limb-body wall complex consists of failure of the anterior abdominal wall to close, short umbilical cord, disruption of the lateral body wall, spinal defects such as dysraphism or scoliosis, limb defects and craniofacial anomalies. The underlying pathology is nonfusion of the amnion and chorion. This disease occurs in 1 in 10,000 live births (TANG et al. 1991). In 95% of cases, cardiac defects, diaphragmatic absence, bowel atresia and renal abnormalities are also seen (HARTWIG et al. 1989). It has been associated with maternal cocaine abuse, and the underlying mechanism is thought to be impaired placental perfusion due to the vasoconstrictive properties of the drug (VISCARELLO et al. 1992, MARTINEZ et al. 1994).

7.6.2
Cause

It is caused by an early vascular disruption that affects many embryonic structures (HARTWIG et al. 1989).

7.6.3
US Findings (Figs. 7.16, 7.17)

- Large anterolateral defect.
- Left side affected 3 times more frequently than the right (MOERMAN et al. 1992).
- Grotesque mass of tissue with few distinguishing features.
- Short umbilical cord adherent to the placental membrane and usually not visualized.
- Scoliosis is prominent (77%) in association with an abdominal wall defect in limb-body wall complex (PATTEN et al. 1986).
- Persistent extraembryonic coelom with separation of the amnion and chorion.

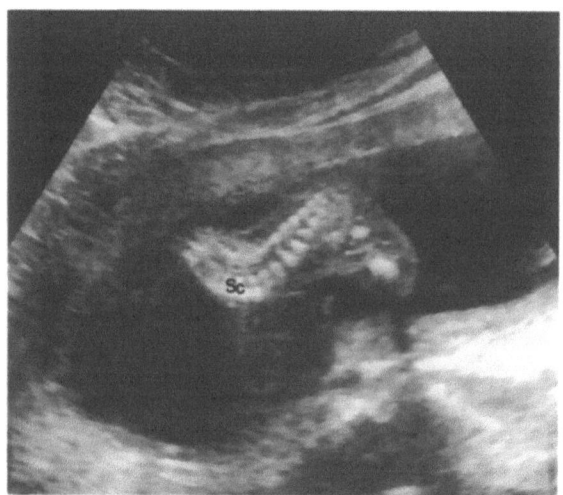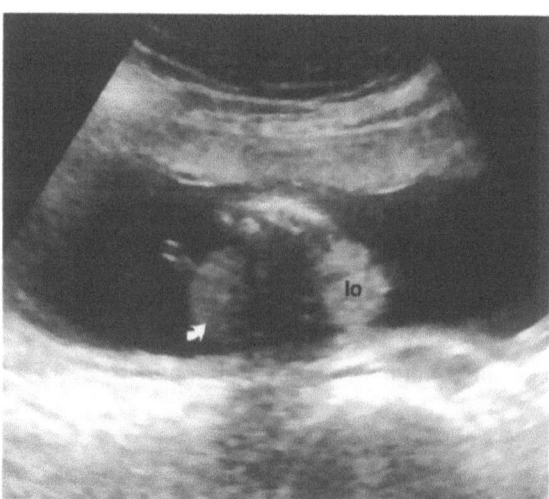

Fig. 7.16. a Eighteen weeks of gestation. Sagittal section. Limb-body wall complex (LBWC). Scoliosis (*Sc*) with severe abdominal wall defect. **b** Same fetus. Transverse section. Exteriorization of liver (*arrow*) and intestinal loops (*lo*)

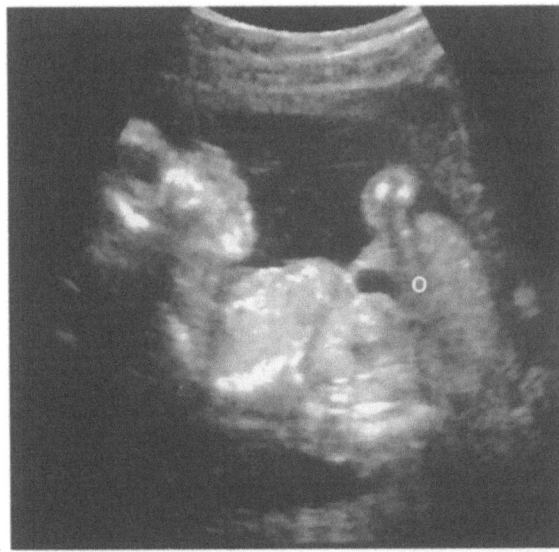

a

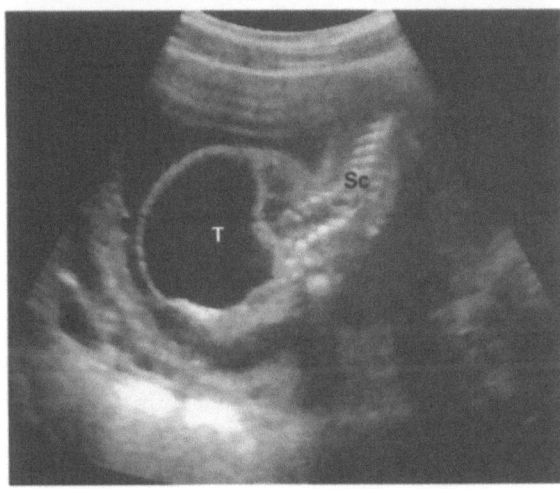

b

17a,b. a Illustration of a LBWC syndrome with a giant ompha-locele (*O*). b Same fetus. Sagittal section. Scoliosis (*Sc*) and sacrococcygeal teratoma (*T*)

7.6.4
Associated Anomalies

- Spinal dysraphism.
- Scoliosis.
- Anencephaly.
- Cephaloceles.
- Facial cleft.
- Limb reduction.
- Heart malformation.
- Diaphragmatic malformation.
- Kidney: agenesis, hydronephrosis, dysplasia.
- Amniotic band: 40% (VAN ALLEN et al. 1987a).
- Chromosomal abnormalities: none reported.

7.6.5
Management

- Antenatal abortion.
- Normal karyotype.
- Lethal in the perinatal period.
- No recurrence risk (PATTEN et al. 1986, VAN ALLEN et al. 1987a,b).

7.7
Amniotic Band Syndrome

7.7.1
Definition

Amniotic band syndrome consists of a congenital malformation ranging from a minor constriction ring to complex multiple congenital anomalies due to amniotic bands that stick to, tangle with and disrupt fetal parts (HIGGINBOTTOM et al. 1979, SEEDS et al. 1982). A few cases are associated with abdominal wall defects The prevalence is 7.8 to 178 in 10,000, with a female to male ratio of 1:1. Some authors claim that amniotic band syndrome and abdominal walls defects together represent coexisting manifestations of limb-body wall complex (MILLER et al. 1981).

7.7.2
Cause

The cause is unknown.

7.7.3
US Findings

- Multiple asymmetric craniofacial abnormalities.
- Limb reduction.
- Restriction of motion of fetal parts.

7.7.4
Associated Anomalies

- Craniofacial anomalies.
- Cleft rib.
- Abdominal wall defect.
- Ambiguous genitalia.
- No chromosomal abnormalities have been reported.

7.7.5
Management

The management depends on the degree of involvement.

7.7.6
Prognosis

The prognosis is related to the extent of the anomalies and the degree of involvement. No recurrence risk has been shown.

7.8
Bladder Exstrophy

7.8.1
Definition

Bladder exstrophy is an eversion and exteriorization of the pelvic viscera on the abdominal surface. Uncommon: 1 in 33,000 live births.

7.8.2
Cause

Bladder exstrophy is caused by inappropriate retraction of the cloacal membrane with subsequent eversion of the bladder mucosa.

7.8.3
US Findings

- Diagnosis is difficult.
- Inferior defect.
- Failure to visualize a normal urinary bladder and pubic diastasis.
- Soft tissue mass protruding from the lower anterior abdominal wall surface.
- Genital anomalies.

7.8.4
Associated Anomalies

Associated anomalies are *uncommon* but most are related to genitourinary aberrations.

7.8.5
Prognosis

- Favorable.
- Urinary incontinence.
- Infertility.
- Pyelonephritis.
- 4% prevalence of bladder carcinoma (MOORE and PERSAUD 1998).

7.9
Cloacal Exstrophy

Cloacal exstrophy is a rare anomaly. The prevalence is 0.05 in 10,000 births (BARTHOLOMEW and GONZALES 1978, TANKS 1986; ERB et al. 1992).

7.9.1
Definition and Cause

The cloaca is a primitive structure from which the rectum and urogenital sinus develop. The urorectal septum serves to separate these organs. Retraction of the cloacal membrane and incomplete descent of the urorectal septum result in failure of the urogenital sinus to separate from the rectum (ERB et al. 1992).

7.9.2
US Findings

- Diagnosis is difficult.
- Inferior defect.
- Ventral wall defect.
- Failure to visualize a normal urinary bladder and pubic diastasis (14–16 weeks).
- Soft tissue mass protruding from the lower anterior abdominal wall surface.
- Myelomeningocele.

7.9.3
Associated Anomalies (Figs. 7.18, 7.19)

- Omphalocele.
- Exstrophy.
- Imperforate anus (Fig. 7.18).
- Genitourinary abnormalities.
- Didelphia.

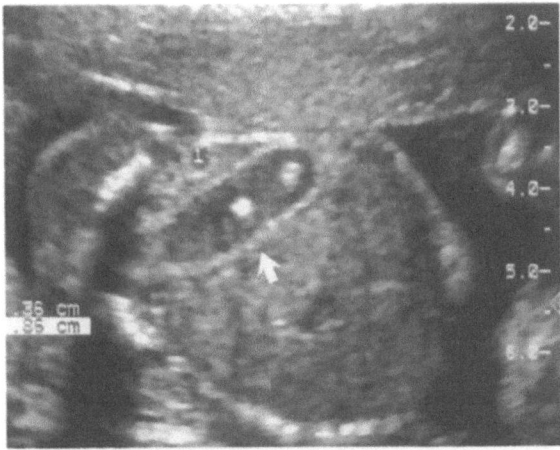

a

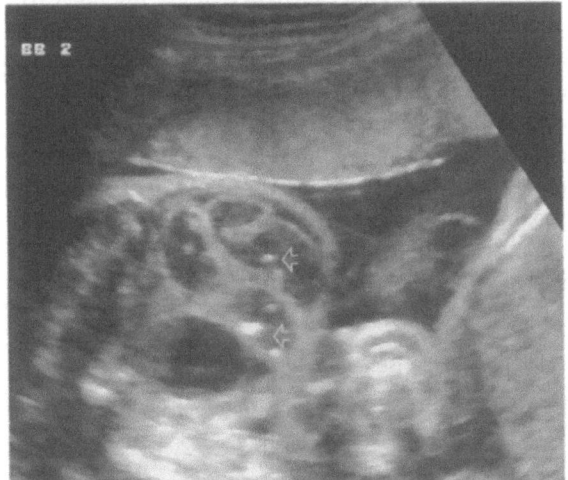

b

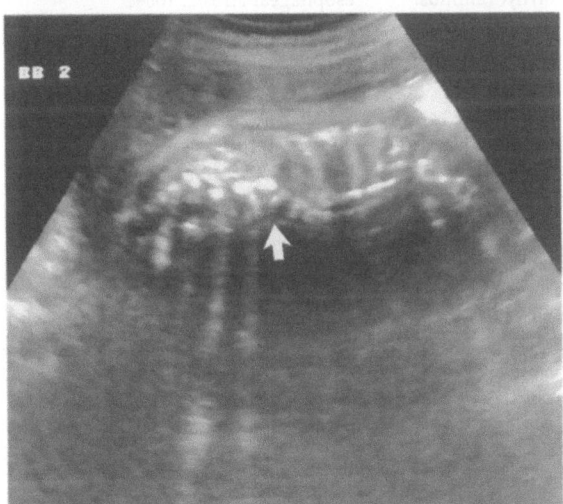

c

Fig. 7.18a-c. a Thirty-seven weeks of gestation. Longitudinal distal section. Imperforate anus with rectovesical fistula and vertebral anomalies. Dilated colon containing calcified meconium (*arrow*) secondary to a rectovesical fistula. **b** Same fetus. Transverse section. Dilated colonic loops containing meconium calcifications (*arrows*). **c** Same fetus. Sagittal section. Vertebral anomalies of segmentation and scoliosis (*arrow*)

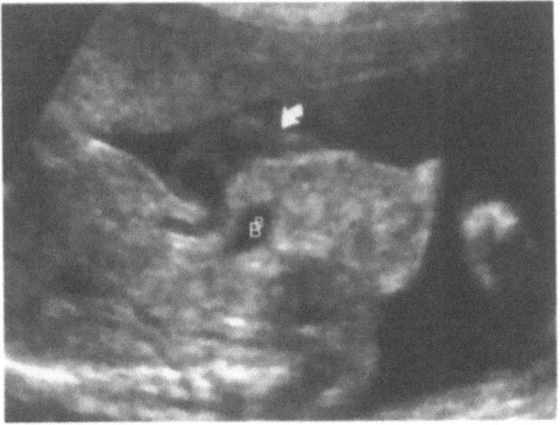

Fig. 7.19. Cloacal exstrophy. Sagittal section. Inferior abdominal wall defect (*arrow*) containing the bladder (*B*) and intestinal loops

- Vaginal absence.
- More severe urogenital anomalies: dysplasia, hydronephrosis.
- Undescended testicles.
- Central nervous system, and chest and vertebral anomalies.
- Chromosomal anomalies: reported with trisomy 21 (GRUNDY et al. 1998) but rare (TANKS 1986).

7.9.4
Management

Antenatal:
- Diagnosis: elevation of maternal serum AFP.
- Increased acetylcholinesterase.

7.9.5
Prognosis

- Poor prognosis.
- 55% mortality (HOWELL et al. 1983).
- Genetic males usually must be reconstructed into females.
- Depends on the severity of the anomalies.
- Multiple surgeries.
- BOYD et al. (1998) reported one case presenting with this anomaly with ileostomy, cystotomy, orthopedic problems with abnormal gait, and repeated urinary infections.

In conclusion, prenatal diagnosis affords opportunities to outline the defect and associated anomalies, allowing parental counseling and intervention. Accurate and detailed parental counseling should be provided as early as possible by a multidisciplinary team. Parents should have opportunities to discuss the prognosis, optional interventions and outcome.

7.10
Gastrointestinal Tract Anomalies

7.10.1
Normal Development, Echoanatomy and Physiology

First Trimester: Foregut division into the esophagus, stomach and duodenum occurs in the 5th week. Herniation of the intestines into the proximal cord develops at 9–12 menstrual weeks with 180° counterclockwise rotation. The stomach may be seen at 11 menstrual weeks. The midgut differentiates into the distal duodenum, the rest of the small bowel as well as the ascending and most of the transverse colon. The midgut is supplied by the superior mesenteric artery. The hindgut develops into the distal transverse colon, descending colon and rectum.

Second Trimester: The fetus can swallow 7 ml/day at 12–13 menstrual weeks, with an increase in volume to 400–500 ml/day at term. Identification of the stomach is possible in 98% of fetuses at 12 weeks. At US the stomach appears as an anechoic structure located in the left hemi-abdomen on the same side of the chest as the heart.

The small bowel is in a central position; it appears hyperechoic compared with the liver, but it contains hypoechoic round areas with a visible lumen ≤1.5 mm.

Meconium consists of desquamated cells, bile pigments and mucoproteins. It is localized in the distal part of the small bowel at 15–16 menstrual weeks. At US it appears as an echogenic mass.

The colon is present peripherally as a discrete tubular structure without any visible lumen.

Third Trimester: Small bowel must be seen after 34 weeks with active peristalsis after 28 weeks.

US findings are of fluid-filled loops in a central position, transient with a diameter £6 mm. They never exceed 15 mm. Valvulae conniventes are rare.

The colon occupies a peripheral position, and appears as a long tubular structure with no peristalsis. The diameter is £23 mm. Haustral folds can be seen. Meconium is propelled by small bowel peristalsis to the colon after 28 weeks. At US, the meconium is hypoechoic and becomes hyperechoic after 39 weeks.

7.11
Foregut Pathology

7.11.1
Introduction

Atresia and secondary obstruction are the most frequent pathology encountered and will induce progressive intestinal obstruction. The role of the sonographic examination is to determine the level and degree of obstruction. Diagnosis is rarely achieved before the end of the second trimester; it is easier in more proximal obstruction. Polyhydramnios is associated in proximal obstructions. Associated pathology of other organs is frequent and should be looked for (Table 7.1) in detail. This will influence the prognosis.

Table 7.1. Comparison of various intestinal obstructions

US diagnosis is successful in 50% for esophageal atresia, 100% for duodenal atresia, 94% for jejunal atresia, 40% for ileal atresia, and 100% for multiple atresia	
Polyhydramnios:	esophageal atresia: 100%
	duodenal: 85.7%
	jejunal: 50%
	ileal: 33%
	multiple: 33%
Intestinal dilatation:	duodenal: 100%
	jejunal: 100%
	ileal: 100%
	multiple: 33%
Meconium peritonitis:	jejunal: 46%
	ileal: 66%
	multiple: 66%
Volvulus:	diagnostic sensitivity: 0
Associated anomalies:	esophageal atresia: VACTERL in 100%
	duodenal: 33% trisomy 21
	jejunal: 25% kidney agenesis
	choledochal cyst
	biliary atresia
	ileal: none
	multiple: 100%
	trisomy 21
	malrotation
	IUGR
	persistent cloacal
	caudal regression syndrome

7.11.2
Absence of Visualization of the Stomach

Non-visualization of the stomach occurs in 2% of cases. The stomach fills regularly with swallowed amniotic fluid and empties by means of peristalsis. The examination should last enough time in order to monitor changes in stomach volume, or be repeated in order to confirm lack of visualization of the stomach.

The differential diagnosis includes conditions of various origins that should be considered systematically in order to assess the correct diagnosis and manage accordingly (Table 7.2). Oligohydramnios is the most common cause. Masses determining meconial obstruction are easily demonstrated whereas depressed fetal swallowing is difficult to assess by US alone.

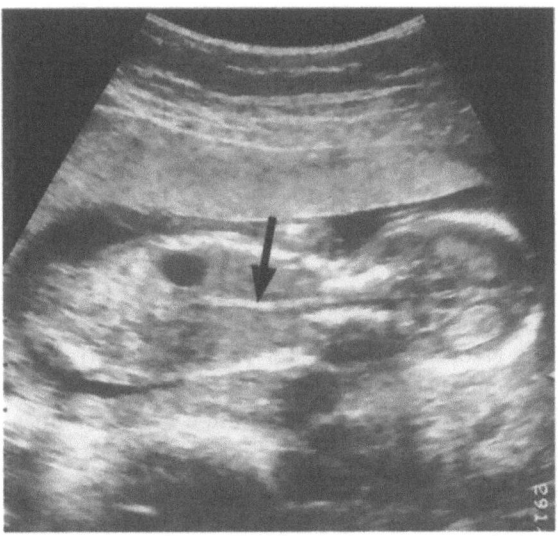

Fig. 7.20. Seventeen weeks of gestation. Normal esophagus (*arrow*)

Table 7.2. Differential diagnosis of absence of stomach

Depressed fetal swallowing:
      neuromotor syndrome (Steinert)
      central nervous system anomalies
      infection
      Pena-Shokeir syndrome
      arthrogryposis
Physical defects: facial clefts
Oligohydramnios is the most frequent cause
Congenital diaphragmatic hernia
Mechanical obstruction: chest mass
Esophageal atresia without fistula

7.11.3
Esophageal Atresia

The incidence of esophageal atresia is 1 in 2,500 live births. The etiology is a failure of early foregut development at 6 menstrual weeks.

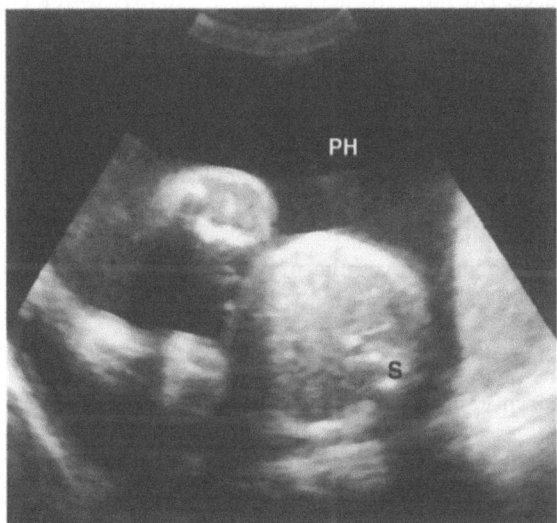

Fig. 7.21. Thirty weeks of gestation. Abdominal transverse section. Esophageal atresia. Absence of stomach with polyhydramnios (*PH*). Spine (*S*)

US Findings

- Normal esophagus: tubular echogenic structure in the posterior part of the fetal chest (AVNI et al. 1994). AVNI et al. reported they were able to visualize the esophagus and thoracic segment in 92% and 87% of fetuses respectively before and after 28 weeks gestation (Fig. 7.20).
- May be seen around 24 weeks.
- The most important feature is absence of the stomach (Fig. 7.21).
- Polyhydramnios is present in the third trimester in 80% (JOLLEYS 1981).
- Because most cases of esophageal atresia coexist with an esophagotracheal fistula, the fetal stomach remains visible and therefore many cases escape an ultrasound diagnosis (over 90% of cases). Occasionally, the upper esophageal pouch can be seen after 26 weeks (KALACHE et al. 1998) and helps to confirm the diagnosis.

Associated Anomalies

There are associated anomalies in 30–70% of cases (GERMAN et al. 1976, DAVID and O'CALLAGHAN 1974, HOLDER et al. 1964):

- Cardiovascular: 27.8%
- Gastrointestinal: 22.6%
- Genitourinary: 18.6%
- Skeletal: 17.7%
- VACTERL (V=vertebral, A=anal, C=cardiac, TE=tracheoesophageal fistula, R=renal, L=limb) is associated in 50–70% of cases with tracheo-esophageal fistulae. (Vertebral anomalies can be diagnosed by the demonstration of supernumerary ossification centers and abnormal cervical curvature)
- Intrauterine growth retardation (IUGR): 40%.

Chromosomal Abnormalities

Chromosomal abnormalities are found in 20% of cases. The most frequent is trisomy 18 (STRINGER et al. 1995).

Prognosis

- Isolated form: good prognosis in 90%.
- Surgery is performed postnatally, but post-surgical stenosis at surgical repair may be a secondary complication.
- Associated form: the prognosis is less favorable, with 50% mortality.

Counseling

Karyotyping should be performed.

Pitfall

The stomach is absent in 2% of fetuses but the amniotic fluid is normal.

7.11.4
Gastric Outlet Obstruction

Gastric outlet obstruction is due to pyloric stenosis or an antral membranous web. The incidence of this congenital anomaly is 1 in 1,000,000 live births (PARRISH et al. 1968). It is secondary to a failure of recanalization of the gastroduodenal canal.

US Findings

- Detected after 22 weeks (WEISSMAN et al. 1994).
- Enlarged stomach.
- Polyhydramnios.

Prognosis

There is a 95.2% survival rate when the antral web is isolated (BELL et al. 1978).

Associated Anomalies

- Cardiovascular.
- Gastrointestinal (duodenal stenosis).

7.11.5
Duodenal Obstruction

The most important US finding is the double bubble sign (Figs. 7.22, 7.23).

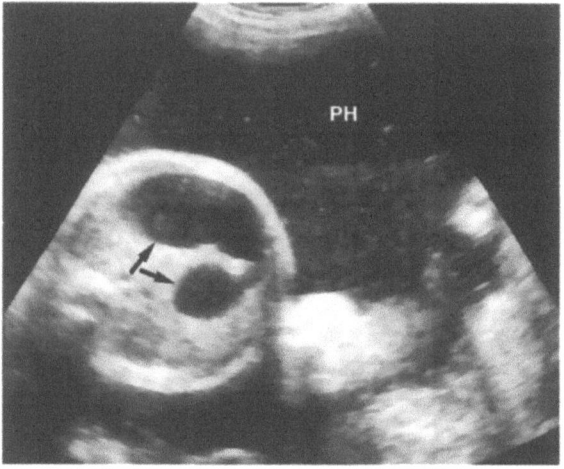

Fig. 7.22. Thirty weeks of gestation. Abdominal transverse section. Duodenal atresia. a Double bubble sign (*arrows*). Polyhydramnios (*PH*). b Gastroesophageal (*GO*) reflux

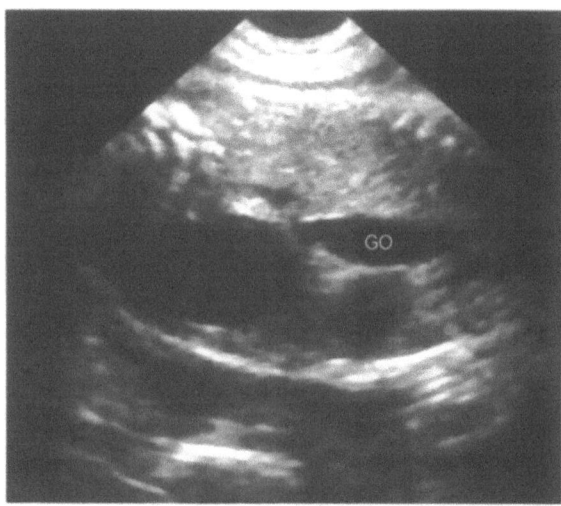

Fig. 7.23. Thirty-six weeks of gestation. Abdominal transverse section. Duodenal web. Dilatation of D2 (*arrow*) without polyhydramnios. Stomach (*S*)

Differential Diagnosis

- Duodenal atresia.
- Duodenal stenosis.
- Annular pancreas.
- Ladd's band.
- Volvulus (malrotation?).
- Intestinal duplication.
- Choledochal cyst.

7.11.6
Duodenal atresia

The most common cause of perinatal intestinal obstruction, with an incidence of 1 in 10,000 live births. It is a failure of recanalization of the primitive duodenum at 10 weeks.

US Findings

- Age at diagnosis after 24 weeks. Appearance of the double bubble is associated with polyhydramnios.
- The persistent fluid-filled duodenum is always abnormal.

Associated Anomalies

- Symmetric growth restriction: 50%.
- Polyhydramnios: 45%.
- Congenital heart defect: 20–36% (ASHCRAFT and HOLDER 1993, NELSON et al. 1982, YOUNG and WILKINSON 1968).
- Gastrointestinal anomalies: 26%.
- Malrotation.
- Tracheoesophageal fistula.
- Hepatobiliary and pancreatic duct anomalies: 1% (GROSFELD et al. 1979).
  Vertebral anomalies: 37%.

Chromosomal Anomalies

Most chromosomal anomalies (30%) are trisomy 21.

Prognosis

- If isolated: excellent.
- If associated anomalies: 36% mortality.

Counseling

- Karyotyping.
- Cardiac US.
- Warning: growth restriction.

Gastric Pseudomass

Most gastric pseudomasses occur in fetuses whose mothers had genetic amniocentesis (FAKHRY et al. 1987).

7.11.7
Small Bowel Pathology

7.11.7.1
Echogenic Small Bowel

Definition: There is hyperechogenicity of the bowel loops when the echogenicity of the loops is comparable to the density of the iliac bone. The incidence is 0.2%. Several studies have been performed on the subject in recent years.

Causes: The causes are unknown. It may be a normal variant or be associated with: (1) viral infections, e.g., cytomegalovirus (PLETCHER et al. 1991, FOROUZAN 1992); (2) toxoplasmosis (MACGREGOR et al. 1995); (3) cystic fibrosis (CF) 25.6% to 50–78% of affected fetuses had hyperechoic bowel on antenatal sonography (DUCHATEL et al. 1993); (4) chromosomal abnormalities: several American studies have described an association with chromosomal abnormalities, particularly trisomy 21, but all of them had a significant bias since they were conducted on a population clearly at risk (advanced maternal age, increased AFP; and (5) IUGR in 18% (NYBERG et al. 1993).

US Findings

The diagnosis is made during the second trimester. The bowel is echogenic, like bone (Fig. 7.24).

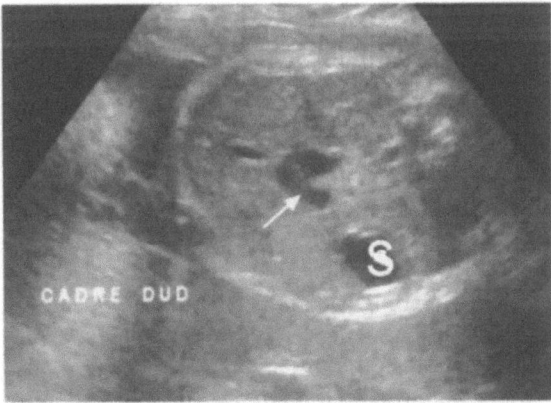

Fig. 7.24. Sixteen weeks of gestation. Abdominal sagittal section. Echogenic dilated bowel loops (EDBL; *arrow*). Stomach (*S*)

Chromosomal Abnormalities

Chromosomal abnormalities are found in 12.4% of cases.

Prognosis

Seventy-six percent of cases with hyperechoic small bowel result in the birth of normal newborns (MAC-GREGOR et al. 1995, MUELLER et al. 1995).

Management

A. Concerning CF: A single study by Dicke and Crane described a potential association with CF, but it was also the only study where systemic DNA analysis was performed. Given that the other studies were relatively recent, it could be that most cases of CF passed unnoticed. Other investigations are needed to draw a conclusion.

B. Concerning a risk of aneuploidy: Three studies, with an evident bias of referral cases (because of advanced maternal age as well as biochemical anomalies such as increased AFP) concluded that amniocentesis should be performed even if the anomaly is isolated: they obviously overestimated the cases of aneuploidy because of the above-mentioned factors. Two studies, by Bromley et al. (1994) and Dicke and Crane (1992), could not clearly show that the hyperechogenic bowel as the sole anomaly was associated with a high risk of aneuploidy. We should also remember that most cases of aneuploidy have other associated echographic anomalies (>60%), which support the score of Benacerraf et al. (1994). In our opinion, hyperechogenic bowel alone should remain a minor criterion for the indication of amniocentesis, except if it is associated with AMA and biochemical abnormalities such as elevated AFP. In addition, other studies should be undertaken on a non-selected population, as in Canada. However, in our hospital echogenic small bowel is an infrequent anomaly, with an incidence well below the 0.6% quoted in the study by Bromley.

C. Concerning pregnancy outcome and the risk of IUGR: All these studies have demonstrated a clear association of IUGR, an increased risk of death in utero and spontaneous abortion with hyperechogenic bowel, in the absence of associated chromosomal abnormalities. Thus, considering this finding, we should be aware of the high level of poor outcomes and proceed with tighter echographic controls. However, it should be remembered that most cases will evolve normally.

D. Consensus: It has been recognized that hyperechogenic bowel as an isolated finding in patients without risk factors (no advanced age, no abnormal AFP levels) remains a minor criterion for amniocentesis, as suggested previously by BENACERRAF, that is, a score of 1. However, if it is an anomaly detected early during the second trimester (about 14–16 weeks), control US at about 18–20 weeks should be performed to exclude other associated abnormalities, particularly a congenital heart disease. Also, these pregnancies should be monitored in a more cautious way with one or more control ultrasounds in the third trimester to detect cases of IUGR, which are strongly increased, as demonstrated in different studies. Finally, with studies proving a possible association with cystic fibrosis, genetic consultation is suggested.

7.11.7.2
Echogenic Dilated Bowel Loops

Definition

The criteria of echogenic dilated bowel loops (EDBL) are a visible lumen >2 mm with echogenic bowel loops as dense as bone before 21 weeks of gestation (Fig. 7.25, 7.26).

Etiology

The cause is probably a vascular insult secondary to transient intestinal occlusion, as proved by low disaccharidase in the amniotic fluid.

Associated Anomalies

- Gastroschisis.
- VACTERL.
- Meconium peritonitis.

Prognosis

- A study of 45 fetuses with EDBL was performed in St. Justine Hospital and reported (GRIGNON et al. 1997).
  - 21 patients had the isolated form. Of these, 91% had a normal outcome, the others had jejunal atresia and hydrops fetalis with no infection.
  - 24 patients had associated anomalies: therapeutic abortion was induced in 14 cases (61%),

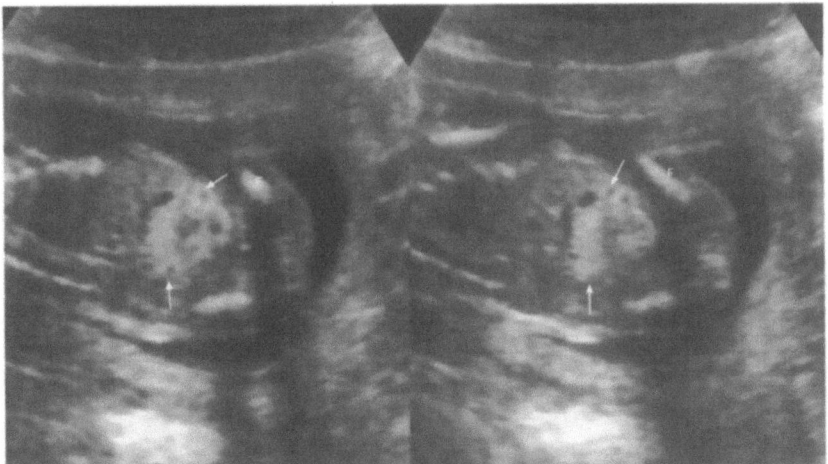

Fig. 7.25. Eighteen weeks of gestation. Sagittal section. EDBL (*arrows*). Femur (*F*)

one death occurred after amniocentesis, and there were nine live births.

- nine fetuses were born alive: six with gastroschisis, two with meconial peritonitis, and one with VACTERL with a good evolution.
- In the two groups, disaccharidase activity was lowered in 10 of 13 cases (77%). No difference was observed in prognosis for the local or diffuse forms or EDBL. No case of cystic fibrosis was documented at birth. Serological infection was found in five cases (11%) antenatally or perinatally.

Counseling

- If isolated, no amniocentesis.
- With other anomalies, amniocentesis is recommended.
- Follow-up: 32 weeks of gestation in order to verify the resolution of EDBL and to assess fetal growth.

7.11.7.3
Small Bowel Atresia

The incidence of small bowel atresia is 1 in 2,700 live births. The etiology is a vascular insult (Louw et al. 1981). Atresias occur in the jejunum, in the ileum and in both, in 50%, 43% and 7% of cases respectively (Osler et al. 1982).

Differences exist between jejunal and ileal atresias. Jejunal atresias are more often multiple compared with ileal atresias. Perforation is more frequent with ileal atresia. Significant dilatation occurs in jejunal atresia and moderate dilatation in ileal atresia. Pre-

maturity is 66% with jejunal atresia compared with 20% with ileal atresia.

US Findings (Figs. 7.27–7.31)

- The diagnosis is made after 28 weeks.
- Polyhydramnios increases with proximal atresia.
- Dilated loops are more obvious and numerous with distal atresia.
- Criteria of obstruction: small bowel >7 mm, mid-abdominal location of the dilated loops, increased bowel dilatation on serial examination, bowel hyperperistalsis, abdominal calcifications, ascites, polyhydramnios.

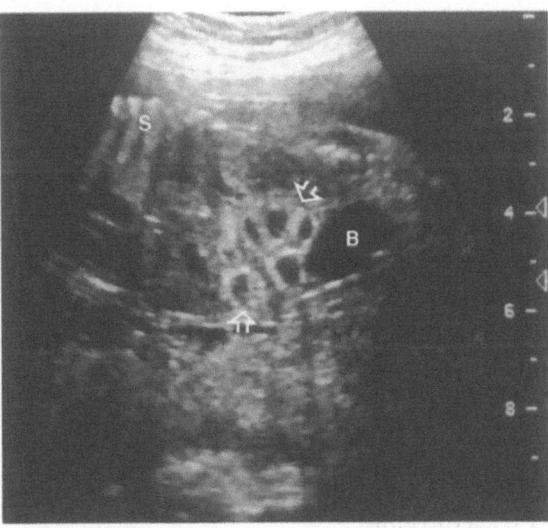

Fig. 7.26. Eighteen weeks of gestation. Sagittal section. EDBL (*arrows*). Bladder (*B*). Spine (*S*)

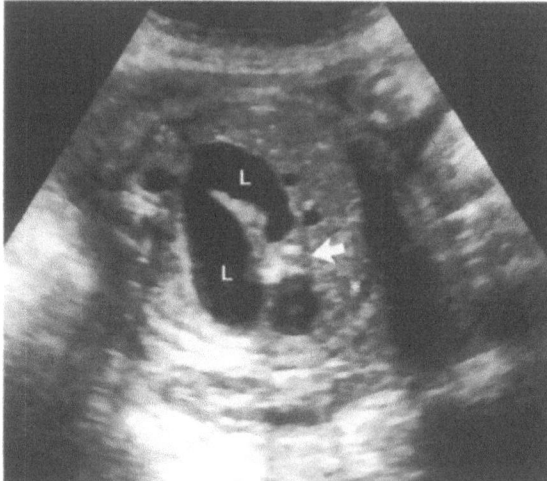

Fig. 7.27. Thirty-three weeks of gestation. Sagittal section. Jejunal atresia. One dilated proximal loop of bowel (*L*). Stomach (*S*)

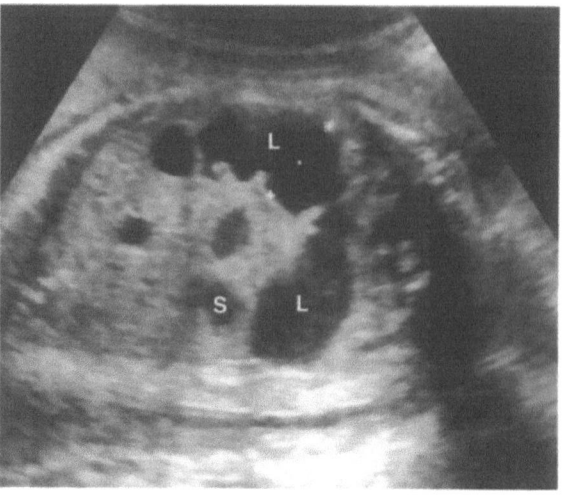

Fig. 7.28. Thirty-two weeks of gestation. Abdominal transverse section. Jejunal atresia. Peritoneal calcifications (*arrow*). Dilated loops of bowel (*L*)

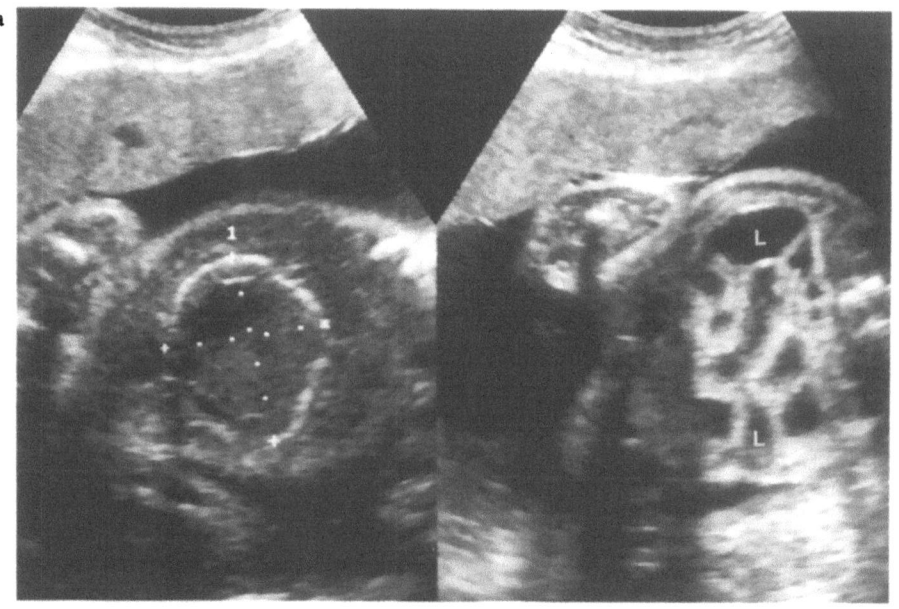

Fig. 7.29. a Thirty weeks of gestation. Sagittal section. Ileal atresia. Peritoneal cyst (between calipers). **b** Same fetus. Transverse section. Dilated loops of bowel (*L*)

Associated Anomalies

- Rare: <10%.
- No chromosomal abnormalities.
- Meconium peritonitis: 6%.

Prognosis

- 88% survival.
- Multiple atresia: poor prognosis. It could be familial.

Counseling

- No karyotyping.
- Preterm labor.
- Prenatal surgery consultation.

Differential Diagnosis: Congenital Chloride Diarrhea

Congenital chloride diarrhea is an autosomal recessive disease with a gene defect on chromosome 7. The typical US findings are a pronounced polyhydramnios and a fetus in the frog position with its abdominal cavity distended by loops of dilated intestine with normal peristalsis. Dilatation of a longer intestinal segment is suggestive of meconium ileus, low intestinal atresia or aganglionosis (LUNDKVIST et al. 1996)

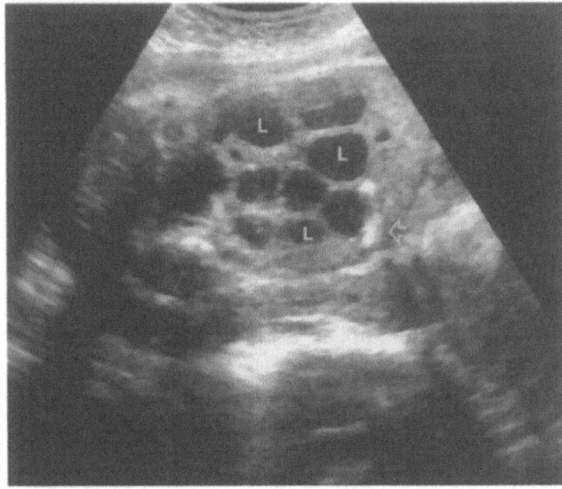

Fig. 7.30. Thirty-one weeks of gestation. Sagittal section. Ileal atresia. Multiple dilated loops of bowel (*L*). Peritoneal calcifications (*arrow*)

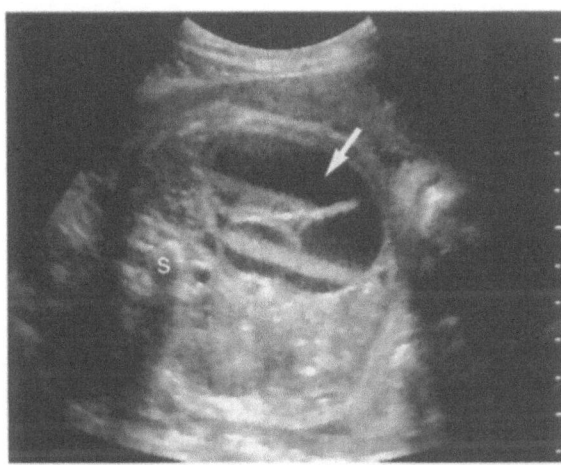

a

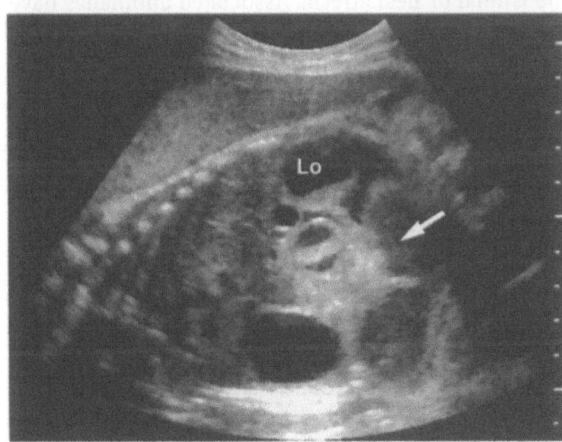

b

Fig. 7.31. a Thirty-three weeks of gestation. Abdominal transverse section. Midgut volvulus. Markedly dilated loop of bowel (*arrow*) with endoluminal echogenic material. Spine (*S*). **b** Same patient. Sagittal view. Proximal dilated loop (*Lo*) and a more distal loop containing echogenic material (*arrow*)

7.11.7.4
Meconium Peritonitis

The incidence of meconium peritonitis is 1 in 30,000 live births (FOSTER et al. 1987). The etiology is vascular. Bowel perforation creates a chemical peritonitis with an intense reaction forming a dense adherent membrane that closes the perforation. When perforation leakage is still present, it creates a cystic space.

Bowel perforation determines a leakage of meconium into the peritoneum. A chemical peritonitis ensues with an intense reaction forming fibrous cicatricial tissue and calcifications. Various evolutions may occur. Cicatricial tissue may close the perforation. In favorable cases, the obstruction resolves and at birth no evidence of the in utero event will be present.

In other cases, obstructions with intestinal dilatation may persist up to birth and a neonatal investigation will be necessary in order to confirm the need for surgical correction.

When the in utero perforation remains for a longer time a virtual space will be created that will contain the meconium limited by the adhesions: the so-called meconium pseudocyst. Typical fine peripheral calcification will be found in utero and after birth (meconium peritonitis with pseudocyst).

US Findings (Fig. 7.32)

- Calcifications appear at least 8 days after the perforation (FOSTER et al. 1987).
- Location: intra-abdominal or scrotal.
- Associated with a cystic mass, ascites or dilated loops.
- Polyhydramnios.

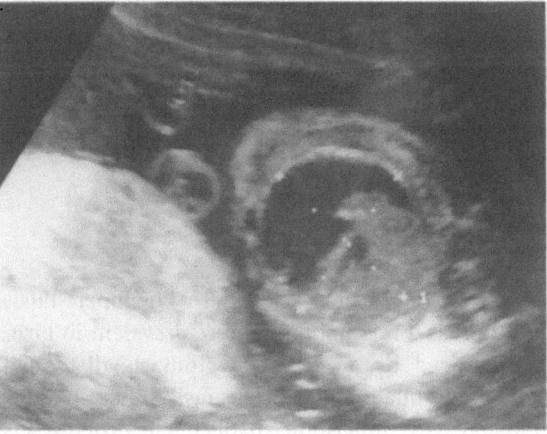

Fig. 7.32. Meconium peritonitis. Abdominal transverse section. Intra-abdominal cystic mass

Associated Anomalies

● Cystic fibrosis: 7.7–40% (FOSTER et al. 1987, PAYNE and NIELSEN 1983, FINKEL and SLOVIS 1982).

Prognosis

● Variable, depending on associated cystic fibrosis or other anomalies.
● In cases of meconium peritonitis with associated abnormalities such as bowel dilatation, meconium cyst, ascites or polyhydramnios, DIRKES et al. (1995) reported a 50% chance that surgical intervention will be required in the newborn period.

7.11.8
Large Bowel Pathology

7.11.8.1
Anorectal Atresia

The incidence of anorectal atresia is 1 in 3,000 live births. Different types are described as the imperforate anus or anorectal atresia.

US Findings

● The diagnosis is made after 29 weeks. A complex anechoic mass is seen.

Different types can be encountered and a diagnosis by US is difficult. It is usually performed after 29 weeks. A complex cystic and echogenic mass can be seen in the fetal pelvis. Intraluminal calcification (enteroliths) of meconium is rare. It is due to a reaction between the urine and meconium. These findings should suggest a rectovaginal fistula (MANDELL et al. 1992).

7.11.8.2
Megacystis-Microcolon-Hypoperistalsis Syndrome

Megacystis-microcolon-intestinal hypoperistalsis syndrome is a rare anomaly, more prevalent in girls, characterized by an enlarged stomach, distended bladder and bilateral pyelocaliectasis. It has an autosomal recessive inheritance pattern. The prognosis is poor and early neonatal death is frequent (PENMAN and LILFORD 1980, CHEN et al. 1998).

7.11.9
Complementary Studies

In cases of intestinal obstructions MR imaging may provide useful information in determining more precisely the level and extent of the obstruction.

In the normal fetus, on T2-weighted sequences the fetal small bowel appears as hyperintense tubular structures whereas the colon is filled with hypointense material. On T1-weighted sequences the fatty meconium will appear as a hyperintense tubular structure.

In the case of obstruction, dilated loops will be visualized easily on T2-weighted sequences; the lack of visualization of the hyperintense colon on T2-weighted images will confirm the ileal level of the obstruction.

MR imaging will also help to differentiate between abdominal masses.

7.11.10
Postnatal Outcome

In our material, the average hospital stay was 31.7 days for jejunal atresia and 22.8 days for ileal atresia. The associated complications, such as volvulus and meconium peritonitis, increase the duration of hospitalization to 39–59 and 33–47 days respectively. Mortality is 50% in esophageal atresia, 0 in duodenal atresia, 11.8% in jejunal atresia (DIU) and 10% in ileal atresia secondary to prematurity.

The important factors to consider for the prognosis are meconium peritonitis and volvulus complicating the jejunal or ileal atresia. Associated anomalies have to be excluded in cases of esophageal and duodenal atresia. However, a small atresia can obscure the diagnosis of multiple atresia with a worse prognosis.

Knowledge of fetal gastrointestinal tract embryology, pathology and associated anomalies is essential for the recognition and management of intestinal abnormalities in utero.

7.12
Intraperitoneal Masses and Calcifications

7.12.1
Abdominal Calcifications

Liver calcifications are detected in 1 in 1,750 second trimester examinations. One large study reported 33 fetuses with isolated intrahepatic calcifications and 56% survival (STEIN et al. 1995). Calcifications may be secondary to: emboli from the portal and umbilical vein (usually unique), ischemia (usually diffuse to one segment) or infection (usually diffuse to a large part of the liver). In cases of meconium peritonitis calcifications may develop around the liver capsule in the peritoneal face.

Management

- Maternal serology for toxoplasmosis, rubella, cytomegalovirus and herpes.
- Trisomy18 reported in two of 52 fetuses (BRONSHTEIN and BLAZER 1995).
- Associated anomalies: 21% gastrointestinal (BRONSHTEIN and BLAZER 1995), cardiovascular and genitourinary malformations.

In the absence of associated anomalies, viral infections and chromosomal abnormalities, liver calcifications are secondary to vascular causes and have an excellent prognosis with a normal neonatal outcome.

Biliary sludge may develop in the gallbladder and constitute a differential diagnosis. Various circumstances favor the development of sludge (twin pregnancies, trisomy 21, cystic fibrosis, hemoglobinopathies) and should be investigated. Without any underlying pathology, sludge disappears after birth once feeding starts.

Another differential diagnosis is the presence of a calcified tumor (see Chap. 13).

7.12.1.1
Meconium Peritonitis and Pseudocyst

Meconium pseudocyst appears as a finely calcified mass that is associated with bowel dilatation (see above). The differential diagnosis should include any calcified mass.

7.12.1.2
Vascular Calcifications

Vascular thrombosis may calcify. This occurs mainly in the inferior vena cava and is associated with renal vein thrombosis (see Chap. 8).

7.12.2
Peritoneal Tumors

7.12.2.1
Organomegaly

Liver or spleen enlargement can be measured on a transverse scan of the fetal abdomen. Liver or spleen enlargement most usually correspond to infection.

7.12.2.2
Cystic Tumors (Table 7.3)

Ovarian cysts are the most commonly encountered mass in the female fetus (see Chap. 8).

Hepatic cysts are benign liver lesions that may develop anywhere around the liver and reach a large diameter. They may resolve spontaneously. Due to their large size some have to be removed after birth.

Choledochal cysts can be diagnosed during the second and third trimesters (BANCROFT et al. 1994). They can be associated with fibrosis, cirrhosis or biliary obstruction.

Sixty-seven percent (67%) will present neonatal jaundice. Surgery must be performed.

Table 7.3. Abdominal cystic tumors

Choledochal cyst
Liver cyst
Splenic cyst
Pancreatic cyst
Ovarian cyst
Duplications
Urachal cyst
(Adrenal cyst)
(Renal cyst)
(Hydrocolpos)
Wolffian duct remnant cyst

7.12.2.3
Mixed-Pattern Tumors (Tables 7.4, 7.5)

Hemangioma (Fig. 7.33)

Hemangioma is the most common vascular tumor in infancy. It may result in high-cardiac output failure and anemia. Doppler US reveals arterial and venous signals. Spontaneous involution may occur during the first few years of life. In cases of cardiac failure, medical treatment, embolization and vincristine can be used.

Table 7.4. Mixed-pattern cystic/solid tumors

Cystic lymphangioma
Cystic teratoma
Hemolymphangioma
Ovarian torsion cyst
Meconium pseudocyst

Table 7.5. Solid-type abdominal tumors

Hepatic hemangioma
Hepatoblastoma
Metastasis (<neuroblastoma)
Teratoma (fetus in fetu)
(Neuroblastoma)
(Sequestration)

In complicated hemangiomas in utero, Mejides et al. (1995) reported that hydrocortisone administration through the umbilical vein resulted in a significant reduction of vascular flow within the tumor.

Neuroblastoma

Patients with neuroblastoma identified by prenatal US follow a clinically favorable course. Survival in a population of 11 infants with neuroblastoma detected on prenatal sonograms was excellent, with no deaths and a mean follow-up of 37 months (Ho et al. 1993).

Teratoma

Fetus in fetu is a fetiform mass in which organ-like tissues are arranged around a vertebral axis (Chitrit et al. 1990). The location is retroperitoneal most of the time. Other locations, such as adrenal, mesenteric, scrotal and cerebral (Chitrit et al. 1990), have been reported. The US findings are a solid, cystic and calcified mass that increases in volume throughout the gestation period. Surgical ablation is required. The prognosis is good but it is potentially malignant, so clinical and radiological follow-up is indicated.

7.12.2.4
Cystic Lesions

Choledochal cysts (Bancroft et al. 1994)
- diagnosis during the second and third trimesters
- associated with fibrosis or cirrhosis and biliary obstruction
- perinatal: 67% neonatal jaundice
- 25% palpable mass
- outcome: surgical exploration
- excellent prognosis.

Hydronephrosis.
Gastrointestinal duplication.
Intestinal atresia.
Mesenteric cyst: lymphangioma.
Ovarian cyst.

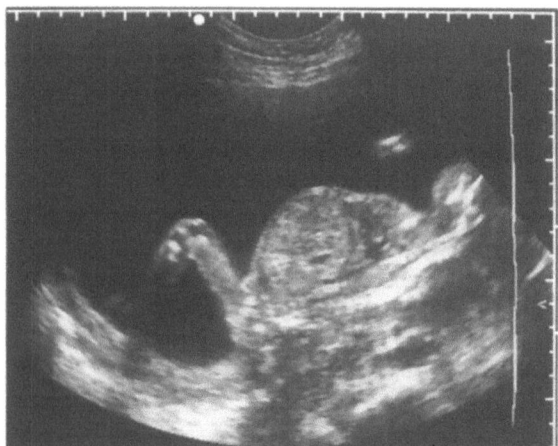

a

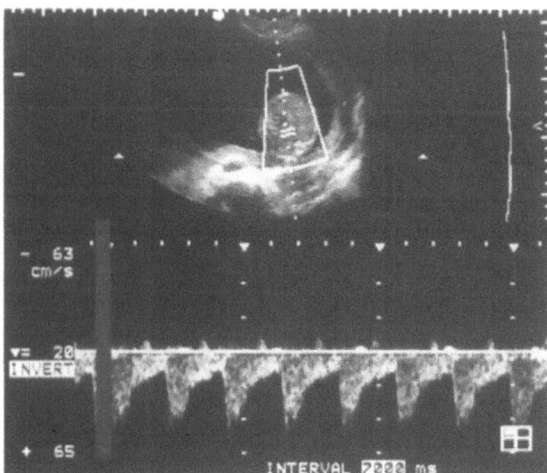

b

Fig. 7.33. a Eighteen weeks of gestation. Sagittal section. Liver hemangioma (*arrow*). **b** Sagittal section. Spectral analysis reveals a high-velocity vascular lesion

References

Abuhamad AA, Mari G, Cortina R, Croitoru DP, Evans AT (1997) Superior mesenteric artery Doppler velocimetry and ultrasonographic assessment of fetal bowel in gastroschisis: a prospective longitudinal study. Am J Obstet Gynecol 176:985–990

Alsulyman OM, Monteiro H, Ouzounian JG, Barton L, Songster GS, Kovacs BW (1996) Clinical significance of prenatal ultrasonographic intestinal dilatation in fetuses with gastroschisis. Am J Obstet Gynecol 175:982–984

Ashcraft KW, Holder TM (1980) Esophageal atresia and tracheoesophageal malformations. In: Holder TM, Ashcraft KW (eds) Pediatric surgery. Saunders, Philadelphia, p 266

Ashcraft KW, Holder TM (1993) Pediatric surgery, 2nd edn. Saunders, Philadelphia

Avni EF, Rypens F, Milaire J (1994) Fetal esophagus: normal sonographic appearance. J Ultrasound Med 13:175–180

Babcook CJ, Hedrick MH, Goldstein RB, et al (1994) Gastroschisis: can sonography of the fetal bowel accurately predict post-natal outcome? J Ultrasound Med 13:701–706

Bair JH, Russ PD, Pretorius DH, Manchester D, Manco-Johnson ML (1986) Fetal omphalocele and gastroschisis: a review of 24 cases. AJR Am J Roentgenol 147:1047–1051

Bancroft JD, Bucuvalas JC, Ryckman FC, Dudgeon DL, Saunders RC, Schwarz KB (1994) Antenatal diagnosis of choledochal cyst. J Pediatr Gastroenterol Nutr 18:142–145

Bartholomew TH, Gonzales ET Jr (1978) Urologic management in cloacal dysgenesis. Urology 11:549–557

Bell MJ, Ternberg JL, Keating JP, Moedjona S, McAlister W, Shackelford GD (1978) Prepyloric gastric antral web: a puzzling epidemic. J Pediatr Surg 13:307–313

Benacerraf BR, Nadel A, Bromley B (1994) Identification of second-trimester fetuses with autosomal trisomy by use of a sonographic scoring index. Radiology 193:135–140

Bond SJ, Harrison MR, Filly RA, Callen PW, Anderson RA, Golbus MS (1988) Severity of intestinal damage in gastroschisis: correlation with prenatal sonographic findings. J Pediatr Surg 23:520–525

Boyd PA, Bhattacharjee A, Gould S, Manning N, Chamberlain P (1998) Outcome of prenatally diagnosed anterior abdominal wall defects. Arch Dis Child Fetal Neonatal Ed 78:F209–F213

Bromley B, Doubilet P, Frigoletto FD Jr, Krauss C, Estroff JA, Benacerraf BR (1994) Is fetal hyperechoic bowel on second-trimester sonogram an indication for amniocentesis? Obstet Gynecol 83:647–651

Bronshtein M, Blazer S (1995) Prenatal diagnosis of liver calcifications. Obstet Gynecol 86:739–743

Chen CP, Wang TY, Chuang CY (1998) Sonographic findings in a fetus with megacystis-microcolon-intestinal hypoperistalsis syndrome. J Clin Ultrasound 26:217–220

Chitrit Y, Zorn B, Scart G, et al (1990) Foetus in foetu surrénalien: un cas évoqué par échographie prénatale. J Gynecol Obstet Biol Reprod 19:1019–1022

Craigo S, Gilieson MS, Cetrulo CL (1992) Pentalogy of Cantrell. Fetus 3: 7548

Crawford DC, Chapman MG, Allan LD (1985) Echocardiography in the investigation of anterior abdominal wall defects in the fetus. Br J Obstet Gynaecol 92:1034–1036

Crawford RA, Ryan G, Wright VM, Rodeck CH (1992) The importance of serial biophysical assessment of fetal wellbeing in gastroschisis. Br J Obstet Gynaecol 99:899–902

David TJ, O'Callaghan SE (1974) Cardiovascular malformations and esophageal atresia. Br Heart J 36:559–564

deVries PA (1980) The pathogenesis of gastroschisis and omphalocele. J Pediatr Surg 15:245–251

Dicke JM, Crane JP (1992) Sonographically detected hyperechoic fetal bowel: significance and implications for pregnancy management. Obstet Gynecol 80:778–782

Di Lorenzo M, Yazbeck S, Ducharme JC (1987) Gastroschisis: a 15-year experience. J Pediatr Surg 22:710–712

Dirkes K, Crombleholme TM, Craigo SD, et al (1995) The natural history of meconium peritonitis diagnosed in utero. J Pediatr Surg 30:979–982

Duchatel F, Muller F, Oury JF, Mennesson B, Boue J, Boue A (1993) Prenatal diagnosis of cystic fibrosis: ultrasonography of the gallbladder at 17–19 weeks of gestation. Fetal Diagn Ther 8:28–36

Dykes EH (1996) Prenatal diagnosis and management of abdominal wall defects. Semin Pediatr Surg 5:90–94

Erb R, Jaffe R, Braren V, et al (1992) Exstrophy of the cloacal sequence. Fetus 2:7515

Fakhry J, Shapiro LR, Schechter A, Weingarten M, Glennon A (1987) Fetal gastric pseudomasses. J Ultrasound Med 6:177–180

Finkel LI, Slovis SL (1982) Meconium peritonitis, intraperitoneal calcifications and cystic fibrosis. Pediatr Radiol 12:92–93

Fitzsimmons J, Nyberg DA, Cyr DR, Hatch E (1988) Perinatal management of gastroschisis. Obstet Gynecol 71:910–913

Forouzan I (1992) Fetal abdominal echogenic mass: an early sign of intrauterine cytomegalovirus infection. Obstet Gynecol 80:535–537

Foster MA, Nyberg DA, Mahony BS, Mack LA, Marks WM, Raabe RD (1987) Meconium peritonitis: prenatal sonographic findings and their clinical significance. Radiology 165:661–665

Fox JE, Gloster ES, Mirchandani R (1988) Trisomy 18 with Cantrell pentalogy in a stillborn infant. Am J Med Genet 31:391–394

German JC, Mabour GH, Woolley M (1976) Esophageal atresia and associated anomalies. J Pediatr Surg 11:299–306

Ghidini A, Sirtori M, Romero R, Hobbins JC (1988) Prenatal diagnosis of pentalogy of Cantrell. J Ultrasound Med 7:567–572

Gilbert WM, Nicolaides KH (1987) Fetal omphalocele: associated malformations and chromosomal defects. Obstet Gynecol 70:633–635

Gray DL, Martin CM, Crane JP (1989) Differential diagnosis of first trimester ventral wall defect. J Ultrasound Med 8:255–258

Greenwood RD, Rosenthal A, Nadas AS (1974) Cardiovascular malformations associated with omphalocele. J Pediatr 85:818–821

Grignon A, Dubois J, Ouellet MC, Garel L, Oligny LL, Potier M (1997) Echogenic dilated bowel loops before 21 weeks' gestation: a new entity. AJR Am J Roentgenol 168:833–837

Grose C, Weiner CP (1990) Prenatal diagnosis of congenital cytomegalovirus infection: two decades later. Am J Obstet Gynecol 163:447–450

Grosfeld JL, Ballantine TV, Shoemaker R (1979) Operative management of intestinal atresia and stenosis based on pathologic findings. J Pediatr Surg 14:368–375

Grundy H, Anderson RI, Goldberg JD (1988) Gastroschisis: prenatal diagnosis and management. Presented at the meeting of the Society of Perinatal Obstetricians, Las Vegas, Nevada, February 3–6

Hagay ZJ, Brian G, Ornoy A, Reece EA (1996) Congenital cytomegalovirus infection: a long-standing problem still seeking a solution. Am J Obstet Gynecol 174:241–245

Hanquinet S, Damry N, Heimann P, Delaet MH, Perlmutter N (1997) Association of a fetus in fetu and two teratomas: US and MRI. Pediatr Radiol 27:336–338

Hartwig NG, Vermeij-Keers C, De Vries HE, Kagie M, Kragt H (1989) Limb body wall malformations complex: an embryologic etiology? Hum Pathol 20:1071–1077

Higginbottom MC, Jones KL, Hall BD, Smith DW (1979) The amniotic band disruption complex: timing of amniotic rupture and variable spectra of consequent defects. J Pediatr 95:544–549

Ho PT, Estroff JA, Kozakewich H, et al (1993) Prenatal detection of neuroblastoma: a ten-year experience from the Dana-Faber Cancer Institute and Children's Hospital. Pediatrics 92:358–364

Hohlfeld P, Daffos F, Costa JM, Thulliez P, Forestier F, Vivaud M (1994) Prenatal diagnosis of congenital toxoplasmosis with a polymerase-chain-reaction test on amniotic fluid. N Engl J Med 331:695–699

Holder TM, Cloud DT, Lewis JE, et al (1964) Esophageal atresia and tracheoesophageal fistula. A survey of its members by the surgical section of the American Academy of Pediatrics. Pediatrics 34:542

Howell C, Caldamone A, Snyder H, Ziegler M, Duckett J (1983) Optimal management of cloacal exstrophy. J Pediatr Surg 18:365–369

Hoyme HE, Higginbottom MC, Jones KL (1981) The vascular pathogenesis of gastroschisis: intrauterine interruption of the omphalomesenteric artery. J Pediatr 98:228–231

Hughes MD, Nyberg DA, Mack LA, Pretorius DH (1989) Fetal omphalocele: prenatal US detection of concurrent anomalies and other predictors of outcome. Radiology 173:371–376

Jolleys A (1981) An examination of the birthweights of babies with some abnormalities of the alimentary tract. J Pediatr Surg 16:160–163

Kalache KD, Chaoui R, Mau H, Bollmann R (1998) The upper neck pouch sign: a prenatal sonographic marker of esophageal atresia. Ultrasound Obstet Gynecol 11:138–140

Knight PJ, Sommer A, Clatworthy HW Jr (1981) Omphalocele: a prognostic classification. J Pediatr Surg 16(Suppl 1): 599–604

Lenke RR, Hatch EL Jr (1986) Fetal gastroschisis: a preliminary report advocating the use of cesarean section. Obstet Gynecol 67:395–398

Louw JH, Cywes S, Davies MR, Rode H (1981) Congenital jejuno-ileal atresia: observations on its pathogenesis and treatment. Z Kinderchir 33:3–17

Lundkvist K, Ewald U, Lindgren PG (1996) Congenital chloride diarrhoea: a prenatal differential diagnosis of small bowel atresia. Acta Paediatr 85:295–298

MacGregor SN, Tamura R, Sabbagha R, Brenhofer JK, Kambich MP, Pergament E (1995) Isolated hyperechoic fetal bowel: significance and implications for management. Am J Obstet Gynecol 173:1254–1258

Mandell J, Lillehei CW, Greene M, Benacerraf BR (1992) The prenatal diagnosis of imperforated anus with rectourinary fistula: dilated fetal colon with enterolithiasis. J Pediatr Surg 27:82–84

Martinez JM, Fortuny A, Comas C, et al (1994) Body stalk anomaly associated with maternal cocaine abuse. Prenat Diagn 14:669–672

Mayer T, Black R, Matlak ME, Johnston DG (1980) Gastroschisis and omphalocele. Ann Surg 192:783–787

Mejides AA, Adra AM, O'Sullivan MJ, Nicholas MC (1995) Prenatal diagnosis and therapy for a fetal hepatic vascular malformation. Obstet Gynecol 85:850–853

Miller ME, Graham JM Jr, Higginbottom MC, Smith DW (1981) Compression-related defects from early amnion rupture: evidence for mechanical teratogenesis. J Pediatr 98:292–297

Moerman P, Fryns JP, Vandenberghe K, Lauweryns JM (1992) Constrictive amniotic bands, amniotic adhesions, and limb-body wall complex: discrete disruption sequences with pathogenesis overlap. Am J Med Genet 42:470–479

Molenaar JC, Tibboel D (1993) Gastroschisis and omphalocele. World J Surg 17:337–341

Moore KL, Persaud TVN (1998) The developing human: clinically oriented embryology, 6th edn. Saunders, Philadelphia

Mueller F, Dommergues M, Aubry MC, et al (1995) Hyperechogenic fetal bowel: an ultrasonographic marker for adverse fetal and neonatal outcome. Am J Obstet Gynecol 173:508–513

Nelson LH, Clark CE, Fishburne JI, Urban RB, Pnery MF (1982) Value of serial sonography in the in utero detection of duodenal atresia. Obstet Gynecol 59:657–660

Nicolaides KH, Snijders RJ, Cheng HH, Gosden G (1992) Fetal gastro-intestinal and abdominal wall defects: associated malformations and chromosomal abnormalities. Fetal Diagn Ther 7:102–115

Novotny DA, Klein RL, Boeckman CR (1993) Gastroschisis: an 18-year review. J Pediatr Surg 28:650–652

Nyberg DA, Mark LA (1990) Abdominal wall defects. In: Nyberg DA, Mahony BS, Pretorius DH (eds) Diagnostic ultrasound of fetal anomalies: text and atlas. Year Book Medical Publishers, Chicago, pp 395–432

Nyberg DA, Fitzsimmons J, Mack LA, et al (1989) Chromosomal abnormalities in fetuses with omphalocele. Significance of omphalocele contents. J Ultrasound Med 8:299–308

Nyberg DA, Dubinsky T, Resta RG, Mahony BS, Hickok DE, Luthy DA (1993) Echogenic fetal bowel during the second trimester: clinical importance. Radiology 188:527–531

Osler GE, Dumaresq L, Becker H (1982) Ultrasonic demonstration in utero of surgically correctable fetal small-bowel obstruction. S Afr Med J 62:83–86

Osuna A, Lindham S (1976) Four cases of omphalocele in two generations of the same family. Clin Genet 9:354–356

Parrish RA Jr, Kanavage CB, Wells SA, Moretz WH (1968) Congenital antral membrane. Surg Gynecol Obstet 127: 999–1004

Patten RM, Van Allen M, Mack LA, et al (1986) Limb-body wall complex: in utero sonographic diagnosis of a complicated fetal malformation. AJR Am J Roentgenol 146:1019–1024

Payne RM, Nielsen AM (1983) Meconium peritonitis. Am Surg 28:22

Penman DG, Lilford RJ (1980) The megacystis-microcolon-intestinal hypoperistalsis syndrome: a fatal autosomal recessive condition. J Med Genet 26:66–67

Perrella RR, Ragavendra N, Tessler FN, Boechat I, Crandall B, Grant EG (1991) Fetal abdominal wall mass detected on prenatal sonography: gastroschisis vs omphalocele. AJR Am J Roentgenol 157:1065–1068

Pletcher BA, Williams MK, Mulivor RA, Barth D, Linder C, Rawlinson K (1991) Intrauterine cytomegalovirus infection presenting as fetal meconium peritonitis. Obstet Gynecol 78:903–905

Pryde PG, Bardicef M, Treadwell MC, Klein M, Isada NB, Evans MI (1994) Gastroschisis: can antenatal ultrasound predict infant outcomes? Obstet Gynecol 84:505–510

Redford DH, McNay MB, Whittle MJ (1985) Gastoschisis and exomphalos: precise diagnosis by midpregnancy ultrasound. Br J Obstet Gynaecol 92:54–59

Richards DS, Cruz AC, Dowdy KA (1988) Prenatal diagnosis of fetal liver calcifications. J Ultrasound Med 7:691–694

Romano KR, Manfredi OL, Farley T, Perez-Guma JE (1988) Omphalocele: sonographic detection at 15 weeks' gestation. NY State J Med 88:596–597

Samuel M, Burge DM (1996) Extra-lobar intra-abdominal pulmonary sequestration. Eur J Pediatr Surg 6:107–109

Schwaitzberg SD, Pokorny WJ, McGill CW, Harberg FJ (1982) Gastroschisis and omphalocele. Am J Surg 144:650–654

Seashore JH (1978) Congenital abdominal wall defects. Clin Perinatol 5:61–77

Seeds JW, Cefalo RC, Herbert WNP (1982) Amniotic band syndrome. Am J Obstet Gynecol 144:243–248

Sermer M, Benzie RJ, Pitson L, Carr M, Skidmore M (1987) Prenatal diagnosis and management of congenital defects of the anterior abdominal wall. Am J Obstet Gynecol 156:308–312

Siles C, Boyd PA, Manning N, Tsang T, Chamberlain P (1996) Omphalocele and pericardial effusion: possible sonographic markers for the pentalogy of Cantrell or its variants. Obstet Gynecol 87:840–842

Sotelo-Avila C, Gooch WM 3rd (1976) Neoplasms associated with Beckwith-Wiedemann syndrome. Perspect Pediatr Pathol 3:255–272

Spirt BA, Gordon LP (1991) The placenta. In: Rumack CM, Wilson SR, Charbonneau JW (eds) Diagnostic ultrasound. Mosby Year Book, St Louis, pp 935–954

Stein B, Bromley B, Michlewitz H, Miller WA, Benacerraf BR (1995) Fetal liver calcifications: sonographic appearance and postnatal outcome. Radiology 197:489–492

Stringer MD, McKenna KM, Goldstein RB, Filly RA, Adzick NS, Harrison MR (1995) Prenatal diagnosis of esophageal atresia. J Pediatr Surg 30:258–263

Tang TT, Oechler HW, Hinke DH, Segura AD, Franciosi RA (1991) Limb-body wall complex in association with sirenomelia sequence. Am J Med Genet 41:21–25

Tanks ES (1986) Urologic complications of imperforate anus and cloacal dysgenesis. In: Campbell F, Walsh PC (eds) Campbell's urology, 5th edn. Saunders, Philadelphia, p 1889

Tibboel D, Kluck P, van der Kamp AW, Vermey-Keers C, Molenaar JC (1985) The development of the characteristic anomalies found in gastroschisis – experimental and clinical data. Z Kinderchir 40:355–360

Tibboel D, Raine P, McNee M, et al (1986) Developmental aspects of gastroschisis. J Pediatr Surg 21:865–869

Toyama WM (1972) Combined congenital defects of the anterior abdominal wall, sternum, diaphragm, pericardium, and heart: a case report and review of the syndrome. Pediatrics 50:778–792

Van Allen MI, Curry C, Gallagher L (1987a) Limb-body wall complex. I. Pathogenesis. Am J Med Genet 28:529–548

Van Allen MI, Curry C, Walden CE, Gallagher L, Patten RM (1987b) Limb-body wall complex. II. Limb and spine defects. Am J Med Genet 28:549–565

van de Geijn EJ, van Vugt JM, Sollie JE, van Geijn HP (1991) Ultrasonographic diagnosis and perinatal management of fetal abdominal wall defects. Fetal Diagn 6:2–10

Viscarello RR, Ferguson DD, Nores J, Hobbins JC (1992) Limb-body wall complex associated with cocaine abuse: further evidence of cocaine's teratogenicity. Obstet Gynecol 80:523–526

Waziri M, Patil SR, Hanson JW, Bartley JA (1983) Abnormality of chromosome 11 in patients with features of Beckwith-Wiedemann syndrome. J Pediatr 102:873–876

Weissman A, Achiron R, Kuint J, Lipitz S, Mashiach S, Avigad I (1994) Prenatal diagnosis of congenital gastric outlet obstruction. Prenat Diagn 14:888–891

Young DG, Wilkinson AW (1968) Abnormalities associated with neonatal duodenal obstruction. Surgery 63:832–836

8 Perinatal Approach to Anomalies of the Urinary Tract, Adrenals and Genital System

FRED E. AVNI, LAURENT GAREL, MICHELLE HALL, FRANÇOISE RYPENS

CONTENTS

8.1 Uro-nephropathies 153
8.1.1 Introduction 153
8.1.2 Imaging the Urinary Tract 153
8.1.3 Normal Sonographic Appearance
of the Urinary Tract 154
8.1.3.1 The Fetus 154
8.1.3.2 The Newborn 155
8.1.4 Abnormal Urinary Tract 156
8.1.4.1 Abnormal Renal Number 156
8.1.4.2 Abnormal Renal Location 156
8.1.4.3 Abnormal Renal Echogenicity 156
8.1.4.4 Abnormal Renal Size 158
8.1.4.5 Urinary Tract Dilatation 158
8.1.4.6 Renal Cysts and Cystic Diseases 168
8.1.4.7 Tumors 171
8.1.4.8 Renal Vein Thrombosis 173
8.1.4.9 Compensatory Renal Growth 174
8.1.4.10 Bladder and Urachus 174
8.1.4.11 Prognosis: In Utero Treatment? 174
8.1.5 Postnatal Investigation 175
8.1.6 Treatment in the Light of the Natural History
of Uro-nephropathies 179
8.1.6.1 Vesico-ureteric Reflux 179
8.1.6.2 Uretero-pelvic Junction Obstruction 180
8.1.6.3 Uretero-vesical Junction Obstruction 180
8.1.6.4 Multicystic Dysplastic Kidney 181
8.1.6.5 Duplex Kidneys 181
8.1.7 Conclusions 181
8.2 Fetal Genitalia 182
8.2.1 Ambiguous Genitalia 183
8.2.2 Male Genital Anomalies 183
8.2.2.1 Scrotum 183
8.2.2.2 Hypospadias and Epispadias 183
8.2.2.3 Urethral Anomalies 185
8.2.3 Female Genital Anomalies 186
8.2.3.1 Hydrocolpos 186
8.2.3.2 Ovarian Cyst 187
8.3 Fetal Adrenals 189
8.3.1 Normal Fetal Adrenals 189
8.3.2 Adreno-genital Syndrome 189
8.3.3 Adrenal Masses 189
References 191

FRED E. AVNI, MD, PhD
Department of Pediatric Imaging, Children's Hospital Queen Fabiola, Avenue J. J. Crocq 15, 1020 Brussels Belgium
LAURENT GAREL, MD
Department of Pediatric Imaging (LG), Sainte Justine Hospital, 3175 Côte-Sainte-Catherine, Montréal, Québec H3T 1C5, Canada
MICHELLE HALL, MD
Department of Pediatric Nephrology, Children's Hospital Queen Fabiola, Avenue J. J. Crocq 15, 1020 Brussels Belgium
FRANÇOISE RYPENS, MD
Department of Pediatric Imaging (LG), Sainte Justine Hospital, 3175 Côte-Sainte-Catherine, Montréal, Québec H3T 1C5, Canada

8.1
Uro-nephropathies

8.1.1
Introduction

In many countries, obstetrical ultrasound (US) is performed routinely during normal pregnancies. In Belgium, three sonographic examinations are performed, one in each trimester. In other countries, only a second mid-trimester examination is performed routinely, first or third trimester examinations being performed only when there is a specific indication. The more systematic use of obstetrical US has led to the discovery of many fetal anomalies, among which the uro-nephropathies represent one of the largest group of congenital anomalies encountered and managed at birth. Furthermore, dramatic changes have occurred in their management since nowadays uropathies are confirmed in mostly asymptomatic patients and the treatment applied is mainly preventive. Also, the antenatal detection and postnatal follow-up have brought new data on the natural history of many pathologies (THOMAS 1990, SCOTT and RENWICK 1999, LIVERA et al. 1989, ZHOU et al. 1999).

8.1.2
Imaging the Urinary Tract

The demonstration of the fetal urinary tract is mainly based on US. In most cases US will be able to differentiate between a normal and abnormal urinary tract. In case of sonographic doubt, MR imaging has proved useful in order to demonstrate the presence of normal or abnormal kidneys (Fig. 8.1) (POUTAMO et al. 2000). Cases with oligohydramnios, maternal obesity and complex uropathies constitute indications for fetal MR imaging. After birth, the imaging armamentarium is much wider; US is still the central technique, a but voiding cysto-urethrogram is also almost routinely performed (see below) in order to detect vesico-ureteric reflux. MR imaging is presently used more often than intravenous pyelography in order to delineate the morphology of the dilated urinary tract (AVNI et al. 2001). Isotopes are still mandatory for the assessment of renal function.

8.1.3
Normal Sonographic Appearance of the Urinary Tract

8.1.3.1
The Fetus

Urine starts to be produced during the 9th week of fetal life. The first US hallmark of a normally functioning urinary tract is the bladder, which is visualized as a cystic structure in the fetal pelvis around the 12th week (Fig. 8.2). The kidneys themselves are visible around the 13th–14th weeks as oval echogenic structures in the two lumbar areas (Fig. 8.3) (ROSATI and GUARIGLIA 1996). During the rest of the pregnancy, their appearance will change and their size will increase progressively. The size measured during an examination can be plotted against nomograms of renal growth (COHEN et al. 1991, SCOTT et al. 1995). The ratio between renal and abdominal circumferences is relatively stable during normal pregnancy (0.27–0.30). Up to the 17th–18th week the kidneys appear "physiologically" hyperechoic compared with the liver or the spleen. The echogenicity of the kidneys decreases with time and simultaneously the cortico-medullary differentiation appears. The final sonographic appearance is demonstrated around the 26th–27th weeks (Figs. 8.4, 8.5).

The fetal bladder fills and empties continuously every 25–30 min and this can be monitored during the US examination (CHAMBERLAIN et al. 1984). These cycles become slower during the third trimes-

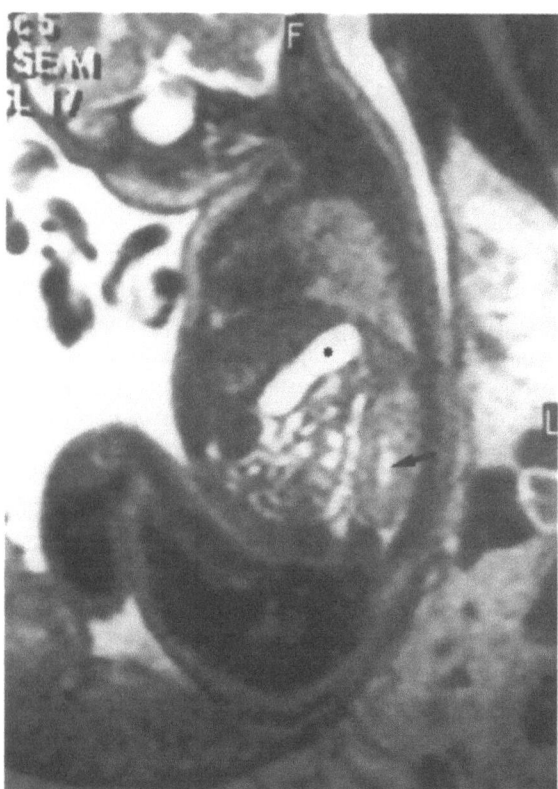

Fig. 8.1. Fetal MR imaging of the kidney. T2-weighted sequence, sagittal view. The kidney can be visualized behind the small bowel loops and stomach (*). Some urine distends the renal pelvis (*arrow*)

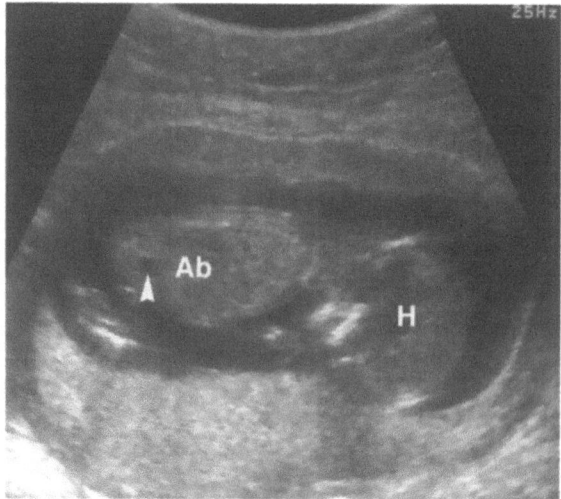

Fig. 8.2. Fetal bladder (first trimester). CRL view. A small bladder (*arrowhead*) can be seen in the pelvis *Ab* fetal abdomen, *H* fetal head

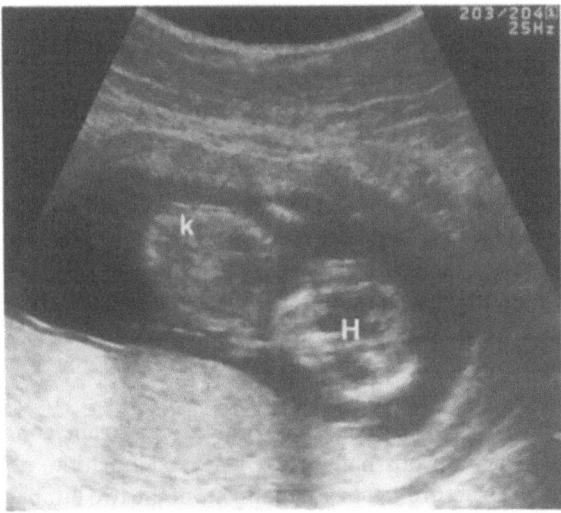

Fig. 8.3. Fetal kidney (first trimester). Sagittal view. The kidney (*k*) appears hyperechoic without cortico-medullary differentiation (CMD). *H* head

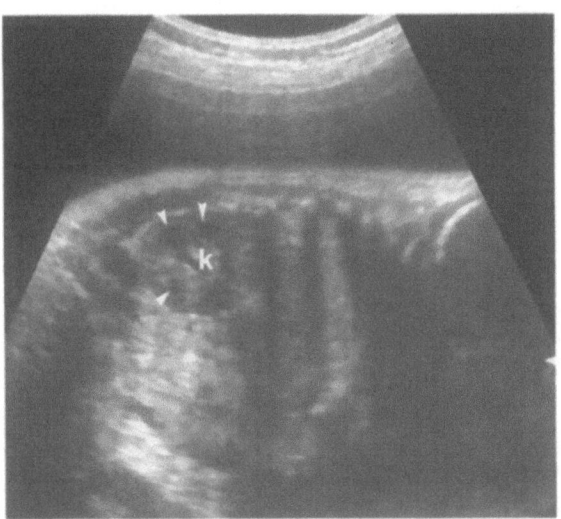

Fig. 8.5. Fetal kidney (third trimester). Sagittal scan of the kidney (*k*). CMD is complete: the medulla appears hypoechoic (*arrowheads*)

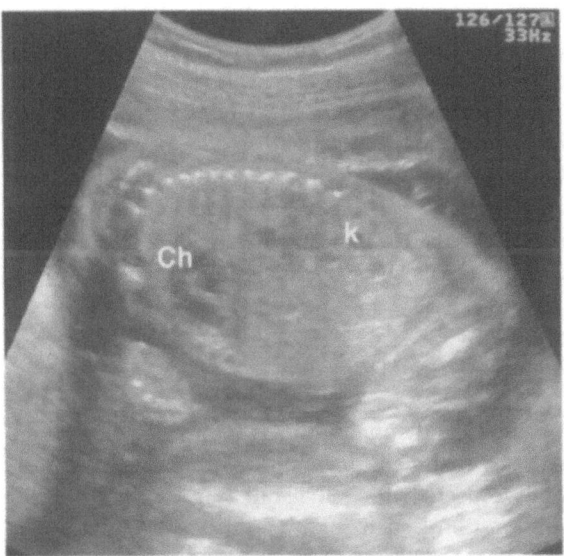

Fig. 8.4. Fetal kidney (*k*) (second trimester). Sagittal view. Cortical echogenicity has decreased somewhat; CMD is appearing. *Ch* chest

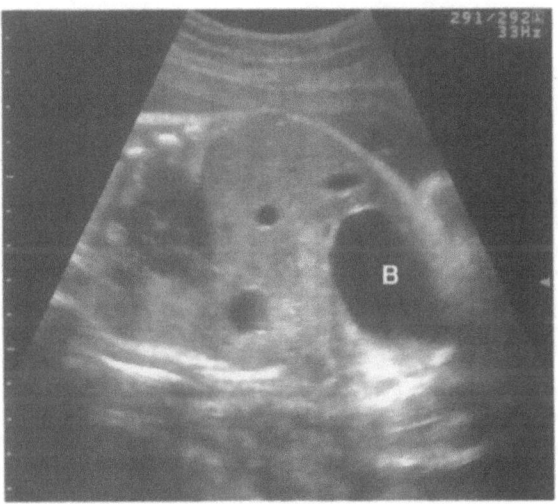

Fig. 8.6. Fetal bladder (third trimester). Sagittal scan of the fetal trunk. Female fetus with a large but normal bladder (*B*)

8.1.3.2
The Newborn

ter, particularly in female fetuses (Fig. 8.6). Under normal conditions, the fetal ureters are not visible.

Besides the visualization of a normal-appearing urinary tract, other indirect evidence of a normal functioning urinary tract is a normal amount of the amniotic fluid (two thirds of which is produced by the fetal kidneys after 15 weeks) and a normal development of the fetal lungs (THOMAS 1990, HILL et al. 1983).

The newborn kidney is similar in appearance to the fetal one, in that a cortico-medullary differentiation (CMD) is obvious (YAMAZAKI 2001). However, in the newborn, the renal cortex appears, transitorily, relatively more hyperechoic and the CMD is increased (Fig. 8.7). This is even more the case in the premature newborn (Fig. 8.8). The origin of this feature is unclear but could be associated with transient neonatal hyperfiltration due to increased fluid turnover. Bladder wall

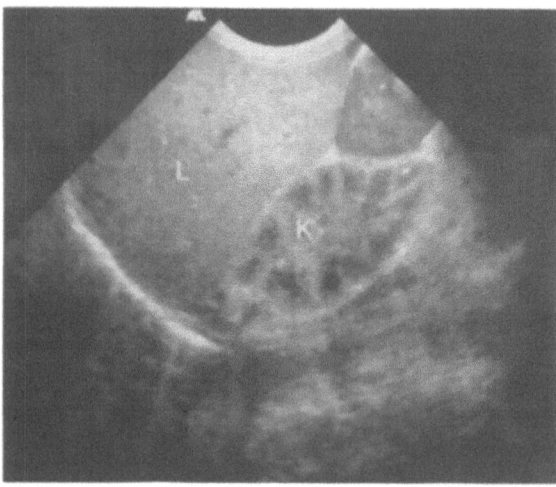

Fig. 8.7. Normal right kidney (*K*) in a full-term neonate. Sagittal scan of the right kidney. CMD is present. The renal cortex is isoechoic or slightly hyperechoic compared with the liver (*L*)

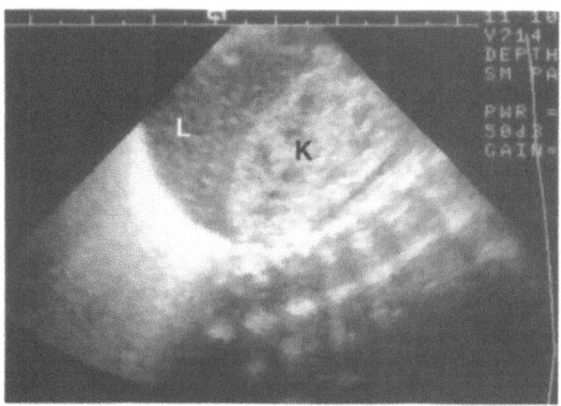

Fig. 8.8. Normal kidney (*K*) in a prematurely born neonate. Sagittal scan of the kidney. CMD is present. The renal cortex is markedly hyperechoic compared with the liver (*L*)

thickening is more often demonstrated in male newborns (YEUNG 1997, YAMAZAKI et al. 2001).

8.1.4
Abnormal Urinary Tract

Anomalies of the urinary tract that can and have been detected in utero are numerous; they include anomalies of the kidney itself, of the collecting system, of the bladder and of the urethra (GUNN et al. 1995, FINE 1992, SCOTT and RENWICK 1988, ROSENDAHL 1990, GLOOR et al. 1995, MANDELL et al. 1991, EURIN et al. 1995, BARAKAT and DROUGAS 1991).

8.1.4.1
Abnormal Renal Number

Bilateral renal agenesis is part of Potter's syndrome and is incompatible with extrauterine life. The diagnosis is based on the absence of renal structure and oligohydramnios after 15 weeks gestation. Pulmonary hypoplasia is invariably associated. Enlarged globular adrenals should not be mistaken for kidneys (BRONSHTEIN et al. 1994, HOFFMAN et al. 1992). The use of color Doppler may help to localize the renal arteries and subsequently the kidneys (BRONSHTEIN et al. 1994).

Unilateral renal agenesis is more common (1/500 pregnancies) and usually without significant consequence on postnatal life. On US examination, no renal structure can be found in one of the two lumbar areas after 15 weeks (SHERER et al. 1990). When the left kidney is missing, the space is occupied by the splenic flexure of the colon. As mentioned above, in the case of renal agenesis the adrenal may look hypertrophied and can be mistaken for a kidney. Renal agenesis is part of the differential diagnosis of the "empty renal fossa" in the fetus that also includes ectopic kidney (JEANTY et al. 1990, MANDELL et al. 1994). An investigation will be necessary after birth to confirm the status of the normal kidney and to look for associated vesico-ureteric reflux (VUR) (ATYEH and HUSMANN 1992, 1993). Associated anomalies must be looked for; among them genital tract malformations are a classical association.

8.1.4.2
Abnormal Renal Location

Whenever only one kidney is found, the second one must be searched for in all the other potential locations, especially the pelvic one (Fig. 8.9). Other ectopic locations, such as horseshoe or crossed fused, can also be detected in utero and the diagnosis is usually aided by the demonstration of a typical CMD (JEANTY et al. 1990, MEIZNER and BERNHARD 1995) (Figs. 8.10, 8.11a). An ectopic kidney is usually smaller and somewhat malrotated. At birth, the anomaly has to be confirmed by US, intravenous pyelography or MR imaging (Fig. 8.11b, c) and associated VUR must be searched by a voiding cystourethrogram (VCUG) (Fig. 8.11d).

8.1.4.3
Abnormal Renal Echogenicity

Kidney hyperechogenicity is diagnosed after 17 weeks gestation, when the kidneys appear more echo-

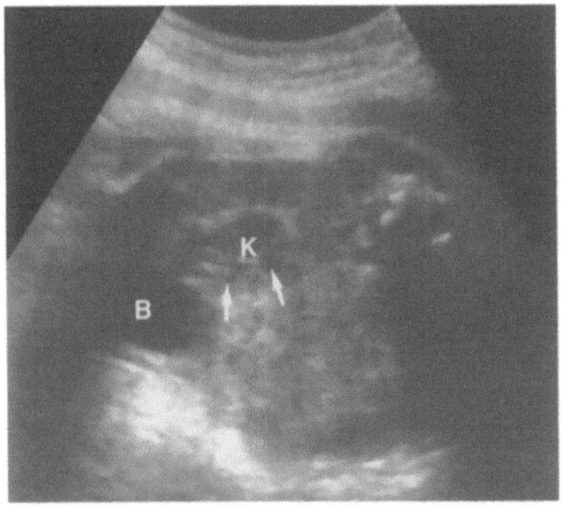

Fig. 8.9. Pelvic kidney (third trimester). Transverse scan of the fetal lower abdomen. The ectopic kidney (*K*) can be recognized behind the bladder (*B*) thanks to its CMD (*arrows*)

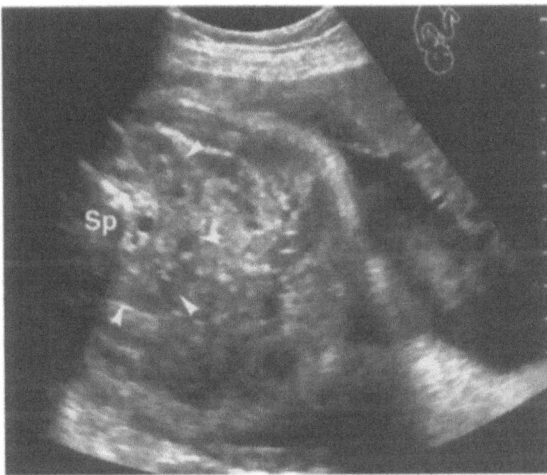

Fig. 8.10. Horseshoe kidney (third trimester). Transverse scan of the lower part of the fetal abdomen; the horseshoe kidney (*arrowheads*) is located in front of the spine (*Sp*) and can be recognized thanks to the CMD

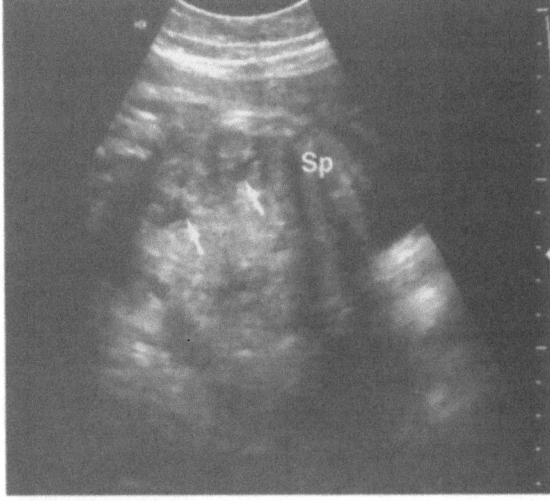

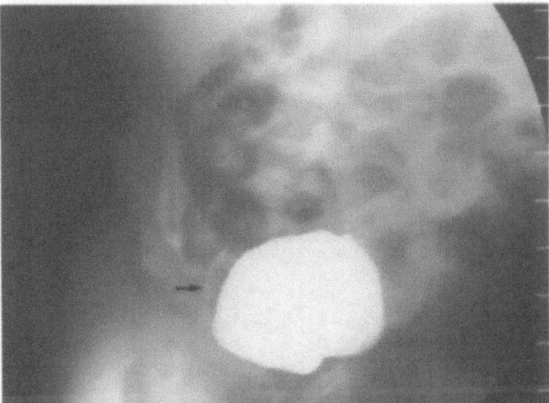

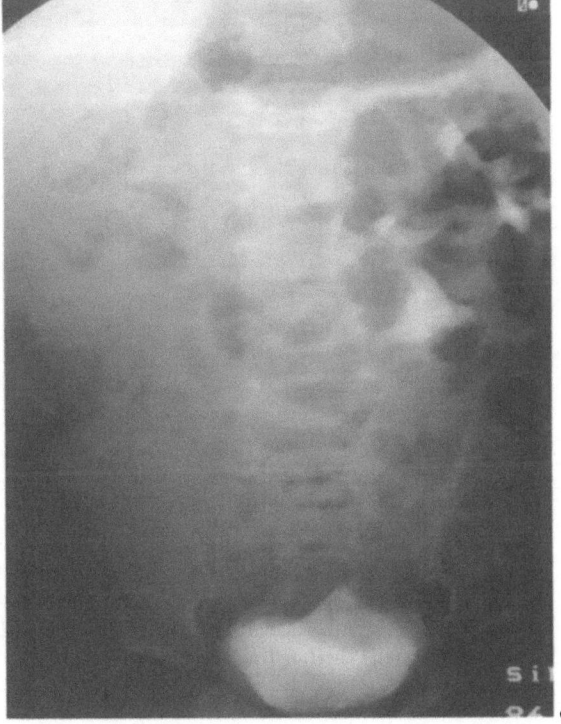

Fig. 8.11a–c. Crossed fused ectopia (third trimester). **a** Transverse scan of the fetal abdomen; both kidneys (*arrows*) are located on the same side of the spine (*Sp*). **b** VCUG at birth demonstrating grade I reflux (*arrow*) into the right ureter. **c** IVP at birth confirming left crossed fused kidneys

genic than the liver or the spleen. Such abnormal echogenicity results either from the presence of multiple cysts (micro- or macroscopic), from dysplasia (or from both = cystic obstructive dysplasia) or from tubular dilatation (Figs. 8.12, 8.13). The detection of hyperechoic kidneys represents a difficult diagnostic challenge. The differential diagnosis must be based on kidney size, CMD, the presence of macrocysts, the degree of dilatation and the amount of amniotic fluid (Table 8.1) (KAEFER et al. 1997, BLANE et al. 1991, CARR et al. 1995). The diagnosis must also take into account the familial history and the presence of associated anomalies. For some patients, the characteristic US patterns will appear after birth or even later

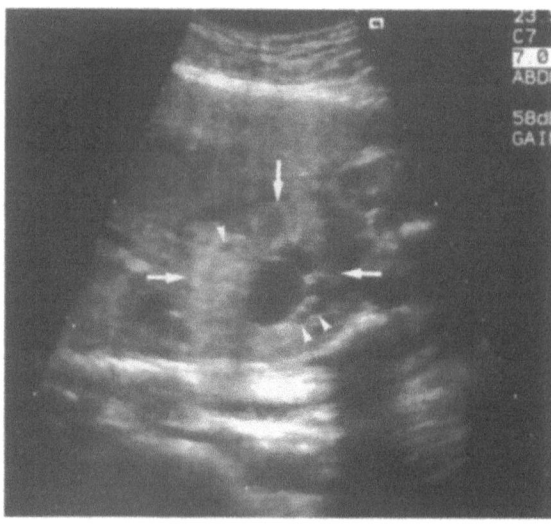

Fig. 8.13. Unilateral obstructive dysplasia (third trimester). Case of an ectopic extravesical ureteral insertion with obstruction. Transverse scan of the left kidney, limited by *arrows*. The cortex is hyperechoic with small cysts within it (*arrowheads*)

(i.e. in the congenital nephrotic syndromes: SARAGA et al. 1995, WAPNER et al. 2001, HOFSTAETTER et al. 1996) or in Bardet-Biedl syndrome (DAR et al. 2001, DIPPELL and VARLAM 1998)). A follow-up is therefore mandatory. It should be stressed that some cases remain unresolved and have to be considered as normal variants (ESTROFF et al. 1991) (Fig. 8.14).

8.1.4.4
Abnormal Renal Size

Measurements of the kidneys must be systematic whenever an anomaly of the urinary tract or of amniotic fluid volume is suspected. Small kidneys most often correspond to hypodysplasia (Fig. 8.15). Their etiology may be primitive or secondary to growth impairment due to VUR (= so-called fetal reflux nephropathy) or obstruction (AVNI et al. 1987). The prognosis depends upon the remaining renal function. Cases with oligohydramnios have the poorest prognosis (OLIVEIRA et al. 999). On the contrary, enlarged kidneys may be related to urinary tract dilatation, renal cystic diseases or tumoral involvement (see below).

8.1.4.5
Urinary Tract Dilatation

Urinary tract dilatation is the most common anomaly detected in utero (ZERIN et al. 1993, TRIPP and HOMSY 1995a, HOMSY et al. 1990, MOURIQUAND

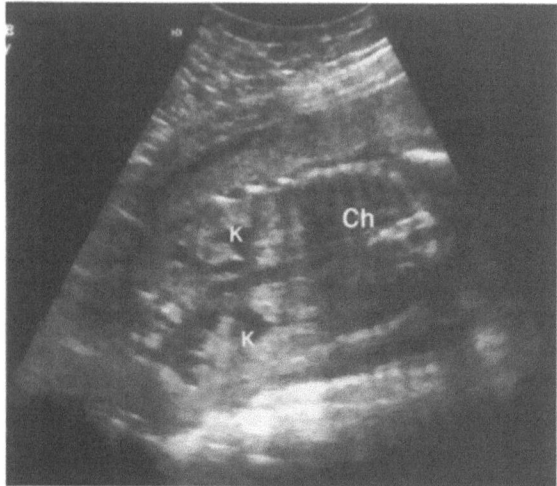

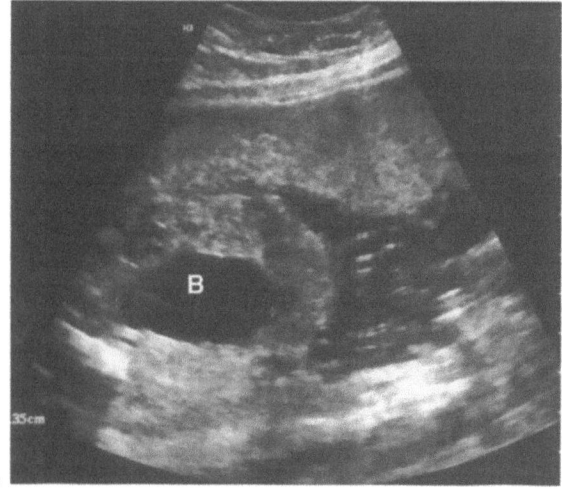

Fig. 8.12. Bilateral obstructive dysplasia secondary to obstructive megabladder (second trimester). a Coronal view of the fetal trunk demonstrating bilateral hyperechoic and dilated kidneys (*K*). *Ch* fetal chest. b Transverse scan through lower fetal abdomen and through the enlarged bladder (*B*) (3.5 cm between crosses)

Table 8.1. Etiologies of hyperechoic kidneys (*CMD* cortico-medullary differentiation, *MDK* multicystic dysplastic kidney, *N* normal, *IVC* inferior vena cava)

	Kidney size	CMD	Cysts	Pyelo-calyceal system	Amniotic volume	Associated findings	After birth
Non-genetically transmitted							
Obstructive dysplasia	–2 to 0 SD	Absent	Cortical <1 cm	Dilated	N or reduced	No	Impaired renal growth
Bilateral MDK	+0 to +4 SD	Absent	Variable sizes, large	Not present	Oligohydramnios	No	Incompatible with life
Normal variant	0 to 2 SD	Present	No	Not seen	Increased	No	N within several weeks
Renal vein thrombosis	0 to 2 SD	Present	No	Not seen	N	Hyperechoic interlobar streaks Thrombus in IVC	Calcified streaks and IVC thrombus
Genetically transmitted							
ARPKD	+2 to +4 SD	Absent or reversed	Small medullary when present	Not seen	Oligohydramnios	Lung hypoplasia	Neonatal death in severe cases
ADPKD, "benign form"	0 to + 2 SD	Increased	No	Not seen	N	No	Cysts appear during childhood
ADPKD, glomerulocystic dysplasia type	+2–+ 4 SD	Absent	Frequent, subcapsular and cortical	Not seen	Oligohydramnios	No	Neonatal renal failure or death
Glomerulocystic dysplasia	+0 to +2 SD	Absent	Small cortical cysts	Not seen	Variable	Isolated: no Syndromic: variable	Isolated: no changes
Medullary cystic dysplasia, syndromic	0 to +2 SD	Absent	Medullary	Not seen	Reduced/ oligohydramnios	Depending on the syndrome	Depending on the syndrome
Medullary cystic dysplasia, Bardet-Biedl	+2–+ 4 SD	Absent	No or medullary	Not seen	Variable	Polydactyly	Hyperechogenicity limited to the medulla
Nephrotic syndrome, Finnish type	??	??	??	??	Polyhydramnios	SGA, large placenta Premature birth	Hyperechoic cortex, small pyramids
Beckwith-Wiedemann syndrome	+2 SD	Present or reversed	No	Not seen	N or increased	Macrosome, omphalocele	Unchanged
Perlman syndrome	+2 SD	Present	No	Not seen	N or increased	Macrosome	Unchanged
Nephro-blastomatosis	+2 SD	Present or absent	No	Not seen	N or increased	No	Wilms' tumor
Renal vein thrombosis	0 to 2 SD	Absent	No	Not seen	N	Hyperechoic streaks, thrombus IVC	Calcified streaks

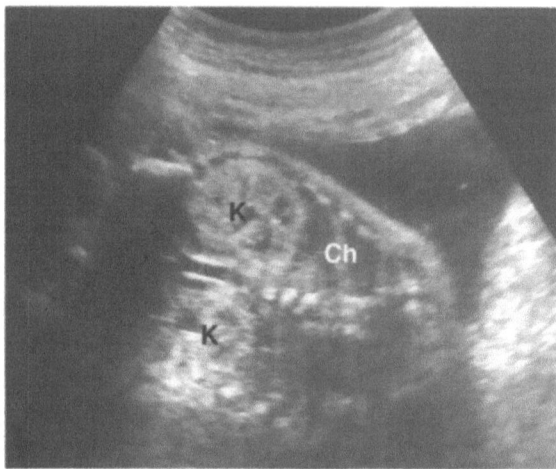

Fig. 8.14. Renal hyperechogenicity with preserved CMD after co-twin embolization (probable ischemic hyperechogenicity). Sagittal scan through both kidneys (*K*). *Ch* fetal chest

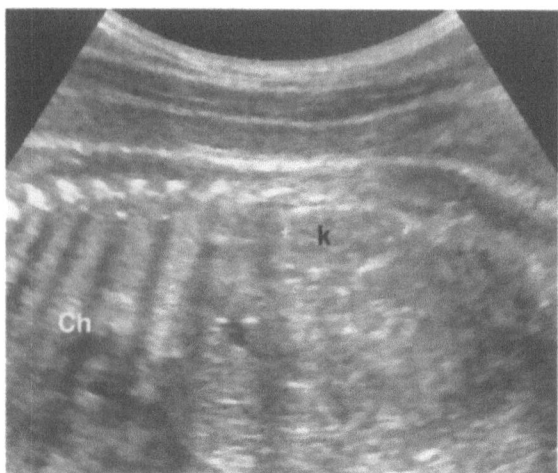

a

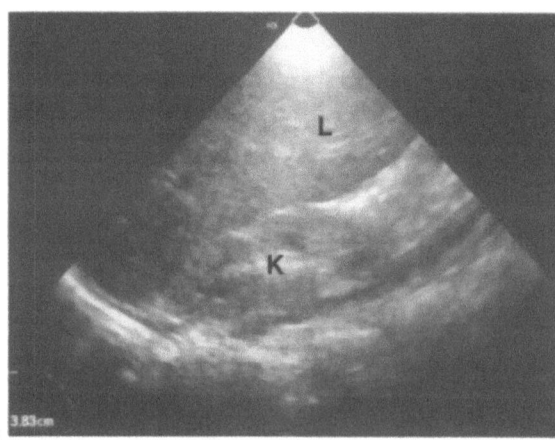

b

Fig. 8.15a, b. (Bilateral) renal hypoplasia. **a** In utero (third trimester). Sagittal scan through the right kidney (*K*) (20 mm between *crosses* = –3SD). *Ch* chest. **b** At 4 years, the kidney (*K*) is still small (38 mm between *crosses*) and a moderate chronic renal failure has developed. *L* liver

1999). it is noteworthy that most cases amenable to treatment are detected during the third trimester. The most common origin for the dilatation is "obstruction" at the uretero-pelvic junction (UPJ). On the basis of the neonatal isotopic findings, authors tend to differentiate between obstructive and non-obstructive UPJ. The other causes of urinary tract dilatation are listed in Table 8.2. The US approach to a dilatation of the fetal urinary tract is similar to the evaluation that is performed after birth. The aim of US is first to differentiate upper from lower urinary tract dilatation.

The basis for the diagnosis of a *UPJ obstruction* is the demonstration of a dilated renal pelvis measured on a transverse scan (Fig. 8.16). Various cut-off diameters have been proposed as abnormal. Most authors accept the limit of 5 mm at 5 months of pregnancy and 8 mm at 8 months. Once a dilatation is detected, the next step is to try to quantify or to grade the "obstruction", and various classifications have been proposed based on the degree of dilatation, and the thickness and echogenicity of the renal parenchyma (Figs. 8.17, 8.18) (GRIGNON et al. 1985, ANDERSON et al. 1995, MAIZELS et al. 1992, STOCKS et al. 1996, DREMSEK et al. 1997). The more dilated the collecting system, the more probable is a decrease in renal function at birth. Unfortunately, there is no direct correlation between the degree of dilatation and renal function. Although classification may be useful in order to determine the prognosis, more and more authors feel that what is most important is to determine which patients will need a postnatal investigation and when.

The best markers of renal obstructive dysplasia and probable poor renal function are hyperechoic parenchyma with macrocysts within it and associated oligohydramnios (BLANE et al. 1991, KAEFER et al. 1997). Another associated finding would be a urinoma that may develop secondary to the obstruction and that appears either as a fluid collection behind and lateral to the kidney or as a hypoechoic rim

Table 8.2. Etiologies of dilatation of the fetal urinary tract

Uretero-pelvic junction (UPJ) (obstructive or not)	45%
Vesico-ureteral reflux (VUR)	30%
Uretero-vesical junction (UVJ) obstruction	10%
Duplex kidneys	7%
Post-urethral valves (PUV)	4%
Multicystic dysplastic kidney (MDK)	4%
Megapolycalycosis	
Infundibular stenosis	

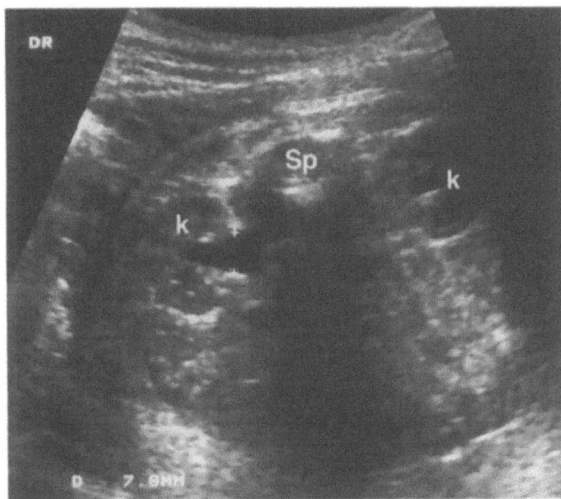

Fig. 8.16. Mild unilateral renal dilatation (third trimester). Transverse scan of the fetal abdomen; the dilated left pelvis measures 7.9 mm (between *crosses*). *k* kidney, *Sp* spine

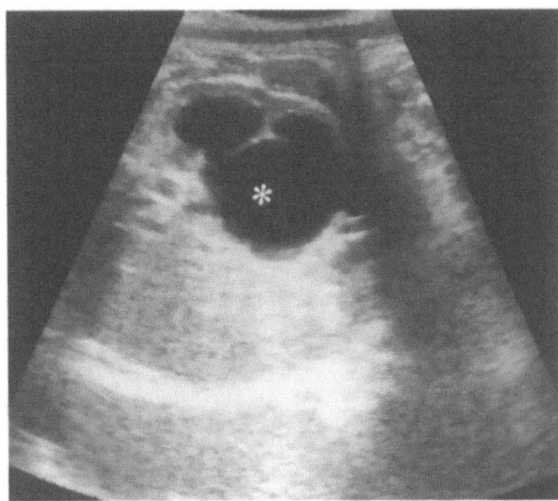

Fig. 8.17. Marked unilateral uretero-pelvic junction obstruction (third trimester). Transverse scan of the fetal abdomen demonstrating the distended renal pelvis (*)

around the kidney (Avni 1985, Kaefer et al. 1995) (see below).

The main differential diagnoses of UPJ obstruction are *multicystic dysplastic kidney (MDK), megacalycosis, uretero-vesical junction (UVJ) obstruction* (Montana et al. 1985) and *vesico-ureteric reflux (VUR)*. The differential diagnosis is not always feasible in utero. Furthermore, there is increasing evidence that urinary tract dilatation is part of a spectrum of obstruction that includes hydronephrosis at one end and MDK at the other; infundibular stenosis lies somewhere in between (Uhlenhut et al. 1990). Antenatal diagnosis provides an opportunity to demonstrate the progression from one form to another (Fig. 8.19).

The sonographic features of *MDK* are described below. In *mega(poly)calycosis* there is a dilatation of the calyces that is related to a probable hypoplasia of the pyramids; on US there are numerous large calyces that contrast with the small dilated renal pelvis (Fig. 8.20). This condition may be associated with a megaureter.

UVJ obstruction and high-grade *VUR* are characterized by the presence of a dilated ureter. Peristaltic waves modify the caliber of the ureter but are not correlated with the degree of obstruction. A tentative classification has also been proposed based on the diameter of the ureter (Maizels et al. 1992) without necessary functional implications. The dilatation may increase progressively in utero then resolve after birth (Fig. 8.21a, b).In the case of a UVJ obstruction, the ureteral dilatation results

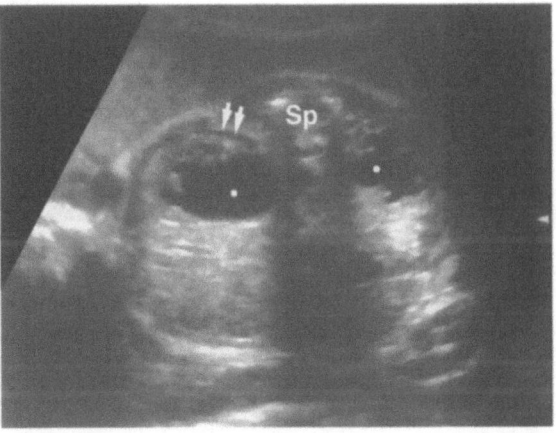

Fig. 8.18. Bilateral uretero-pelvic junction obstruction (third trimester). Transverse scan of the fetal abdomen showing a bilateral dilatation (*). A small amount of free fluid is visible around the left kidney (*arrows*) *Sp* spine

from obstruction (obstructive or primary megaureter) or from an associated obstructive orthoptic ureterocele (Fig. 8.22). Obstructive megaureter may be associated with VUR that will be demonstrated after birth only (Fig. 8.21c). It is noteworthy that a variability in renal pelvis dilatation during one examination seems more specific for VUR (Fig. 8.23). An enlarged fetal bladder (above 6 cm height) can be the result of massive VUR with dilated ureters (the so-called megacystis-megaureter syndrome) (Fig. 8.24) (Mandell et al. 1992). This condition has to be differentiated from other

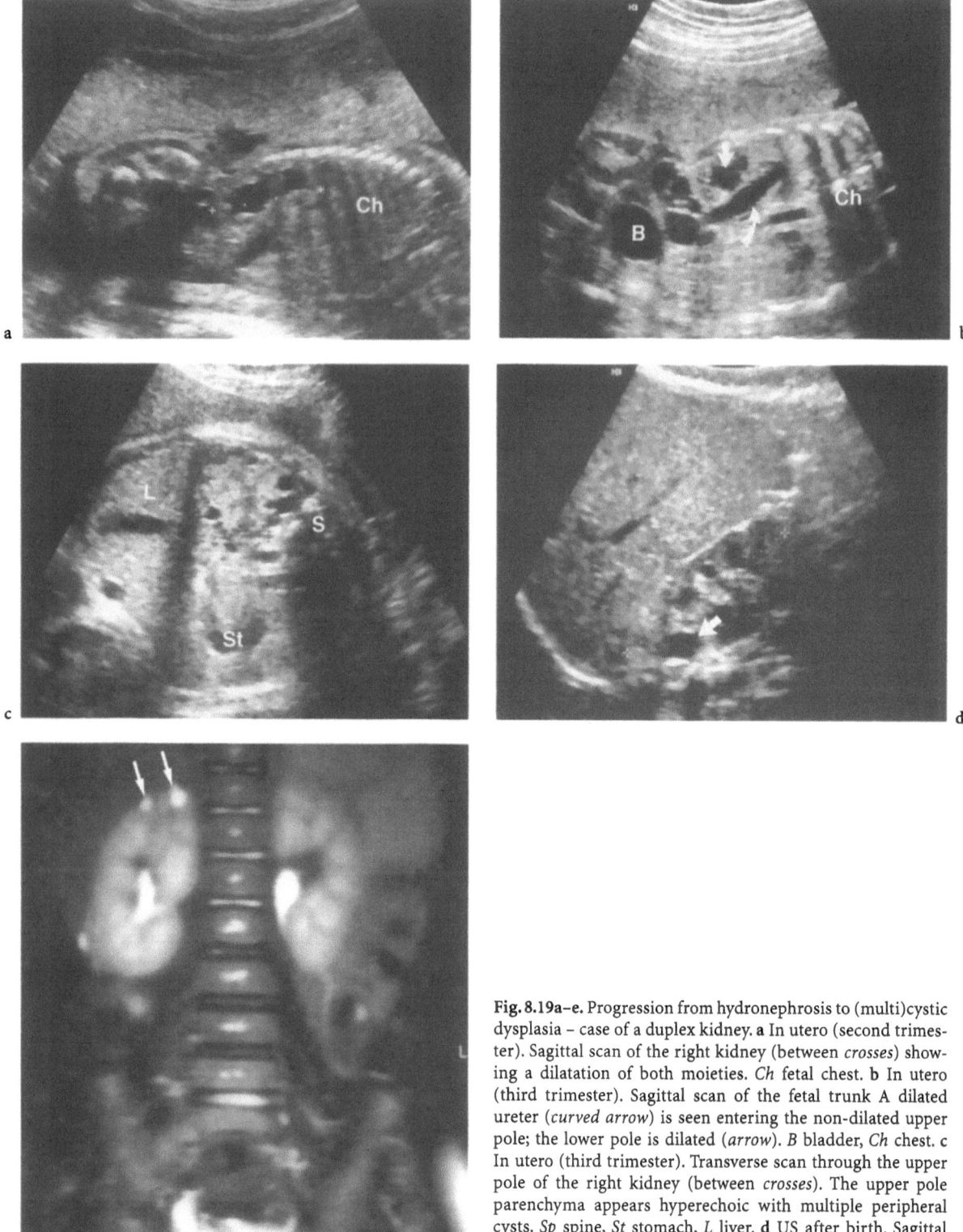

Fig. 8.19a–e. Progression from hydronephrosis to (multi)cystic dysplasia – case of a duplex kidney. **a** In utero (second trimester). Sagittal scan of the right kidney (between *crosses*) showing a dilatation of both moieties. *Ch* fetal chest. **b** In utero (third trimester). Sagittal scan of the fetal trunk A dilated ureter (*curved arrow*) is seen entering the non-dilated upper pole; the lower pole is dilated (*arrow*). *B* bladder, *Ch* chest. **c** In utero (third trimester). Transverse scan through the upper pole of the right kidney (between *crosses*). The upper pole parenchyma appears hyperechoic with multiple peripheral cysts. *Sp* spine, *St* stomach, *L* liver. **d** US after birth. Sagittal scan of the right kidney. A single cyst (*arrow*) remains in the upper pole. **e** MR imaging at age 4 years. Small cysts are still visible in the upper pole (*arrows*) and are in association with the dilated ureter (*curved arrow*) that has an ectopic lower insertion (*arrowhead*). At that time the child was dribbling urine and the upper pole was removed

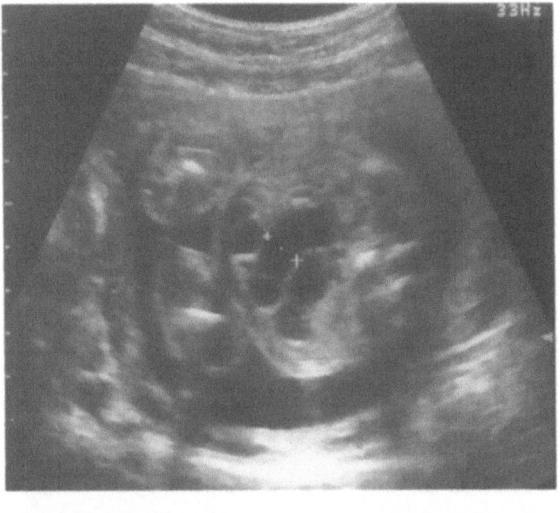

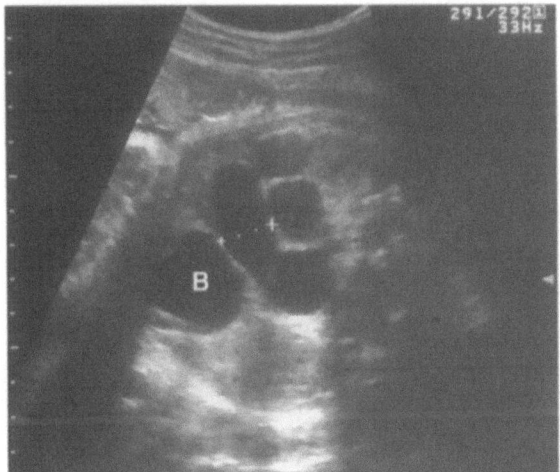

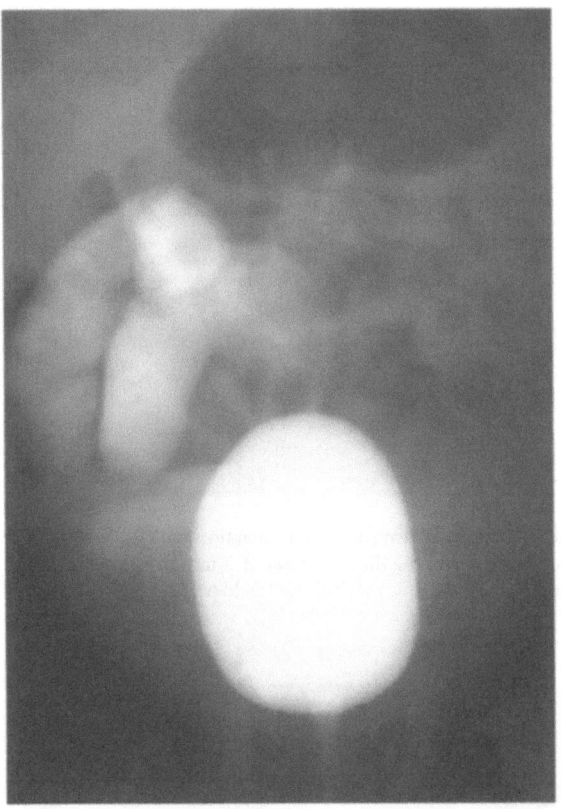

Fig. 8.21a–c. Refluxing megaureter. **a** In utero (second trimester). Transverse scan of the fetal abdomen showing the dilated ureter (7 mm between *crosses*). **b** In utero (third trimester). Transverse scan of the fetal abdomen. The dilatation has increased (14 mm between *crosses*). *B* bladder. **c** VCUG after birth. There is massive reflux into a right megaureter

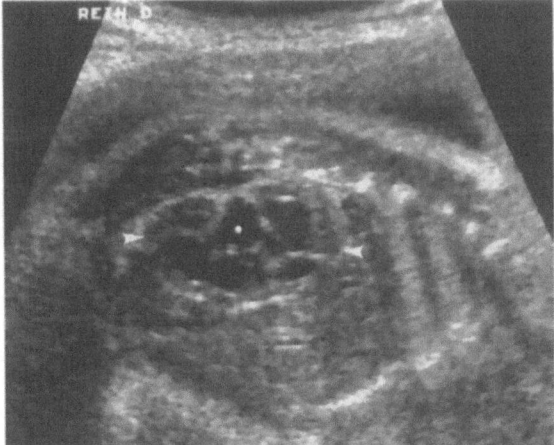

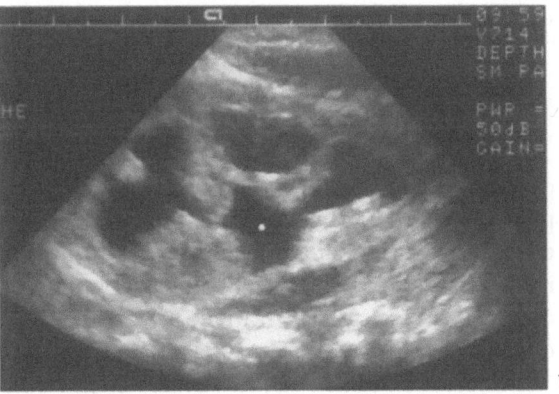

Fig. 8.20a, b. Megacalycosis. **a** US in utero (third trimester). Sagittal scan through the kidney (between *arrowheads*). All calyces are even more dilated than the renal pelvis (*). **b** US after birth. Sagittal scan of the kidney. The calyceal dilatation contrasts with the non-dilated renal pelvis (*)

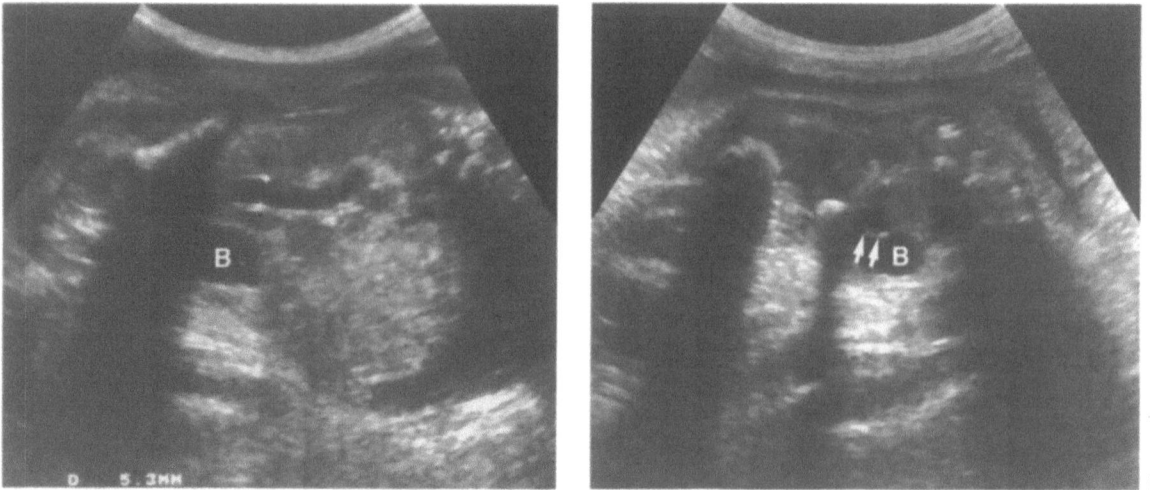

Fig. 8.22a, b. Hydroureter in association with an orthoptic ureterocele (third trimester). **a** Sagittal scan of the fetal abdomen demonstrating the dilated ureter (5.3 mm between *crosses*). *B* bladder. b Transverse scan of the fetal pelvis demonstrating the ureterocele (*arrows*) within the bladder (**B**)

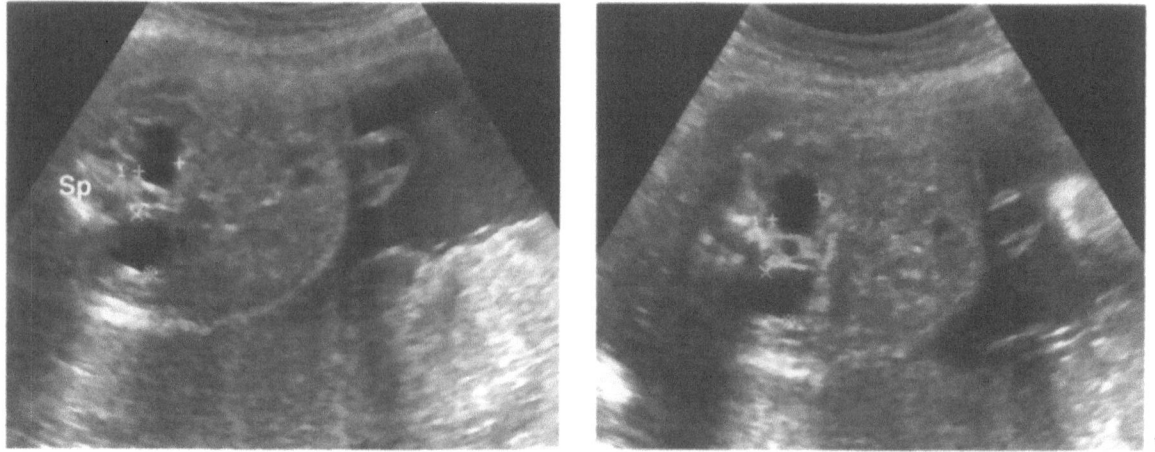

Fig. 8.23a, b. Vesico-ureteric reflux in utero (third trimester). Transverse scans of the fetal abdomen taken a few seconds apart. a The dilated pelves measure 10 and 14 mm (between *crosses*). *Sp* spine. b The dilatation measured 13 mm bilaterally

causes of large bladders in utero; in male fetuses, posterior urethral valves (*PUV*) (Fig. 8.25) produce a large thickened bladder, bilateral uretero-hydro-nephrosis, lung hypoplasia and oligohydramnios in the most severe cases (DINNEEN et al. 1993). The dilated posterior urethra may even be visualized. *Megacystis-microcolon-hypoperistalsis syndrome* is another potential differential diagnosis of megabladder in female or male fetuses (Fig. 8.26) (CARLSSON et al. 1992, MANDELL et al. 1992). It is noteworthy that, as mentioned above, during the last weeks of the pregnancy, female fetuses tend to

have a larger bladder than males due to slow emptying of their bladder (Fig. 8.5).

Another cause for urinary tract dilatation is *duplex kidney* complicated by an anomaly of its upper or lower poles (JEE et al. 1993, ABUHAMAD et al. 1996, VERGANI et al. 1999). The upper pole may be dilated and enlarged because of obstruction, or small and completely dysplastic. Dilatation of the lower pole is usually related to VUR. The anomalies of the upper pole can be associated with an ectopic insertion of an extravesical ureter or an ectopic ureterocele that can be demonstrated already in

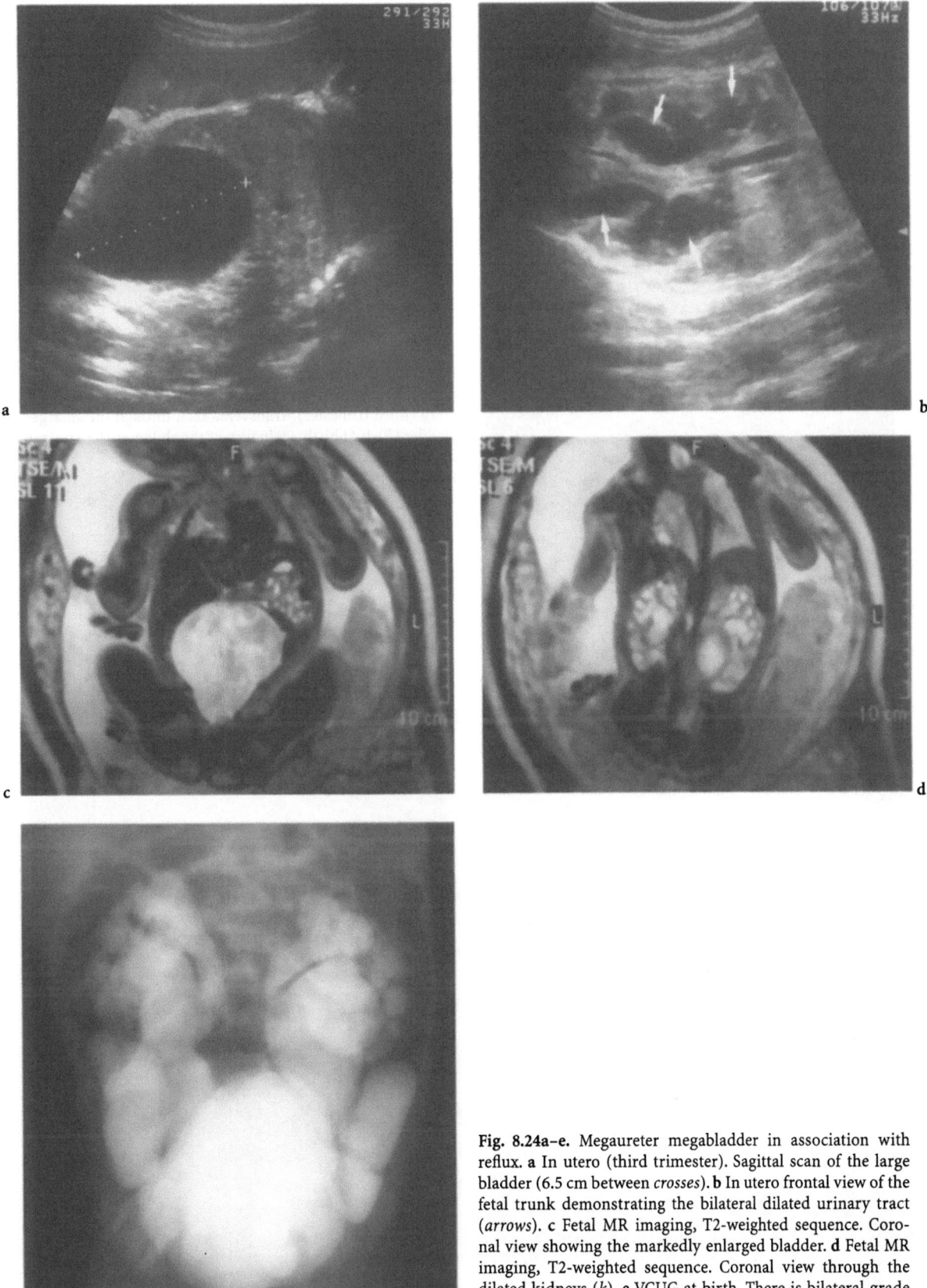

Fig. 8.24a–e. Megaureter megabladder in association with reflux. **a** In utero (third trimester). Sagittal scan of the large bladder (6.5 cm between *crosses*). **b** In utero frontal view of the fetal trunk demonstrating the bilateral dilated urinary tract (*arrows*). **c** Fetal MR imaging, T2-weighted sequence. Coronal view showing the markedly enlarged bladder. **d** Fetal MR imaging, T2-weighted sequence. Coronal view through the dilated kidneys (*k*). **e** VCUG at birth. There is bilateral grade V reflux

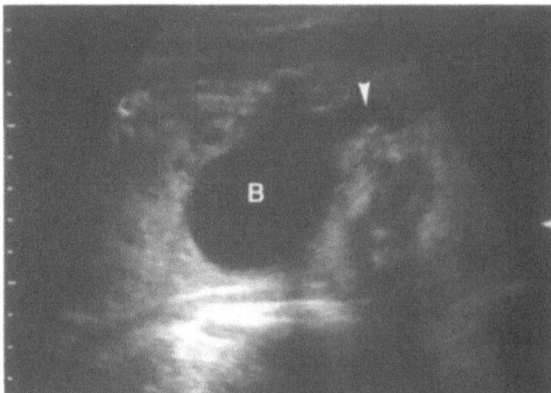

Fig. 8.25. Posterior urethral valves (third trimester). Mid-sagittal scan through the bladder (*B*) and the dilated posterior urethra (*arrowhead*). Bilateral ureterohydronephrosis was also present (not shown)

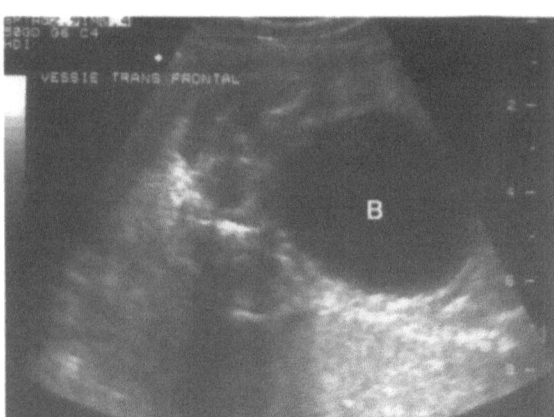

Fig. 8.26a–c. Megabladder–microcolon–hypoperistalsis syndrome (courtesy of Danielle EURIN, MD, Rouen, France). **a** In utero (third trimester). Transverse scan through the enlarged bladder (*B*). **b** At birth. Plain film of the abdomen demonstrating intestinal obstruction (due to hypoperistalsis). **c** At birth. Partially opacified microcolon

a

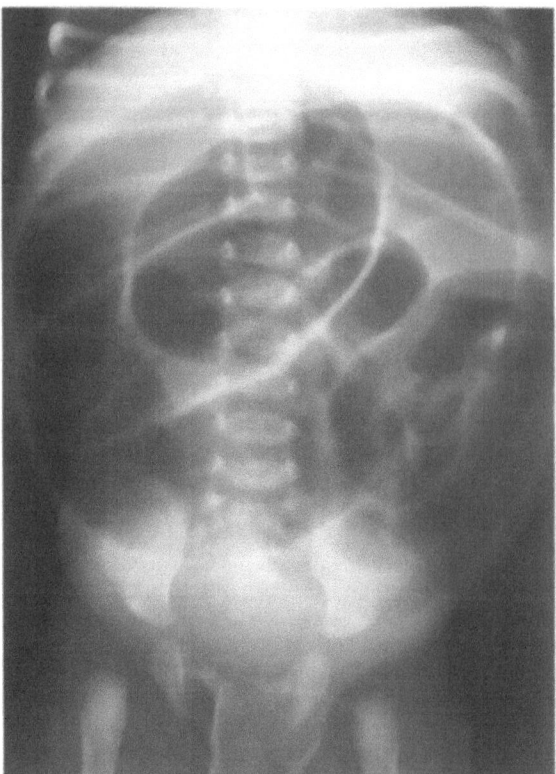

b

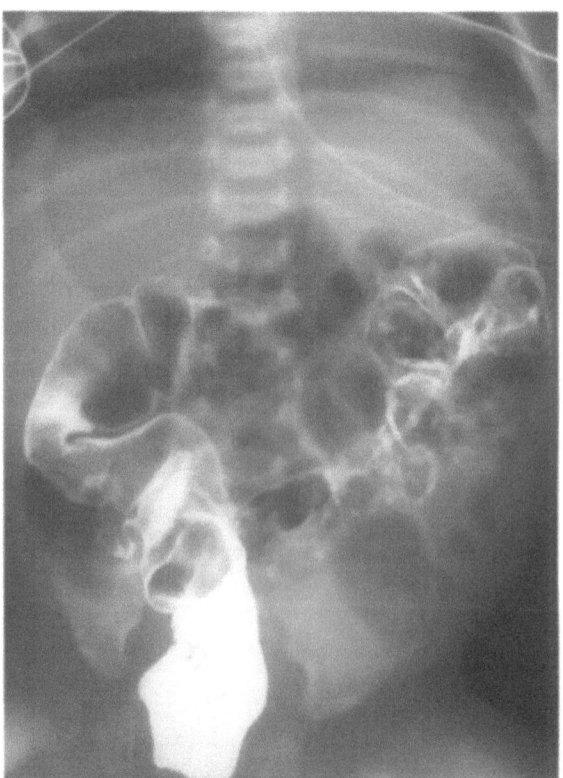

c

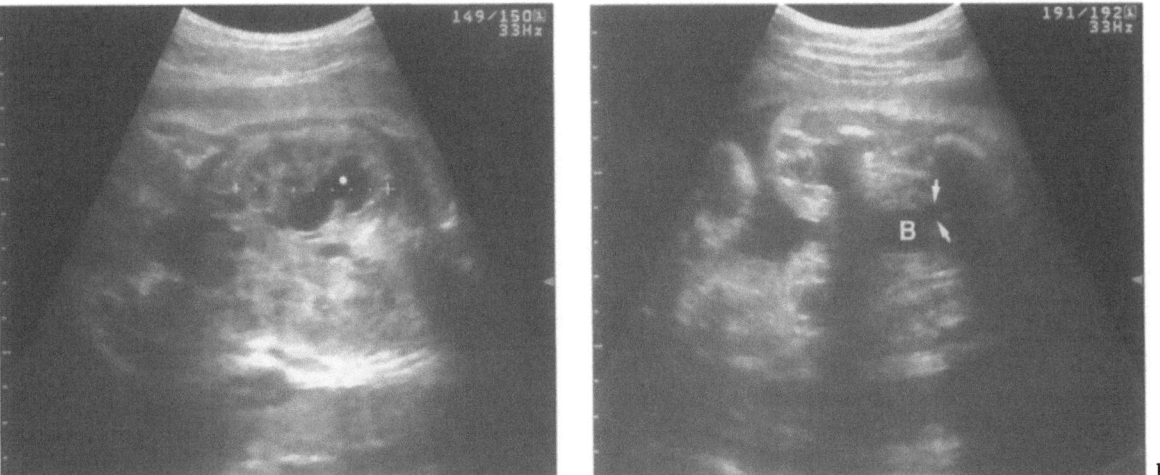

Fig. 8.27a, b. Duplex kidney with ectopic extravesical insertion of the upper pole ureter (second trimester). **a** Sagittal scan of the kidney (4 cm between *crosses*). Dilatation of the upper pole (*). **b** Transverse scan of the pelvis demonstrating the ectopic ureter (*arrows*) behind the bladder (*B*)

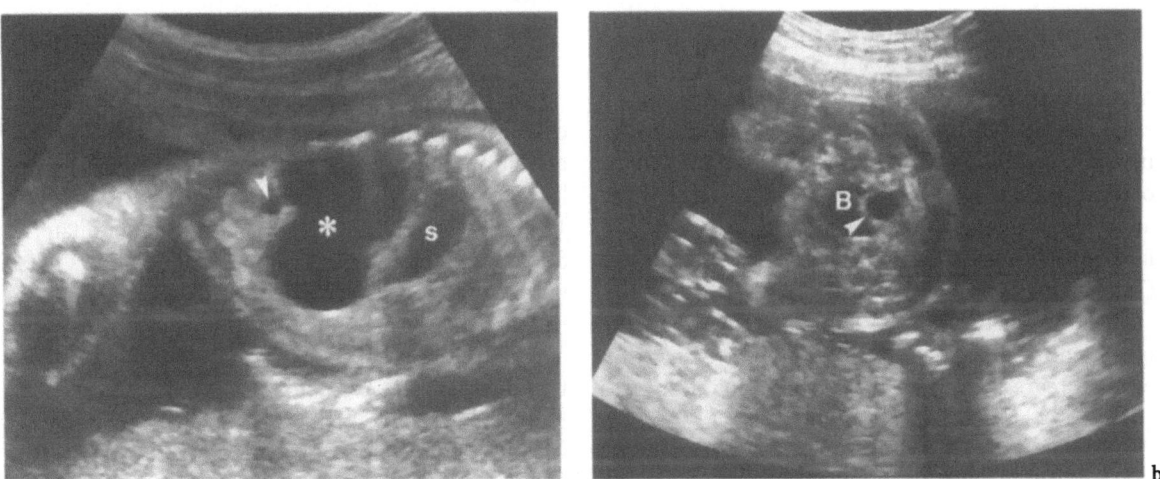

Fig. 8.28a, b. Duplex left kidney with ectopic ureterocele (third trimester). **a** Sagittal scan of the kidney demonstrating a huge dilatation of the upper pole (*) and minimal dilatation of the lower pole (*arrowhead*). *s* stomach. **b** Transverse scan of the renal pelvis showing a ureterocele (*arrowhead*) protruding within the bladder (*B*)

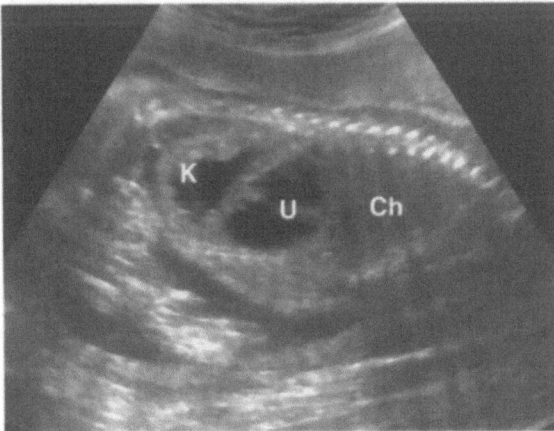

Fig. 8.29. Perirenal urinoma (second trimester). Case of urethral obstruction. Sagittal scan of the fetal trunk. *Ch* chest. A urinoma (*U*) is displacing the dilated kidney (*K*)

utero but is more easily demonstrated after birth
(Fig. 8.27, 8.28). The ureterocele may prolapse into
the urethra during micturition and induce acute
bladder outlet obstruction (AUSTIN et al. 1998).

As mentioned above, perirenal *urinomas* can be
encountered in association with a number of urinary tract malformations that cause obstruction
(Fig. 8.29). PUV and UPJ obstruction are the most
common causes; urinomas have been also encountered after a ureterocele prolapse in the urethra
in fetuses with duplex kidneys (AVNI et al. 1985,
CALLEN et al. 1983). In some instances, urinomas
constitute a protective mechanism for the kidney
in order to prevent the deleterious effect of acute
obstruction (RITTENBERG et al. 1988). The urinomas
may resolve in utero or persist after birth.

8.1.4.6
Renal Cysts and Cystic Diseases

Renal cystic diseases should be suspected not only in
the case of obvious macrocysts but also in the case of
hyperechoic kidneys (Table 8.3) (GUAY-WOODFORD
et al. 1998, REUSS et al. 1991). Cysts may be present
in one or both kidneys. Their origin may be genetic
or non-genetic, and they may occur as an isolated
anomaly or part of a syndrome (Table 8.3). Familial history is of great importance for the diagnosis
(FRIEDMANN et al. 2000).

Isolated cortical cysts, although rare, may be
observed in utero (Fig. 8.30); they may persist after
birth or regress spontaneously, in utero or after birth
(BLAZER et al. 1999).

Obstructive cystic dysplasia and *MDK* are the
most common entities in which macrocystic renal
disease can be detected in utero. Obstructive cystic
dysplasia is associated with urinary tract obstruction (Figs. 8.12, 8.13). The obstruction may have
"resolved" at the time of diagnosis and the cystic

Table 8.3. Syndromes with cystic renal disease

Meckel-Gruber
Trisomy 9, 13, 18
Bardet-Biedl
Short ribs polydactyly
Zellweger
Glutaric aciduria
Ivemark
Jeune
Beckwith-Wiedemann
Tuberous sclerosis

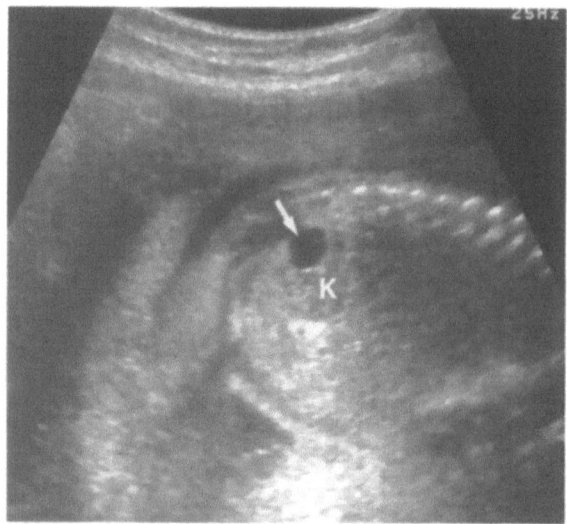

Fig. 8.30. Isolated renal cyst (third trimester). Sagittal scan of
the kidney (*K*) demonstrating a cyst (*arrow*) within the renal
cortex

changes must be considered as the sequelae. In this
condition, the cysts measure less than 1 cm and are
located within the hyperechoic cortex (BLANE et al.
1991, KAEFER et al. 1997). MDK is usually unilateral.
Sonographically, the typical pattern includes a mass
with multiple cysts of varying sizes without connections between them and without normal renal parenchyma (Fig. 8.31). The main differential diagnosis is
UPJ obstruction (AVNI et al. 1987, STRIFE et al. 1993,
PEDICELLI 1986). Bilateral cases are incompatible
with extrauterine life. In some patients with MDK,
the diagnosis may be difficult because of a peculiar
pattern or location. In such instances, MR imaging
may contribute to an accurate diagnosis (Fig. 8.32).

The most frequent genetically transmitted cystic
renal diseases are represented by the recessive and
dominant polycystic kidney diseases. The classical
pattern of autosomal recessive polycystic kidney
disease (ARPKD) includes markedly enlarged (+4
SD) hyperechoic kidneys without CMD. Many other
patterns can be encountered: less significantly
enlarged kidneys, medullary cysts or reversed CMD
(Fig. 8.33). The liver involvement typical of the condition is usually impossible to demonstrate in utero.
The differential diagnosis includes the dominant
polycystic kidney disease glomerulo-cystic kidneys
and Bardet-Biedl syndrome, in which polydactyly
is present (Fig. 8.34). One of the main difficulties in
diagnosing ARPKD results from the variability of the
in utero appearances and timing of occurrence of the

kidney anomalies. These variations occur even in the offspring of a single family (FITCH and STAPLETON 1986, BRONSHTEIN et al. 1992, ZERRES et al. 1998, REUSS et al. 1990, BARTH et al. 1992, BERNSTEIN 1993, LILFORD et al. 1992, WISSER et al. 1995, GERSHONI-BARUCH et al. 1992).

In cases of autosomal dominant polycystic kidney disease (*ADPKD*), the kidneys may be enlarged but to a lesser extent than with ARPKD. There may be two different presentations of the disease in utero. In most cases, the kidneys are not enlarged but

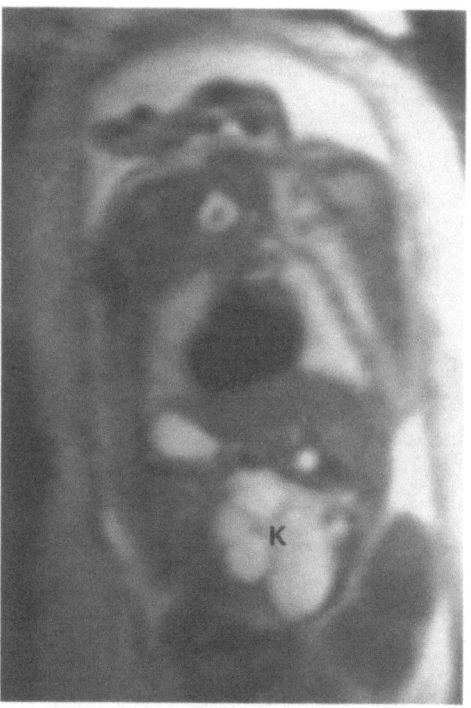

Fig. 8.32. Fetal MR imaging of a pelvic multicystic kidney (*K*) that was thought on US to represent a dilated ureter. T2-weighted sequence. Coronal view

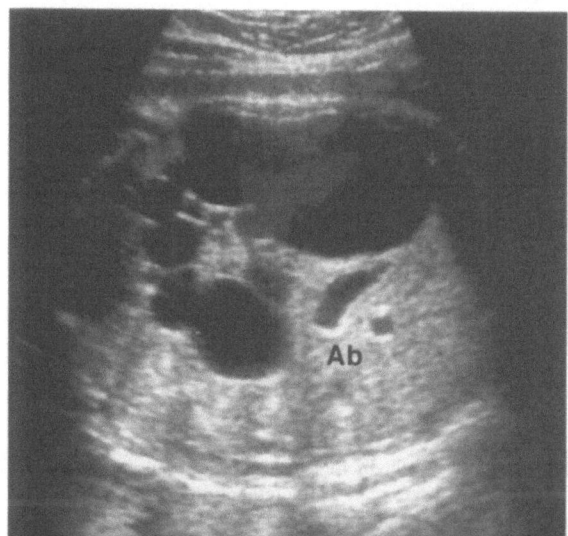

a

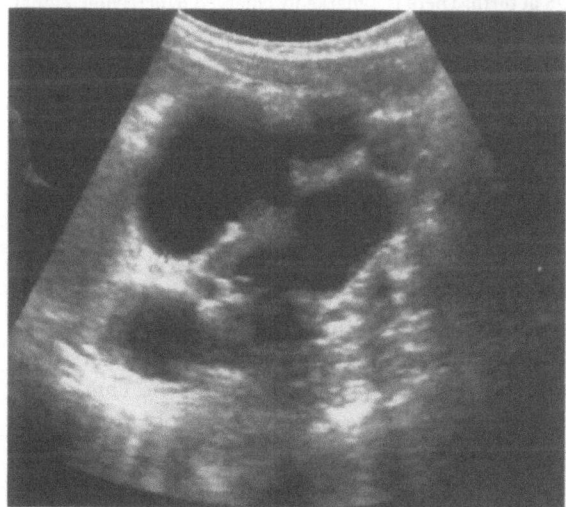

b

Fig. 8.31a, b. Multicystic dysplastic kidney. **a** In utero (third trimester). Transverse scan of the fetal abdomen (*Ab*) demonstrating cysts of variable sizes not connected to each other (5 cm between the *crosses*). **b** US at birth. Sagittal scan of the left kidney. It has the same appearance as on the in utero scan of the dysplastic kidney

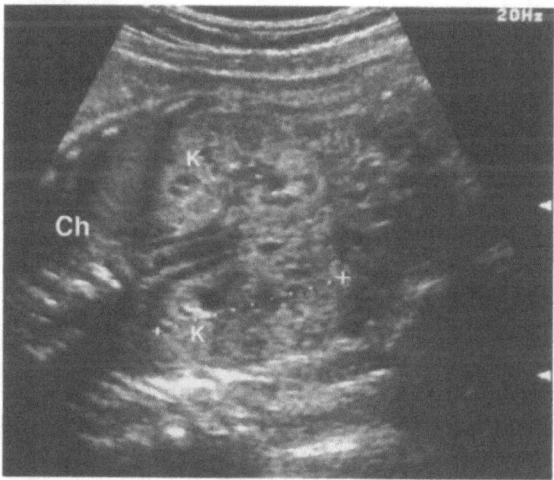

Fig. 8.33. Autosomal recessive polycystic kidney disease (third trimester). Coronal view of both kidneys (*K*) that appear hyperechoic but with a cystic medulla. The kidneys measured 7 cm at 32 weeks. *Ch* chest

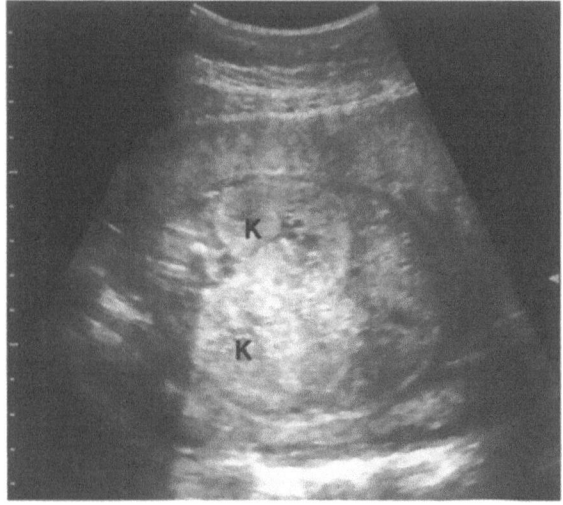

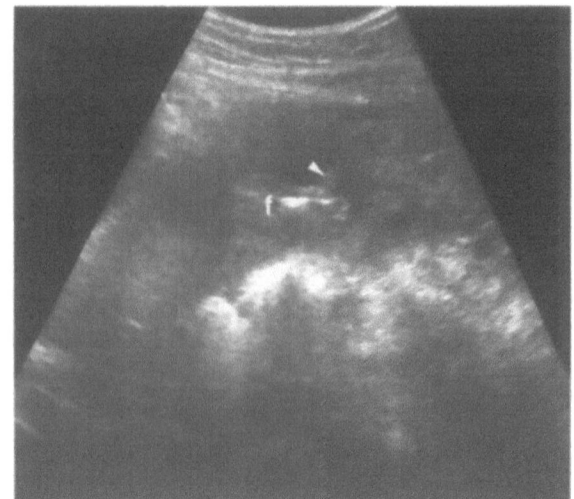

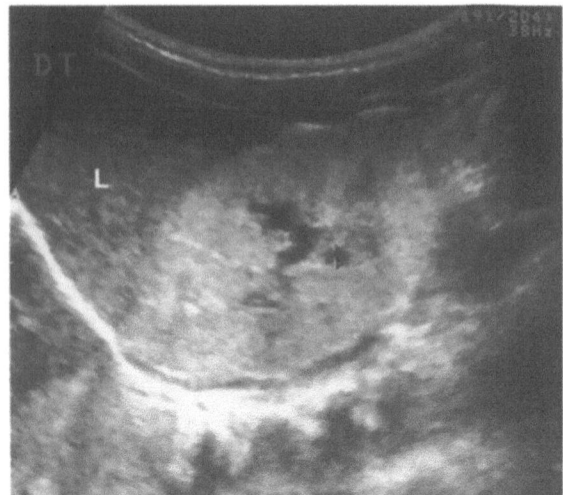

Fig. 8.34a–c. Bardet-Biedl syndrome. a In utero (third trimester). Transverse scan of the fetal abdomen demonstrating enlarged (+ 4SD) hyperechoic kidneys (K) without clear CMD. b In utero. Fetal foot (f) with a supernumerary toe (arrow). c US at birth. There is a markedly enlarged hyperechoic kidney without CMD but with a small cyst (between crosses). L liver

the CMD is increased due to cortical hyperechogenicity (Fig. 8.35) (JOURNEL et al. 1989). In this type of ADPKD, cysts are unusual in utero; they will develop after birth only. Markedly enlarged kidneys resembling ARPKD are another pattern that can be encountered in utero and that suggests the glomerulocystic type of ADPKD. In this presentation of the disease, some subcortical cysts may be present in utero and renal failure may develop at birth (GREER et al. 1998) (Fig. 8.36). This type carries a poorer prognosis. Another difficulty in diagnosing ADPKD is that at the time of the examination familial history is unknown in over 50% of cases. Conversely, examination of the parents and grandparents is mandatory for the investigation of such fetuses (ZERRES 1998, MCDERMOT et al. 1998, MICHAUD

et al. 1994, CECCHERINI et al. 1989, EDWARDS and BALDINGER 1989, FICK et al. 1994).

Cystic kidneys are part of many syndromes (Table 8.3) that may present many associated anomalies (LEHMAN et al. 1995, NYBERG et al. 1990). At pathological examination, glomerulocystic type and (medullary) cystic dysplasia anomalies are commonly found (GREER et al. 1998). The clue to the diagnosis, will be the demonstration of an associated malformation typical of the diagnosis (e.g. central nervous system anomaly, polydactyly and medullary cystic dysplasia in the case of Meckel-Gruber syndrome (Fig. 8.37) (NYBERG et al. 1990). Another illustration would be Jeune's syndrome with associated small chest dwarfism and medullary cystic kidneys (Fig. 8.38).

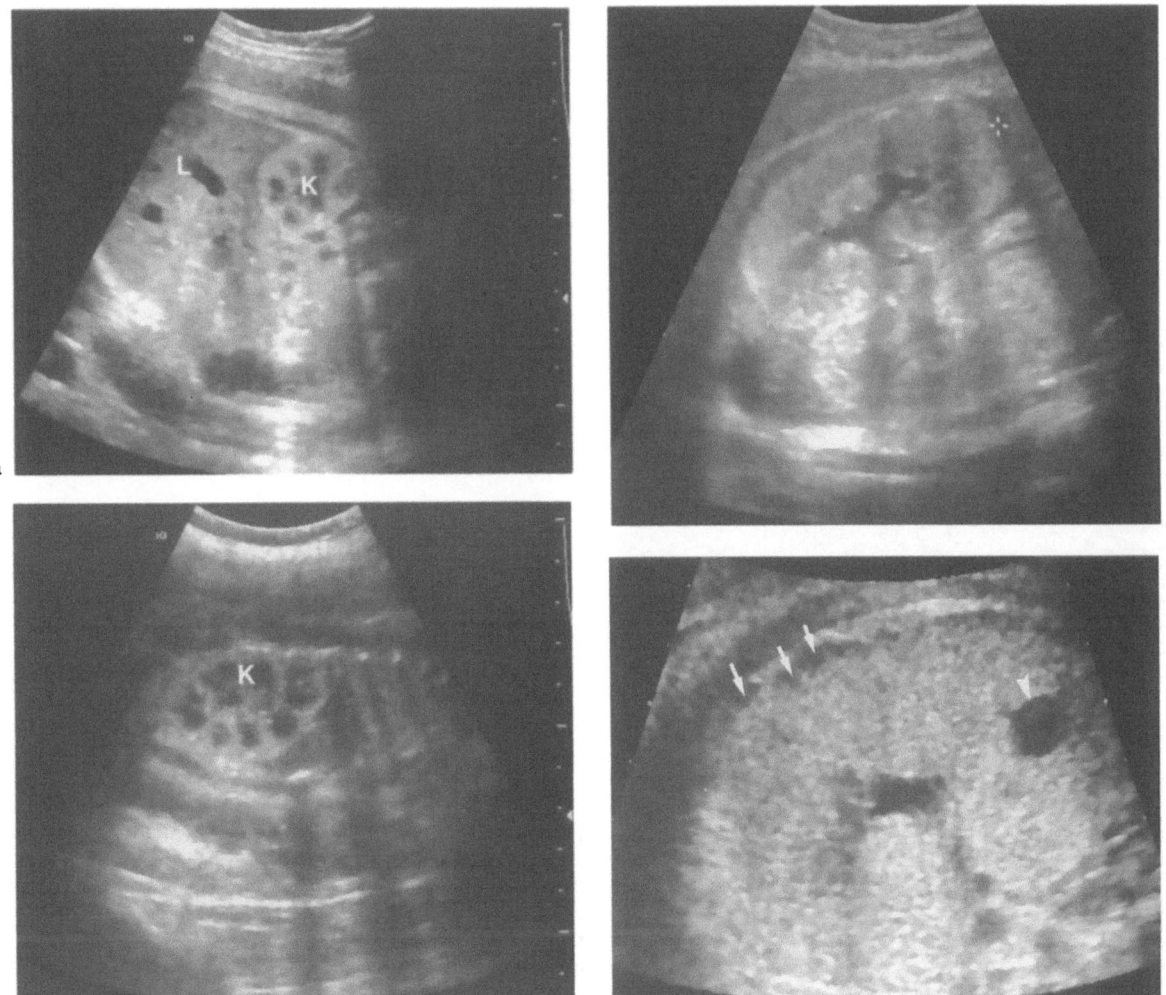

Fig. 8.35a, b. Autosomal dominant polycystic kidney disease (third trimester), classical type. The mother was affected. **a** Transverse scan of the fetal abdomen. CMD is visible in the right kidney (*K*) but the cortex appears hyperechoic compared with adjacent liver (*L*). **b** Sagittal scan of the kidney (46 mm between *crosses;* =+1.5 SD). The cortex is hyperechoic. *K* kidney)

Fig. 8.36a, b. Autosomal dominant polycystic kidney disease (third trimester), glomerulocystic type (courtesy of Danielle EURIN, MD, Rouen, France). **a** Bilateral enlarged fetal kidneys (between *crosses;* + 4 SD), without CMD. **b** Sagittal scan of the kidney. Enlarged hyperechoic kidney without CMD but with peripheral tiny cysts (*arrows*) and one cortical cyst (*arrowhead*)

8.1.4.7
Tumors

Fetal renal tumors are rare. In the case of a tumor with multiple cysts, a multicystic dysplastic kidney should be considered first. Mesoblastic blastoma and Wilms' tumor may also appear as a partially cystic tumor but are usually more localized (BOVE 1999, SHIBAHARA et al. 1999, APPLEGATE et al. 1999, IRSUTTI et al. 2000). Both appear more frequently as solid-type masses difficult to separate from the normal renal parenchyma; fetal MR imaging may contribute to this differential diagnosis (POUTAMO et al. 2000) (see Chap. 13). Another differential diagnosis to be included is nephroblastomatosis, which appears either as hypoechoic nodule(s) or as a diffusely enlarged hyperechoic kidney (AMBROSINO et al. 1990). Renal tumors have to be differentiated from adrenal tumors and from intra-abdominal sequestrations (DANEMAN et al. 1997) (see Chap. 13).

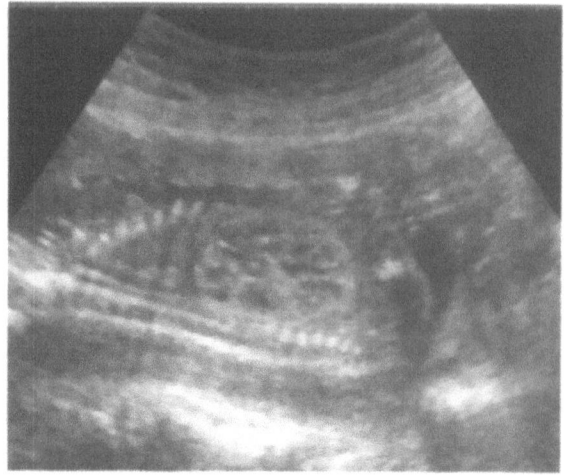

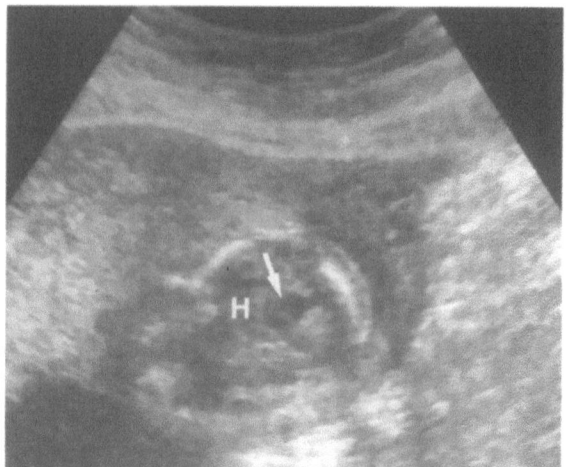

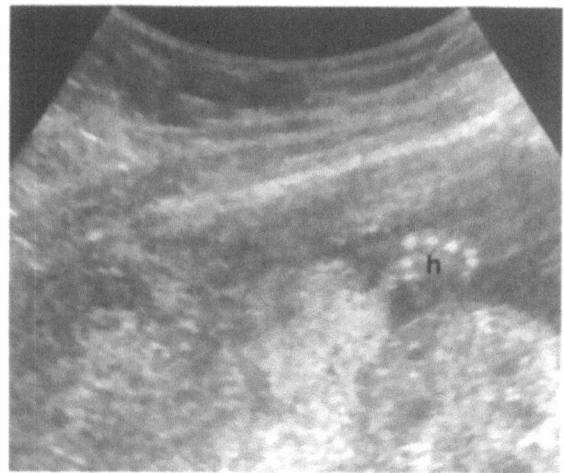

Fig. 8.37a–c. Meckel-Gruber syndrome (second trimester). a Sagittal scan through one kidney (32.7 mm between *crosses*; + 3 SD) demonstrating enlarged hypoechoic pyramids. b Transverse scan of the fetal posterior fossa showing a cystic dilatation of the fourth ventricle (*arrow*). *H* head. c View of the fetal hand demonstrating polydactyly

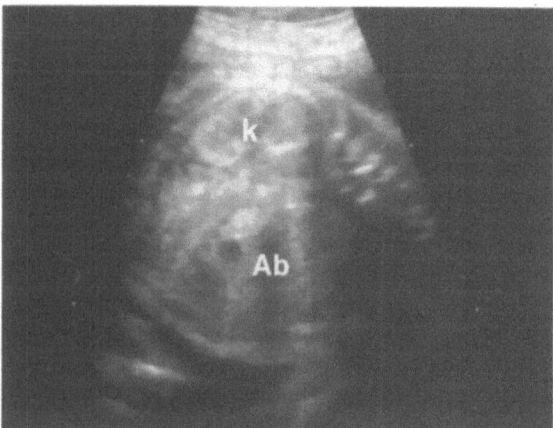

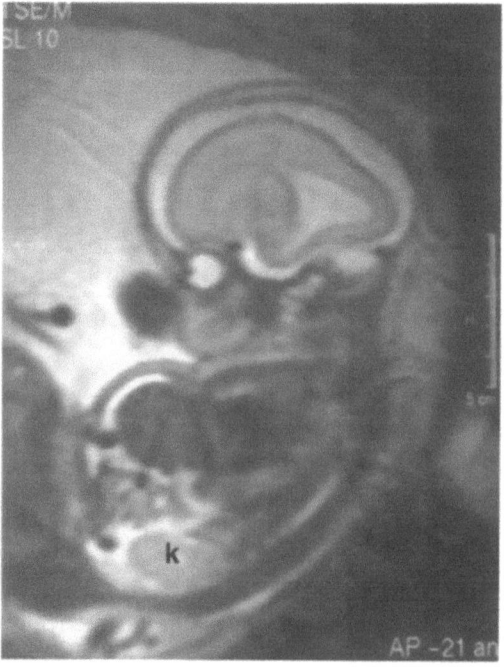

Fig. 8.38a, b. Cystic kidneys in a case of Jeune syndrome (asphyxiating thoracic dysplasia), end of second trimester. a Transverse /oblique scan of the fetal abdomen (*Ab*) The kidneys (*k*) are moderately enlarged with increased echogenicity of the cortex and large pyramids. b Fetal MR imaging, T2-weighted sequence. The small chest is relatively to the abdomen. The kidney (*) appears globular with a hypointense rim possibly corresponding to the cortex

8.1.4.8
Renal Vein Thrombosis

Renal vein thrombosis (RVT) may occur in utero; the origin of the thrombosis is not always obvious. Placental emboli or slowing of the blood flow within the inferior vena cava (IVC) are usually suspected. Sonographically, the kidney appears somewhat enlarged or of normal size; the cortex may appear hyperechoic and without CMD. Hyperechoic stripes may be visible in the interlobar areas. Thrombus in the IVC is a usual association (Fig. 8.39a, b). Collateral vessels develop very rapidly and in most cases there are no consequences on further renal development (LALMAND et al. 1990, WRIGHT et al. 1996, FISHMAN and JOSEPH 1994). After birth, the hyperechoic stripes and the thrombus within the IVC are usually calcified (Fig. 8.39c, d). This feature helps to differentiate antenatal from postnatal onset of the RVT (LALMAND et al. 1990).

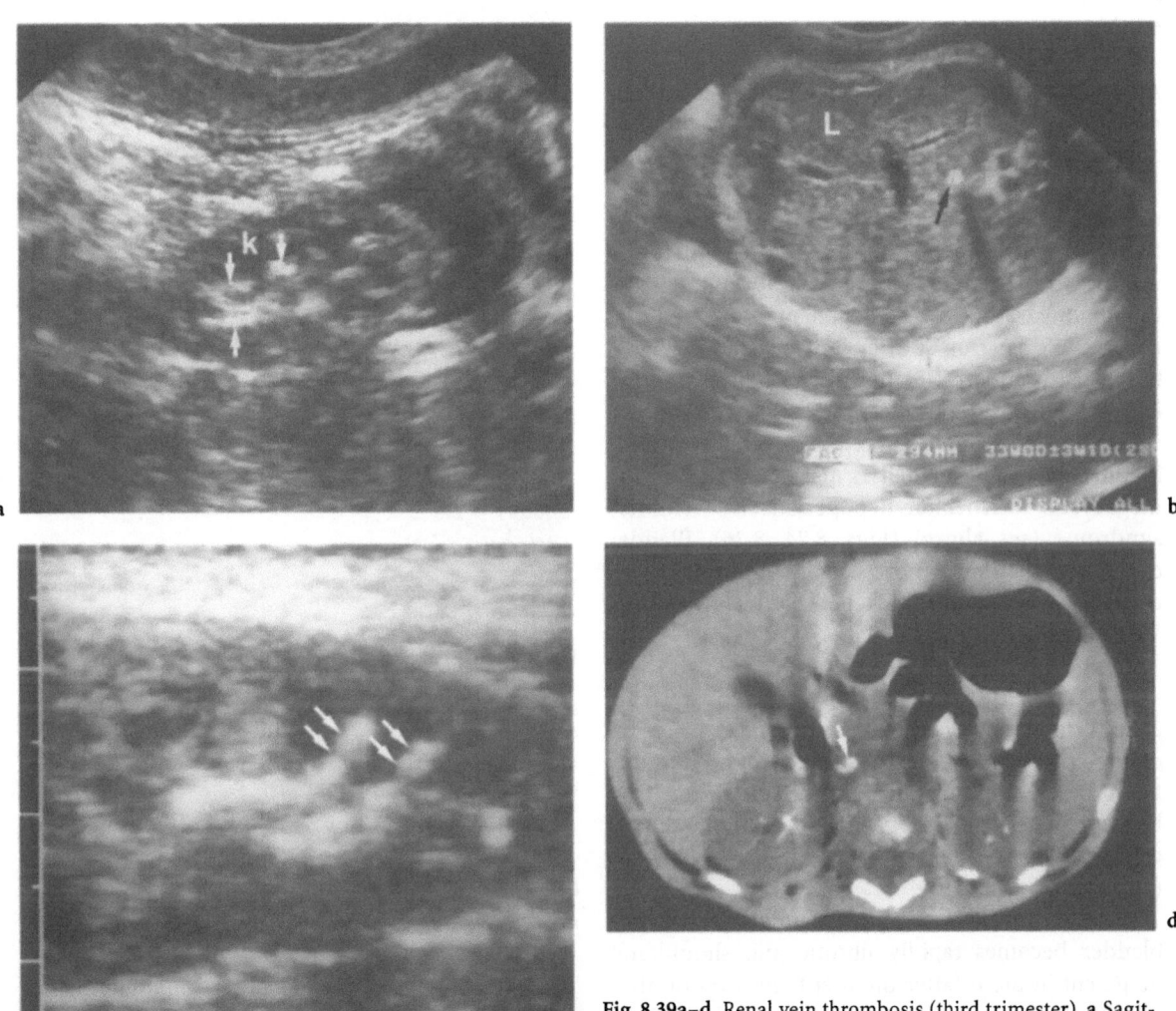

Fig. 8.39a–d. Renal vein thrombosis (third trimester). **a** Sagittal scan of the left kidney (*k*) containing hyperechoic streaks (*arrows*). **b** Transverse scan of the fetal abdomen demonstrating a calcified thrombus (*arrow*) within the inferior vena cava. *L* liver. **c** Neonatal US of the left kidney. Sagittal scan demonstrating the hyperechoic streaks (*arrows*). **d** Neonatal CT without contrast enhancement confirming calcifications within the inferior vena cava (*arrow*) and the renal veins

8.1.4.9
Compensatory Renal Growth

Compensatory hypertrophy of a solitary functioning kidney seems to occur already in utero; however,
it does not happen in every type of uropathy. It is
evaluated by measurement of the length of the kidney
(MANDELL et al. 1993, GLAZEBROOK et al. 1993). The
mechanism by which the phenomenon occurs is
unclear and has yet to be demonstrated.

8.1.4.10
Bladder and Urachus

An enlarged bladder (above 3 cm in the second trimester, above 6 cm in the third trimester) suggests
a bladder outlet obstruction. During the second
trimester, a bladder enlargement may result from
urethral atresia or stenosis. It may be part of a Prune
Belly sequence (Fig. 8.25). The more complete the
urethral obstruction the more important will be
the oligohydramnios. The degree of associated urinary tract dilatation and renal dysplasia is variable
but usually underestimated by US. The prognosis
is poor. During the third trimester, an obstructive
origin has to be differentiated from other causes of
bladder enlargement such as massive VUR and the
megacystis–microcolon–hypoperistalsis   (MMH)
syndrome (see above) (Figs. 8.24, 8.26). Bladder
outlet obstruction is more usually associated with
oligohydramnios and thickened bladder wall than
VUR or MMH.

In the case of bladder exstrophy, no bladder is
seen between the two umbilical arteries and, instead,
a small mass is seen below the umbilical insertion
of the cord (Fig. 8.40). Bladder exstrophy is a difficult sonographic diagnosis since some fluid may
be trapped between the open bladder and the thighs;
this may be misinterpreted as a normal bladder
(GEARHART et al. 1995).

Urachus canal connecting the umbilicus and the
bladder becomes rapidly fibrotic and should not
be patent in utero (after the first trimester) or after
birth. Anomalies of the urachus may be detected in
utero. Urachal cyst should be included in the differential diagnosis of a cystic abdominal mass developed on the midline. Patent dilated urachus may also
be a feature of bladder outlet obstruction (Fig. 8.41)
(PERSUTTE et al. 1988, HILL et al. 1990, GOBET et al.
1998). Allantoid remnant cyst can be detected as a
cystic mass within the umbilical cord in connection
with the bladder (Fig. 8.42). It disappears spontaneously in utero (ruptures?).

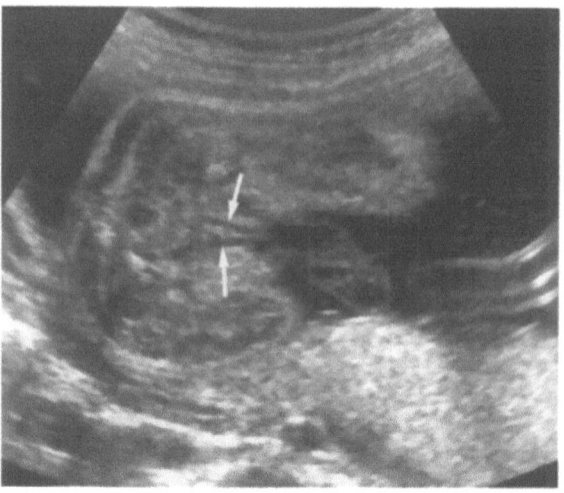

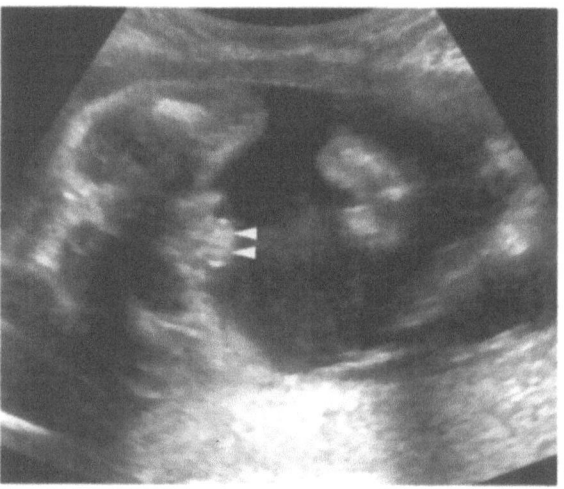

Fig. 8.40a, b. Bladder exstrophy (third trimester). **a** Transverse
scan at the level of the fetal pelvis. No cystic structure can be
seen between the two umbilical arteries (*arrows*). **b** Transverse
scan above the level in **a**; a small mass (*arrowheads*) is bulging out the fetal abdomen; it corresponds to the malformed
bladder

8.1.4.11
Prognosis: In Utero Treatment?

The prognosis in utero is based on the time of
diagnosis, the degree of urinary tract dilatation, the
presence of a uni- or bilateral dilatation, the amount
of amniotic fluid, signs of renal dysplasia and the
consequences on pulmonary development. Factors
indicating a poor prognosis are listed in Table 8.4.
The lethal uropathies are mainly detected during
the first half of the pregnancy (BLACHAR et al.
1994). Non-lethal renal anomalies are mainly diagnosed during the second half of pregnancy (ECONO-
MOU et al. 1994, OLIVEIRA 1999, FUGELSEH 1994). A

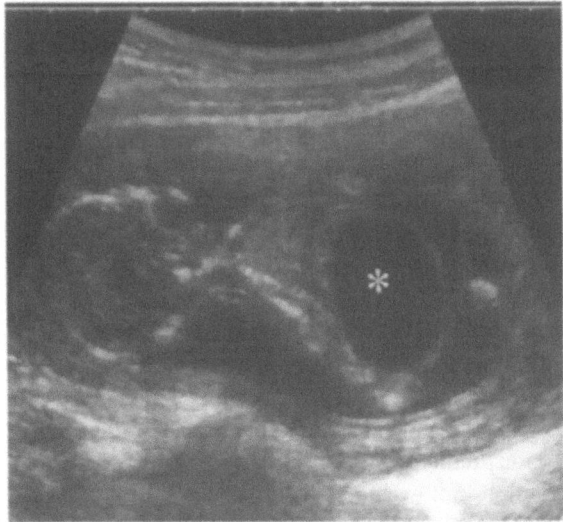

a

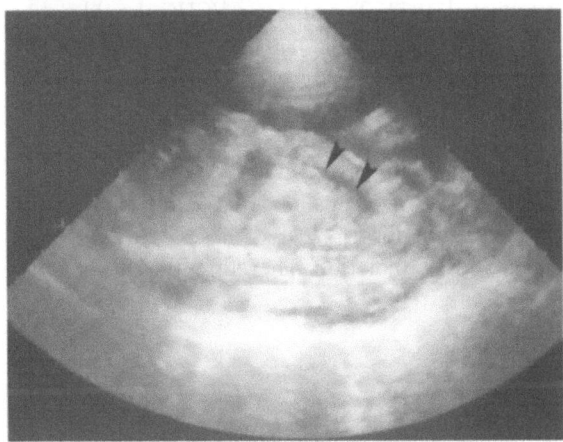

b

Fig. 8.41a, b. Patent urachus. **a** US scan at the beginning of the second trimester demonstrates an obstructed megabladder (*); it disappeared subsequently and amniotic fluid volume increased. **b** US scan during the third trimester demonstrates a small bladder and a patent urachus (*arrowheads*). Perinatal death occurred due to lung hypoplasia

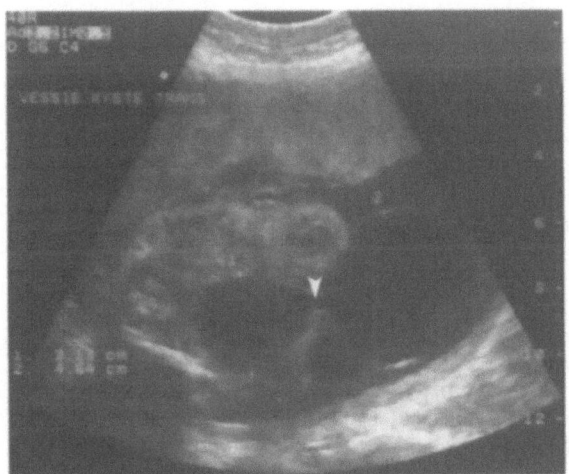

a

Table 8.4. Factors of poor prognosis for uropathies detected in utero

Early diagnosis (<20 weeks)
Oligohydramnios
Bilateral uretero-hydronephrosis
Bilateral cystic dysplasia
Other systems anomalies
Chromosomal anomalies

systematic chromosomal analysis in the case of fetal uropathies has been controversial. Some authors advocate a systematic analysis, especially in the case of bilateral pyelectasis of the second trimester, which they consider an important marker for trisomy 21. For others, chromosomal analysis is indicated mainly in bilateral obstructive anomalies and when other systems anomalies are demonstrated. Analysis of fetal urine is possible and has led several teams to obtain urine by puncture (BUSSIÈRES et al. 1995, SPITZER 1996, ELDER et al. 1990, MULLER et al. 1993) . To date there is no convincing evidence that such measures have had beneficial consequences on fetal outcome (JOHNSON et al. 1994, FREEDMAN et al. 1996, MAKKINO et al. 2000, McLORIE et al. 2001).

It is noteworthy that, unless there is evidence of fetal distress, no uropathy justifies advancing the date of delivery.

The main advantage of an in utero diagnosis is to induce an optimized neonatal investigation and management of the uropathy so that no supplementary damage occurs to the kidney (CENDRON et al. 1994, ELDER 1992, et al. SKARI 1998, WOODWARD 1993).

> A wide spectrum of uropathies can be detected in utero with increasing diagnostic accuracy. UPJ obstruction and VUR are the two most common causes for fetal dilatation.

8.1.5
Postnatal Investigation

After birth, severe bilateral renal diseases such as PUV and ARPKD can be associated with pneumothorax, lung hypoplasia and life-threatening respiratory distress (PERLMAN and LEVIN 1973). This respiratory failure constitutes an emergency and respiratory assistance is mandatory even before any

Fig. 8.42. Urachal-allantoid cyst (third trimester) (courtesy of Danielle Eurin, MD, Rouen, France). Transverse scan of the fetal abdomen. A cyst (*crosses 2*) is present anterior to the abdominal wall and connecting with the bladder (*crosses 1*) through a narrow channel (*arrowhead*)

treatment can be considered for the urinary tract anomaly. Conversely, whenever a neonate presents a "spontaneous" pneumothorax, a US examination should be performed in order to verify the status of the urinary tract.

No other uropathy constitutes a real emergency. Nevertheless, several conditions could necessitate early management and an investigation in the immediate neonatal period. For instance, in the case of posterior urethral valves, the rapid placement of a catheter within the bladder is necessary in order to drain the urine and to reduce the dilatation (NAKAYAMA et al. 1986). Ectopic ureterocele associated with an obstructed upper pole of a duplex kidney is prone to prolapse into the urethra during micturition and to induce an acute bladder outlet obstruction and obstructive anuria (AVNI et al. 1991, AUSTIN et al. 1998). Unroofing of the ureterocele under cystoscopy is therefore advocated by several teams as the first step in the management of this type of complicated duplex kidneys (VANSAVAGE and MESROBIAN 1995, HAGG et al. 2000).

For all the uropathies, the investigation has been tentatively standardized (Diagram 8.1). Nowadays, the major workload of an imaging department dealing with neonatal pathology is related to the inves-

tigation of an antenatal diagnosis of a urinary tract dilatation, trying to define its significance (OWEN et al. 1996, DACHER et al. 1995, DEVAUSSUZENET et al. 1997). The extensive neonatal investigations performed in recent years by many teams have mainly increased the detection of neonatal VUR (ZERIN et al. 1993, PALTIEL and LEBOWITZ 1989, AVNI et al. 1998). The main question has been, and remains, to determine which patients with an in utero urinary tract dilatation should be investigated postnatally.

Several approaches have been proposed. For some authors, whatever the result of a neonatal US, a VCUG should be performed in the case of any antenatal diagnosis of a urinary tract dilatation. For them, US is a poor predictor of VUR and a normal US examination does not exclude VUR (TIBBALS and DE BRUYN 1996, WALSH and DUBBINS 1996, SCOTT et al. 1991, BLANE et al. 1993). For others, a VCUG should not be performed in all the neonates as there would be too many false negative studies, partly because spontaneous resolution of VUR is frequent. At Sainte Justine Hospital, only 5% of mild fetal pyelectasis showed evidence of VUR on postnatal VCUG (unpublished data). There they consider that extrarenal pelves, which account for 15–20% of cases, should not be considered as dilatation. Therefore, they favor post-

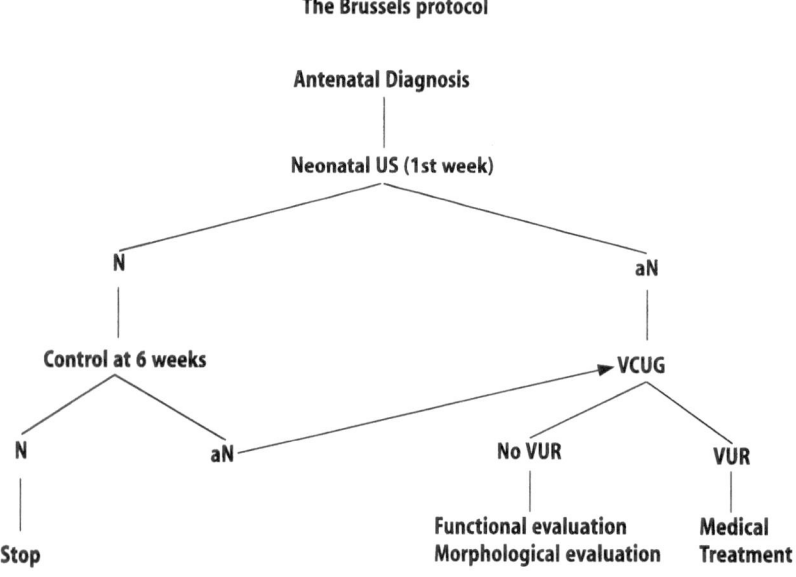

Diagram 8.1. Proposed neonatal investigation of fetal uropathies. *N* normal. *aN*, abnormal, *VCUG* voiding cystourethrogram, *VUR*, vesico-ureteric reflux

natal investigations only if there is prenatal evidence of pyelectasis >10 mm, caliectasis whatever the renal pelvis measurement, ureterectasis or bladder distension. Other authors rely on postnatal US to decide whether a VCUG is indicated. A VCUG should be performed only in those patients in which the anomaly had been confirmed after birth (YERKES et al. 1999). Therefore, among most teams, US is performed first in order to confirm the anomaly (MARRA et al. 1994, AVNI et al. 1997a, HULBERT et al. 1992). In the case of a clinical emergency, it can even be performed as soon as the clinical condition permits. For all other cases, it should be delayed until after the physiological dehydration period, namely after the 5th day. At that time, the US examination should be as detailed as possible in order to detect every anomaly that would justify continuing the investigation . The presence of a urinary tract dilatation is the most important landmark; 7 mm (anteroposterior diameter, measured on a transverse scan) is the most widely accepted upper limit of normal (preferably with an empty bladder), though others prefer 5 mm, and some 10 mm (Fig. 8.43). Dilatation of the pelvis is not the only anomaly that should be looked for. Other anomalies can be associated with VUR (Table 8.5). Loss of CMD is a good predictor of high-grade VUR. One should not forget to visualize the bladder during the examination; a large bladder could be a sign of VUR. With a meticulous US examination, one should be able to detect over 85% of cases of VUR. Cases that are missed are non-dilating grades I–II VUR (MARRA et al. 1994, AVNI et al. 1997a, WEINBERG and YEUNG 1998).

According to these authors, if the US examination is entirely normal, no further examination is necessary. A control examination should be performed at 1

or 3 months in order to detect cases that would have escaped the neonatal screening (DEJTER and GIBBONS 1989, CLAUDICE-ENGEL 1994) (Table 8.5).

Table 8.5. US findings that may be associated with vesico-ureteric reflux

Pelvic dilatation above 7 mm (bladder empty)
Variable dilatation
Calyceal dilatation
Ureteral dilatation above 3 mm
Pelvic wall thickening
Loss of cortico-medullary differentiation
Small kidney
Signs of dysplasia
Enlarged bladder

If the US examination is abnormal, a VCUG should be performed, preferably during the first 2 weeks of life. Cyclic filling of the bladder increases the rate of detection of VUR. The use of pulsed fluoroscopy reduces the radiation doses (PALTIEL et al. 1992, CLEVELAND et al. 1992). The examination should be performed under antiseptic chemotherapy. The aim of the examination is to detect VUR, bladder or urethral anomalies (Figs. 8.11c, 8.44).

If VUR is demonstrated, the patient is put under prophylactic antibiotic therapy and followed-up clinically and by imaging for 2 years hoping that the VUR will resolve spontaneously. During this period, renal growth is monitored every 3 months by US and renal function every 6 months by isotopes. The resolution of VUR is verified every year on isotopic or radiological VCUG.

If no VUR is present, the dilatation is probably related to obstruction and the investigation must be

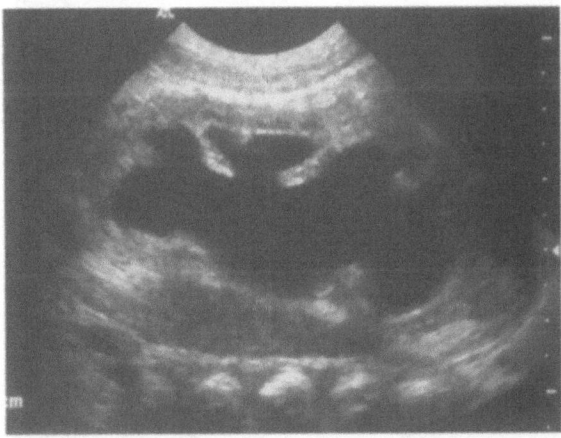 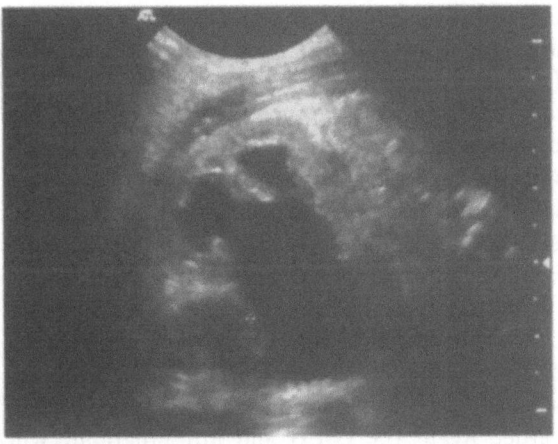

a b

Fig. 8.43a, b. Neonatal US of a uretero-pelvic junction obstruction. **a** Sagittal scan of the kidney (between *crosses*) with typical pyelo-calyceal dilatation. **b** Transverse scan showing a 13 mm anteroposterior dilatation of an extrarenal pelvis

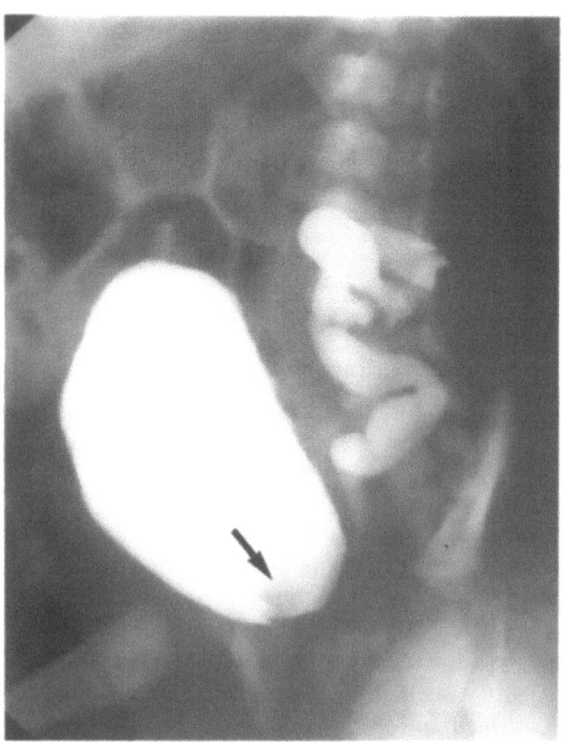

Fig. 8.44. VCUG in the case of a left duplication. There is reflux grade IV into the lower pole and ureterocele (*arrow*) connected to the upper pole

ureter (AVNI et al. 1998, 2001). Isotopic studies using Tc-DTPA or MAG3 are also mandatory in order to evaluate the remaining function of the two poles.

For all the other anomalies, especially MDK, renal ectopia or unilateral agenesis, the investigation should also include US and a VCUG in order to detect ipsi- or contralateral VUR that would require prophylactic chemotherapy (ATIYEH 1992, 1993, FLACK and BELLINGER 1993, SELZMAN and ELDER 1995, CASCIO et al. 1999). In the case of hereditary renal cystic disease, the postnatal investigation will depend upon the type of cystic disease and the clinical condition. US is usually the first procedure performed (Fig. 8.48). Patients who survive the neonatal period will require long-term and close clinical and imaging follow-up. In the case of a renal tumor, a classical investigation will determine the type of tumor and its extent. A nephrectomy will usually be required.

> A US examination has to be performed at birth in all patients with an antenatal diagnosis. A VCUG should follow in the case of a US abnormality. The presence or absence of VUR will determine the rest of the neonatal investigation.

completed by isotopic studies including a furosemide nephrogram (CHUNG et al. 1993).

If surgery is decided on, the morphology of the urinary tract must be assessed preoperatively. Excretory urography (EU) used to be performed for this purpose. However, it is an irradiating technique and contrast material injection is needed. Also, the poorer the function, the poorer will be the opacification of the dilated urinary tract. Therefore, more and more authors advocate the use of MR urography for the assessment of a dilated urinary tract (Figs. 8.45–8.47) (BORTHNE 1999, AVNI et al. 2001). Furosemide is usually injected in order to increase the diuresis and to optimize the visualization of the urinary tract. T2-weighted, inversion recovery and post-gadolinium enhancement T1-weighted sequences allow a good evaluation of the urinary tract. The drawback of the method is that it necessitates sedation. In the case of an abnormal duplex collecting system, the investigation is similar to that of obstruction. However, the morphological assessment must be more rapid since a therapeutic decision might have to be made earlier. Again US, VCUG and MR urography will optimally assess the morphology. MR urography is the best method to visualize an ectopic extravesical

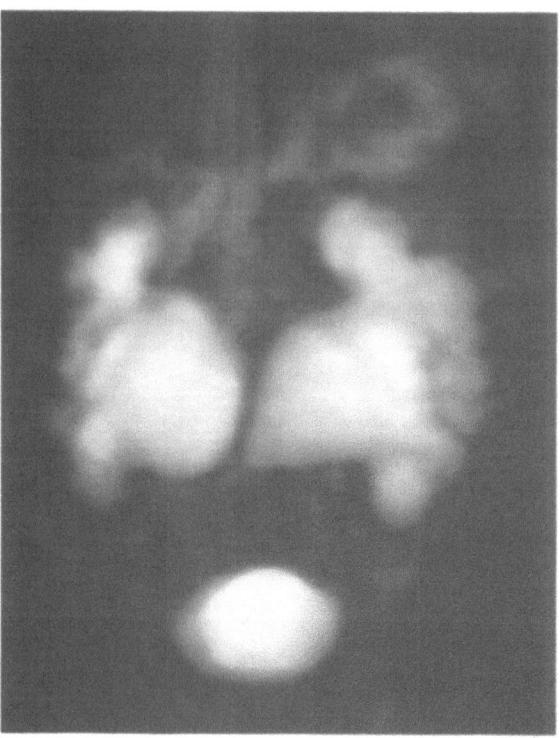

Fig. 8.45. MR imaging of a bilateral uretero-pelvic junction, T2-weighted sequence. Coronal view

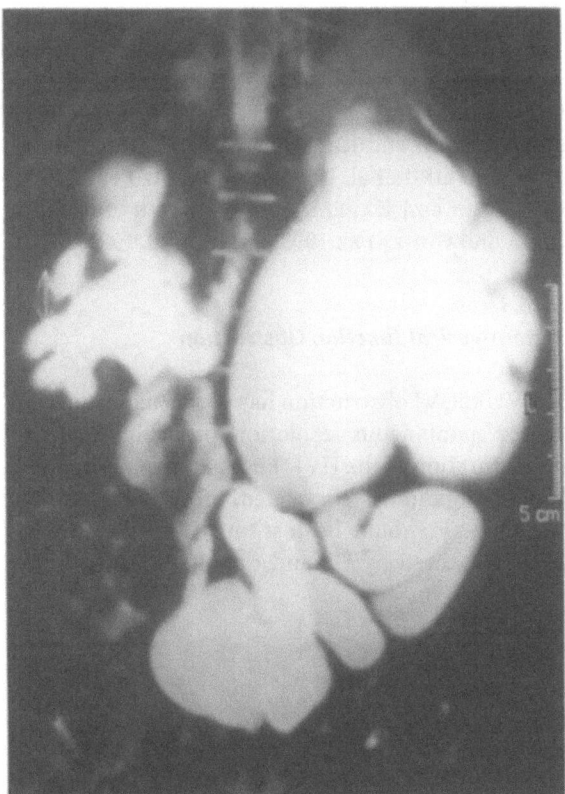

Fig. 8.46. MR imaging of a bilateral uretero-vesical junction obstruction more important on the left side, T2-weighted sequence. Coronal view

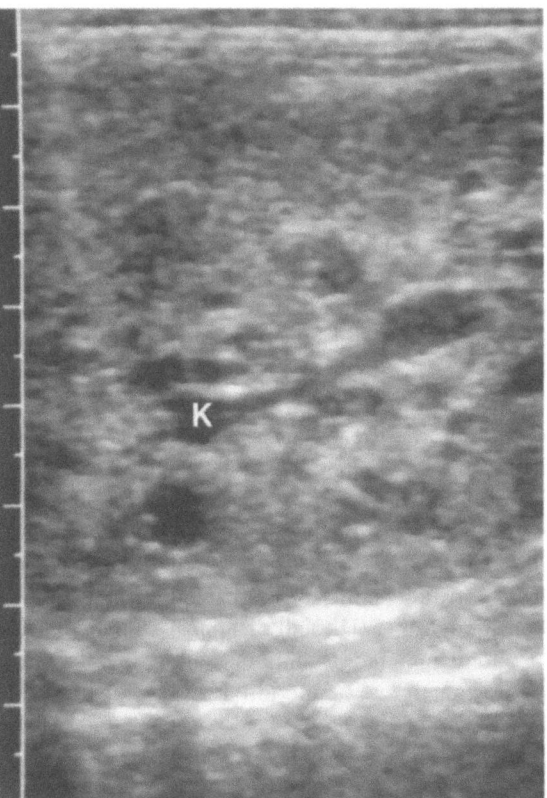

Fig. 8.48. US of autosomal recessive polycystic disease in a newborn with bilateral pneumothoraces (not shown). Large kidney (*K*) with a cystic-appearing medulla

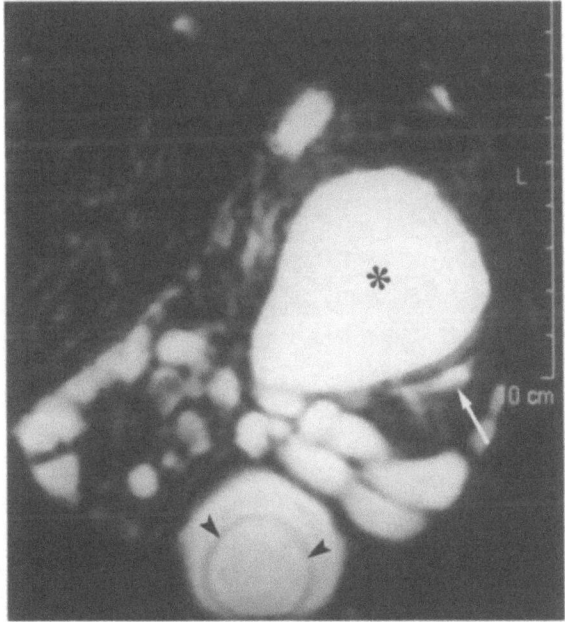

Fig. 8.47. MR imaging of a left duplex kidney demonstrating an obstructed upper pole (*) in association with an ectopic ureterocele (*arrowhead*) and a non-dilated lower pole (*arrow*)

8.1.6
Treatment in the Light of the Natural History of Uro-nephropathies

As mentioned above, antenatal diagnosis has led to dramatic changes in the management of uropathies. First, the patients are mostly asymptomatic; second, the medical follow-up of many pathologies has shown their potential to resolve spontaneously. Consequently, surgery has been less and less advocated. The main goal of prophylactic treatment is to prevent further renal damage during the period in which spontaneous resolution is expected. There are cases of infection despite the antibiotic prophylactic therapy; these cases render an alternative treatment necessary (DACHER et al. 1992, JASWON et al. 1999, MORIN et al. 1996).

8.1.6.1
Vesico-ureteric Reflux

The vast majority of cases of dilating neonatal vesico-ureteric reflux (VUR) occur in male neonates, possibly related to an embryological difference between the sexes (ANDERSON and RICKWOOD 1991, AVNI and SCHULMANN 1996, BAILEY et al. 1992, YEUNG 1997). Many series have shown that two thirds of neonatal VUR, whatever its grade, is likely to resolve or at least to improve during an observation period of 2 years. Therefore, once the anomaly is detected the patient is put under prophylactic antibiotic therapy and followed clinically and by imaging as described above. In some circumstances another therapeutic approach (surgery or Teflon injection) should be proposed, i.e. in cases of infection despite therapy, in cases of failure to thrive or in cases of familial problems with continuing the treatment (HERNDON et al. 1999, GORDON et al. 1990, BURGE et al. 1992, BOUACHRINE et al. 1996, DUDLEY et al. 1997, ASSAEL et al. 1998). Fetal reflux nephropathy is another factor that may alter the prognosis; here parenchymal lesions exist already in utero and are associated with the VUR. Even though the VUR will disappear in many cases, the parenchymal loss will persist and will determine the postnatal renal function (MARRA et al. 1994, NAJMALDIN et al. 1990).

8.1.6.2
Uretero-pelvic Junction Obstruction

The therapeutic management of UPJ obstruction has been much more controversial than for VUR. Advocates and opponents of neonatal surgery have published much scientific material showing opposite or contradictory results. For some, early surgery is safe and notably improves renal function. Other advocate the use of double-J stenting of the UPJ obstruction. For others, the UPJ obstruction has been present for a long time and there is only a faint chance of improving it by surgery, which does not justify operating on a neonate. Furthermore the dilatation may resolve spontaneously. Yet others suggest following renal function and operating on only those who will show functional deterioration. Finally, some suggest following renal growth on US and operating when the contralateral kidney displays compensatory growth. Also, the criteria used to diagnose obstruction are not clear-cut, either on US or on many isotopic studies.

From all the data accumulated up to now, conservative management seems the most adequate in mild or moderate cases. The clinical status and renal function must be monitored closely. In most cases the dilatation will be stable or even resolve. Surgery must be proposed if clinical symptoms appear or if renal function deteriorates. In the more severe cases, spontaneous resolution is less likely to occur

and symptoms related to abdominal discomfort are more frequent. For these patients, surgery may be beneficial (KOFF and CAMPBELL 1992, 1994, DOCIMO and SILVER 1997, BLACHAR et al. 1994, DUCKETT 1993, ARNOLD and RICKWOOD 1990, RANSLEY et al. 1990, DOWLING et al. 1988, CAPOLICCHIO et al. 1999, MCALLEER and KAPLAN 1999, CHERTIN et al. 1999, TAPIA and GONZALEZ 1995, SALEM et al. 1995).

8.1.6.3
Uretero-vesical Junction Obstruction

Like VUR, UVJ obstruction has shown a great potential for spontaneous resolution, probably thanks to the maturation of the UVJ (Fig. 8.49). Therefore, after the investigation is completed, prophylactic antibiotic therapy should be instituted and the urinary tract monitored by US and eventually isotopes. US

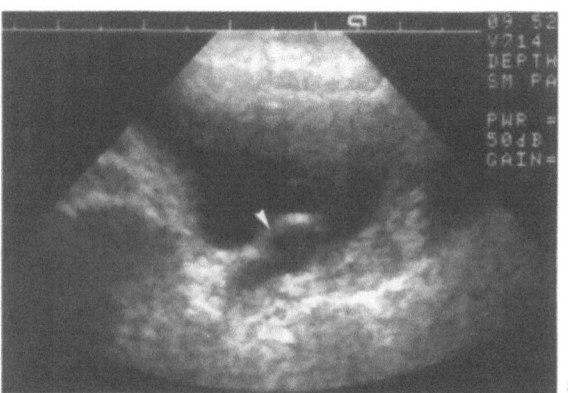

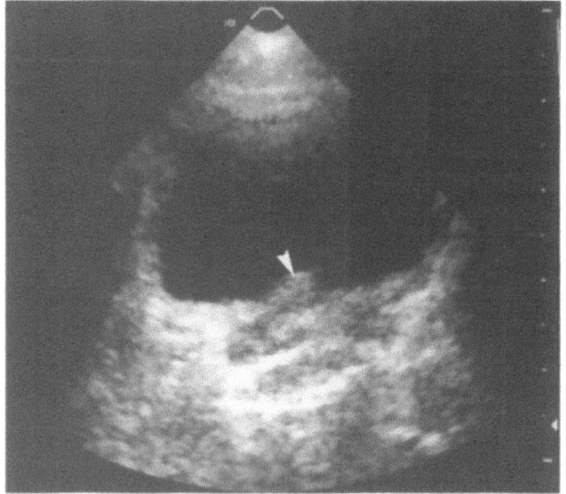

Fig. 8.49a, b. Spontaneous resolution of a megaureter with an orthoptic ureterocele. **a** At birth. Transverse scan of the bladder demonstrating the ureterocele (*arrowhead*). **b** At 12 months the ureterocele has "collapsed" (*arrowhead*) and there is no longer any ureteral dilatation

may underestimate the dilatation, especially since the renal pelvis may not be dilated. Therefore, before confirming that complete resolution has occurred, a morphological assessment of the urinary tract may be necessary (by EU or, better, by MR urography) (BASKIN et al. 1994, LIU et al. 1994, PETERS et al. 1989, AVNI et al. 1992).

8.1.6.4
Multicystic Dysplastic Kidney

Once the diagnosis of MDK appears highly probable (on the basis of the neonatal US examination and on the lack of function demonstrated by isotopes), a clinical and imaging follow-up by US is the most widely accepted course of action. Two thirds of MDK cases diagnosed in utero will involve spontaneously within the first 2 years of life; the involution may start already in utero (Fig. 8.50). Complications are very unusual. Only very large that cause abdominal discomfort and do not resolve on control examinations will necessitate surgical removal (PEDICELLI et al. 1986, STRIFE et al. 1993, VINOCUR and SLOVIS 1988, HRAIR et al. 1993, AVNI et al. 1987).

8.1.6.5
Duplex Kidneys

In the case of duplex collecting systems, one of the aims of imaging is to differentiate between ectopic ureteral insertion and ectopic ureterocele. In the case of an extravesical ectopic ureter, if no function

is demonstrated, an upper pole heminephrectomy is proposed; ureteral reimplantation and modeling are performed if some renal function is preserved. In the case of ectopic ureterocele causing an important obstruction, incision of the ureterocele is performed under cystoscopy in order to relieve the high-pressure obstruction. Resection of the ureterocele with heminephrectomy is performed secondarily according to the degree of remaining renal function (HULSMAN et al. 1999, BLYTH et al. 1993).

> Apart from acute conditions necessitating immediate treatment, the therapeutic approach towards congenital uropathies is less and less surgical. Prophylactic antibiotic therapy is usually instituted in the immediate neonatal period.

8.1.7
Conclusions

Many changes have occurred in the management of perinatal uro-nephropathies. US plays the central role in the diagnosis, investigation and follow-up of these cases. Further information will be provided by the results of prospective studies, in order to determine which attitude is optimal.

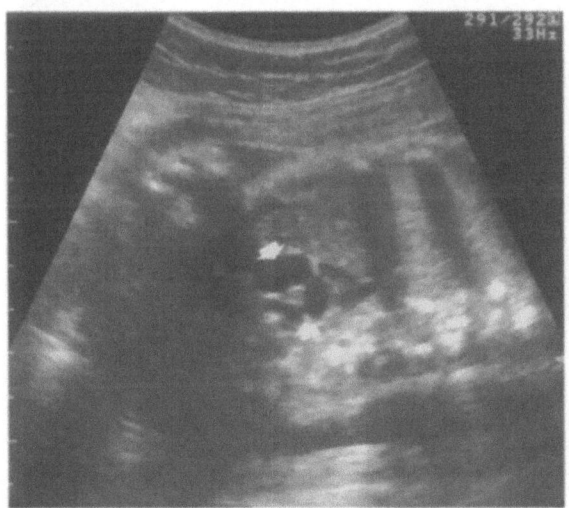 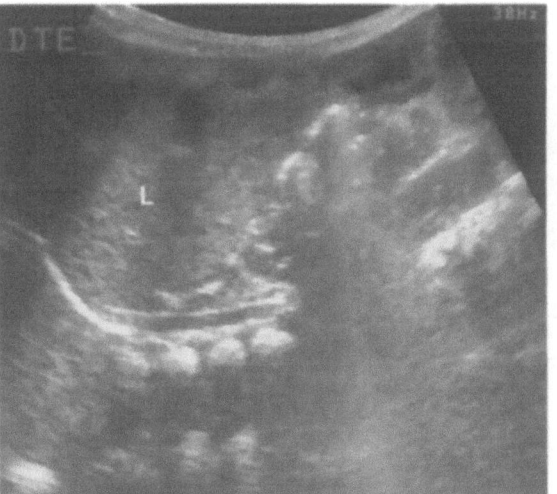

a   b

Fig. 8.50a, b. Spontaneous involution of a multicystic kidney. **a** In utero (third trimester). Sagittal scan of the fetal trunk. A right multicystic kidney is present (*arrows*). **b** After birth. No cysts are visible any longer in the right lumbar fossa. *L* liver, *arrow* adrenal gland

8.2
Fetal Genitalia

The determination of fetal gender is part of each sonographic examination; it is feasible at around 14–15 weeks. Before then, a hypertrophied clitoris can be misinterpreted as a penis. At that time a good method allowing the differentiation between penis and clitoris is the so-called sagittal sign: on a sagittal scan of the fetal pelvic area the penis points upwards, where as the clitoris points downwards (EMERSON et al. 1989).

Later, during the second trimester, the difference between the penis (Fig. 8.51) and the labia in the female (Fig. 8.52) becomes obvious. At the end of the second trimester and during the third trimester, the testes can now be seen within the scrotum and the penis has grown (Fig. 8.53) (SHAPIRO 1999). In the female fetus, the differentiation of the external genitalia is also more obvious (Fig. 8.54a). Furthermore, the uterus hypertrophies progressively due to materno-placental hormonal stimulus. It can be identified in the fetal pelvis and should not be misinterpreted as a pelvic tumor (Fig. 8.54b) (SORIANO et al 1998, SHAPIRO 1999).

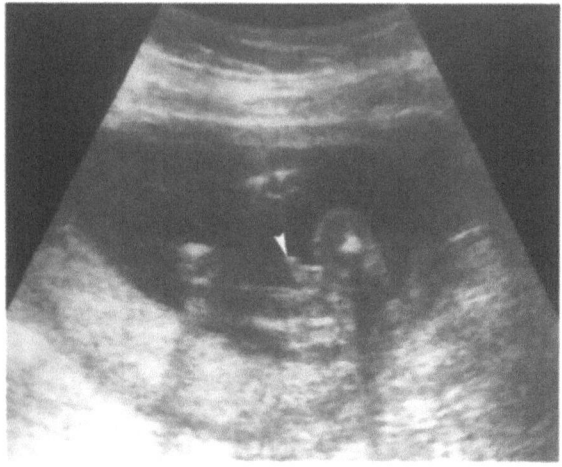

Fig. 8.51. Male sex (second trimester). The penis (*arrowhead*) points between the fetal thighs

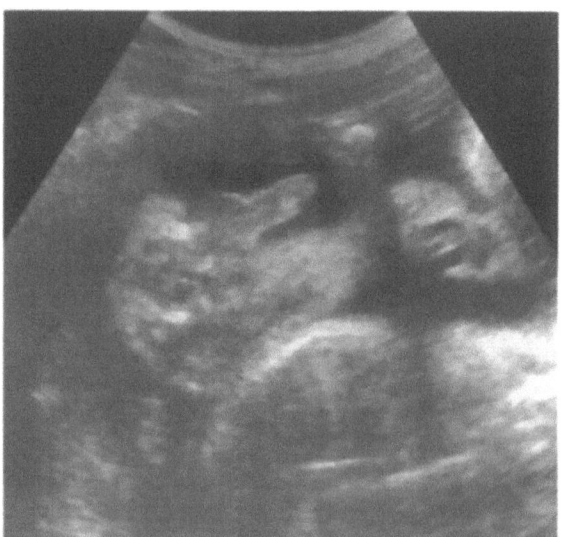

a

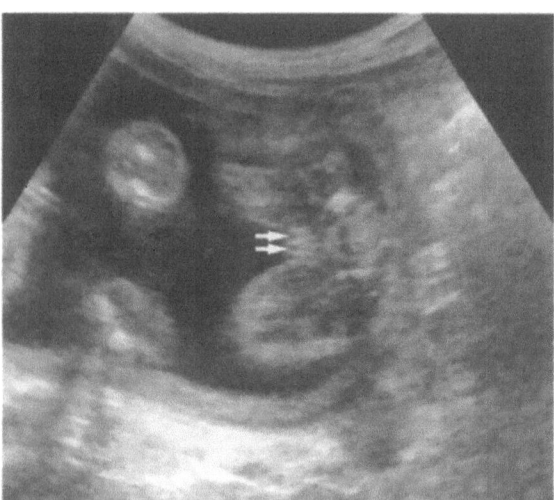

Fig. 8.52. Female sex (second trimester). The labia are visible (*arrows*) between the thighs

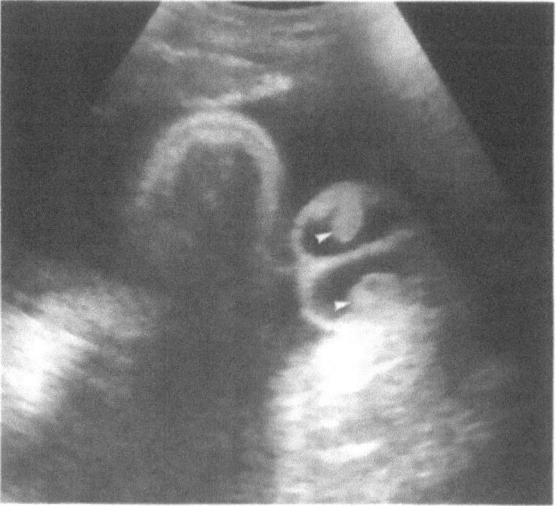

b

Fig. 8.53a, b. Male sex (third trimester). **a** Sagittal scan of the penis. **b** Transverse scan of the scrotum containing the two testes (*arrowheads*) and a small amount of free fluid (hydrocele)

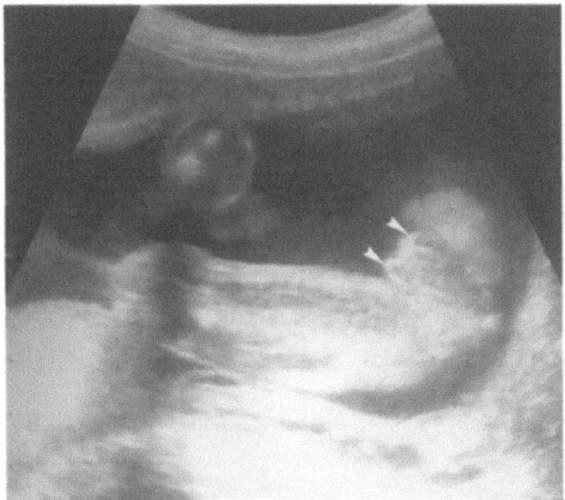

a

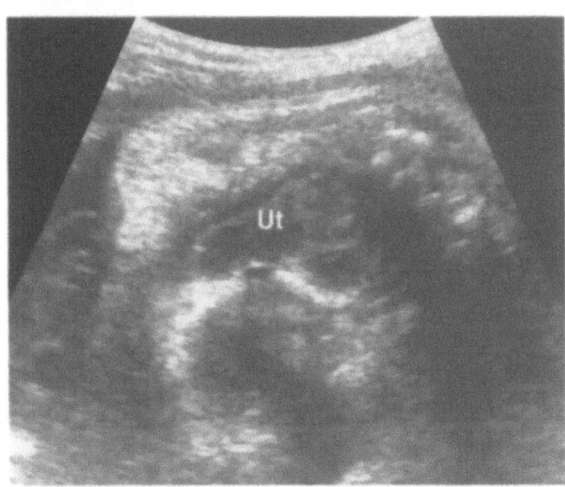

b

Fig. 8.54a, b. Female sex (third trimester). **a** View from the buttocks demonstrating the labia majora (*arrows*). **b** Transverse/oblique view of the lower fetal pelvis demonstrating the uterus (*Ut*)

8.2.1
Ambiguous Genitalia

Ambiguous genitalia is associated with various anomalies, mainly adreno-genital syndrome (AGS). In the female fetus affected by AGS, the genitalia are virilized and the clitoris is hypertrophied; it cannot be differentiated from a penis. Furthermore, according to the degree and type of disease, the effects on the external genitalia and urethra vary. In extreme cases, a vagino-urethral fistula may occur. In the male fetus, no significant changes occur. An aid to the diagnosis of AGS can be the size and pattern of the adrenals, which hypertrophy and appear cerebriform during the third trimester (CHAMBRIER et al. 2002) (see below).

Ambiguous genitalia may be an isolated finding or part of various malformation syndromes; therefore, a careful sonogram has to be performed in order to find associated anomalies. In cases of ambiguity, the penis is short and the scrotum split, while the testicles cannot be demonstrated (Figs. 8.55, 8.56) (AVNI et al. 1993, BASKIN 1999, BRONSHTEIN et al. 1995, CHEILHELAND et al. 2000, MANDELL et al. 1995, SIVAN et al. 1995, PRESTON et al. 1996).

> Ambiguous gender is a challenging US diagnosis; making such diagnosis is important since it is part of many syndromes.

8.2.2
Male Genital Anomalies

8.2.2.1
Scrotum

The fetal testes can be visualized in utero at the end of the second trimester as a small echogenic mass measuring less than 1 cm. Hydrocele and/or undescended uni- or bilateral testis should be considered as normal findings during the third trimester (Fig. 8.53). Hydrocele can persist up to the postnatal period. It must be differentiated from ascites, associated or not with meconium peritonitis. The latter appears as echogenic effusion into the scrotum; it may even calcify; both can be associated with intra-abdominal digestive anomalies (MEIZNER et al. 1983, RING 1989).

Torsion of the testis may occur in the perinatal period. In the acute phase, the testis and the scrotum are swollen; the enlarged testis is hypoechoic (Fig. 8.57) (CARTWRIGHT et al. 1995, DRIVER 1998, RYKEN et al. 1990, TRIPP and HOMSY 1995b). In the sequelar stage, the testis will appear shrunken and calcified.

Testicular tumors are extremely rare. The differential diagnosis should include intrascrotal hernia (Fig. 8.58) (SHIPP and BENACERAFF 1995, OBER and SMITH 1991).

8.2.2.2
Hypospadias and Epispadias

Hypospadias is a frequent malformation of the penis. The urethral opening lies on the inferior face of the penis on the midline. The penis appears shortened and broadened (Fig. 8.59). During micturition, the jet is directed downwards. Hypospadias can be part of many syndromes; it is usually an accessory sign

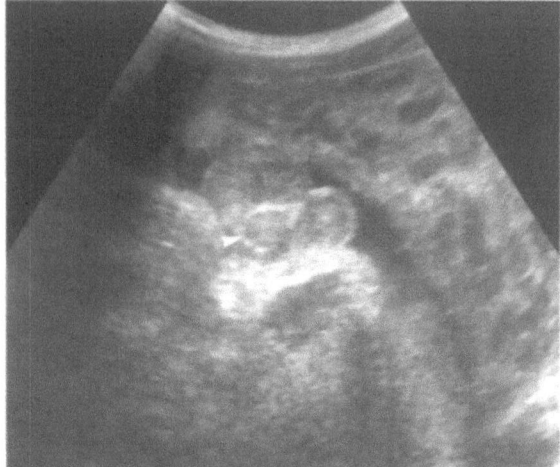

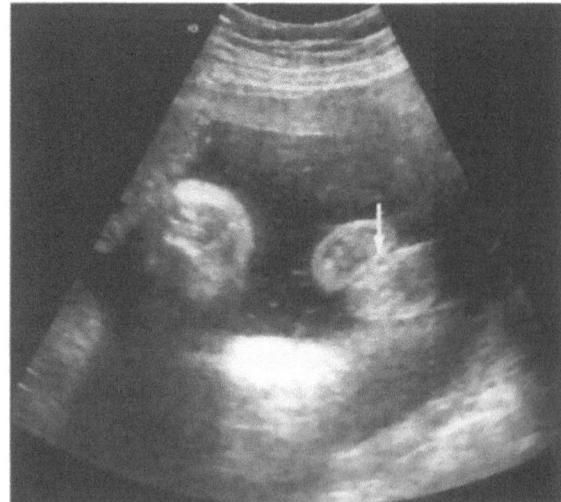

Fig. 8.56. Ambiguous genitalia (third trimester). Case of a polymalformed fetus. Transverse scan through the scrotum demonstrates with difficulty the micropenis (*arrow*)

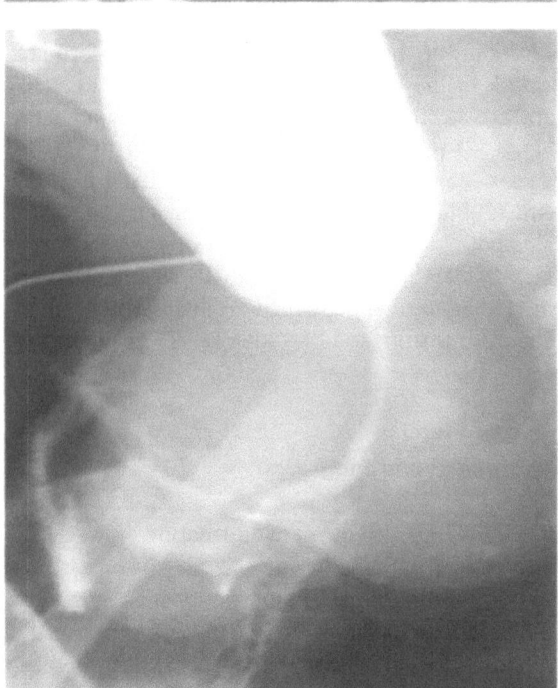

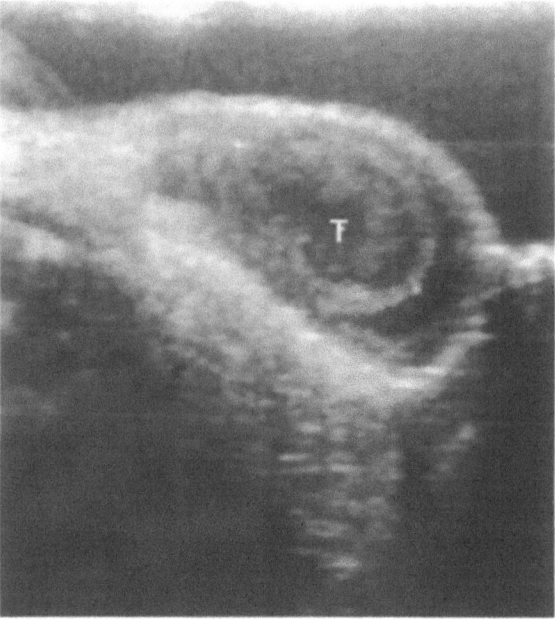

Fig. 8.57. Testicular torsion, acute phase. US scan at birth demonstrating an enlarged hypoechoic left testis (*T*) (2 cm between *crosses*)

Fig. 8.55a–c. Ambiguous genitalia. **a** In utero (third trimester). Transverse scan through the "scrotum". The penis (*arrowhead*) is short and difficult to visualize. **b** In utero (third trimester). A tangential view makes this ambiguous genitalia (*arrowheads*) resemble a female sex. *B* bladder. **c** VCUG after birth. The voiding phase demonstrates a marked shortening of the urethra in association with a balanic hypospadias

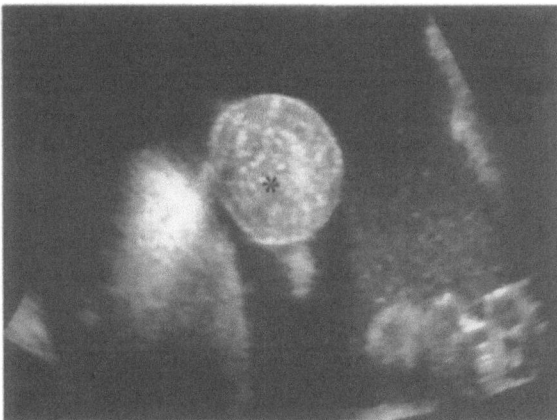

Fig. 8.58. Scrotal hernia (third trimester). Transverse scan of the scrotum, which is filled with herniated small bowel (*)

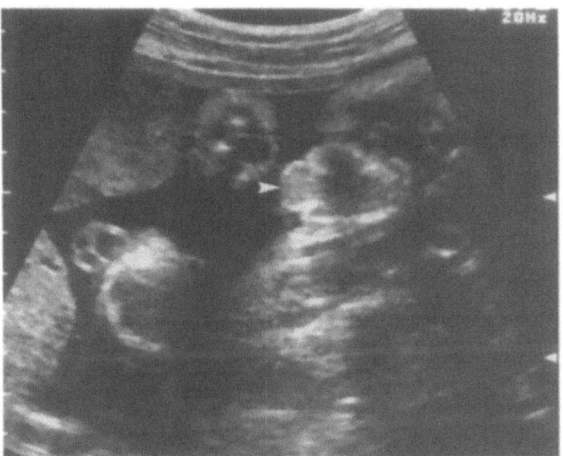

a

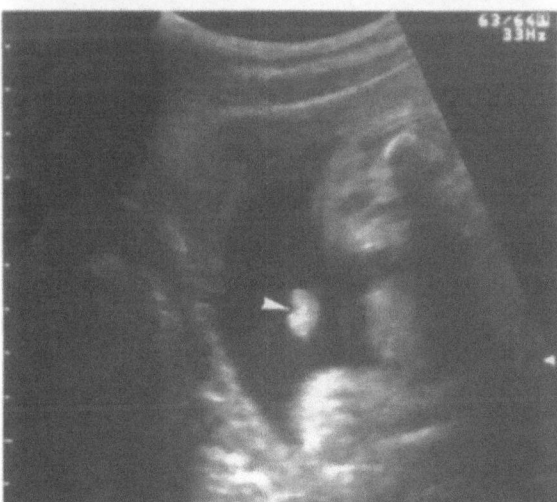

b

Fig. 8.59a, b. Hypospadias (third trimester). **a** Transverse scan of the scrotum. The penis (*arrowhead*) is shortened and broadened. **b** Closer view of the tip of the penis. The abnormal ventral opening of the penis can be visualized (*arrowhead*)

(BRONSHTEIN et al. 1995, MANDELL et al. 1995). In the case of epispadias the urethral opening lies on the superior face of the penis (SMULIAN et al. 1996). The condition can theoretically be diagnosed using the site and direction of the micturition jet.

8.2.2.3
Urethral Anomalies

In the male fetus, malformations may also involve specifically the urethra.

The most classical malformation is posterior urethral valves (PUV), which may cause bladder outlet obstruction and hydronephrosis (see above). The bladder wall is thickened and the dilated posterior urethra may be visualized when the fetus lies in a favorable position (Fig. 8.60). Another anomaly is urethral atresia, in which the urethra is completely atretic without any urine flow. This condition is detected somewhat earlier than PUV, during the early second trimester, because of bladder enlargement and associated oligohydramnios. This finding is associated with the Prune Belly sequence. The prognosis is poor. Sonographically, in some cases the dilated urethra may be visualized. The differential diagnosis of classical urethral obstructions includes megalourethra. In the latter, the penis is elongated and loose and the anterior urethra is dilated (Fig. 8.61). Ureterohydronephrosis and megabladder are usually present in all conditions with significant urethral obstruction (FISK et al. 1990, STEPHENS and FORTUNE 1993).

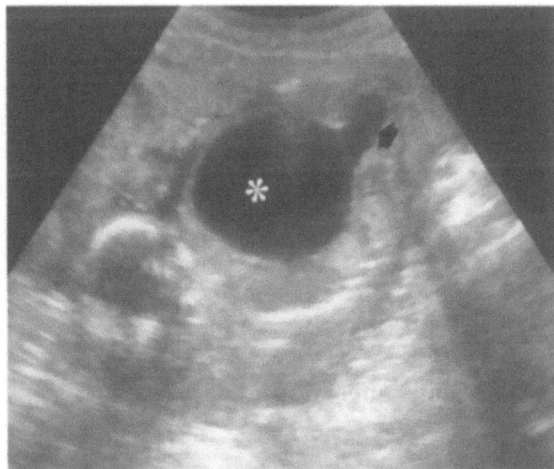

Fig. 8.60. Urethral atresia (second trimester). Sagittal view through the fetal megabladder (*) and dilated posterior urethra (*arrow*). Bilateral ureterohydronephrosis and oligohydramnios were also present

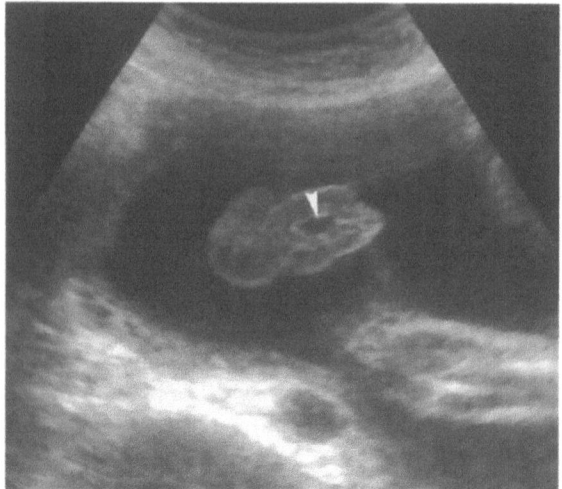

a

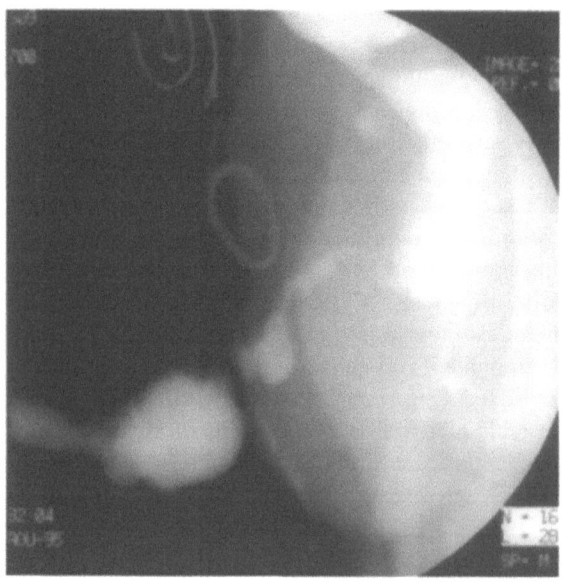

b

Fig. 8.61a, b. Megalourethra. **a** In utero (third trimester). View of the large penis and segmental dilated urethra (*arrowhead*). **b** Neonatal VCUG. Micturating phase demonstrating the abnormal urethra with segmental dilatation

In the male fetus, the commonest anomalies are related to urethral obstruction. Widening and shortening of the penis is suggestive of hypospadias. Hydrocele is a normal finding.

8.2.3
Female Genital Anomalies

8.2.3.1
Hydrocolpos

Urethral anomalies are uncommon in the female fetus. Internal genital anomalies are more classical. Imper-

forate hymen or vaginal atresia lead to hydrocolpos, which is visualized during the third trimester as a large midline cystic (sometimes echogenic) mass (Fig. 8.62) (WINDERL and SILVERMAN 1995). The uterus, distended to a lesser extent, should be demonstrated at the top of the dilated vagina (Fig. 2.12).

Differential diagnosis of such a midline mass should include urachal cyst, duplication cyst and megabladder. Hydrocolpos may be associated with urinary tract malformations, such as renal agenesis or dilatation (due to compression) (WINDERL and SILVERMAN 1995, HILL et al. 1990, AWAD et al. 1994).

Hydrocolpos may also be part of the OEIS complex (see Chap. 7) or cloacal exstrophy (Fig. 8.63).

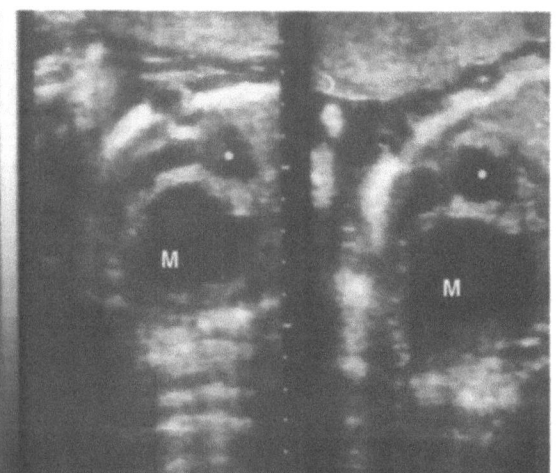

a

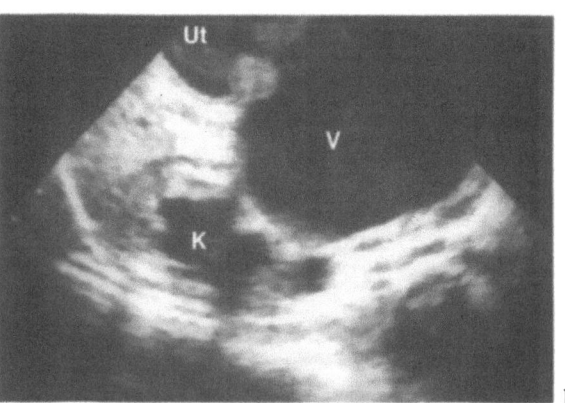

b

Fig. 8.62a, b. Hydrocolpos. **a** In utero (third trimester). Sagittal/oblique scan of the fetal abdomen. There is a centrally located cystic mass (*M*) and a dilated urinary tract (*). **b** After birth. Sagittal scan of the abdomen and pelvis. The cystic mass appears bilobed; the mass on top corresponds to the distended uterine cavity (*Ut*), the lower mass to the distended vagina (*V*). *K* dilated right kidney

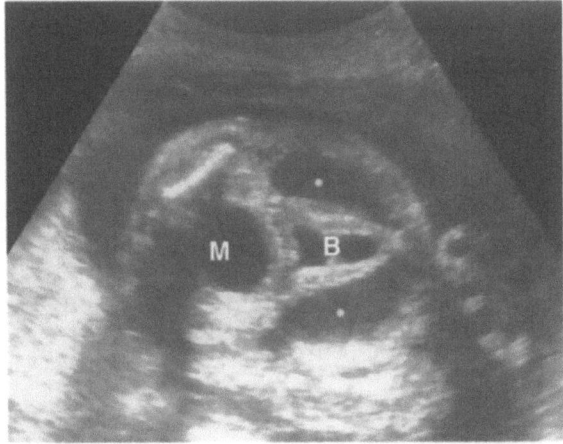

a

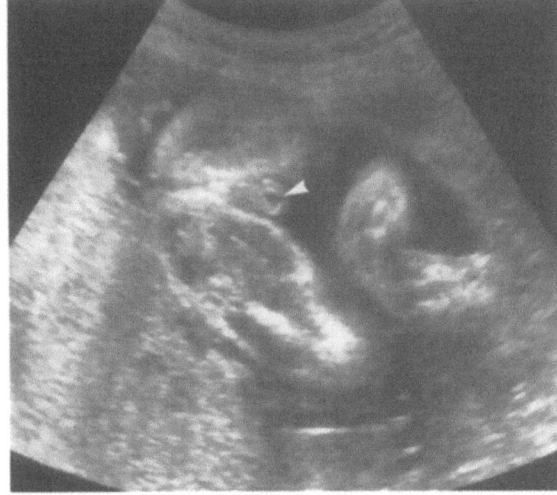

b

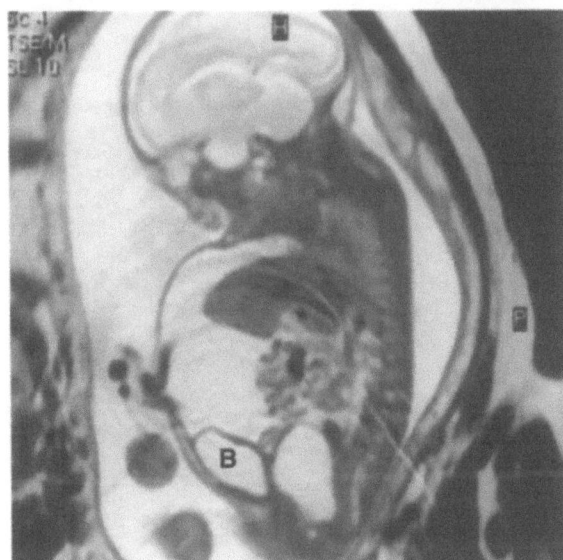

c

Fig. 8.63a–c. Hydrocolpos in a case of cloacal exstrophy (third trimester). **a** US transverse scan of the fetal pelvis. A cystic mass (*M*) is visible behind the bladder (*B*). Ascites (*) is also present. **b** US transverse scan through the perineum showing abnormal, ambiguous genitalia (*arrowhead*). **c** MR imaging demonstrating the bladder (*B*), the distended vagina (*V*) and the small uterus on top of it (*arrow*). A large amount of ascites is seen on the T2-weighted sequence

8.2.3.2
Ovarian Cyst

Ovarian "cyst" is a common finding in the female fetus and the detection of small cysts has increased since the use of high-resolution transducers. These cysts may be very large (10–12 cm) and occupy a large part of the abdomen (Fig. 8.64). They can be bilateral (Fig. 8.65). They result from materno-placental hormonal impregnation and are equivalent to follicles. They can be associated with maternal diabetes and hypothyroidism. They are usually completely cystic and a sign that may be helpful for the diagnosis is the presence within the cyst of a smaller one, attached to the wall (the so-called daughter cyst sign) (Figs. 8.64, 8.65) (HEE-JUNG 2000). Complications such as bleeding and/or torsion occur in utero. The content of the cyst will then appear hyperechoic and hetero-

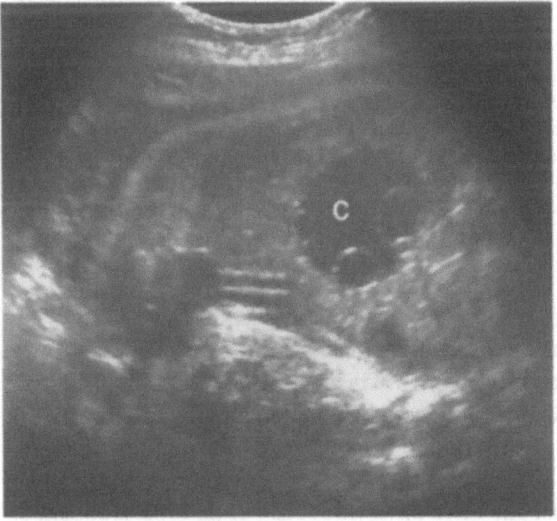

Fig. 8.64. Ovarian cyst with the daughter cysts sign (third trimester). Oblique view of the fetal abdomen demonstrating the cyst (*C*) with small cysts within it

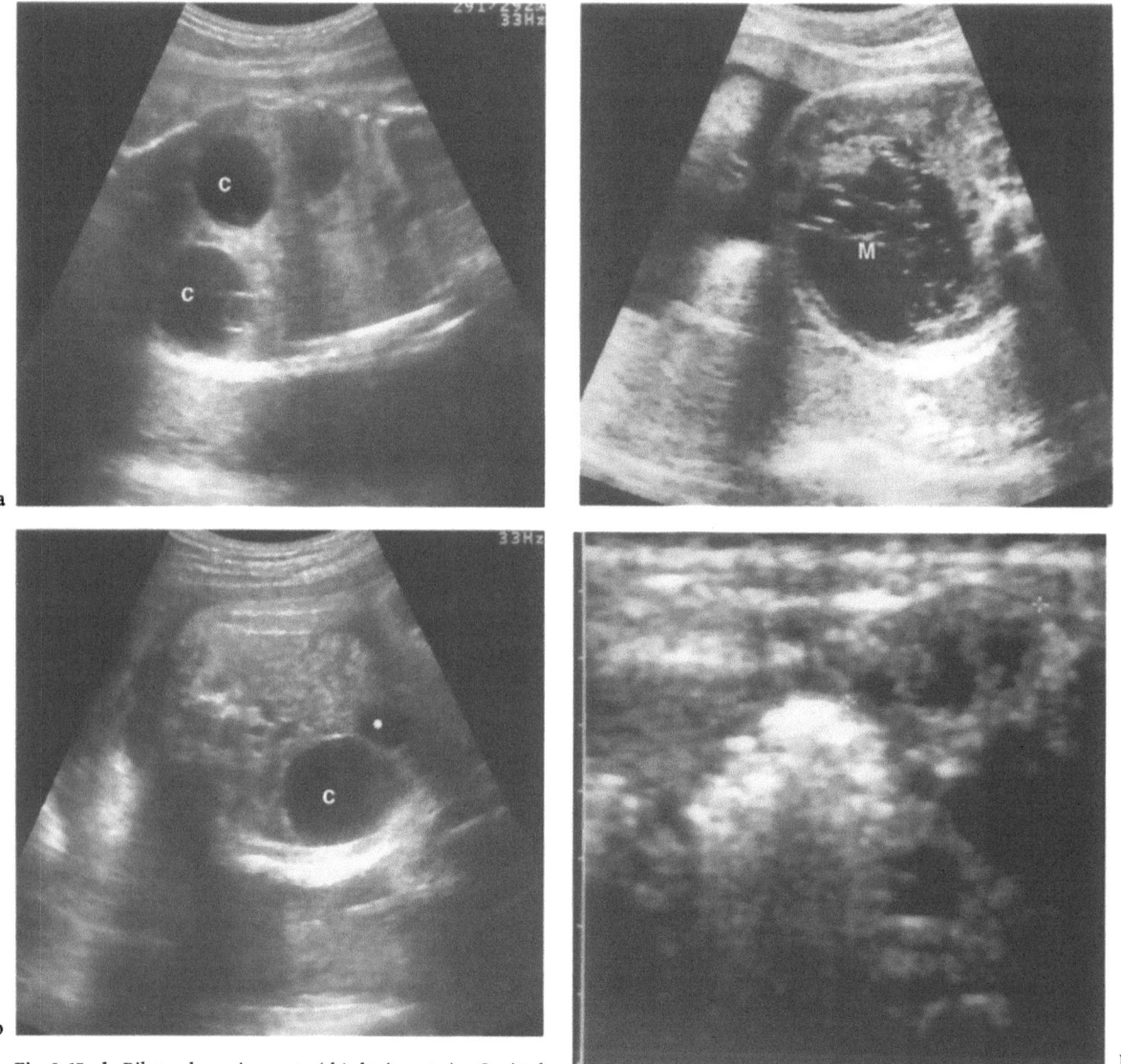

Fig. 8.65a, b. Bilateral ovarian cysts (third trimester). **a** Sagittal scan of the fetal trunk demonstrating the two cysts (*c*; one of them with the daughter cyst sign). *Ch* chest. **b** A few weeks later. Transverse scan of the fetal abdomen. Only one cyst (*c*) remains. *Asterisk* indicates the top of the bladder

Fig. 8.66a, b. Complicated ovarian cyst. **a** In utero (third trimester). A large mass (*M*) occupies the left fetal abdomen It is mainly cystic but contains echoes within it. **b** At birth the left ovary (between *crosses*) appears somewhat enlarged but no mass is visible

geneous (Fig. 8.66). Torsion can also induce tearing of the ovarian ligament and the ovary may wander in the abdomen. This ligament is loose and this too favors mobilization and torsion of the ovary (AVNI et al. 1983, D'ADDARIO et al. 1990, PREZZIOSI 1986).

Spontaneous involution may or not occur, most usually after birth (JOUPPILA et al. 1982, NUSSBAUM et al. 1988) (Fig. 8.66). Therefore, the management of ovarian cysts after birth is controversial : some advocate neonatal surgery. Others suggest clinical and US follow-up only, since many cysts will resolve (or rupture) without known sequelae. Furthermore, some authors have suggested a role for in utero decompression (CROMBEHOLME et al. 1997, GAREL et al. 1991, IKEDA et al. 1988, NUSSBAUM 1987, PERROTIN et al. 2000).

> Ovarian cyst is a common finding in the female fetus. It is usually a cystic mass but the content may be echogenic. Management is controversial.

8.3
Fetal Adrenals

8.3.1
Normal Fetal Adrenals

Using vaginal probes, fetal adrenals are visualized by obstetrical US at the end of the first trimester. They appear as hypoechoic round masses at the top of the kidneys. Their size is half that of the kidney. They will progressively flatten as the kidney grows. CMD appears during the second trimester: hypoechoic cortex and hyperechoic medulla (Fig. 8.67) (JEANTY et al. 1984, SCOTT et al. 1990). At that time, they have the same echogenicity and size as in the immediate postnatal period.

The adrenals remain round in the case of homolateral renal agenesis and should not be mistaken for a dysplastic kidney (BRONSHTEIN et al. 1994).

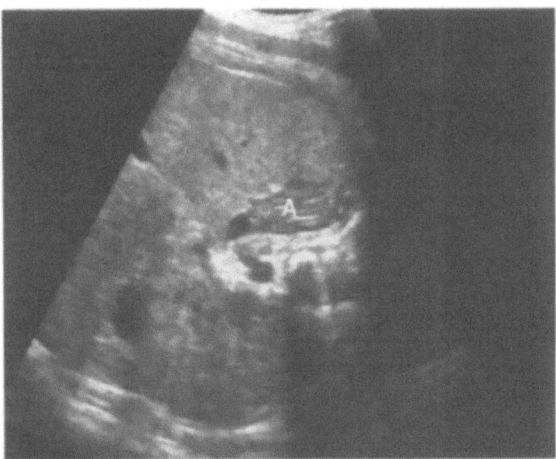

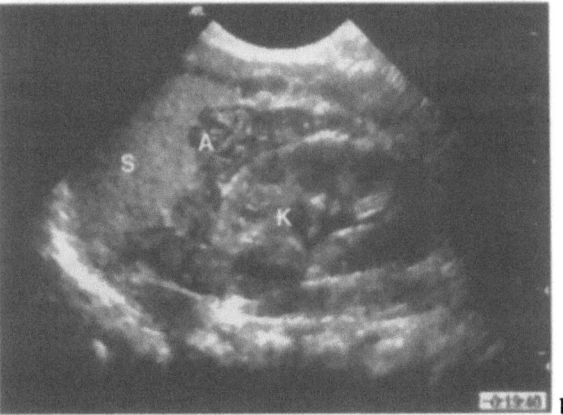

Fig. 8.68a, b. Adreno-genital syndrome. **a** In utero (third trimester). Transverse scan of the abdomen. Multilayered-appearing adrenal gland (*A*) (compare with Fig. 8.67). **b** At birth. Sagittal scan. Cerebriform hypertrophied pattern of the left adrenal (*A*). *K* left kidney, *S* spleen

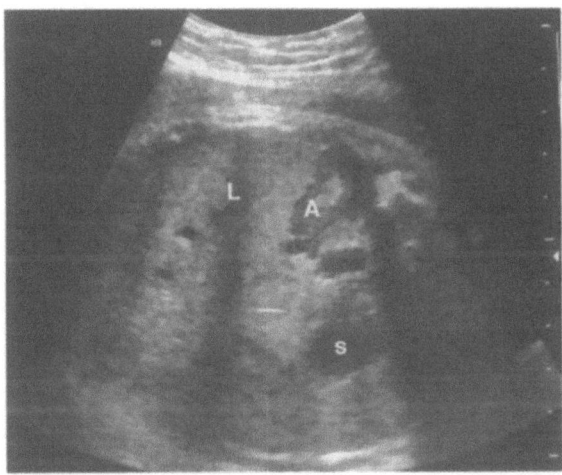

Fig. 8.67. Normal adrenal in utero (third trimester). Transverse scan of the fetal abdomen. The adrenals (*A*) are characterized by a hypoechoic cortex and hyperechoic medulla. *L* liver, *s* stomach

8.3.2
Adreno-genital Syndrome

In the case of adreno-genital syndrome, the adrenals enlarge during the third trimester and present a characteristic cerebriform pattern (AVNI et al. 1993b, BROOK 2000, CHAMBRIER et al. 2002) (Fig. 8.68). The condition may be associated with ambiguous genitalia (see above).

8.3.3
Adrenal Masses

Adrenal masses can be found during the second and third trimesters. Simple adrenal cysts are uncommon findings (Fig. 8.69). However, they may develop and even resolve spontaneously in utero. They may also enlarge markedly due to a hemorrhage, and in such cases an association with Beckwith-Wiedemann syndrome should be suspected (Fig. 8.70) (MORGANTY and ANDERSON 1991, PATTI et al. 1993).

Most adrenal tumors are neuroblastomas. In utero they appear as a solid mixed or cystic type mass above the kidney (Fig. 8.71, 8.72) (FERRARO et al. 1988, GOLDSTEIN et al. 1994, JAFFA et al. 1993). The differential diagnosis should include other adrenal or non-adrenal masses (DANEMAN et al. 1997) (see Chap. 13).

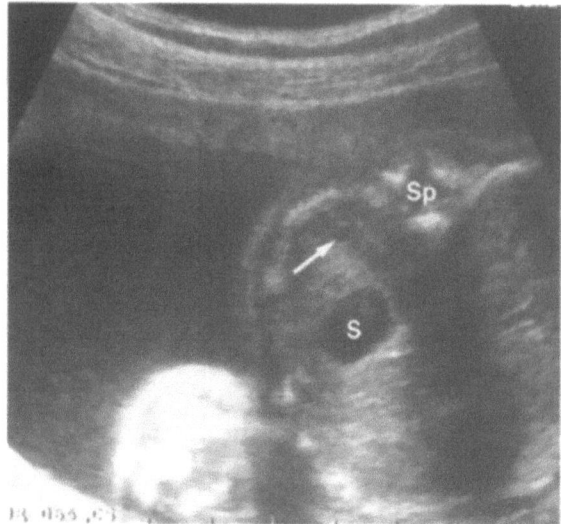

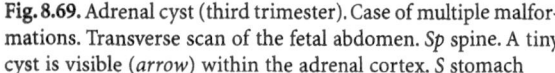

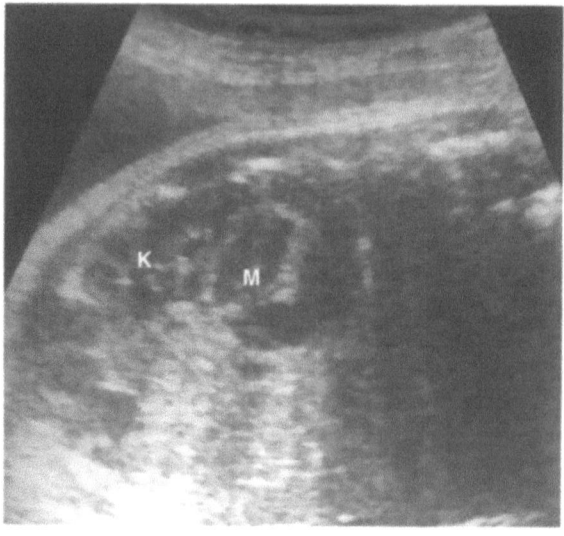

Fig. 8.69. Adrenal cyst (third trimester). Case of multiple malformations. Transverse scan of the fetal abdomen. *Sp* spine. A tiny cyst is visible (*arrow*) within the adrenal cortex. *S* stomach

Fig. 8.71. Neuroblastoma (third trimester). Sagittal scan of the left kidney A solid-type mass (*M*) is visible in front of the kidney (*K*)

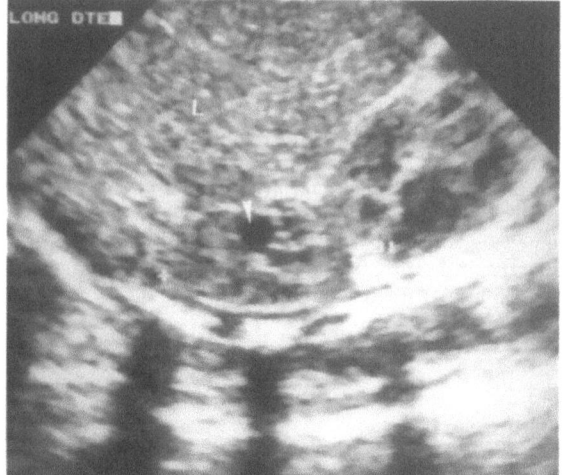

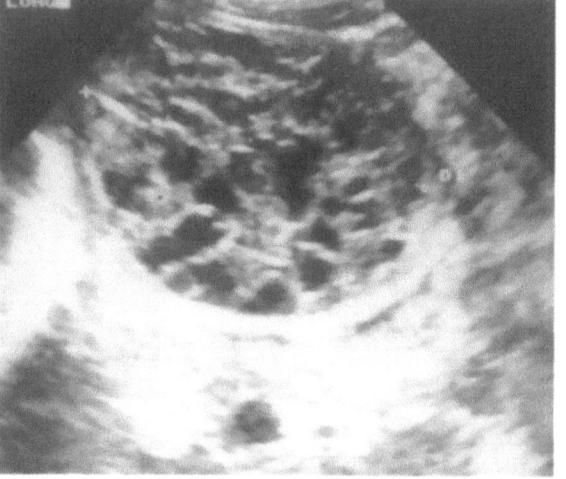

a   b

Fig. 8.70a, b. Massive enlargement of adrenals in a case of Beckwith-Wiedemann syndrome (courtesy of G. Kalifa, MD). US at birth. **a** Sagittal scan of the enlarged right adrenal with one cyst within it (*arrowhead*). *L* liver. **b** Sagittal scan of left adrenal containing a large cyst (between *crosses*) and with a mixed pattern (corresponding to hemorrhage within it)

Adrenal hemorrhage may also occur in utero and the differential diagnosis with a cystic neuroblastoma may be difficult since neuroblastomas themselves may bleed. As a rule, a fetal adrenal mass should be considered to be a neuroblastoma until proven otherwise (BURBRIGE 1993, STROUSE et al. 1995). Neuroblastoma may metastasize already in utero, especially in the liver. Metastasis should therefore be considered as a differential diagnosis of a liver mass (VAN DER SLIKKE and BALK 1980, LIYANAGE and KATOCH 1992, TOMA et al. 1994).

The prognosis of prenatally detected neuroblastoma is usually good, even with metastasis. Therefore, some have advocated conservative management. Some neuroblastomas have shown a potential for spontaneous involution (FORMAN et al. 1990, HO et al. 1993, SAYLORS et al. 1994) (see Chap. 13).

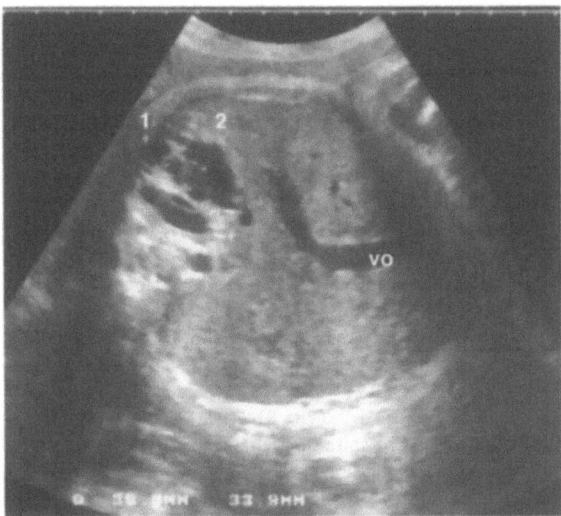

Fig. 8.72. Cystic neuroblastoma (third trimester). Transverse scan of the fetal abdomen demonstrating a mixed-type mass (between *crosses*) that was removed after birth and corresponded to a cystic neuroblastoma. *vo* umbilical vein

References

Abuhamad AZ, Horton CE, Horton SH, Evans AT (1996) Renal duplication anomalies in the fetus: clues for prenatal diagnosis. Ultrasound Obstet Gynecol 7:174–177

Allen TD (1992) The swing of the pendulum. J Urol 148:534–535

Ambrosino MM, Hernanz-Schulman M, Horii SC, Raghavendra BN (1990) Prenatal diagnosis of nephroblastoma in two siblings. J Ultrasound Med 9:49–51

Anderson N, Clautice-Engle T, Allan R, et al (1995) Detection of obstructive uropathy in the fetus. AJR Am J Roentgenol164:719–723

Anderson PAM, Rickwood AMK (1991) Features of primary VUR detected by prenatal US. Br J Urol67:267–271

Applegate KE, Ghei M, Perez-Atayde AR (1999) Prenatal detection of a Wilms' tumor. Pediatr Radiol 29:65–67

Arnold AJ, Rickwood AMK (1990) Natural history of pelviureteric obstruction detected by prenatal sonography. Br J Urol65:91–96

Assael BM, Guez S, Marra E, et al (1998) Congenital reflux nephropathy: a follow-up of 108 cases diagnosed perinatally. Br J Urol82:252–257

Atiyeh B, Husmann D, Baum M (1992) Contralateral renal abnormalities in MDKD. J Pediatr121:65–67

Atiyeh B, Husmann, D Baum M (1993) Contralateral renal abnormalities in patients with renal agenesis and noncystic renal dysplasia. Pediatrics91:812–815

Austin PF, Cain MP, Casale AJ, et al (1998) Prenatal outlet obstruction secondary to ureterocele. Urology52:1132–1135

Avni EF, Schulmann CC (1996) The origin of VUR in male newborns. Br J Urol 78:454–459

Avni EF, Godart S, Israël C, Schmitz C (1983) Ovarian torsion cyst presenting as a wandering mass in a newborn. Pediatr Radiol13:169–171

Avni EF, Thoua Y, VanGansbeke D, et al (1985) The development of hypodysplastic kidney. Radiology164:123–123

Avni EF, Thoua Y, Lalmand B, et al (1987) Multicystic dysplastic kidney: natural history from in utero diagnosis and postnatal followup. J Urol138:1420–1424

Avni EF, Dacher JN, Stallenberg B, et al (1991) Renal duplications the impact of perinatal ultrasound on diagnosis and management. Eur Urol 20:43–48

Avni EF, Pichot E, Schulman CC (1992) Neonatal congenital megaureters: trends in diagnosis and management. World J Urol10:90–93

Avni EF, Rypens F, Smet MH, Galetty E (1993a) Sonographic demonstration of congenital adrenal hyperplasia in the neonate: the cerebriform pattern. Pediatr Radiol 23:88–90

Avni EF, Rypens F, Smet MH, Galetty E (1993b) Sonographic demonstration of congenital adrenal hyperplasia. Pediatr Radiol 23:88–90

Avni EF, Ayadi K, Rypens F, et al (1997a) Can careful ultrasound examination of the urinary tract exclude vesicoureteric reflux in the neonate? Br J Radiol 170:977–982

Avni FE, Matos C, Rypens F, et al (1997b) Ectopic vaginal insertion of an upper pole ureter: demonstration by MR imaging, J Urol 158:1931–1932

Avni FE, Hall M, Schulman CC (1998) Congenital uronephropathies: is routine VCUG always warranted? Clin Radiol53:247–250

Avni FE, Nicaise N, Hall M, et al (2001) The role of MR imaging for the assessment of complicated duplex kidneys in children. Pediatr Radiol 31:215–223

Awad J, Azar G, Soubra M (1994) US diagnosis of urachal cyst in utero. Acta Obstet Gynecol Scand 73:156–157

Baskin LS (1999) Society for Fetal Urology: prenatal diagnosis and treatment of genital anomalies. Urology 53:1029–1031

Bailey RR, Lynn KL, Smith AH (1992) Long term follow-up of infants with gross VUR. J Urol 148:1709–1711

Barakat AJ, Drougas JG (1991) Occurrence of congenital abnormalities of the kidney and urinary tract in 13775 autopsies. Urology38:347–350

Barth RA, Filly RA, Sondheimer FK (1990) Prenatal US findings in bladder exstrophy. J Ultrasound Med9:359–361

Barth RA, Guillot AP, Capeless EL, Clemmons JJW (1992) Prenatal diagnosis of ARPKD: variable outcome in one family. Am J Obstet Gynecol 166:560–1

Baskin LS, Zderic SA, Snyder HM, Duckett JW (1994) Primary dilated megaureter: long term followup. J Urol 152:618–621

Bernstein J (1993) Glomerulocystic kidney disease: nosological considerations. Pediatr Nephrol7:464–470

Blachar A, Blachar Y, Pinhas M, et al (1994) Clinical outcome and follow up of prenatal hydronephrosis. Pediatr Nephrol8:30–35

Blane CE, DiPietro MA, Zerin M, Sedman AB, et al (1990) Renal US is not a reliable screening examination for VUR. J Urol152:752–755

Blane CE, Barr M, DiPietro MA, et al (1991) Renal obstructive dysplasia: ultrasound diagnosis and therapeutic implications. Pediatr Radiol21:274–277

Blane CE, DiPietro M, Zerin JM, et al (1993) Renal US is not a reliable screening examination for vesico-ureteral reflux. J. Urol 150:752–755

Blazer S, Zimmer EZ, Blumenfeld Z, et al (1999) Natural history of fetal simple cysts detected in early pregnancy. J Urol162:812–814

Blyth B, Passerini Glazel G, Camuffo C, et al (1993) Endoscopic incision of ureteroceles: intravesical versus ectopic. J Urol149:556–560

Borthne A, Nordshus T, Reiseter T, et al (1999) MR urography the future gold standard in paediatric urogenital imaging? Pediatr Radiol29:694–701

Bouachrine H, Lemelle JL, Didier F, Schmitt DA (1996) Follow-up study of pre-natally detected primary VUR: a review of 61 patients. Br J Urol78:936–939

Bove KE (1999) Wilms tumor and related abnormalities in the fetus and newborn. Semin Perinatol23:310–318

Bronshtein M, Bar-Havat I, Blumenfeld Z (1992) Clues and pitfalls in the early prenatal diagnosis of late onset infantile polycystic disease. Prenat Diagn12:293–298

Bronshtein M, Amit A, Achiron R, et al (1994) The early prenatal diagnosis of renal agenesis. Prenat Diagn 14:291–297

Bronshtein M, Riechler A, Zimmer EZ (1995) Prenatal US signs of possible fetal genital anomalies. Prenat Diagn 15:215–219

Brook CGD (2000) Antenatal treatment of a mother bearing a fetus with congenital adrenal hyperplasia. Arch Dis Child Fetal Neonatal Ed 82:F176–F181

Burbrige KA (1993) Prenatal adrenal hemorrhage confirmed by postnatal surgery. J Urol 150:1867–1869

Burge DM, Griffiths MD, Malone PG, Atwell JD (1992) Fetal VUR outcome following conservative management. J Urol148:1743–1745

Bussieres L, Laborde K, Souberbielle JC, et al (1995) Fetal urinary insulin like growth factor I and binding protein 3 in bilateral obstructive uropathies. Prenat Diagn15:1047–1055

Callen PW, Bolding D, Filly RA, Harrison MR (1983) US evaluation of fetal paranephric pseudocysts. J Ultrasound Med2:309–312

Capolicchio G, Leonard MP, Wong C, et al (1999) Prenatal diagnosis of hydronephrosis: impact on renal function. J Urol162:1029–1032

Carlsson SA, Hokegard KH, Mattson LA (1992) Megacystis microcolon hypoperistalsis syndrome. Acta Obstet Scand 71:645–648

Carr MC, Benaceraff BR, Estroff JA, Mandell J (1995) Prenatally diagnosed hyperechoic kidneys with normal amniotic fluid: postnatal outcome. J Urol153:442–444

Cartwright PC, Snow BW, Reid BS, Schulz PK (1995) Color Doppler US in newborn testis. Urology45:667–670

Cascio S, Paran S, Puri P (1999) Associated urological anomalies in children with unilateral renal agenesis. J Urol162:1081–1083

Ceccherini I, Lituania M, Cordoni MS, et al (1989) ADPKD: prenatal diagnosis by DNA analysis and US at 14 weeks. Prenat Diagn9:751–758

Cendron M, D'Alton M, Crombleholme TM (1994) Prenatal diagnosis and management of the fetus with hydronephrosis. Semin Perinatol18:163–181

Chamberlain PF, Manning FA, Morrison I, Lange IR (1984) Circadian rhythm in bladder volume in the term human fetus. Obstet Gynecol64:64:657–660

Chambrier D, Heinrich C, Avni EF (2002) Adrenal hyperplasia in a fetus. J Ultrasound Med (in press)

Cheikheland A, Lheton D, Philippe Chonette P, et al (2000) How accurate is the prenatal diagnosis of abnormal genitalia? J Urol 164:984–987

Chertin B, Fridman A, Knizhnik M, et al (1999) Does early detection of UPJ obstruction improve surgical outcome? J Urol162:1037–1040

Chung S, Majd M, Gil-Rushdon H, Belman BA (1993) Diuretic renography in the evaluation of neonatal hydronephrosis: is it reliable? J Urol150:765–768

Clautice-Engle T, Anderson NG, Allan RB, Abbott GD (1995) Diagnosis of obstructive hydronephrosis in infants: comparison sonograms performed 6 days and 6 weeks after birth. AJR Am J Roentgenol164:963–967

Cleveland RH, Constantinou C, Blickman JG, et al (1992) VCUG in children: value of digital fluoroscopy in reducing radiation dose. AJR Am J Roentgenol 152:137–142

Cohen HL, Cooper J, Eisenberg P, et al (1991) Normal length of fetal kidneys. AJR Am J Roentgenol 157:545–548

Crombleholme TM, Craigo SD, Gaomal S, D'Alton ME (1997) Fetal ovarian cyst decompression to prevent torsion. J Pediatr Surg 32:1447–1449

Dacher JN, Mandell J, Lebowitz RL (1992) Urinary tract infection in infants in spite of prenatal diagnosis of hydronephrosis. Pediatr Radiol22:401–405

Dacher JN, Eurin D, Mitrofanoff P, LeDosseur P (1995) Imagerie et prise en charge postnatales après diagnostic anténatal d'une uropathie. Feuil Radiol35:220–227

D'Addario V, Volpe G, Kurjak A et al (1990) US diagnosis and perinatal management of complicated and uncomplicated fetal ovarian cyst. J Perinat Med 18:375–381

Daneman A, Baunin C, Lobo E, et al (1997) Disappearing suprarenal masses in the fetus and neonate. Pediatr Radiol 27:675–681

Dar P, Sachs GS, Carter JC, et al (2001) Prenatal diagnosis of Bardet Biedl syndrome by targeted second trimester US, Ultrasound Obstet Gynecol 17:354–356

Dejter SW, Gibbons MD (1989) The fate of infant kidneys with fetal hydronephrosis but initially normal postnatal sonography. J Urol 142:661–662

Devaussuzenet V, Dacher JN, Eurin D, et al (1997) Echographie et cystographie postnatales après diagnostic prénatal. J Radiol 78:27–31

Dinneen MD, Dhillon DK, Ward HC, Duffy PG, Ransley PG (1993) Antenatal diagnosis of PUV. J Urol 72:364–369

Dippel J, Varlam DE (1998) Early US aspects of kidney morphology in Bardet-Biedl syndrome. Pediatr Nephrol 12:559–563

Docimo SG, Silver RI (1997) Renal ultrasonography in newborns with prenatally detected hydronephrosis: why wait? J Urol 157:1387–1389

Dowling KJ, Harmon EP, Ortenberg J, et al (1988) UPJ obstruction: the effect of pyeloplasty on renal function. J Urol 140:1227–1230

Dremsek PA, Gindi K, Voitl P, et al (1997) Renal pyelectasis in fetuses and neonates. AJR Am J Roentgenol 168:1017–1019

Driver CP, Losty PD (1998) Neonatal testicular torsion. Br J Urol 82:855–858

Duckett JW (1993) When to operate on neonatal hydronephrosis. Urology43:617–619

Dudley JA, Haworth JM, McGraw ME, et al (1997) Clinical relevance and implications of antenatal diagnosis of antenatal hydronephrosis. Arch Dis Child 76:F31–F34

Economou G, Egginton IA, Brookfield DSK (1994) The importance of late pregnancy scans for renal tract abnormalities Prenat Diagn 14:177–180

Edwards OP, Baldinger S (1989) Prenatal onset of ADPKD. Urology 34:265–270

Elder JS (1992) Commentary: importance of antenatal diagnosis of VUR. J Urol148:1750–1754

Elder JS, O'Grady P, Ashmead G, et al (1990) Evaluation of fetal renal function: unreliability of fetal urinary electrolytes. J Urol 144:574–578

Emerson DS, Fleker RE, Brown DL (1989) The sagittal sign: an early trimester US indicator of fetal fender. J Ultrasound Med 8:293–297

Estroff JA, Mandell J, Benaceraff BR (1991) Increased renal echogenicity in the fetus. Radiology 181:135–139

Eurin D, Dacher JN, LeDosseur P (1995) Diagnostic antenatal des uropathies. Feuil Radiol 35:212–219

Ferraro EM, Fakhry J, Ammy JE, Bracero L.A (1988) Prenatal adrenal neuroblastoma. J Ultrasound Med 7:725–728

Fick GM, Duley IT, Johnson JD, et al ,(1994) The spectrum of ADPKD in children. J Am Soc Nephrol 4:1654–1660

Fine RN (1992) Diagnosis and treatment of fetal urinary tract abnormalities. J Pediatr 121:333–341

Fishman JE, Joseph RC (1994) Renal vein thrombosis: in utero duplex US. Pediatr Radiol 24:135–136

Fisk NH, Dhillon HK, Ellis C.E, et al (1990) Antenatal diagnosis of megalourethra in a fetus with the PBS. J Clin Ultrasound 18:124–128

Fitch SJ, Stapleton SB (1986) US features of glomerulocystic diseases in infancy: similarity to IPKD. Pediatr Radiol 16: 400–403

Flack CE, Bellinger MF (1993) The multicystic dysplastic kidney and contralateral vesicoureteral reflux protection of the solitary kidney. J Urol 150:1873–1874

Flaschner SC, Mesrobian HG, Flatt JA, et al (1993) Nonobstructive dilatation of the upper urinary tract may later convert to obstruction. Urology 42:569–573

Forman HP, Leonidas JL, Berdon W, et al (1990) Congenital neuroblastoma: evaluation with multimodality imaging. Radiology 175:365–368

Freedman AL, Bukowski TP, Smith CA, et al (1996) Fetal therapy for obstructive uropathy: specific outcomes diagnosis. J Urol 156:720–724

Friedmann W, Vogel M, Dimer JS, et al (2000) Prenatal differential diagnosis of cystic renal disease and urinary tract obstruction. Obstet Gynecol 89:127–133

Fugelseth D, Lindermann R, Sande HA, et al (1994) Prenatal diagnosis of urinary tract anomalies: the value of two US examinations. Acta Obstet Gynecol Scand 73:290–293

Garel L, Filiatrault D, Brandt M, et al (1991) Antenatal diagnosis of ovarian cysts. Pediatr Radiol. 21:182–184

Gearhart JP, Ben-Chaim J, Jeffs RD, Sanders RC (1995) Criteria for the prenatal diagnosis of classic bladder exstrophy. Obstet Gynecol 85:961–964

Gelfand MJ, Koch BL, Eleazzar AH, et al (1999) Cyclic cystography: diagnostic yield in a selected pediatric population. Radiology 213:118–120

Gershoni-Baruch R, Nachlieli T, Leibo R, et al (1992) Cystic kidney dysplasia and polydactyly in 3 sibs with the Bardet-Biedl syndrome. Am J Med Genet 44:269–273

Glazebrook KN, McGrath FP, Steele BT (1993) Prenatal compensatory renal growth: documentation with US. Radiology 189:733–735

Gloor JM, Ogburn PL, Robert MD, et al (1995) Urinary tract anomalies detected by prenatal ultrasound examination at Mayo Clinic, Rochester. Mayo Clin Proc 70:526–531

Gobet R, Bleakley J, Peeters GA (1998) Premature urachal closure induces hydronephrosis in the fetus. J Urol 160:1463–1467

Goldstein I, Gomez K, Copel JA (1994) The real time and color Doppler appearance of adrenal neuroblastoma. Obstet Gynecol 83:854–856

Gordon AC, Thomas DFM, Arthur RJ, et al (1990) Prenatally diagnosed reflux: a follow up study. Br J Urol 65:407–412

Greer ML, Danin J, Lamont AC (1998) Glomerulocystic disease with hepatoblastoma in a neonate. Pediatr Radiol 28:703–705

Grignon A, Filion R, Filiatrault D, et al (1985) Urinary tract dilatation in utero: classifications and clinical applications. Radiology 160:645–647

Guay-Woodford LM, Galliani CA, Musulman-Mroczek E, et al (1998) Diffuse renal cystic disease in children. Pediatr Nephrol 12:173–182

Gunn TR, Dermot MD, Mora J, et al (1995) Antenatal diagnosis of urinary tract abnormalities by ultrasonography after 28 weeks gestation: incidence and outcome. Am J Obstet Gynecol 172:479–486

Hagg MJ, Mourachov PV, Snyder HM, et al (2000) The modern endoscopic approach to ureterocele. J Urol 163:940–943

Hee-Jung L (2000) Daughter cysts sign: a US finding of ovarian cyst in children. AJR Am J Roentgenol 174:1013–1015

Herndon CDA, McKenna PH, Kolon TF, et al (1999) A multicenter outcomes analysis of patients with neonatal reflux presenting with prenatal hydronephrosis. J Urol 162: 1203–1208

Hill LM, Breckle R, Ellefson RD, et al (1983) The contribution of the fetal kidney to the amniotic fluid lung profile. Am J Obstet Gynecol 146:709–710

Hill LM, Kislak S, Belfar HS (1990) The US diagnosis of urachal cyst in utero. J Clin Ultrasound 18:434–437

Ho P, Estroff J., Kozakewich H, et al (1993) Prenatal detection of neuroblastoma. Pediatrics 92:358–364

Hoffman CK, Filly RA, Callen PW (1992) The lying down sign: a US indicator of renal agenesis or ectopia. J Ultrasound Med 11:533–536

Hofstaetter C, Neuman I, Lennert T, et al (1996) Prenatal diagnosis of diffuse mesangial sclerosis by US. Fetal Diagn Ther 11:126–131

Homsy YL, Saad F, Laberge I, et al (1990) Transitional hydronephrosis of the newborn and infant. J Urol 144:579–583

Hrair-Georges JM, Rushton HG, Bulas D (1993) Unilateral agenesis may result from in utero regression of MDK. J Urol 150:793–794

Hulbert WC, Rosenberg HK, Cartwright PC, et al (1992) The predictive value of ultrasonography in evaluation of infants with posterior urethral valves. J Urol 148:122–124

Hulsman D, Strand B, Ewalt D, et al (1999) Management of ectopic ureterocele associated with renal duplication. J Urol 162:1406–1409

Ikeda K, Snita S, Nakano H (1988) Management of ovarian cyst detected antenatally. J Pediatr Surg 23:432–435

Irsutti M, Puget C, Baunijn C, et al (2000) Mesoblastic nephroma: prenatal US and MRI features. Pediatr Radiol 30:147–150

Jaffa AJ, Many A, Hartoor J, et al (1993) Prenatal US diagnosis of metastatic neuroblastoma. Prenat Diagn 13:73–77

Jaswon MS, Dibble L, Puri S, et al (1999) Prospective study of outcome in antenatally diagnosed renal pelvis dilatation. Arch Dis Child Fetal Neonatal Ed 80:F135–F138

Jayanti VR, Koff SA (1999) Long term outcome of transurethral puncture of ectopic ureteroceles. J Urol 162:1077–1079

Jeanty P, Chevenak F, Grannum P, Hobbins JC (1984) Normal US size and characteristics of the fetal adrenal glands. Prenat Diagn 4:21–28

Jeanty P, Romero R, Kepple D, et al (1990) Prenatal diagnoses in unilateral empty renal fossa. J Ultrasound Med9: 651–654

Jee LD, Rickwood AMK, Williams ML, Anderson PAM (1993) Experience with duplex system anomalies detected by prenatal US. J Urol149:808–810

Johnson MP, Bukowski TP, Reitelman C, et al (1994) In utero surgical treatment of obstructive uropathy. Am J Obstet Gynecol 170:1770–1775

Jouppila P, Kirkinen P, Tuowonen S (1982) US detection of bilateral ovarian cysts in the fetus. Eur J Obstet. Gynecol 13:87–92

Journel H, Guyot C, Barc RM, et al (1989) Unexpected US prenatal diagnosis of autosomal dominant polycystic kidney disease. Prenat Diagn9:663–671

Kaefer M, Keating MA, Adams MC, et al (1995) PUV, pressure pop-offs and bladder function. J Urol 154:708–711

Kaefer M, Peters CA, Retik AB, Benacerraf BB (1997) Increased renal echogenicity: a sonographic sign for differentiating between obstructive and nonobstructive etiologies of in utero bladder distension. J Urol158:1026–1029

Kangarloo H, Diament MJ, Gold PH (1986) US of adrenal glands in neonates and children: changes in appearance with age. J Clin. Ultrasound 14:43–47

Kapoor R, Saha M, Mandal AK (1988) Antenatal detection of wolffian duct cyst. J Clin Ultrasound17:515–517

Koff SA, Campbell K (1992) Nonoperative management of unilateral neonatal hydronephrosis. J Urol148:525–531

Koff SA, Campbell KD (1994) The nonoperative management of unilateral neonatal hydronephrosis: natural history of poorly functioning kidneys. J Urol152:593–595

Koff SA, Peller PA, Young DC, Pollifrone DL (1995) The assessment of obstruction in the newborn with unilateral hydronephrosis using the renal growth chart. J Urol154:662–666

Lalmand B, Avni EF, Nasr A, et al (1990) Perinatal renal vein thrombosis: US demonstration. J Ultrasound Med9: 437–442

Lehman CD, Nyberg DA, Winter TC, et al (1995) Trisomy 13 syndrome: prenatal US findings in a review of 33 cases. Radiology194:217–222

Lilford RJ, Irving HC, Alliborne EB (1992) A tale of two prior probabilities. Br J Obstet Gynecol99:216–219

Liu HYA, Dhillon HK, Yeung CK, et al (1994) Clinical outcome of prenatally diagnosed primary megaureters. J Urol152:614–617

Livera LN, Brookfield DSK, Egginton JA, Hawnaur JM (1989) Antenatal ultrasonography to detect fetal renal abnormalities: a prospective screening programme. BMJ298: 1421–1423

Liyanage IS, Katoch D (1992) US prenatal diagnosis of liver metastases from adrenal neuroblastoma. J Clin Ultrasound 20:401–403

MacDermot KD, Saggar AK, Economides DL, Jeffery S (1998) Prenatal diagnosis of ADPKD presenting in utero. J Med Genet 35:13–16

Maizels M, Reisman ME, Flom LS, et al (1992) Grading nephroureteral dilatation detected in the first year of life: correlation with obstruction. J Urol148:609–614

Makino Y, Kobayashi H, Kyono K, et al (2000) Clinical results of fetal obstructive uropathy treated by vesico-amniotic shunting. Urology55:118–122

Mandell J, Blyth BR, Peters CA, et al (1991) Structural genitourinary defects detected in utero. Radiology178:193–196

Mandell J, Lebowithz RL, Peters CA, et al (1992) Prenatal diagnosis of the megacystis megaureter association. J Urol148: 1487–1489

Mandell J, Peters CG, Estroff JA, et al (1993) Human compensatory renal growth. J Urol150:790–792

Mandell J, Paltiel HJ, Peters CA, Benacerraf (1994) Prenatal findings associated with a unilateral nonfunctioning or absent kidney. J Urol152:176–178

Mandell J, Bromly B., Peters CA, Benaceraff BR (1995) Prenatal US detection of genital malformation. J Urol 153: 1994–1996

Marra G, Barbieri G, Dell'Agnola CA, et al (1994) Congenital renal damage associated with primary vesicoureteral reflux detected prenatally in male infants. J Pediatr124:726–730

Marra G, Barbieri G, Moioli C, et al (1994) Mild fetal hydronephrosis indicating VUR. Arch Dis Child Dis70:147–150

McAleer IM, Kaplan GW (1999) Renal function before and after pyeloplasty: does it improve? J Urol162:1041–1044

McLorie G, Farhat W, Khoury A, et al (2001) Outcome analysis of vesico-amniotic shunting. J Urol 166:1036–1040

Meizner I, Bernhard Y (1995) Bilateral fetal pelvic kidneys. J Ultrasound Med14:487–489

Meizner I, Katz M, Zmora E, Insler V (1983) In utero diagnosis of congenital hydrocele. J Clin Ultrasound 11:449–450

Menzel D, Hanffa BP (1990) Changes in size and US characteristics of the adrenal glands during the first year of life and the US diagnosis of adrenal hyperplasia. J Clin Ultrasound 18:619–625

Michaud J, Russo P, Grignon A, et al (1994) ADPKD in the fetus. Am J Med Genet51:240–246

Montana MA, Cyr DR, Lenke RR, et al (1985) Sonographic detection of fetal ureteral obstruction. AJR Am J Roentgenol145:595–596

Morganti VJ, Anderson NG (1991) Simple adrenal cysts in the fetus, resolving in neonate. J Ultrasound Med 10:521–524

Morin L, Cendron M, Crombleholme M, et al (1996) Minimal hydronephrosis in the fetus: clinical significance and implications for management. J Urol155:2047–2049

Mouriquand PDE, Troisfontaines E, Wilcox DT (1999) Antenatal and perinatal uronephrology: current questions and dilemmas. Pediatr Nephrol13:938–944

Muller F, Dommerguez M, Mandelbrot L (1993) Fetal urinary biochemistry. Obstet Gynecol 82:813–820

Najmaldin A, Burge AM, Atwell JD (1990) Fetal VUR. J Pediatr65:403–406

Najmaldin A, Burge AM, Atwell JD (1990) Reflux nephropathy secondary to intrauterine VUR. J Pediatr Surg25:387–390

Nakayama DK, Harrison MR, DeLorimier AA (1986) Prognosis of PUV presenting at birth. J Pediatr Surg21:43–45

Nussbaum AR, Sanders RC, Benator R.M, et al (1987) Spontaneous resolution of neonatal ovarian cysts. AJR Am J Roentgenol148:175–177

Nussbaum AR, Sanders RC, Hartman DS, et al (1988) Neonatal ovarian cysts : US-pathologic correlation. Radiology 168: 817–821

Nyberg DA, Hallesy D, Mahony BS, et al (1990) Meckel-Gruber syndrome. J Ultrasound Med9:691–696

Ober KJ, Smith CV (1991) Prenatal US diagnosis of fetal inguinal hernia containing small bowel. Obstet Gynecol 78:905–906

O'Flynn KJ, Gough DCS, Gupta S et al (1993) Prediction of recovery in antenatally diagnosed hydronephrosis. Br J Urol71:478–480

Oliveira EA, Diniz JSS, Cabral ACV, et al (1999) Prognostic factors in fetal hydronephrosis: a multivariate analysis. Pediatr Nephrol13:859–864

Owen RJT, Lamont AC, Brookes J (1996) Early management and postnatal investigation of prenatally diagnosed hydronephrosis. Clin Radiol51:173–176

Paltiel HJ, Lebowitz RL (1989) Neonatal hydronephrosis due to primary vesicoureteral reflux: trends in diagnosis and treatment. Radiology170:787–789

Paltiel HJ, Rupich RC, Kiruluta HG (1992) Enhanced detection of VUR in infants and children with use of cyclic VCUG. Radioliogy184:753–755

Patti G, Fiocca G, Latini T, et al (1993) Prenatal diagnosis of bilateral adrenal cysts. J Urol 150:1189–1191

Pedicelli G, Jecquier S, Bowen A, Boisvert J(1986) MDK: spontaneous regression demonstrated with US. Radiology160:23–26

Perlman M, Levin M (1973) Fetal pulmonary hypoplasia, anuria and oligohydramnios. Am J Obstet Gynecol 118:1119–1123

Perrotin Ray F, Potin J, et al (2000) US diagnosis and prenatal management of fetal ovarian cysts. J Gynecol Obstet Biol Reprod 29:161–169

Peters CA, Mandell J, Lebowitz RL, et al (1989) Congenital obstructed megaureters in early infancy: diagnosis and treatment. J Urol142:641–645

Peters CA, Carr CA, Lay A, et al (1992) The response of fetal kidney to obstruction. J Urol148:403–408

Peters CA (1995) Urinary tract obstruction in children. J Urol154:1874–1884

Perlman M,Levin M (1974) Fetal pulmonary hypoplasia,anuria and oligohydramnios: clinicopathologic observations and review of the literature. Am J Obstet Gynecol15:1119–1123

Persutte WH, Lenke RR, Kropp K, Ghareeb C (1988) Antenatal diagnosis of patent urachus. J Ultrasound Med7:399–403

Poutamo J, Vanninen R, Partanen K, Kirkinen P (2000) Diagnosing fetal urinary tract anomalies: benefits of MRI compared to US. Acta Obstet Gynecol Scand79:65–71

Preston Smith D, Felker RE, Noe N, et al (1996) Prenatal diagnosis of genital anomalies. Urology 47:114–117

Preziosi P, Fariello G, Maiorana A, et al (1986) Antenatal US diagnosis of complicated ovarian cysts. J Clin Ultrasound 14:196–198

Ransley PG, Dhillon HK, Gordon I, et al (1990) The postnatal management of hydronephrosis diagnosed by prenatal US. J Urol144;584–587

Reuss A, Wladimiroff JW, Stewart PA, Niermeijer MF (1990) Prenatal diagnosis by US in pregnancies at risk for ARPKD.Ultrasound med Biol 16:355–359

Reuss A, Wladimoroff JW, Niermeyer MF (1991) US, clinical and genetic aspects of prenatal diagnosis of cystic kidney disease. Ultrasound Med Biol17:687–694

Ring KS, Axelrod SL, Burbige K.A., Hensle TW (1989) Meconium hydrocele: an unusual etiology of a scrotal mass in the newborn. J Urol 141:1172–1173

Rittenberg MH, Hulbert WC, Snyder HM, Duckett JW (1988) Protective factors in PUV. J Urol140:993–996

Rosati P, Guariglia L (1996) Transvaginal sonographic assessment of the fetal urinary tract in early pregnancy. Ultrasound Obstet Gynecol7:95–100

Rosendahl H (1990) Ultrasound screening for fetal urinary tract malformations: a prospective study in general population. Eur J Obstet36:27–33

Ryken TC, Turner J.W, Haynes T (1990) Bilateral testicular torsion in a preterm neonate. J Urol 140:102–103

Salem YH, Majd M, Rushton HG, Belman AB (1995) Outcome analysis of pediatric pyeloplasty as a function of patient age at presentation and differential renal function. J Urol154:1889–1893

Saraga M ,Jaaskilaaien J, Koskimies O (1995) Diagnostic US changes in the kidneys of 20 infants with congenital nephrotic syndrome of the Finnish type. Eur Radiol 5: 49–54

Saylors RL, Cohn SL, Morgan ER, Brodeur L (1994) Prenatal detection of neuroblastoma by fetal US. Am J Pediatr Hematol Oncol 16:356–360

Scott EM, Thomas A, McGanigle HHG, et al (1990) Serial US in normal neonates. J Ultrasound Med 9:279–283

Scott JES, Lee REJ, Hunter EW, et al (1991) Ultrasound screening of newborn urinary tract. Lancet338:1571–1573

Scott JES, Renwick M (1988) Antenatal diagnosis of congenital abnormalities in the urinary tract. Br J Urol62:295–300

Scott JES, Wright B, Wilson G, et al (1995) Measuring the fetal kidney with ultrasonography. Br J Urol76:769–774

Scott JES, Renwick M (1999) Screening for fetal urological abnormalities: how effective? BJU Int84:693–700

Selzman AA, Elder JS (1995) Contralateral vesicoureteral reflux in children with a multicystic kidney. J Urol153:1252–1254

Shapiro E (1999) The US appearance of normal and abnormal fetal genitalia. J Urol 162:530–533

Sherer DM, Thompson HO, Armstrong B, et al (1990) Prenatal US diagnosis of unilateral renal agenesis. J Clin Ultrasound18:648–652

Shibahara H, Mitsuo M, Fujimoto K, et al (1999) Prenatal US diagnosis of fetal mesoblastic nephroma. Hum Reprod 14:1324–1327

Shipp TD, Benaceraff BR (1995) Scrotal inguinal hernia in a fetus. AJR Am J Roentgenol 165:1494–1495

Sivan E, Koch S, Reece EA (1995) US prenatal diagnosis of ambiguous genitalia. Fetal Diagn Ther 10:311–314

Skari H, Bjornland K, Bjornstad Ostensen A, et al (1998) Consequences of prenatal ultrasound diagnosis: a preliminary report on neonates with congenital malformations. Acta Obstet Gynecol Scand77:635–642

Smulian JC, Scorza WE, Guzman ER, et al (1996) Prenatal diagnosis of midshaft hypospadias. Prenat Diagn 16:276–280

Song JT, Ritchey ML, Zerin JM, Bloom DA (1995) The incidence of VUR in children with unilateral renal agenesis. J Urol 153:1249–1251

Soriano D, Lipitz S, Seidman DS, et al (1998) Development of the fetal uterus between 19 and 38 weeks gestation. Hum Reprod 14:215–218

Spitzer A (1996) The current approach to the assessment of fetal renal function: fact or fiction? Pediatr Nephrol10:230–235

Stephens FD, Fortune DW (1993) Pathogenesis of megalourethra. J Urol. 149:1512–1516

Stocks A, Richards D, Frentzen B, et al (1996) Correlation of prenatal renal pelvic antero-posterior diameter with outcome in infancy. J Urol155:1050–1052

Strife JL, Souza AS, Kirks DR, et al (1993) MDK in children: US follow-up. Radiology186:785–788

Strouse PJ, Boweman RA, Schlenizer AE (1995) Antenatal findings of fetal adrenal hemorrhage. J Clin Ultrasound 23:442–446

Sukthankar S, Watson AR (2000) Unilateral MDKD: defining the natural history. Acta Paediatr89:811–813

Tapia J, Gonzalez R (1995) Pyeloplasty improves renal function and somatic growth in children with ureteropelvic junction obstruction. J Urol154:218–222

Thomas DFM (1990) Fetal uropathy. Br J Urol66:225–231

Tibballs JM, De Bruyn R (1996) Primary vesicoureteric reflux: how useful is postnatal ultrasound? Arch Dis Child75:444–447

Toma P, Lucigrai G, Marzoli A, Litranici M (1994) Prenatal diagnosis of metastasis of adrenal neuroblastoma with US and MRI. AJR Am J Roentgenol 162:1183–1184

Tripp BM, Homsy YL (1995a) Neonatal hydronephrosis: the controversy and the management. Pediatr Nephrol9: 503–509

Tripp BJ, Homsy Y (1995b) Prenatal diagnosis of bilateral neonatal torsion: a case report. J Urol 153:1990–1991

Uhlenhuth E, Amin M, Harty JI, Howerton LW (1990) Infundibulopelvic dysgenesis: a spectrum of obstructive renal disease. Urology35:334–337

Van der Slikke JW, Balk AG (1980) Hydramnios with hydrops fetalis and disseminated fetal neuroblastoma. Obstet Gynecol 55:250–253

Van Savage JG, Mesrobian HG (1995) The impact of prenatal US on the morbidity and outcome of patients with duplication anomalies. J Urol 153:768–770

Vergani P, Ceruti P Locatelli A, et al (1999) Accuracy of prenatal US diagnosis of duplex renal system. J Ultrasound Med18:463–467

Vinocur L, Slovis TL, Perlmutter AD, et al (1988) Follow-up studies of MDK. Radiology167:311–315

Walsh G, Dubbins PA (1996) Antenatal renal pelvis dilatation: a predictor of vesicoureteral reflux? AJR Am J Roentgenol167:897–900

Wapner RJ, Jenkind TM, Silverman N, et al (2001) Prenatal diagnosis of congenital nephrosis by in utero biopsy. Prenat Diagn 21:256–261

Weinberg B, Yeung N (1998) US sign of intermittent dilatation of the renal collecting system in 10 patients with VUR. J Clin Ultrasound26:65–68

Winderl LM, Silverman RK (1995) Prenatal diagnosis of congenital imperforate hymen. Obstet Gynecol 85:857–860

Wisser J, Hebisch G, Foster U, et al (1995) Prenatal US diagnosis of ARPKD during the early second trimester. Prenat Diagn15:868–871

Wladimoroff JW, Heydanus R, Stewart PA, et al (1993) Fetal renal artery flow velocity waveforms in the presence of congenital renal tract anomalies. Prenat Diagn13:545–549

Woodward JR (1993) Hydronephrosis in the neonate. Urology 42:320–321

Wright NB, Blanch G, Walkinson S Pilling DW (1996) Antenatal and neonatal renal vein thrombosis. Pediatr Radiol26:686–689

Yamazaki Y, Yago Rie Toma H (2001) US characteristics of the urinary tract in healthy neonates. J Urol 166:1054–1057

Yerkes EB, Adams MC, Pope JC, et al (1999) Does every patient with prenatal hydronephrosis need voiding cystourethrography? J Urol162:1218–1220

Yeung CK, Godley ML, Dhillon HK, et al (1997) The characteristics of primary VUR in male and female infants with prenatal hydronephrosis. Br J Urol80:119–127

Zerin JM, Ritchey ML, Chang ACH (1993) Incidental vesicoureteral reflux in neonates with antenatally detected hydronephrosis and other renal abnormalities. Radiology187: 157–160

Zerres K, Rudnig-Schönbron S, Deget F (1993) Childhood onset ADPKD in sibs. J Med Genet30:583–588

Zerres K, Mücher G, Becker J, et al (1998) Prenatal diagnosis of ARPKD. Am J Med Genet 76:137–144

Zhou Q, Cardoza JD, Barth R (1999) Prenatal US of congenital renal malformations. AJR Am J Roentgenol 173:1371–1376

9 Perinatal Diagnosis of Musculoskeletal Anomalies

FRANÇOISE RYPENS, FRANCE ZIEREISEN, FRED E. AVNI

CONTENTS

9.1 General Considerations 197
9.1.1 Circumstances of Discovery 197
9.1.2 How to Study the Fetal Musculoskeletal System 198
9.1.3 Management 198
9.2 Development and Appearance
of the Normal Skeleton 199
9.2.1 The Skull and Face 199
9.2.2 The Spine, Clavicles, Ribs and Sternum 199
9.2.3 The Limbs 201
9.3 Skeletal Dysplasias 202
9.3.1 Very Short Femur (Second Trimester) 203
9.3.2 Short Femur (Second Trimester) 209
9.3.3 Very Short Femur (Third Trimester) 210
9.3.4 Short Femur (Third Trimester) 210
9.3.5 Attitude 211
9.4 Focal Limb Anomalies 212
9.4.1 Limb Transverse Distal Amputation 212
9.4.2 Intermediate-Type Malformation 213
9.4.3 Longitudinal-Type Malformation 214
9.4.3.1 Radial Hypoplasia 214
9.4.3.2 Fibular Hypoplasia 214
9.5 Hand and Foot Malformations 216
9.5.1 Common Foot Anomalies 216
9.5.2 Clubhand Anomalies 218
9.5.3 Complex Malformations of Hands and Feet 218
9.6 Fetal Immobility or Akinesia Syndrome 220
9.7 Axial Skeletal Anomalies 221
9.7.1 Vertebral Malformations 221
9.7.2 Caudal Regression Syndrome 222
9.7.3 Sacrococcygeal Teratoma 223
References 224

FRANÇOISE RYPENS, MD
Department of Medical Imaging, Sainte Justine Hospital, 3175
Côte-Sainte-Catherine, Montréal, Québec H3T 1C5, Canada
FRANCE ZIEREISEN, MD; FRED E. AVNI, MD, PhD
Department of Pediatric Imaging, University Children's
Hospital Queen Fabiola, Avenue J. J. Crocq 15, 1020 Brussels,
Belgium

9.1
General Considerations

Skeletal malformations constitute a heterogeneous group of anomalies affecting the axial and peripheral skeleton. They include generalized disorders of the skeleton, characterized by abnormal cartilage and bone formation (skeletal dysplasias or osteochondrodysplasias), and focal musculoskeletal malformations. Malformations may be diffuse or localized. They occur in 0.4–0.6% of all pregnancies (WEINTROUB et al. 1999).

Skeletal and limb anomalies are underdiagnosed compared with other organ malformations (only 18.5% of limb malformations are detected in utero) (WEINTROUB et al. 1999, STOLL et al. 1995). Their detection is important since limb anomalies may be part of more complex syndromes (BROMLEY and BENACERRAF 1995). The systematic measurement of fetal long bones during routine sonographic (US) examinations leads also to the detection of skeletal dysplasias. One of the most difficult tasks for the sonographer is to determine the type of dysplasia and its prognosis. Therefore, a good knowledge of normal skeletal and limb development as well as of the pathological entities is mandatory in order to improve the US score.

Nevertheless, some malformations will remain impossible to diagnose during pregnancy due to their natural history, while the characteristic anomalies will develop after birth only.

9.1.1
Circumstances of Discovery

Fetal skeletal malformations may be discovered incidentally during a routine US survey of the fetus. In other cases, the skeletal anomaly is detected due to the presence of another malformation discovered by US (polyhydramnios, oligohydramnios, hydrops, small thorax, facial cleft, etc.). Also, in selected circumstances (previous family history, maternal diabetes mellitus, drugs), the attention will be specifically focused on a possible skeletal defect (EVANS et al. 1994). In high-risk patients, some skeletal dysplasias may be diagnosed already during the first trimester of pregnancy, using endovaginal US and genetic diagnosis on chorionic villous sampling (DIMAIO et al. 1993). For instance, endovaginal US may allow an early diagnosis of some severe skeletal dysplasias such as short-rib polydactyly dysplasia, osteogenesis imperfecta or achondrogenesis when there is a known family history. Yet, in less severe cases of skeletal dysplasia, an early biometric evaluation seems to be of no value (GABRIELLI et al. 1999, HILL and LEARY 1998).

Fetuses of insulin-dependent diabetic mothers have a 3- to 10-fold increased risk for malformations including congenital heart disease, renal anomalies and skeletal malformations (caudal regression sequence and inferior limb malformations), particularly when glycemia is poorly controlled at the time of conception (EVANS et al. 1994). Warfarin (which may induce a syndrome identical to chondrodysplasia punctata), phenytoin (digital hypoplasia), alcohol (fetal alcohol syndrome), methotrexate, aminopterin, anesthetics, and other drugs have been involved in some skeletal malformations (KOREN et al. 1987).

Finally, some malformations may escape even a detailed antenatal examination, and will be discovered after birth (i.e. rib and clavicle anomalies).

9.1.2
How to Study the Fetal Musculoskeletal System

The detection of skeletal malformation in a fetus relies mostly upon conventional US, which provides both static and dynamic information. The best time to study the fetal musculoskeletal system is between 14 and 18 weeks gestation. At this time the fetus, although very mobile, can easily be seen as a whole and the fingers are often extended allowing clear depiction of the extremities. Each limb must be evaluated from the girdle to the distal part. The spine must be systematically studied from the base of the skull to the coccyx by the use of multiple planes. The ribs, shoulder and pelvic bones are best studied along with the spine.

Measurement of the femoral diaphysis is a systematic part of a routine examination (see Chap. 1). Ideally, both femurs should be measured in order to detect malformations with asymmetrical involvement. If the result is abnormal, measurement of the other long bones of the limbs will help to determine the type of malformation. Reference values are available for

most bony structures. Assessment of the fetal skeleton includes evaluation of active movements of the fetus.

Beside traditional two-dimensional (2D) US, other imaging modalities can be used in selected circumstances in order to study the fetal skeletal system. Three-dimensional (3D) US may be useful in order to provide complementary information in selected indications. It has been shown to provide additional information in depicting the thoracic skeleton (ribs and scapula), the spatial orientation of fetal structures in positional limb anomalies and in malformations of fingers (GARJIAN et al. 2000, BABA et al. 1999).

In the case of skeletal dysplasia or complex spinal malformation, fetal radiographs may be useful in order to study the degree of mineralization of the fetal skeleton, and to detect fractures or specific deformations of bones. Due to poor mineralization at the early stage of development, radiography is not useful before the 27th week of gestation. In some rare circumstances, some teams have used abdominal CT, particularly in cases of complex spinal malformations or difficult cases of undermineralization (BRUNELLE et al. 1999). The radiation hazards severely limit the indications of CT.

Fetal MRI may be useful in some rare cases of complex spinal malformations and in order to determine the intrapelvic extent of sacrococcygeal teratoma (AVNI, in press).

9.1.3
Management

Discovery of a skeletal malformation implies a complete US survey of the fetus (in order to detect associated malformations), a karyotype analysis, and multidisciplinary panel consultation (including obstetrician, pediatrician, neonatologist, geneticist, orthopedic surgeon, psychologist) in order to explain to the parents the diagnosis, the prognosis and the therapeutic possibilities.

As mentioned, a precise diagnosis of skeletal dysplasia is sometimes not possible in utero and a complete postnatal investigation or even pathological study will be necessary to confirm the diagnosis. Postnatal radiographs of the affected neonate must be performed systematically. They should include frontal and lateral views of the skull and of the whole spine (with the ribs and clavicles), frontal view of the bony pelvis and frontal views of both limbs up to the extremities (possibly on separate films in the case of very small neonates or fetuses).

9.2
Development and Appearance of the Normal Skeleton

Ossification of the fetal skeleton progresses through two different processes: cartilaginous ossification for appendicular and axial skeletal structures, and membranous ossification for bone formation of the skull, facial bones, and portions of the clavicles and mandible.

9.2.1
The Skull and Face

Ossification of the skull starts at the level of the occipital bones around the 10th week of gestation. The remainder of the cranial bones ossify around the 14th week and at this stage when measuring the biparietal diameter, the entire vault must appear hyperechoic (except for sutures and fontanelles, which remain unossified throughout gestation) (Fig. 9.1). Ossification of the maxilla and mandible starts around 10–11 weeks (Fig. 9.2). These structures are clearly visualized around 18–20 weeks including the developing teeth (van Zalen-Sprock et al. 1997). Nasal bones can also be identified and measured.

9.2.2
The Spine, Clavicles, Ribs and Sternum

Chondrification centers appear in each mesenchymal vertebra during the 6th week of embryological development. By 8–9 weeks, three ossification centers have appeared in each vertebra (one in the centrum and one in each half of the neural arch) (Russ et al. 1986). Earlier on, each vertebral body has two primary ossification centers, one dorsal and one ventral, which fuse precociously to form one centrum (Zelop et al. 1993). On US, the faint outlines of the spine are first visible at 10–11 weeks gestation. At this stage, the spine looks like two hyperechoic discontinuous lines (Fig. 9.3). Ribs are not yet visible; they will appear 1–2 weeks later. Ossification of the vertebral bodies begin at the thoracolumbar junction and progresses in cephalic and caudal directions. In the lower fetal spine, ossification of the centra and the neural arches proceeds in a cephalocaudal direction (Budorick et al.1991). Starting at 16 weeks gestation, the three primary ossification centers are visible in each vertebra up to the fifth lumbar vertebra. An additional vertebral level then becomes ossified every 2–3 weeks

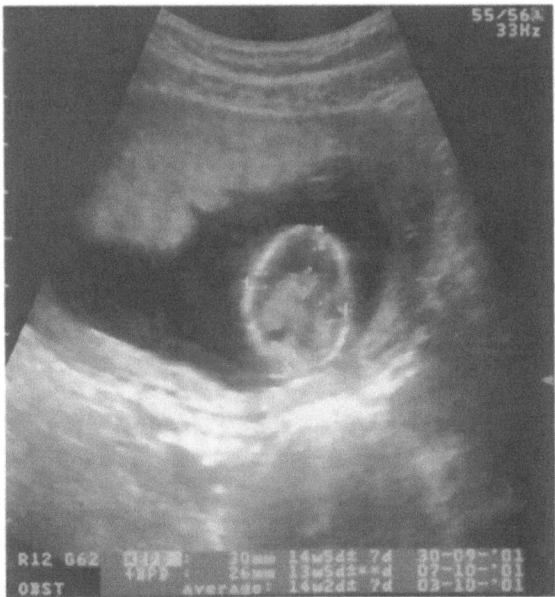

Fig. 9.1. Bony skull (end of the first trimester). Biparietal diameter view (26 mm between *crosses*). The fronto-occipital diameter is also measured (between *XX*)

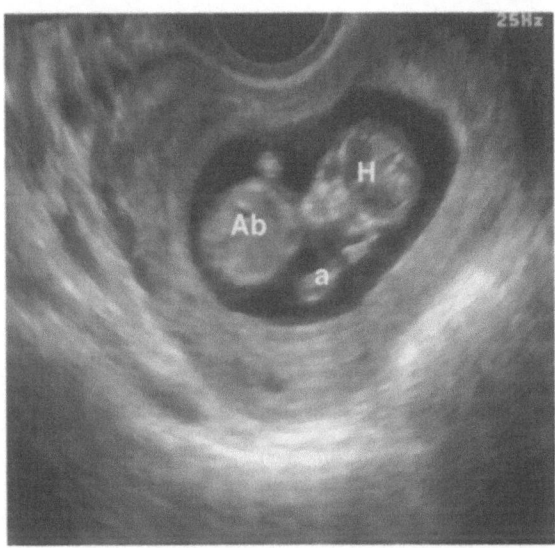

Fig. 9.2. Facial bony structures (end of the first trimester). Frontal view of the maxillae and orbits. *a* arm, *Ab* abdomen, *H* fetal head

from L5 to S5. By week 22, S2 is ossified (Budorick et al. 1991). At birth, the ossification has usually reached the first coccygeal vertebra. Supplementary paired ossification centers appear laterally in the three first sacral vertebrae at 40 weeks of gestation. The alignment of the ossification centers is regular and the only fixed normal curvature is the sacral one (Figs. 9.4–9.6).

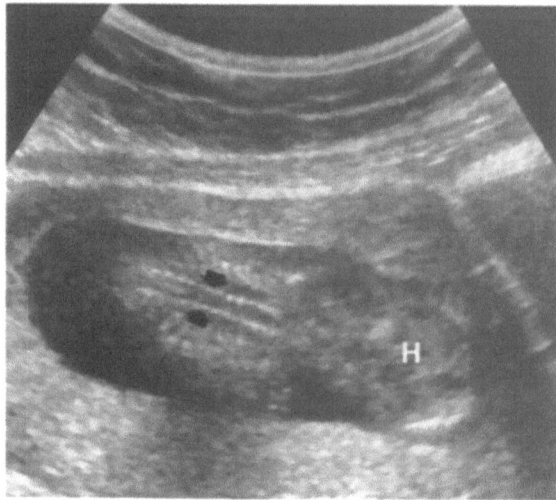

Fig. 9.3. Spine and ribs (first trimester). (Faint) parallel lines correspond to the lateral ossification centers of the spine (*arrows*). Some ribs are seen perpendicular to the spine. *H* head

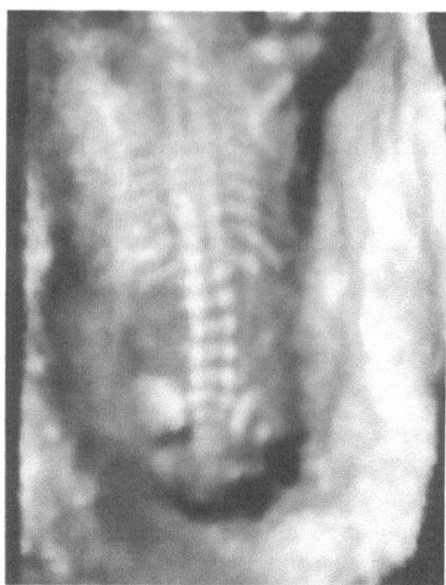

Fig. 9.5. Spine 3D analysis (second trimester)

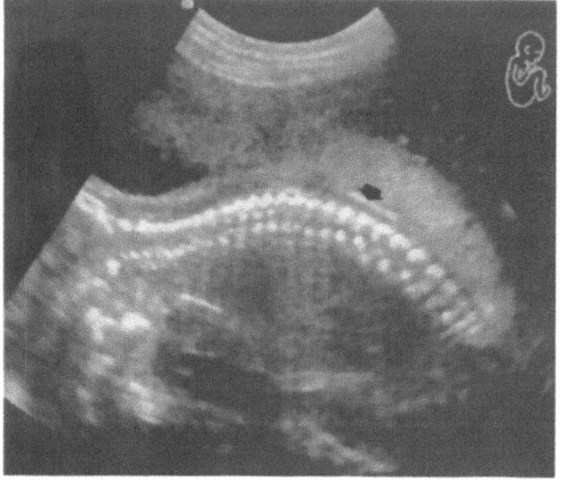

Fig. 9.4. Spine (second trimester). Sagittal views of the entire spine. The ossification centers are ossified and appear as two parallel lines. The skin surface is visualized as a hyperechoic uninterrupted line (*arrow*)

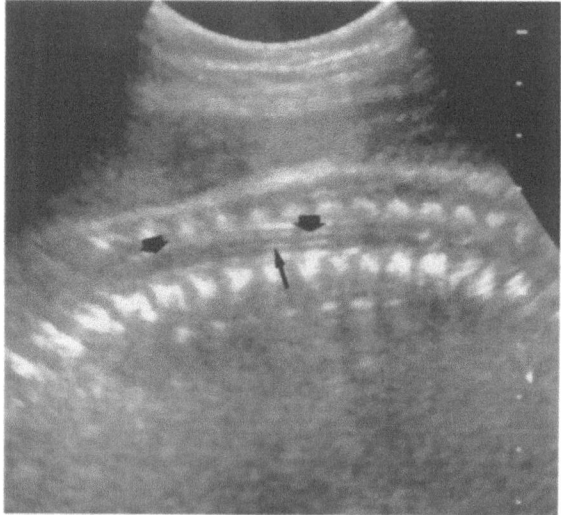

Fig. 9.6. Spine (third trimester). Visualization of the skin, the ossification centers and the cord (*wide arrows*), which appears as a hypoechoic tubular structure with a hyperechoic central line (*arrow*) (corresponding to the central ependymal canal complex)

The entire bony chest wall is clearly visible at 14 weeks gestation. The ribs are best evaluated on parasagittal and axial views. They are regularly positioned with smooth regular curvature but are difficult to measure due to their oblique orientation.

The rest of the shoulder girdle is more difficult to evaluate due to its particular morphology. Clavicles are the first structures to ossify from the 9th ges-

tational week. They appear at least partially at the upper level of the chest around the trachea. The scapula starts to be ossified around the 14th week and is best studied on the sagittal view that includes the upper arm. The sternum arises from two bands of somatopleural mesenchyme near the median plane of the thorax at about 6 weeks. These bilateral sternal bands become cartilaginous at about 7 weeks. They are continuous with the ribs and fuse with each other, beginning cranially. The fusion is more or less complete at the end of the embryonic period. A series of median ossification centers develop progressively, first in the manubrium, then in the body and finally in the xyphoid process (McCormick and Nichols 1981) (Fig. 9.7). The process of ossification can be followed sonographically from about the 20th gestational week (Zalel et al. 1999). On US, the sternum is best visualized either on an anterior frontal view or on a midsagittal view of the fetal chest. The ossification centers will appear as echogenic foci within the hypoechoic sternal cartilage. Each ossified center will grow throughout the rest of gestation but the fusion of the manubrium, body and xyphoid process ossification centers occurs after birth only (McCormick and Nichols 1981, Odita et al. 1985).

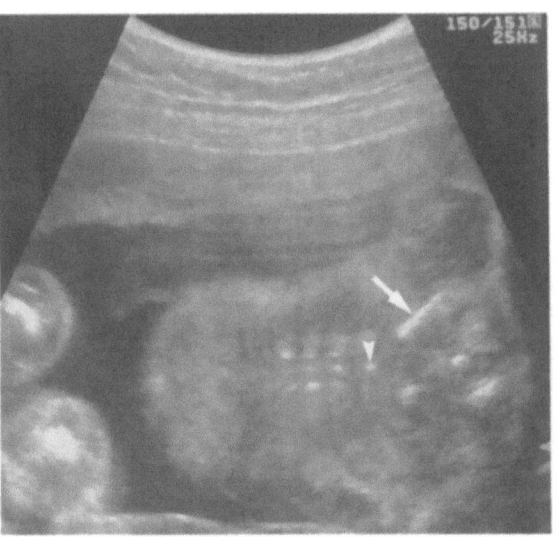

Fig. 9.7. Sternum (±20 weeks LMP). Frontal view. The ossification centers start to appear; the earliest and largest is that of manubrium (*arrowhead*). The *arrow* indicates the clavicle

9.2.3
The Limbs

Embryological development of the limbs includes cellular interactions between the ectoderm and the mesenchymal cells forming the limb buds. The position of the cells in the limb bud at the beginning of the development determines how the cells will develop and what sort of cartilaginous elements will be formed. The positional value of the cells is acquired in the progress zone, located at the tip of the bud. Lesion of this zone leads to truncations or phocomelia. Muscle cells have a different origin, migrating from the somites (Wolpert 1999).

The osteogenesis of the appendicular skeleton starts at the end of the embryonic period (about 8–9 weeks). Ossification centers develop centrally in the middle of the cartilaginous tissue of the diaphysis of the long bones and the ossification progresses towards the extremities of the bone. These centers become echogenic and distinct from the cartilage around 10–11 weeks. Thanks to the improvements in transducers and to the use of endovaginal probes, the extremities are more rapidly and more precisely identified (Reiss et al. 1995). At this stage they can be measured, preferably by endovaginal US (Van Zalen-Sprock et al. 1997).

At age 10–11 weeks, the differentiation in bone, articulations and muscles is completed and during the rest of the pregnancy all the structures will grow and become more complex (Figs. 9.8–9.11) (Moore and Persaud 1993, Bromley and Benacerraf 1995).

Later on and progressively, similar processes will occur and convert all cartilaginous epiphyses into bony ossification centers sometime after birth. Cartilaginous epiphyses appear as hypoechoic finely striated areas whereas ossification centers appear as echogenic round areas. The ossification of the epiphyseal centers progresses in a centrifugal way and their growth can be monitored and compared with normal gestational values (Gentili et al. 1984, Mahony 1984b).

Thanks to the monitoring of the development of the ossification centers, it is possible to determine the approximate gestational age. For instance, the talus and calcaneus ossification centers starts to be visualized around 23 and 25 weeks, the distal femoral center around 32 weeks, the proximal tibial center around 34 weeks and the proximal humeral center around 37 weeks (Fig. 9.12).

An evaluation of the gestational age can also be obtained through measurements of the length of the long bones, usually of the femur (Fig. 9.13). Their growth is linear from 13 to 25 weeks, more irregular thereafter (Merz et al. 1987). All the values express the diaphyseal length. In daily practice the measurements obtained are compared with reference values established longitudinally in normal populations. Tables comparing the growth of each long bones against gestational age are available (Brons et al. 1990). Nowadays, thanks to better equipment, more details of the cartilage, of the

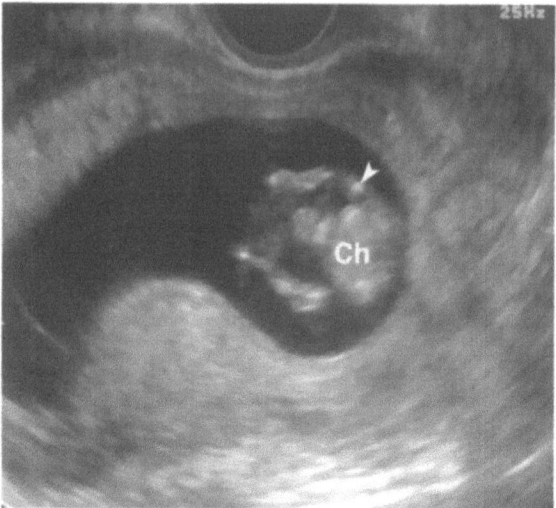

Fig. 9.8. Upper limbs (first trimester). The arms are visible lateral to the chest (*Ch*). Some ossification processes are visible (*arrowhead*)

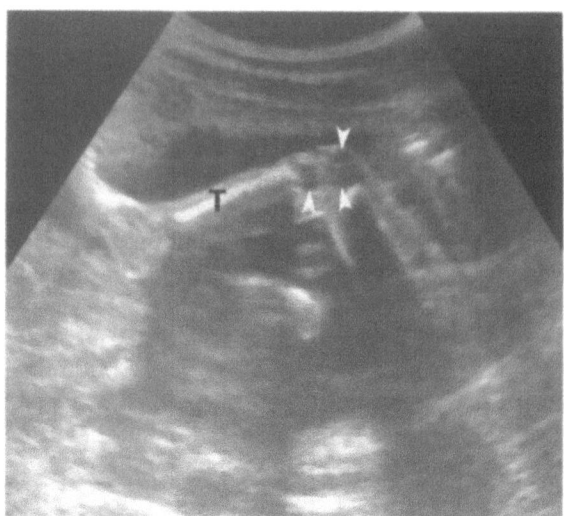

Fig. 9.9. Lower limbs (first trimester). Both limbs are visible (*arrowheads*)

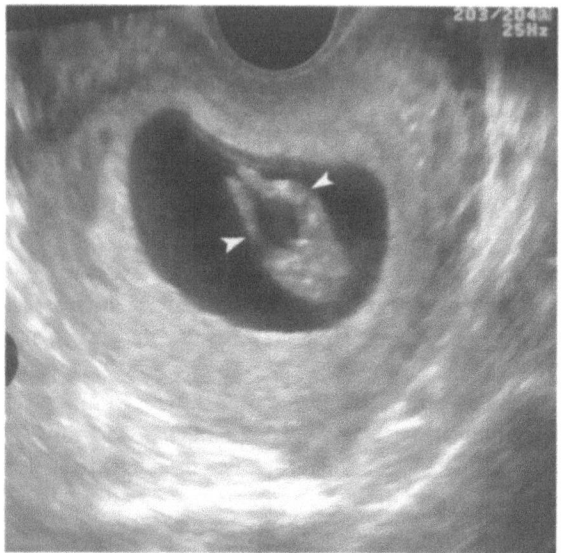

Fig. 9.10. Lower limb (second trimester). Hyperechoic ossified tibia (*T*) and hypoechoic cartilaginous epiphyses are visualized (distal femoral, proximal tibial, patella, etc.) (*arrowheads*)

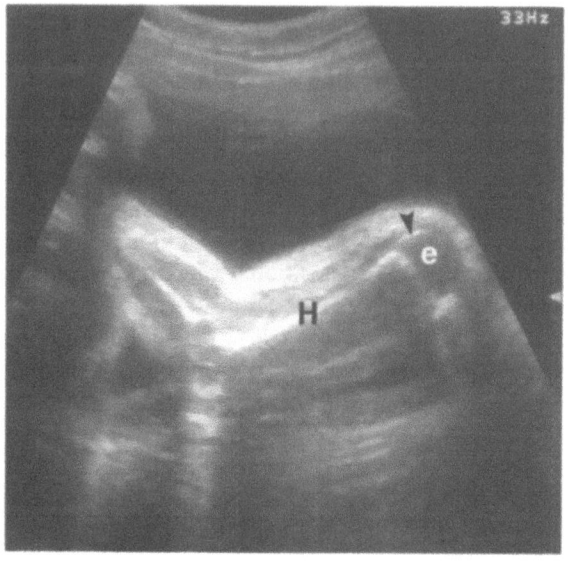

Fig. 9.11. Upper limb (third trimester). Hyperechoic humerus (*H*), muscles and soft tissues are visible. Hypoechoic proximal humerus cartilaginous epiphysis (*e*) and hyperechoic capsule (*arrowhead*) are present as well

muscles and of articulations are identified (RYPENS and AVNI 1994).

Evaluation of the ossification of the pelvic girdle has gained popularity since the demonstration of an increased iliac angle in cases of trisomy 21. In such patients the angle between the two iliac wings measures above 90° on a symmetrical axial scan. This measurement is best achieved around 18–22 weeks (KLIEWER et al. 1996; SHIPP et al. 1997).

9.3
Skeletal Dysplasias

Skeletal dysplasias occur in 0.024–0.07% of births. Several of these disorders are associated with a poor prognosis for postnatal life (KURTZ et al. 1990, GONCALVES and JEANTY 1994, DRISCOLL 1991, SPIRT et al. 1990, SANDERS and BLAKEMORE 1989). Prenatal detection of these disorders may influence the obstet-

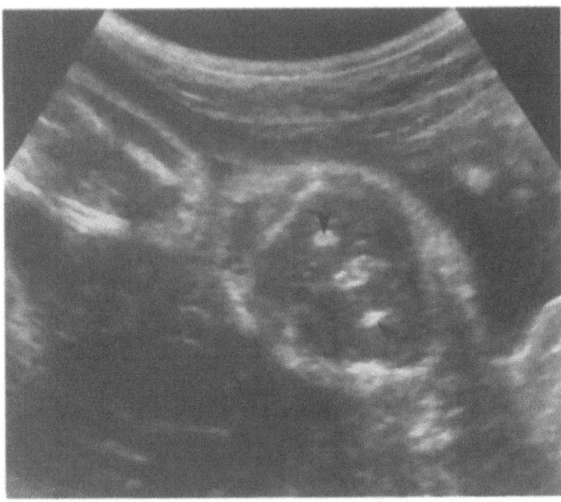

Fig. 9.12. Knee epiphyseal ossification centers (third trimester). Transverse scan through a bended knee. Echogenic epiphyseal ossification centers (*arrowheads*) are visible within the tibial and femoral cartilages. Gestational age can therefore be evaluated as around 34 weeks

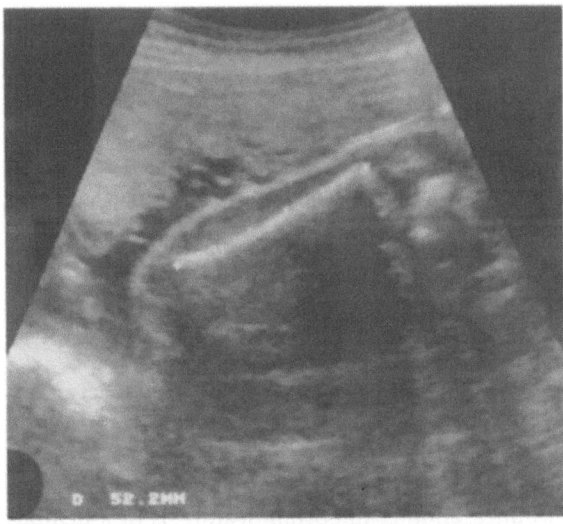

Fig. 9.13. Measurement of the femoral diaphysis (second trimester). There is 52.2 mm between the *crosses*

ric and perinatal management of affected fetuses. Obstetric US offers a unique opportunity for an antenatal diagnosis of a bone dysplasia that is suspected either by the detection of shortened long bones or because of family history. The time of detection can be as early as the end of the first trimester, but is more often during the second and third trimesters (GONCALVES and JEANTY 1994, BRONSHTEIN et al. 1993).

In Belgium, in the course of most uncomplicated pregnancies, three US examinations are routinely performed (one per trimester), and the femur is systematically measured during the second and the third trimester examinations, so a shortened femur is easily detected. However, a short femur does not necessarily imply a bone dysplasia. Therefore, a tailored approach must be applied after the detection of a short femur, based on the time of discovery, the degree of shortness, previous family history and the skeletal anomalies observed by US.

KURZ et al. (1990) have shown that the number of millimeters below the 2 SD line is an accurate and easy criterion for evaluating femoral shortening. On this basis, two groups of patients can be defined: the group with femoral length 1–4 mm below the 2 SD line (short femur) and the group with femoral length more than 5 mm below the 2 SD line (very short femur).

9.3.1
Very Short Femur (Second Trimester)

During the second trimester, a very short femur is highly suggestive of dwarfism (PRETORIUS et al. 1986, ROMERO et al. 1990) (Figs. 9.14–9.16). The only alternative diagnosis is that of an early growth-retarded fetus, a condition that can mimic bone dysplasia (PATTARELLI et al. 1990). In this type of growth retardation the outcome is poor, and karyotype anomalies can be encountered. In families with a previous history of bone dysplasia, the detection of a very short femur means recurrence of the disease and, if the disorder is lethal, parents may elect at this stage to terminate the pregnancy (SANDERS and BLAKEMORE 1989). In the case of an unexpected detection, a systematic fetal survey should be undertaken in order to find additional information that could ascertain the diagnosis and prognosis of the dwarfism and help to differentiate it from a growth-retarded fetus (PATTARELLI et al. 1990). First, all long bones should be measured in both extremities and compared with reference values in order to confirm the degree of shortening and determine its form (mainly rhizomelic or micromelic; mesomelic dwarfism would not be detected by the measurement of the femur only) (SPIRT et al 1990, ROMERO et al. 1990).

The long bones should be analyzed thereafter for any shape or contour abnormalities: long bone bowing, angulation, fracture or thickening secondary to callus formation (Figs. 9.17, 9.18; Table 9.1). Bone fractures appear as an interruption in the bone con-

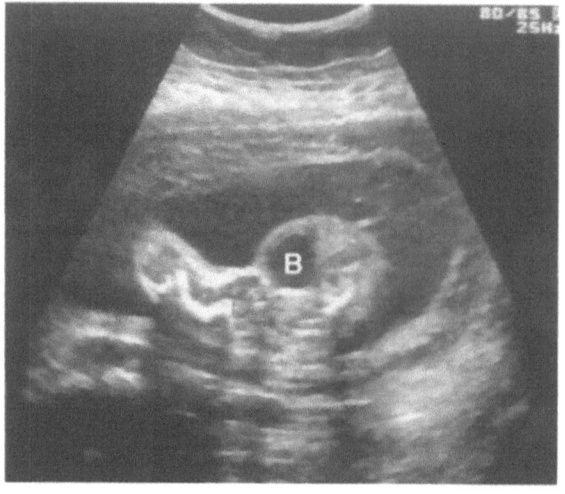

a

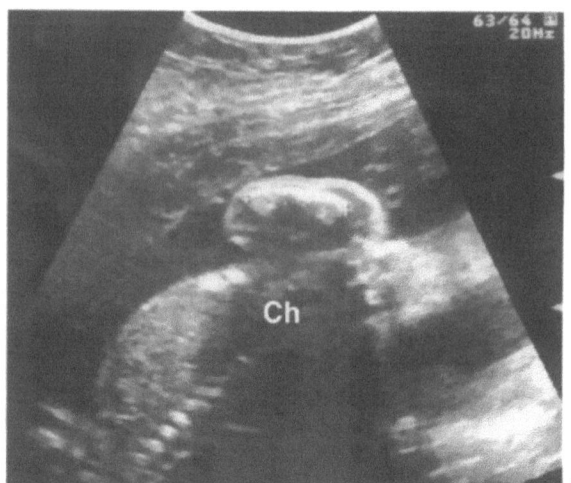

b

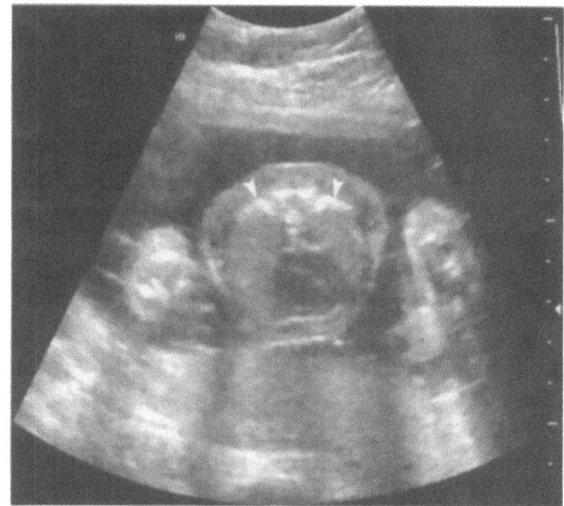

c

Fig. 9.14a–c. Very short femur (second trimester). Case of osteogenesis imperfecta (OI). **a** The curved femoral diaphysis measures 22 mm between crosses (50th percentile for age = 36 mm). *B* bladder. **b** Very short and curved humerus (28 mm between *crosses*). *Ch* chest. **c** Transverse scan of the chest demonstrating very short ribs (*arrowheads*)

tours; localized thickening or irregular contours may correspond to callus formation. Fractures strongly suggest osteogenesis imperfecta (OI) of type II, but other diagnoses are possible (Munoz et al. 1990, Brons et al. 1988) (Table 9.2). Bowed or angulated femurs may correspond to several dysplasias (Maroteaux 1982) (Table 9.1). Stippled epiphysis along with femoral asymmetry suggest Conradi-Hünermann syndrome (Taybi and Lachman 1996) (Fig. 9.19; Table 9.3). If possible the hands and feet should also be studied in order to find any associated malformation (Fig. 9.16).

The fetal spine is the second skeletal area that can help in narrowing the differential diagnosis: the presence of all ossification centers, the size of each vertebra and the degree of ossification of all vertebral segments have to be checked (Figs. 9.16, 9.20). The lack of ossification of segments of the cervical and lumbosacral spine facilitated the diagnosis of achondrogen-

esis type I (Mahony 1984a) (Table 9.4). Platyspondyly is less easy to appreciate and can be missed on fetal US; it is better demonstrated on an abdominal radiograph (Table 9.5). Diffuse undermineralization of bones, another important feature, is best demonstrated at the level of the calvaria bones. It may be suspected when the brain structures appear too clear and when the skull appears thin or even absent on the biparietal view (Fig. 9.21). Furthermore, in undermineralization the skull is too easily compressed by the transducer (Berge et al. 1995).

Such findings are of utmost importance in confirming dysplasias such as OI type II or hypophosphatasia. Conversely, normal ossification of the skull helps to exclude such syndromes (Munoz et al. 1990, Bulas et al. 1994, Brons et al. 1988).

Furthermore, the skull is an important landmark in cases of thanatophoric dwarfism, one of the most frequent lethal forms of dysplasia detected in utero

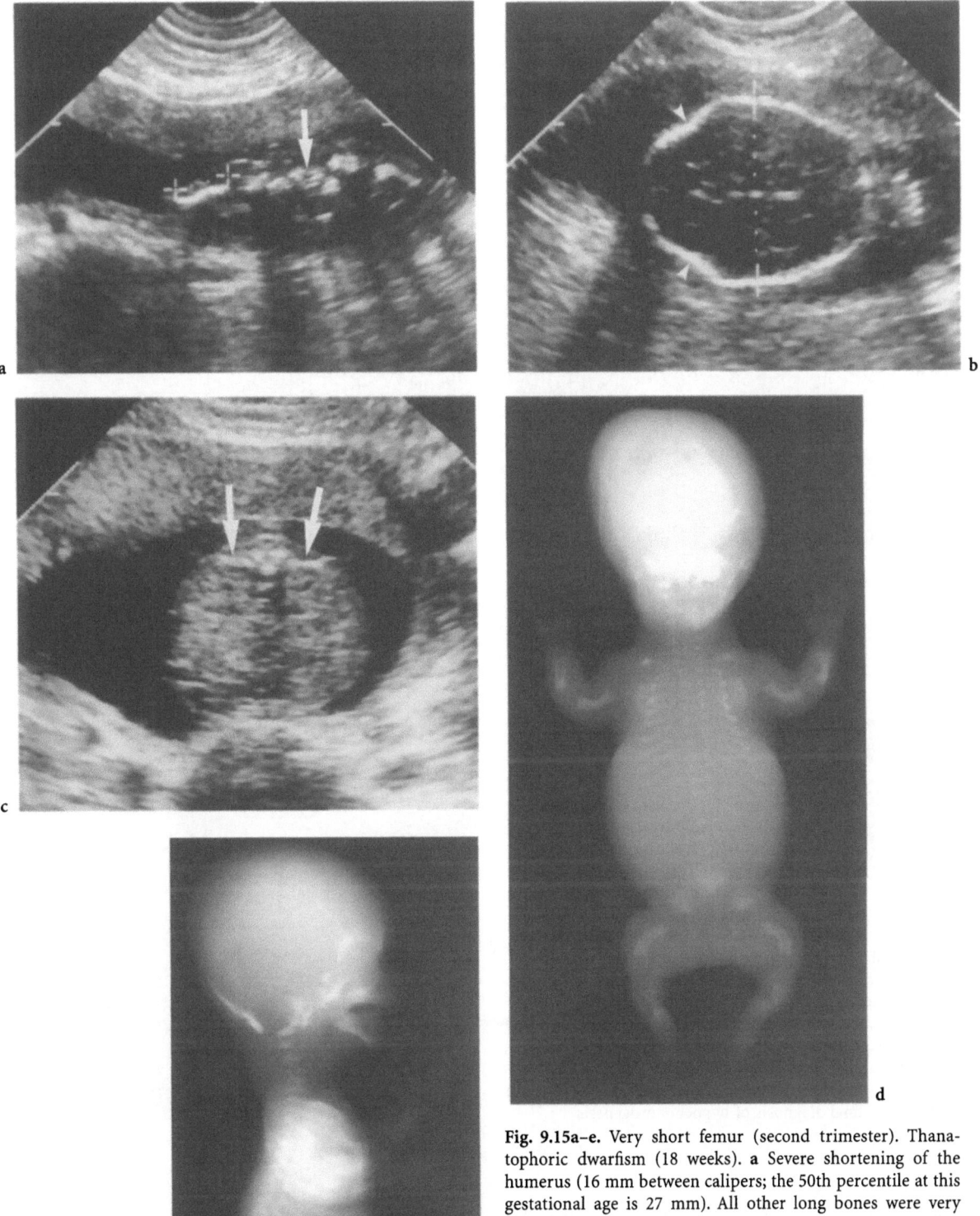

Fig. 9.15a–e. Very short femur (second trimester). Thanatophoric dwarfism (18 weeks). **a** Severe shortening of the humerus (16 mm between calipers; the 50th percentile at this gestational age is 27 mm). All other long bones were very short. The *arrow* points to the thoracic vertebrae. **b** Axial view of the skull shows deformation of the frontal bones (*arrowheads*). **c** Axial view of the upper abdomen demonstrating short ribs (*arrows*). **d, e** Corresponding fetograms obtained after termination of the pregnancy, showing platyspondyly, short ribs with wide-cupped costochondral junctions and a narrow chest. The metaphyses are irregular and flared. Final diagnosis was thanatophoric dysplasia

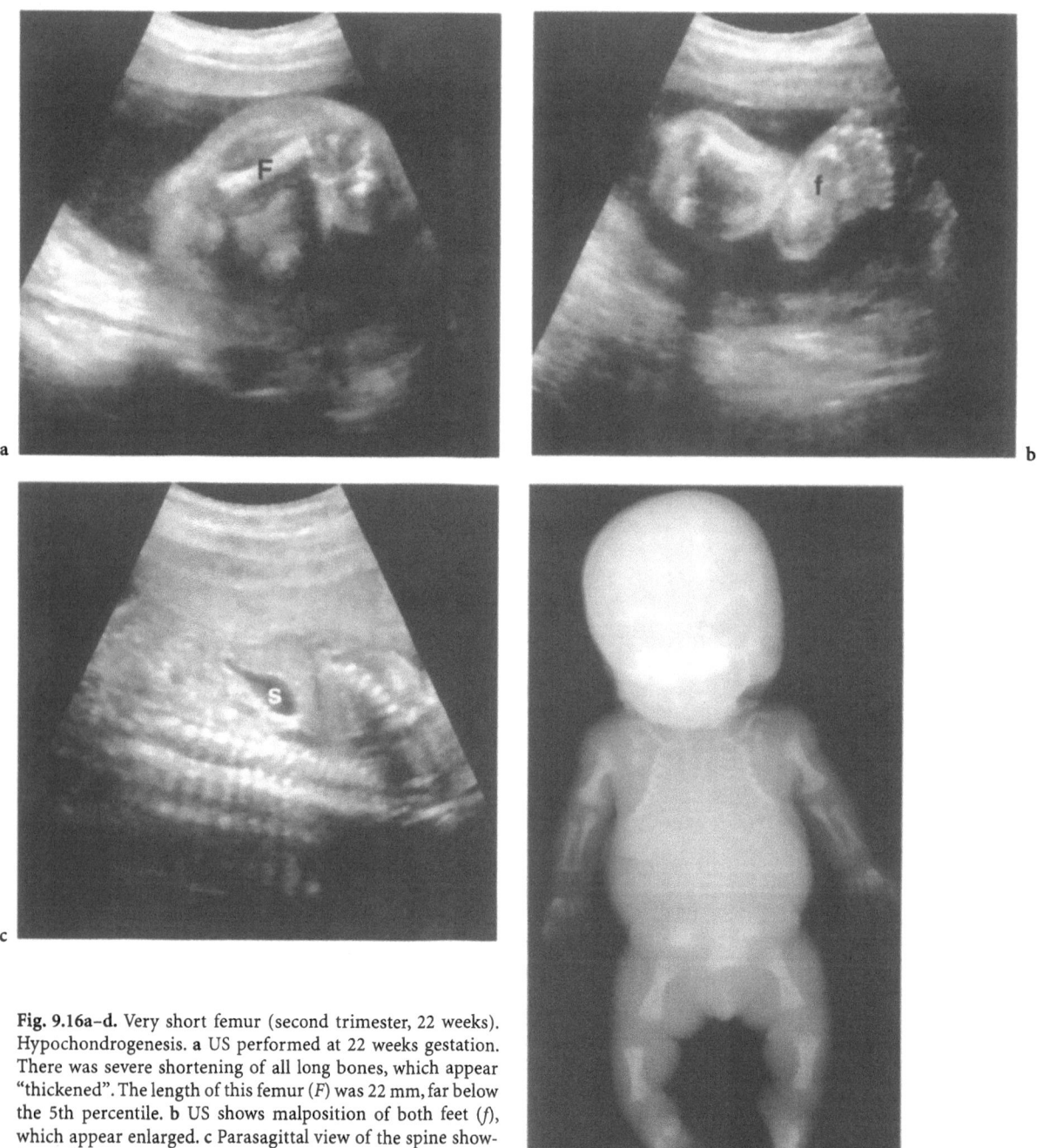

Fig. 9.16a–d. Very short femur (second trimester, 22 weeks). Hypochondrogenesis. **a** US performed at 22 weeks gestation. There was severe shortening of all long bones, which appear "thickened". The length of this femur (*F*) was 22 mm, far below the 5th percentile. **b** US shows malposition of both feet (*f*), which appear enlarged. **c** Parasagittal view of the spine showing diffuse small ossification centers. *S* stomach. **d** Fetogram confirms the final diagnosis of hypochondrogenesis

(1/30,000 births); in this dysplasia, the skull has a peculiar cloverleaf appearance (also named "Kleeblattschädel deformity") (Fig. 9.15). In this dwarfism, as well as in other dysplasias (achondroplasia and achondrogenesis for example), hydrocephalus and other brain malformations may be present. As mentioned already, many of the dysplasias detected during the second trimester are lethal, and most fetuses die at birth, mainly because of associated lung hypoplasia with respiratory failure; this can be predicted in utero by measuring the thoracic diameter or circumference (SKIPTUNAS AND WEINER 1987, DUGOFF et al. 1997).

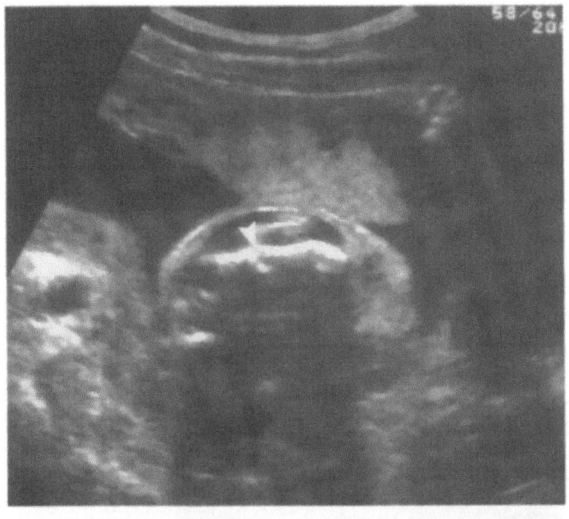

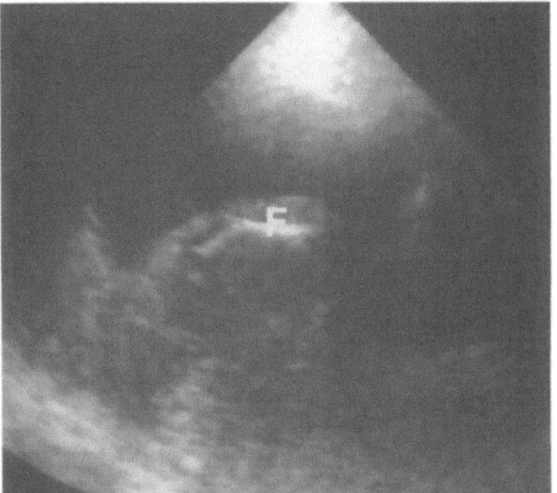

a

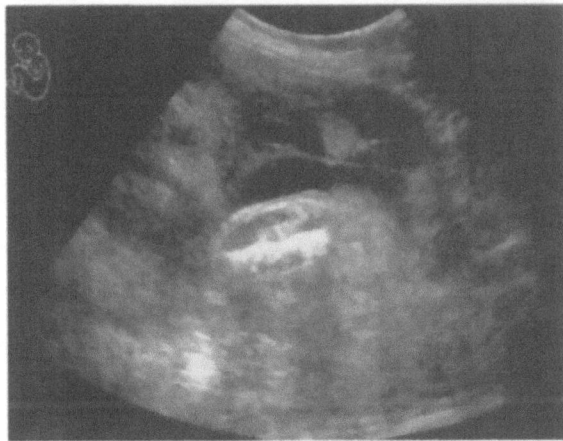

b

Fig. 9.17a, b. Fracture in utero. Case of osteogenesis imper-fecta. **a** Longitudinal US of one femur that shows shortening (femoral length below the 5th percentile) and interruption of the bone suggesting fracture (*arrowhead*). **b** Deformation of the contralateral femur

Table 9.1. Bowed tubular bones

Achondroplasia
*Camptomelic dysplasia
Chondroectodermal dysplasia
*Diastrophic dysplasia
Dyssegmental dysplasia
Fibrochondrogenesis
Hydrolethalus syndrome
Hypophosphatasia
Larsen syndrome
*Osteogenesis imperfecta
Oto-palato-digital syndrome type II
Short-rib polydactyly syndromes
*Thanatophoric dwarfism

*Most frequent

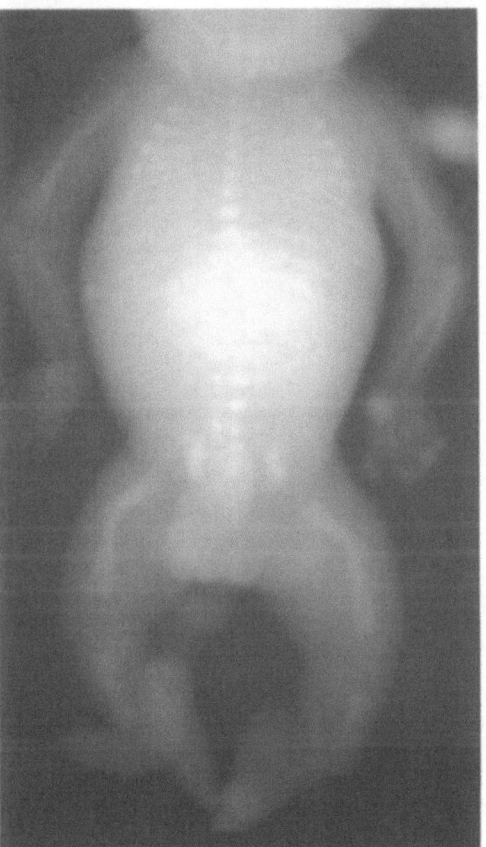

b

Fig. 9.18a, b. Bowed femurs. Case of camptomelic dwarfism. **a** In utero. Bowed femur (*F*). **b** Radiograph of the stillbirth confirms the dysplasia

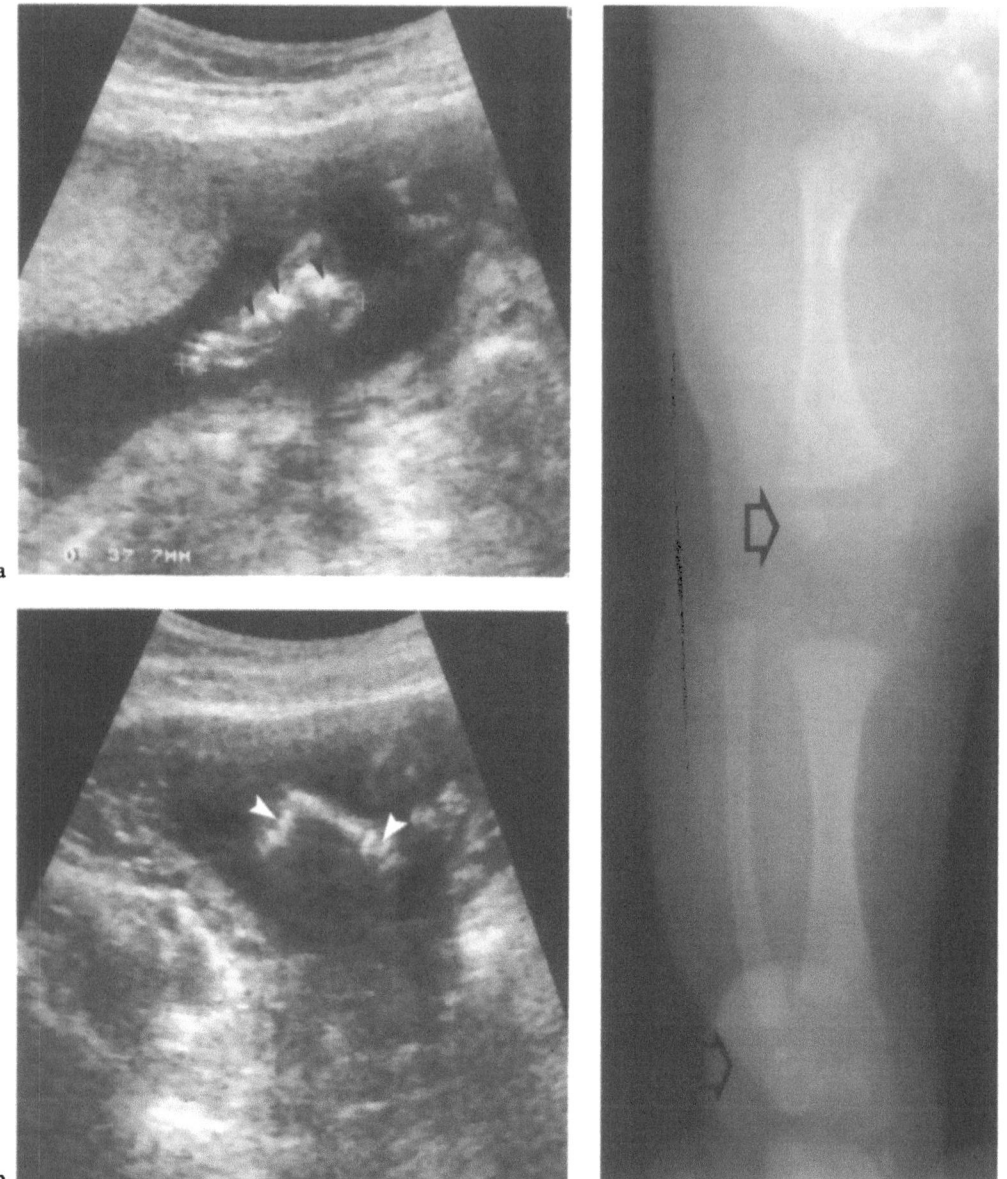

Fig. 9.19a–c. Stippled epiphysis. **a** Profile US view of the foot (between *crosses*) of a 25-week-old fetus showing the abnormal appearance of multiple tarsal ossification centers (*arrowheads*). Normally at this stage of development, only the calcaneus and talus already have their centers ossified. **b** Longitudinal US scan of the inferior limb shows multiple ossification centers in the tibial epiphysis (*arrowheads*). **c** Corresponding radiograph of the leg of this neonate shows disseminated stippled epiphyseal calcifications (*arrow*) as observed in chondrodystrophia punctata (also known as Conradi-Hünermann disease). With aging, these calcifications disappear progressively

Table 9.2. Fractures in utero
Achondrogenesis type I
Hypophosphatasia
Mucolipidosis II
*Osteogenesis imperfecta
Osteopetrosis

*Most frequent

Table 9.3. Stippled epiphysis
Acrodysostosis
*Chondrodysplasia punctata
Fetal alcohol syndrome
Warfarin embryopathy
*Zellweger syndrome

*Most frequent

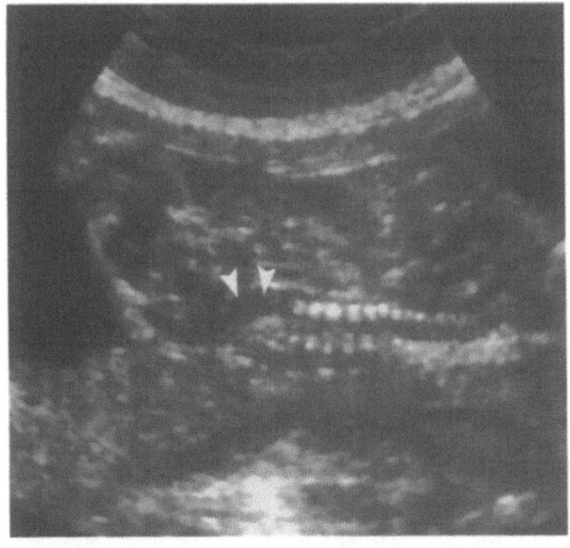

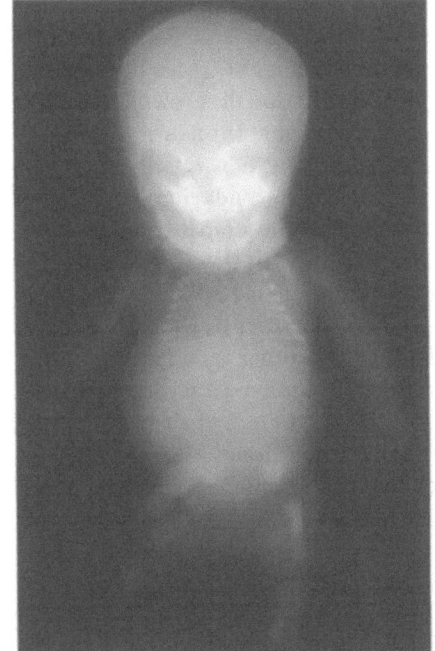

Fig. 9.20a, b. Achondrogenesis (second trimester). **a** Lumbar spine: hypoechoic unossified spine centers (*arrowheads*). **b** Corresponding stillbirth radiograph confirms the lack of ossification of the lumbar and sacral spine

Table 9.4. Vertebrae: absent or minimal ossification

*Achondrogenesis type I
Achondrogenesis type II
Hypochondrogenesis

*Most frequent

Table 9.5. Vertebrae: platyspondyly

Fibrochondrogenesis
*Hypochondrogenesis
*Hypophosphatasia
Metatropic dysplasia
Thanatophoric dysplasia
Thanatophoric variant

*Most frequent

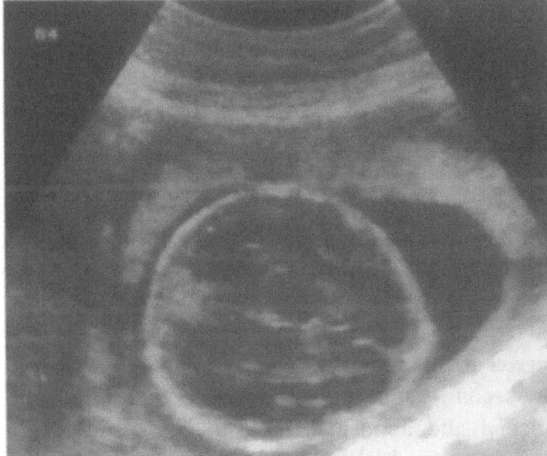

Fig. 9.21. Demineralization in bone dysplasia (second trimester). Case of osteogenesis imperfecta (courtesy of E. Cohen, MD, Brussels, Belgium). Unossified cranial bones result in a "too visible" brain

9.3.2
Short Femur (Second Trimester)

The significance of a short femur (2 SD below the mean) detected during the second trimester appears less straightforward as it may correspond to various pathologies. In the study by KURZ et al. (1990), many patients with a short femur had a favorable outcome and no case of bone dysplasia was found. Yet such a finding could suggest the progressive development of a dwarfism and successive control examinations are mandatory to monitor the growth curve of the long bones. For example, OI may develop differently within a same family during successive pregnancies ; the shortening sometimes appearing early and sometimes late in the second trimester. Therefore in a family with previous history, this finding indicates the recurrence of the disease and, consequently, a family with a previous history of OI can be reassured only if after 28 weeks gestation the growth of the long bones continues to be normal (BULAS et al. 1994).

Most commonly the question raised by a short femur detected during the second trimester is that of a possible indicator of chromosomal anomaly. It has been shown that patients with Down syndrome may have a short femur and an expected femur/measured femur length ratio below 0.91. However, it is never an isolated finding and other abnormalities must be present in order to suggest a karyotype analysis (BENACERAFF et al. 1989, LYNCH et al. 1989). Finally, a short femur very often indicates a growth-retarded fetus for which follow-up examination will be necessary.

9.3.3
Very Short Femur (Third Trimester)

During the third trimester a very short femur most probably corresponds to a short-limbed dwarfism, and therefore the investigation should be the same as during the second trimester. The whole fetal skeletal system, must be checked for associated anomalies (Fig. 9.22).

9.3.4
Short Femur (Third Trimester)

The significance of a short femur in the third trimester is much more difficult to appreciate than in the second trimester, and various conditions, both normal and abnormal, have to be considered. It can correspond to a short-limbed dwarfism of late development, usually a non-lethal type. Heterozygous achondroplasia is typically detected during the third trimester after femoral growth has slowed down (SANDERS and BLAKEMORE 1989, GONCALVES and JEANTY 1994). More commonly a short femur detected during the third trimester expresses intrauterine growth retardation (IUGR) of asymmetrical type, where the growth of the cranial bones is preserved but the femur is shortened (ZIMMER and DIVON 1992). The femur/foot ratio may help to differentiate between bone dysplasia and IUGR: the value is 0.99±0.06 in normal or growth-retarded fetuses but is markedly decreased in dwarfism (Fig. 9.23) (CAMPBELL et al. 1988). Constitutional shortness must also be included in the differential diagnosis for a short

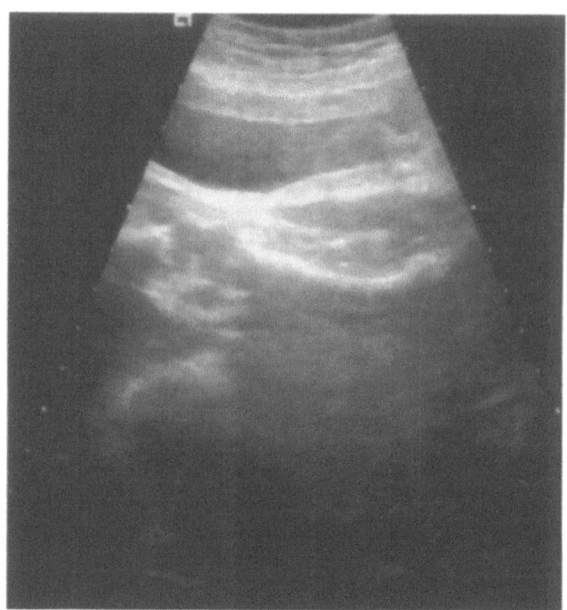

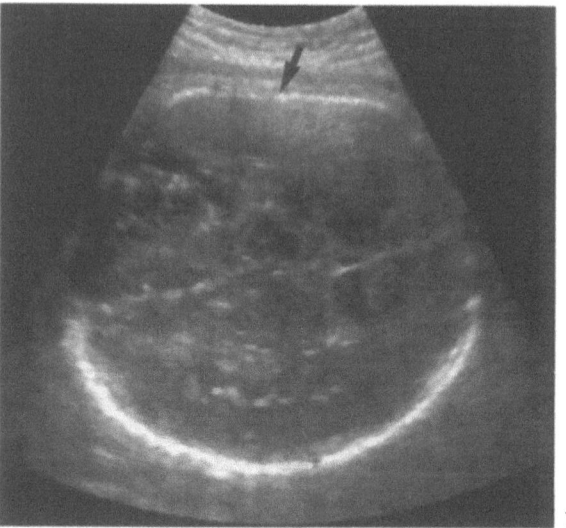

Fig. 9.22a, b. Very short femur (third trimester). Case of osteogenesis imperfecta. **a** Femoral length is 56 mm (between *crosses*), far below the 5th percentile for gestational age. The bone is bowed. The shortening of the long bones was diffuse but predominated in the proximal parts of the limbs. **b** Axial US of the fetal head at 36 weeks gestation shows abnormally good visualization of the hemisphere located close to the probe and depression (*arrow*) of the skull (due to hypomineralization). Final diagnosis was osteogenesis imperfecta with a specific mutation of the *col1A1* gene

femur detected during the last weeks of pregnancy: a family inquiry may help. Finally, one should be aware of possible error in measuring the long bones and therefore a control examination should be carried out in doubtful cases.

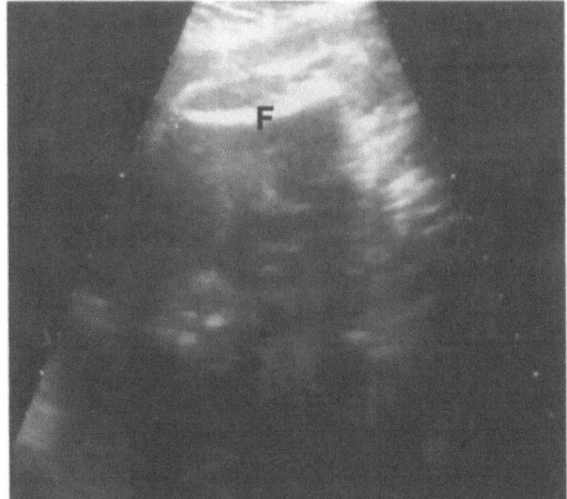

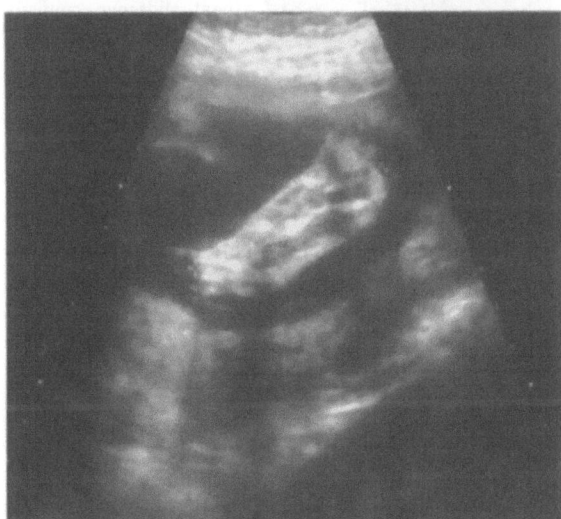

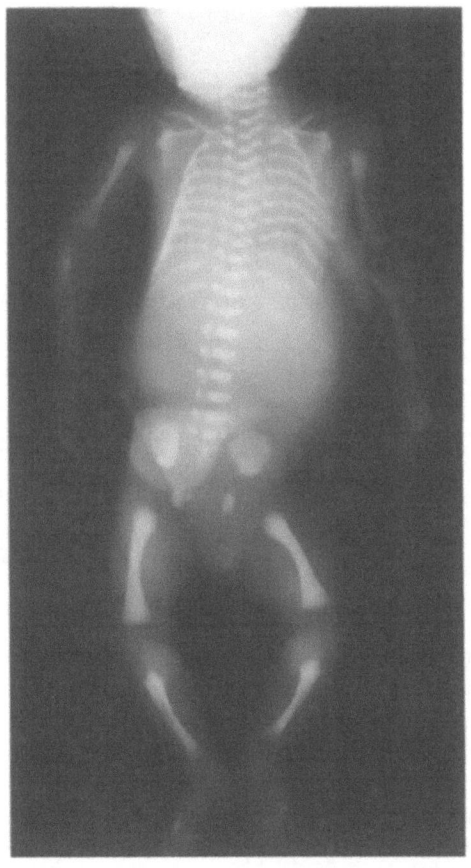

Fig. 9.23a–c. Short femur (third trimester). Case of asphyxiating thoracic dysplasia. **a** The femur (*F*) length was at the 5th percentile for the estimated age (4.2 cm between *crosses*). **b** The foot was 5.2 cm (between *crosses*). Thus the femur/foot ratio was 0.8 instead of 1. (There were also cystic kidneys and a relatively small chest.) **c** Radiograph of the stillbirth confirms the small chest and iliac wing anomalies

9.3.5
Attitude

Obviously it is impossible to identify every dysplasia. Many will remain unclassified even with skeletal radiographs at birth, and for some the characteristic features will appear only later, sometimes later in childhood. Early detection will allow a long-term follow-up and a full investigation at birth.

Although a precise antenatal diagnosis of a bone dysplasia may be difficult in some cases, differentiation between lethal and non-lethal diseases is usually easier (Azouz et al. 1998). The US findings that are suggestive of lethal skeletal dysplasia include an early second trimester diagnosis, femur length <1st centile, a small thorax, decreased mineralization, femur length-to-abdominal circumference ratio <0.16, vertebral anomalies, other structural malformations as well as chromosomal anomalies (Hersh et al. 1998, Ramus et al. 1998).

Whatever the type of anomaly and the time of detection, it is mandatory to obtain confirmation of the sonographic findings either in utero by plain film of the mother's abdomen or after delivery by skeletal radiographs of the newborn (or of the stillborn) (Figs. 15–19, 24) (Winter et al. 1984). Each case should be managed individually with the help of pediatric radiologists, fetopathologists and geneticists. An antenatal diagnosis of dwarfism carries many questions and much anxiety for parents and, therefore, a multidisciplinary team should inform and counsel the parents so they can choose the most appropriate attitude.

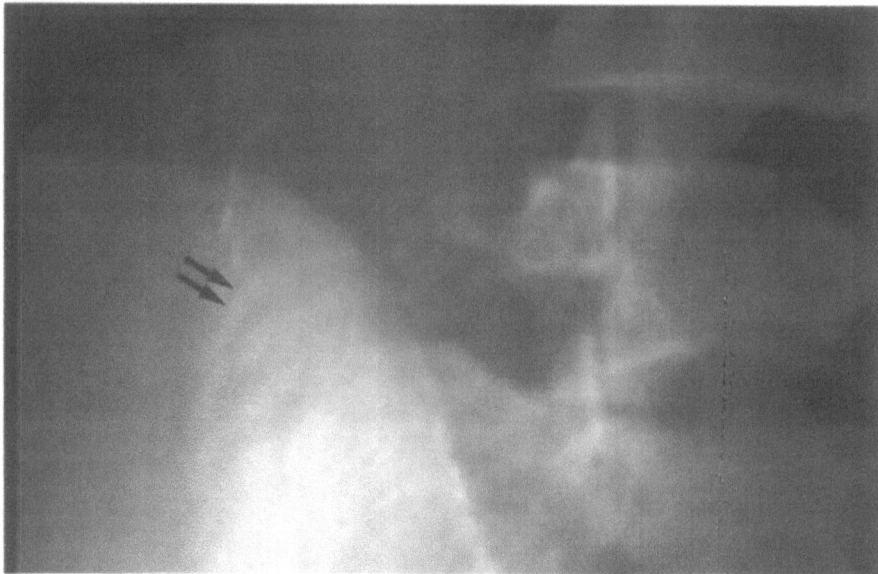

Fig. 9.24. Short femur (third trimester). Case of osteogenesis imperfecta. Radiograph of the pregnant abdomen confirming fractures (*arrows*)

In conclusion, many skeletal dysplasias may be accurately identified by US. A careful assessment of the fetal skeleton should be performed when the fetus is at risk or when the screening examination identifies a skeletal disorder. The main differential diagnosis for bone dysplasia is a growth-retarded fetus. Each case should be cautiously approached, focusing the analysis on the time of diagnosis, severity of shortness and associated findings.

This approach should provide sufficient information to counsel the family not only for the current pregnancy but also for subsequent ones.

The investigation of skeletal dysplasias has to be systematic, taking into account US findings (age at diagnosis, bones involved, associated anomalies) as well as family history. Pre- or postnatal confirmation is essential to obtain by means of imaging or pathology.

9.4
Focal Limb Anomalies

Focal skeletal defects range from extensive and diffuse malformations to subtle focal findings (BOWERMAN 1995, BROMLEY and BENACERRAF 1995). Their incidence is estimated at 6.5/10,000 births (STOLL et al. 1994). The rate of detection still remains poor, particularly for distal lesions (ANDERSON et al. 1995).

Focal limb anomalies may be isolated findings, may be associated with other skeletal malformations, or may be part of syndromes or associated with aneu-

ploidies (BROMLEY and BENACERAFF 1995). Most limb reduction deformity disorders are not genetically transmitted. However, complete sonographic examination is mandatory in order to detect associated malformations that will induce the search for acronymic or syndromic association or chromosomal anomaly.

9.4.1
Limb Transverse Distal Amputation

The group of limb transverse distal amputations includes the so-called amniotic band sequence that is the most common type. Its incidence varies from 1/15,000 to 1/1,200 live births or even to 1/56 previable fetuses (TAYBI and LACHMAN 1996). Its etiology is still unknown. Two different theories explain the anomalies encountered: the "constrictive amniotic bands" theory or the vascular disruption event (VAN ALLEN et al. 1992, MOERMAN et al. 1992). Absence of fusion between the amniotic membrane and the chorion or early rupture of the amnion can lead to acute oligohydramnios and to abnormal contact between the chorionic side of the amnion and the fetus (FROSTER and BAIRD 1993). Such an acute decompression would be associated with amniotic constrictions that determine ischemic lesions localized at the level of the fetal structures entrapped by the mesodermal bands. The spectrum of resulting anomalies is wide. It includes limb ring constrictions ranging from simple grooves to complete amputation (Fig. 9.25), syndactyly, limb deformities, pterygium,

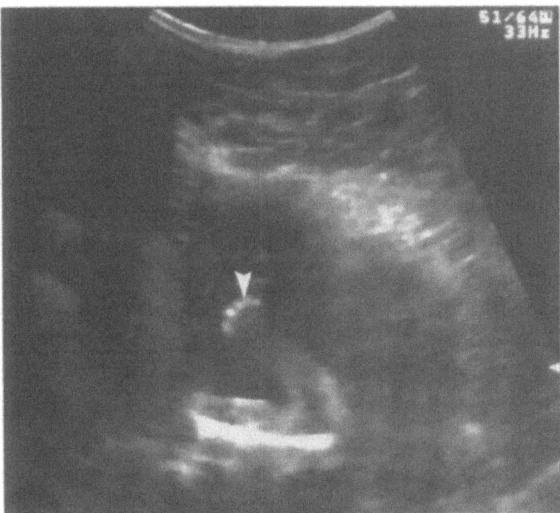

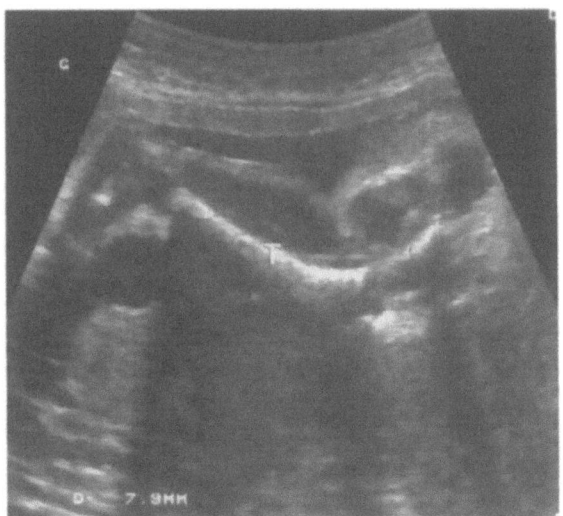

Fig. 9.25. Amniotic band syndrome. Amputation of the distal end of the hand (arrowhead)

facial clefts, cranial defects (encephalocele, anencephaly, acrania, ocular defects) and laparoschisis (TADMOR 1997, TAYBI and LACHMAN 1996). Chromosomal anomalies are usually not associated with the sequence. Most cases are sporadic but associations have been described with epidermolysis bullosa and Ehlers-Danlos syndrome.

Prenatal diagnosis relies upon the discovery of limb, trunk or cranial defects associated with loose amniotic bands close to the abnormal structure. The lesions are characteristically asymmetrically distributed. Diagnosis may be achieved early during the first trimester in severe forms. These most severe forms are lethal.

9.4.2
Intermediate-Type Malformation

Intermediate-type malformation involves the proximal segment of the limb. Congenital short femur, or proximal femoral focal deficiency, illustrates this type of malformation (Fig. 9.26). This rare anomaly (0.2/10,000 births) is characterized by variable shortening of the proximal part of the femur. There may be a simple shortening associated or not with proximal pseudarthrosis or complete femoral aplasia (JEANTY et al. 1985). The acetabulum and proximal part of the femur are always abnormal. The malformation may be unilateral (most often on the right side) or rarely bilateral. In the more severe cases it may be associated with fibular hemimelia, agenesis of the lateral tarsal bones and lateral toes and even hypo-

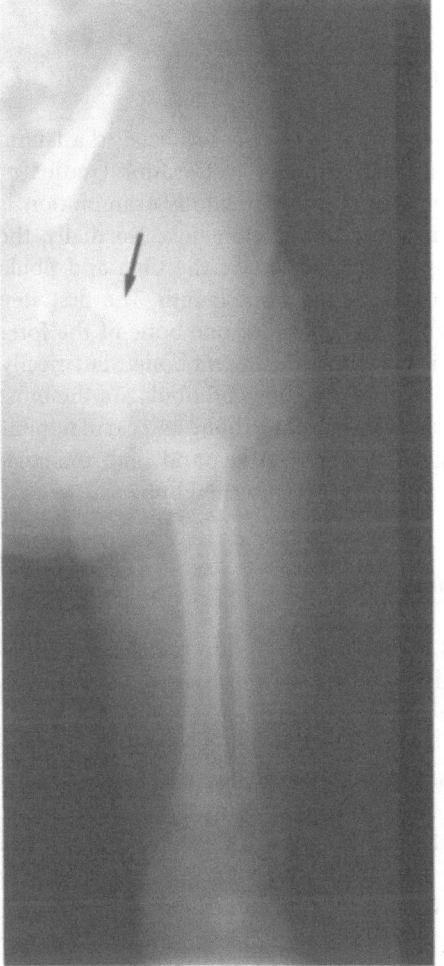

Fig. 9.26a,b. Intermediate-type malformation: congenital short femur (third trimester). **a** Severe shortening of the femur (between *crosses*), corresponding to proximal femoral deficiency. This illustrates the importance of bilateral measurement and systematic study of the limbs. *T* tibia. **b** Postnatal appearance of a congenital focal femoral deficiency (*arrow*)

plasia of the ipsilateral pubic bone as part of a fibular developmental spectrum (SEPULVEDA et al. 1994, SORGE et al. 1995). Most cases are sporadic and non-syndromal but association with maternal diabetes mellitus (JEANTY et al. 1985, ROMERO et al. 1990) and familial transmission have been described. The occurrence of such malformations emphasizes the need for bilateral femoral measurement (CAMERA et al. 1993).

After birth, the malformation is characterized by limb-length discrepancy, malrotation, and deficiency of the iliofemoral articulation (Fig. 9.26b). Treatment and surgical planning rely upon postnatal imaging. X-rays, US and MRI are necessary to precise the extent of the malformation and the presence and location of the femoral head.

9.4.3
Longitudinal-Type Malformation

Longitudinal-type is primarily localized to a lateral (or rarely medial) segment of the limb (radius or cubitus, fibula or tibia). Meticulous examination is necessary to detect such anomalies. Normally, the ulna is longer than the radius; the tibia and fibula have approximately the same length. The first step in the diagnosis of aplasia of one bone of the forearm or leg is to identify the absent bone. Statistically, malformations of the radius and fibula are the most frequent. Careful study of the bone and cartilaginous morphology, articular relations and limb malposition help to identify the abnormal bone.

9.4.3.1
Radial Hypoplasia

Congenital radius deficiency (or radial hemimelia) corresponds to hypoplasia or absence of the radius (GECK et al. 1999). The incidence of this malformation varies from 1/30,000 to 1/100,000 live births. The anomaly is bilateral in 38–58% of cases and presents with a 3:2 male to female ratio (GECK et al. 1999). Radial hypoplasia is a part of a spectrum of entities that affect the radial side of the extremity and may include deficiency of the radius, carpal bones and hypoplastic thumbs (Fig. 9.27; Table 9.6) (JAMES et al. 1999) When the malformation is significant, it is characteristically associated with a radial clubhand deformity. The discovery of such a radial hypoplasia implies a careful and complete sonographic survey, fetal blood sampling and determination of complete fetal blood cell count and karyotypic determination.

Associated conditions are numerous, the commonest being Fanconi anemia, TAR syndrome, Holt Oram syndrome and VATER association (ROMERO et al. 1990). Fanconi anemia is an autosomal recessive pancytopenia due to bone marrow failure and is associated with radial clubhand, absent thumb and radial hypoplasia. Other malformations of the skeletal system (scoliosis), the heart, the lungs and the gastrointestinal system, and intrauterine growth retardation, may be observed. In the autosomal recessive TAR syndrome (Thrombocytopenia Absent Radius), thumbs and metacarpals are present but the radius is absent. Absence of ulna and humerus and clubfoot may be associated. In 33% of cases, cardiac malformations (tetralogy of Fallot and septal defects) are present. Due to the risk of fetal cerebral hemorrhage, cesarean section is recommended (ROMERO et al. 1990). Forty percent of affected infants die in infancy following hemorrhage precipitated by viral illness. The severity of thrombocytopenia decreases with age. In Holt-Oram syndrome (autosomal dominant), congenital heart disease (atrial and ventricular septal defects) are associated with aplasia or hypoplasia of the radius. The limb defects are frequently asymmetrical and there is often a positive family history. Radial clubhand associated with vertebral segmental anomalies suggests VATER association or Goldenhar syndrome (associating hypoplasia of the maxillary and/or mandibular region, microtia). Finally, radial hypoplasia is found in various karyotypic anomalies, including trisomy 18 and 21, and may be seen in exposure conditions (fetal valproate syndrome) (ROMERO et al. 1990).

9.4.3.2
Fibular Hypoplasia

Absence of the fibula is the most common mesomelic para-axial hemimelia (SEPULVEDA et al. 1994, SORGE et al. 1995). The malformation is frequently associated with anteromedial bowing and shortening of the tibia and equinovarus deformation of the foot (Fig. 9.28). The anomaly is part of the spectrum of malformation affecting the entire lateral part of the inferior limb, including defects of the pubic bone, femoral proximal part, patella, fibula, and a variable number of lateral tarsal bones and toes (the so-called fibular developmental field concept) (SEPULVEDA et al. 1994, SORGE et al. 1995). Considering the associated anomalies of the lower extremities, some orthopedic teams prefer to use the term of "postaxial hypoplasia" for these defects (STEVENS and ARMS 2000). Most cases are sporadic, due to disruption or terato-

Fig. 9.27a–c. Longitudinal-type malformation (second trimester). Radial hypoplasia. **a** US: only one bone is visible in the forearm; the hand (*h*) is abnormal as well. *H* humerus. **b** Radiograph of stillbirth confirms the radial aplasia. **c** Fetal CT 3D reconstruction

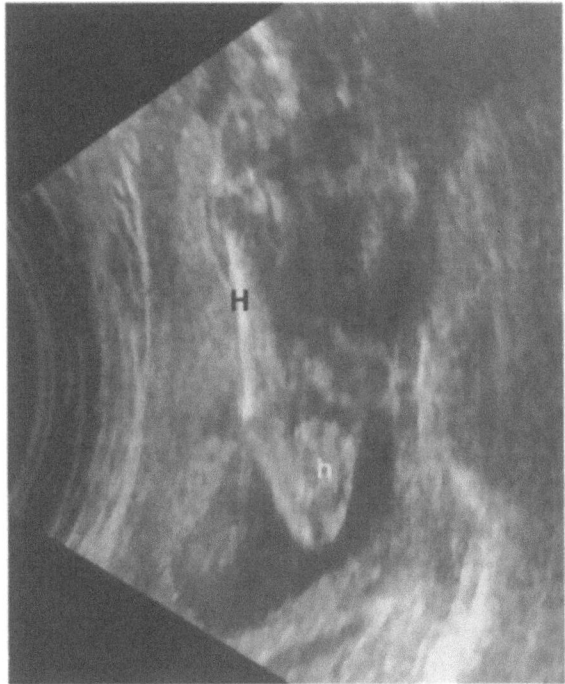

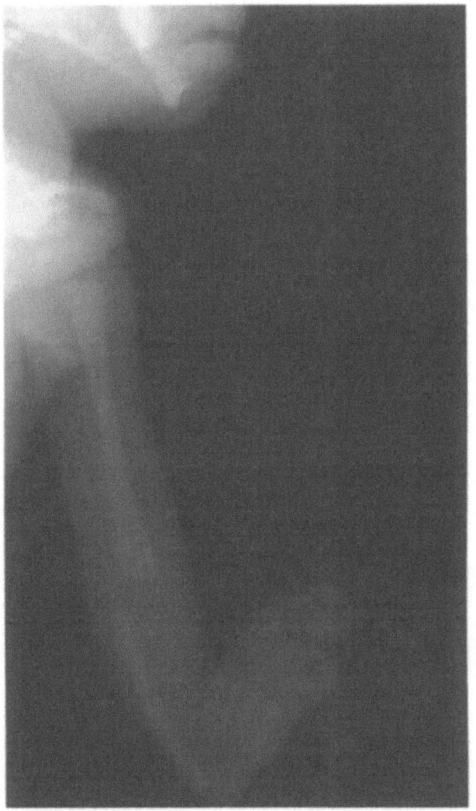

Table 9.6. Radius/radial ray: aplasia, hypoplasia

Dyschondrosteosis
*Fanconi anemia
*Holt-Oram syndrome
Roberts syndrome
TAR syndrome
Thalidomide embryopathy
VATER association

*Most frequent

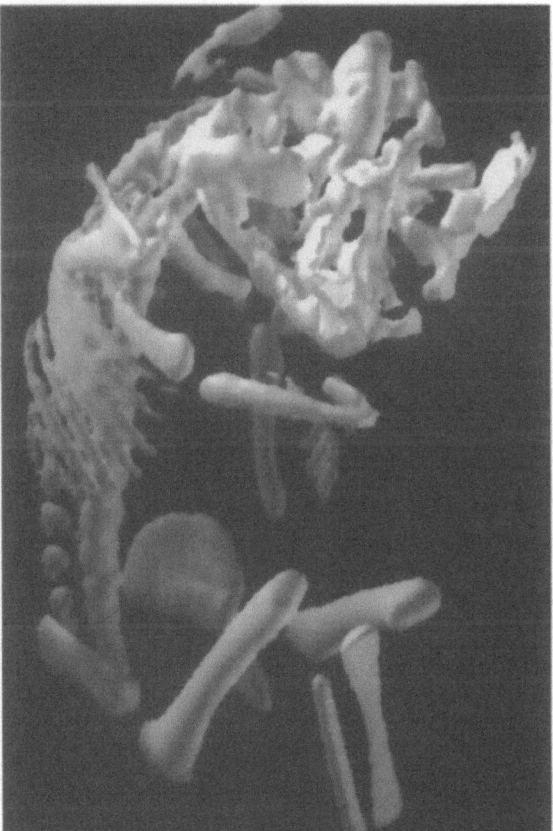

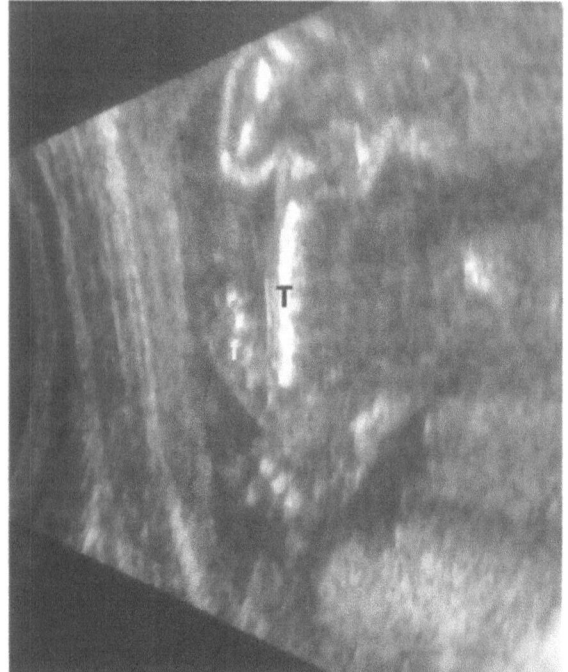

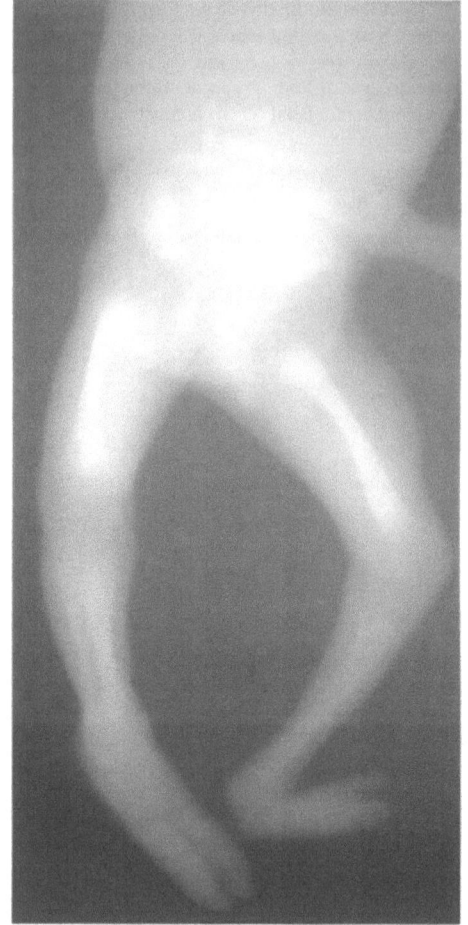

Fig. 9.28a, b. Fibular agenesis. **a** US (third trimester). Only the tibia (*T*) is visible. The foot (*f*) is malpositioned. **b** Radiograph of the stillbirth confirms the anomaly

genic insults. Bilateral fibula hypoplasia or agenesis may be associated with complex dysostosis (camptomelic dysplasia), rare syndromes and some aneuploidies (Table 9.7). Non-skeletal anomalies are rarely associated. The discovery of such a malformation implies a careful search for associated anomalies and karyotypic analysis. The orthopedic prognosis is poor in polymalformation syndromes.

The spectrum of focal limb malformations is wide and sometimes complex. Such (difficult) diagnoses

Table 9.7. Fibular ray defect: aplasia, hypoplasia

Atelosteogenesis
Camptomelic dysplasia
Chondroectodermal dysplasia
Femur-fibula-ulnar dysplasia
Mesomelic dysplasia, Langer type
Oto-palato-digital syndrome type II
Proximal femoral deficiency
Short-rib polydactyly syndrome type I

necessitate a meticulous examination of all four limbs with systematic measurements of all bones. Family history can provide helpful information.

9.5
Hand and Foot Malformations

9.5.1
Common Foot Anomalies

Foot positional anomalies are quite common and occur in 3/1,000 births. The US diagnosis is based upon the simultaneous visualization of the leg in a longitudinal axis and the foot in a frontal view (Figs. 9.29, 9.30) (CHERVENAK et al. 1985, JEANTY ET AL. 1985). Clubfoot is one of the most common musculoskeletal malformations. Its incidence varies according to the ethnic origin of the patient; it is found in 0.09–0.12% of the newborn population and 0.43% of

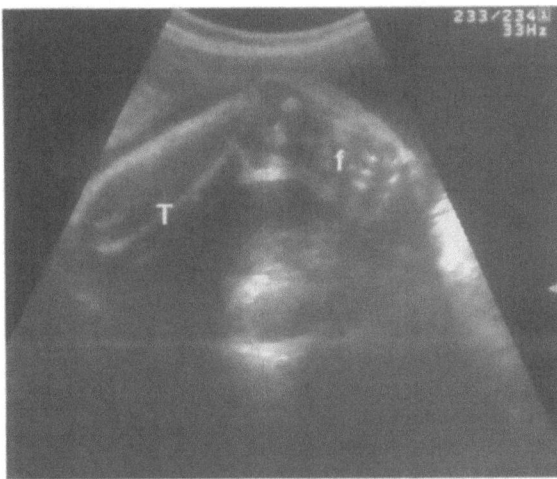

Fig. 9.29. Unilateral clubfoot. Frontal view of the ankle in this 30-week-old fetus demonstrated fixed deformation of the ankle. The foot (*f*) is seen frontally in the same plane as the tibia (*T*)

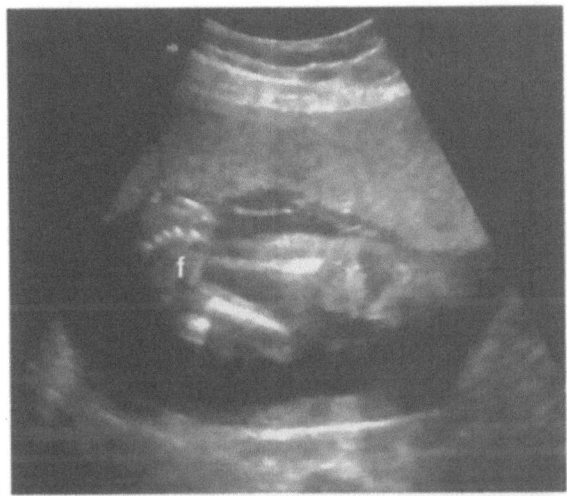

a

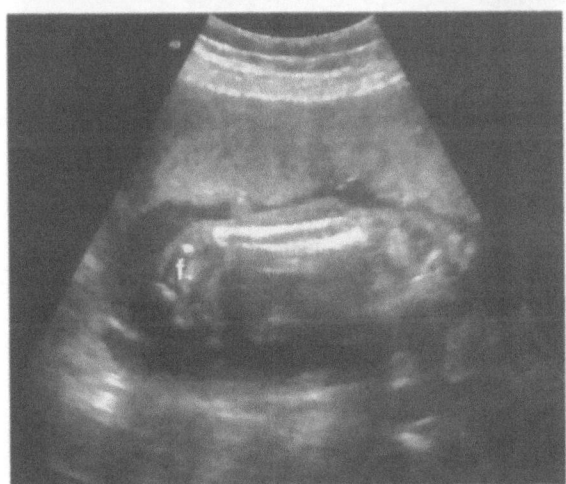

b

Fig. 9.30a, b. Bilateral clubfoot. **a** Typical deformity of the right foot (*f*). **b** Same typical deformity of the left foot (*f*)

fetuses (WEINTROUB et al. 1999, TREADWELL et al. 1999).

In the clubfoot malformation, an abnormal relationship exists between the tarsal bones and the calcaneus. The appearance in utero depends on the severity of the deformation. In the most severe cases, the foot appears persistently malpositioned in equinovarus; the metatarsals are visible in the same plane as the tibia and fibula in a frontal view and the heel is inverted with an abnormal relation between the talus and calcaneus and both bones of the leg. The angle of the junction between the foot and the lower leg is rounded (JEANTY et al. 1985). The plantar surface appears angled. In order to be considered abnormal, these relations must persist during the entire examination. This diagnosis may be not so easy in utero. False positive diagnoses of clubfoot have been reported at the end of the first trimester and during the third trimester of pregnancy (WEINTROUB et al. 1999). True clubfoot must be differentiated from metatarsus adductus (simple deformation) in which the forefoot is simply adducted, while the relations of the hindfoot with the lower leg are normal. Another differential diagnosis is the rarer rocker-bottom foot deformity where the talus is in a vertical position. The appearance is typical: the plantar surface is convex and the calcaneus bulges posteriorly. This malformation is frequently associated with karyotypic anomalies (such as trisomy 13) or other malformations (Fig. 9.16). However, in rare cases it may be isolated (JEANTY et al. 1985, TAYBI and LACHMAN 1996).

The sonographer and the orthopedic surgeon must be aware of the limits of the prenatal diagnosis and differential diagnosis for accurate counseling. There are no predictive US criteria to determine prenatally the severity of the foot malformation. No correlation exists between the severity and rigidity of the clubfoot and the sonographic findings in utero (TILLETT et al. 2000, WEINTROUB ET AL. 1999).

Prenatal diagnosis is important in order to search for associated anomalies. In neonates, associated malformations are found in 10–14% of cases. This percentage rises when the malformation is detected in utero (Budorick 2000). Most commonly, the associated anomalies involve the central nervous system and the genitourinary system but all organs may be affected. The need for karyotype analysis is controversial. Some teams propose systematic karyotypic determination in cases of clubfoot detection (BROMLEY and BENACERRAF 1995, PAGNOTTA et al. 1996). Karyotypic determination is absolutely indicated if additional abnormalities are found (BROMLEY and BENACERRAF 1995, TREADWELL et al. 1999, MALONE et al. 2000).

The risk of recurrence is approximately 2–8% in the case of isolated clubfoot when both parents are normal.

9.5.2
Clubhand Anomalies

The prognosis of clubbed hands is worse than for clubfeet and chromosomal anomaly must be suspected (trisomy 13 or 18). It may also be the result of central nervous system lesions. On US, it is impossible to obtain an open hand at any time during the examination. Two types of clubhand are encountered. Ulnar clubhand is rare but usually isolated (ROMERO et al. 1990). In contrast, radial clubhand usually occurs in association with the radial hypoplasia sequence (JAMES et al. 1999). It is frequently syndromic. Discovery of a clubhand implies a complete US examination of the fetus, fetal echocardiography and fetal blood sampling (complete blood cell count and fetal karyotype). The association of vertebral anomalies induces the search for other malformations observed in the VACTERL association (vertebral segmentation anomalies, anal atresia, tracheoesophageal fistula, defects of the radius, esophageal atresia, renal and radial anomalies) or in Goldenhar syndrome. Associated cardiac malformations are suggestive of Holt-Oram and TAR syndromes. In the case of fetal hematologic anomalies, TAR syndrome or Fanconi anemia must be suggested (see Sect. 9.4.3.1). The most common karyotypic anomalies associated with radial clubhand are trisomy 18 or 21 and anomalies of chromosomes 13 and 4 (ROMERO et al. 1990).

9.5.3
Complex Malformations of Hands and Feet

Other anomalies of the hand include polydactyly (Fig. 9.31) (isolated or part of a syndrome), brachyphalangism and syndactyly (Fig. 9.32) (BROMLEY and BENACERRAF 1995, JEANTY et al. 1985, REISS et al. 1995). Hand and foot malformations may be isolated but are also part of many congenital syndromes, including karyotype anomalies and skeletal dysplasias (REISS et al. 1995) (Tables 9.8, 9.9). Detection relies upon careful and systematic study of all extremities in the fetus. A precise diagnosis of the malformation is not always possible in utero. In each case, the discovery of a hand malformation induces a careful and complete survey

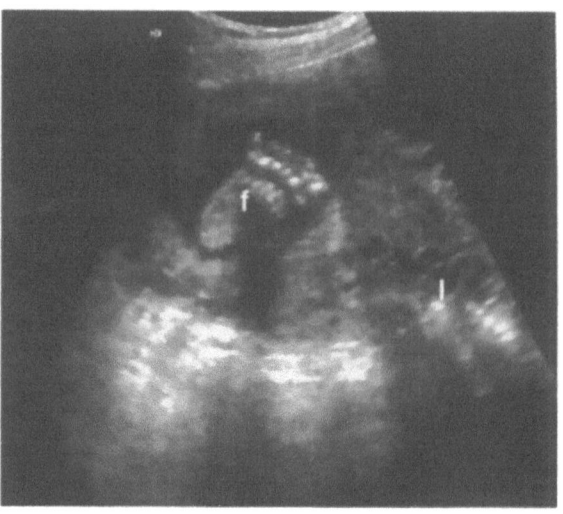

a

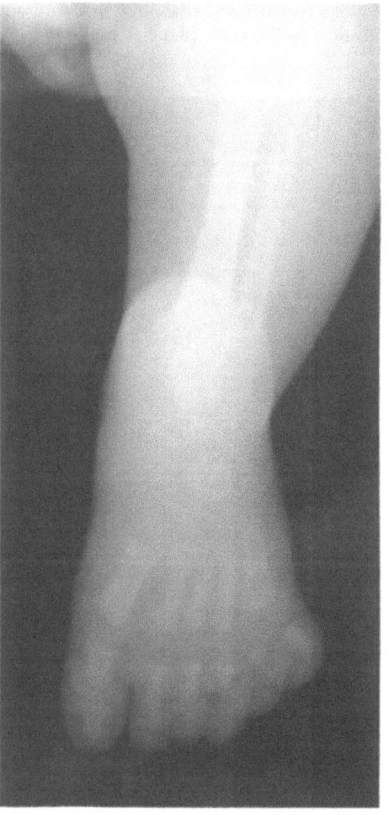

b

Fig. 9.31a, b. Polydactyly. **a** Both feet of this 20-week-old fetus show postaxial hexadactyly. This anomaly was isolated and familial. *f* foot, plantar view. **b** Radiograph at birth confirms hexadactyly

of the fetus and karyotypic determination (REISS et al. 1995).

Polydactyly corresponds to the presence of an additional more or less complete digit (Fig. 9.31). The most common form is postaxial (on the ulnar or fib-

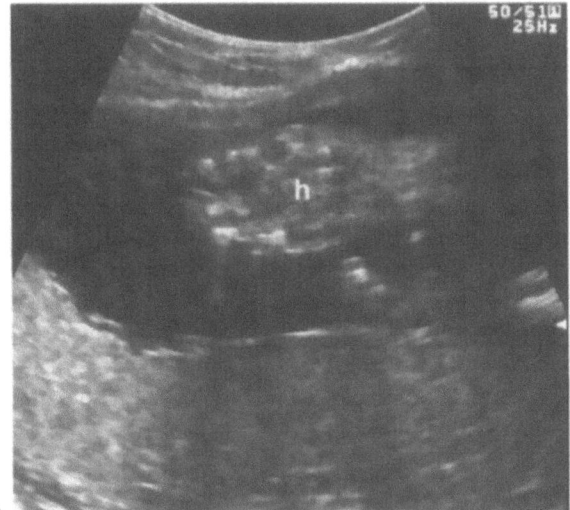

a

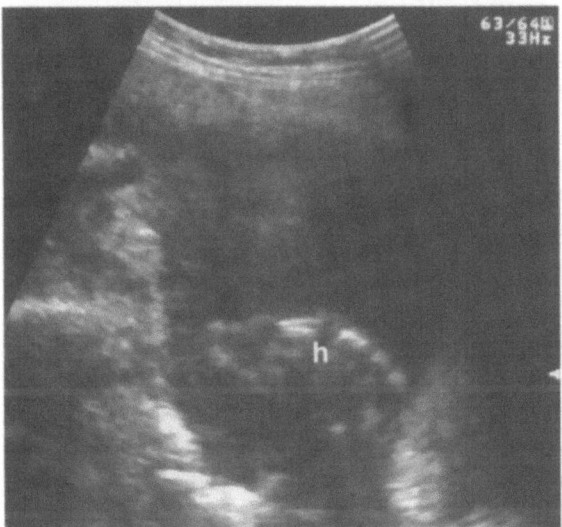

b

Fig. 9.32a, b. Syndactyly. **a, b** US views of the fetal hands (*h*) at 27 weeks gestation show bilateral syndactyly. At no time could the digits be seen independently. This anomaly was present in several members of the mother's family

Table 9.8. Polydactyly

Acrocallosal syndrome
Asphyxiating thoracic dysplasia
Bardet-Biedl syndrome
Chromosome 13 trisomy
Cerebro-reno-digital syndrome
Goltz syndrome
Kaufman-McKusick syndrome
Meckel syndrome
Mesomelic dysplasia
Oto-facial-digital syndrome
Pallister-Hall syndrome
Rubinstein-Taybi syndrome
Smith-Lemli-Opitz syndrome
Short-rib polydactyly syndromes

ular side). In the majority of cases, this malformation is isolated with autosomal dominant transmission and its prognosis is favorable (ROMERO et al. 1990, STEVENS and ARMS 2000). However, this anomaly may be associated with trisomy 13 (with neural and cardiac malformations), Meckel-Gruber syndrome (polycystic kidneys, posterior encephalocele), Bardet-Biedl syndrome (medullary cystic kidneys), and various dysplasias including short-rib polydactyly syndrome (narrow thorax, short limbs). In these circumstances, other anomalies are usually found in the fetus (BROMLEY and BENACERRAF 1995). If the anomaly is preaxial, and especially if a triphalangeal thumb is present, a multisystem syndrome must be suspected (ROMERO et al. 1990). Other malformations may suggest a specific diagnosis. Syndactyly in the early second trimester of gestation can be detected in triploidy. This anomaly is usually associated with intrauterine growth retardation and abnormal placenta. Syndactyly associated with craniosynostosis is observed in Apert's syndrome (BROMLEY and BENACERAFF 1995). Clenched hands with overlapping of index fingers suggest trisomy 18, Pena–Shokeir syndrome or Smith–Lemli–Opitz syndrome (BROMLEY and BENACERRAF 1995, TAYBI and LACHMAN 1996). Trident hand (all the digits the same length) suggests chondrodysplasia (such as achondroplasia). Hitchhiker thumb is a characteristic feature of diastrophic dystrophy (BROMLEY and BENACERRAF 1995). Isolated thumb hypoplasia represents radial deficiency in its mildest form (JAMES et al. 1999).

In claw-type hands and feet, the middle segment of the hand is missing; this anomaly may be difficult to detect in utero depending on the position of the hand (Fig. 9.33).

Anomalies of the hands and feet are quite common; the spectrum varies from benign and isolated clubfoot to much more complex malformations (syndactyly, lobster claw hands) that are more difficult to diagnose.

Table 9.9. Digital defects

Acrorenal syndrome
Amniotic band syndrome
Brachman–de Lange syndrome
Goltz syndrome
Holt-Oram syndrome
Oromandibular-limb hypogenesis
Poland sequence
Postaxial acrofacial dysostosis
Pterygium syndromes
Roberts syndrome

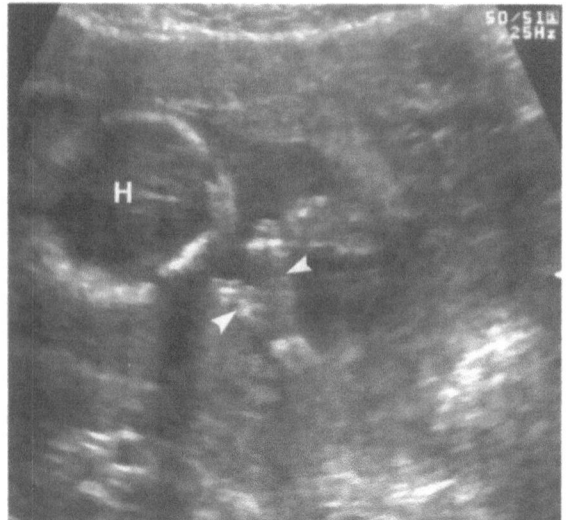

a

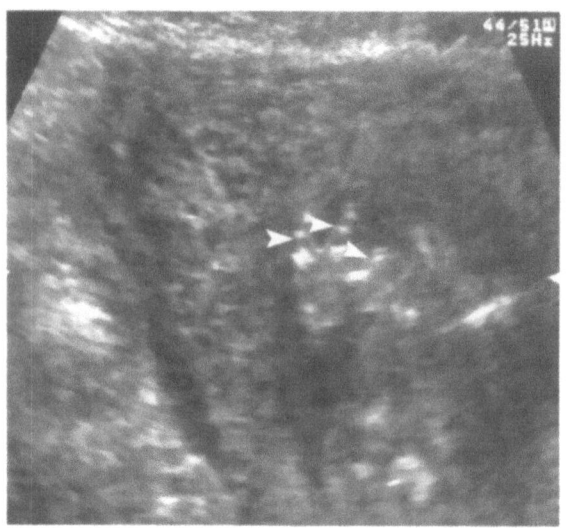

b

Fig. 9.33a, b. Lobster claw hand deformity (second trimester). US. **a** Left hand: only two rays are visible (*arrowheads*). *H* fetal head. **b** Right hand: three rays are visible (*arrowheads*)

9.6
Fetal Immobility or Akinesia Syndrome

Active intrauterine fetal motion plays a key role in normal development. Prolonged decrease or absence of fetal movements results in a group of deformational anomalies, characterized by abnormal limb positions (immobility, arthrogryposis, pterygia), craniofacial malformations, growth restriction, polyhydramnios, lung hypoplasia and short umbilical cord (Fig. 9.34). This fetal akinesia or hypokinesia deformation sequence (FADS), or Pena–Shokeir phenotype, can be due to different etiologies, including

neurogenic diseases (hypoxic-ischemic injuries), myogenic anomalies (congenital muscular dystrophy) and restrictive dermopathies (HOFFMANN et al. 1993). The most common pattern of transmission is autosomal recessive. However, since various etiologies have to be considered, prediction of recurrence is difficult, varying from 10–15% (when associated with primary cerebral malformations) to 25% (myogenic etiology) (Ho 2000). The disease is usually lethal. Most neonates are prematurely delivered and the survivors die within a few weeks of life from respiratory insufficiency (HALL 1986). The differential diagnosis includes trisomy 18, which shares some of the craniofacial, limb and thoracic anomalies.

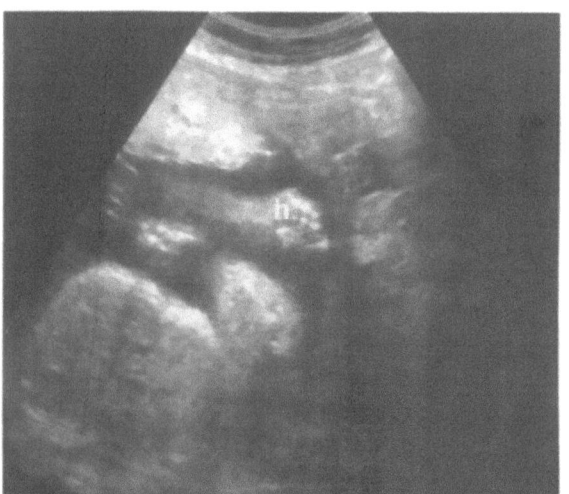

a

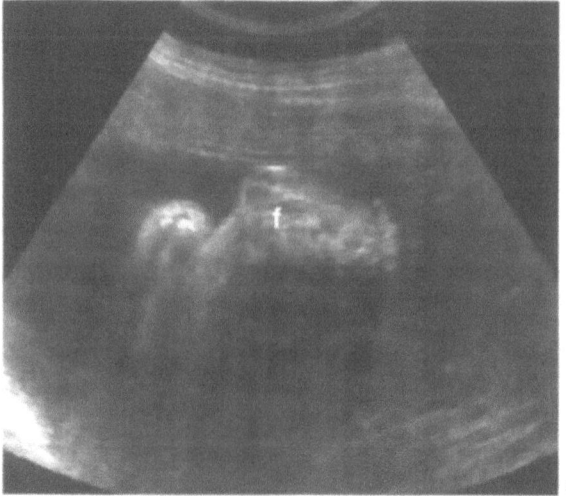

b

Fig. 9.34a, b. Pena-Shokeir syndrome (30 weeks old). **a** During the whole examination, the fetal hands remained closed (*h*). **b** Coronal US of the legs showing a permanently immobile varus position of both ankles. *f* foot

9.7
Axial Skeletal Anomalies

9.7.1
Vertebral Malformations

Abnormal development or segmentation of the spine is responsible for various vertebral malformations (hemivertebrae, butterfly vertebra, fused vertebra, bars, blocks) (Figs. 9.35, 9.36) associated with sco-

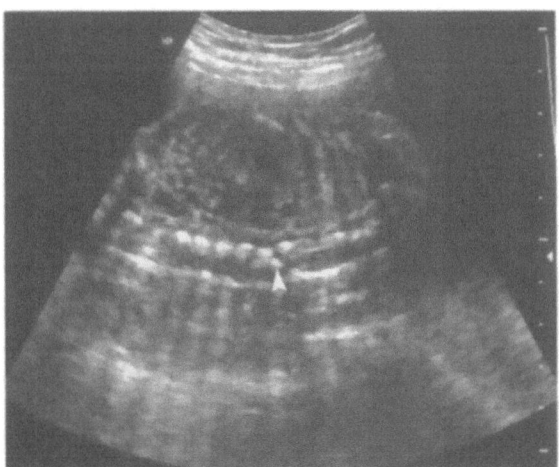

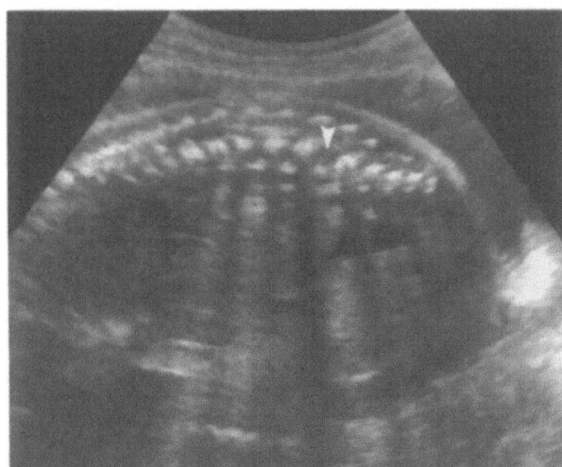

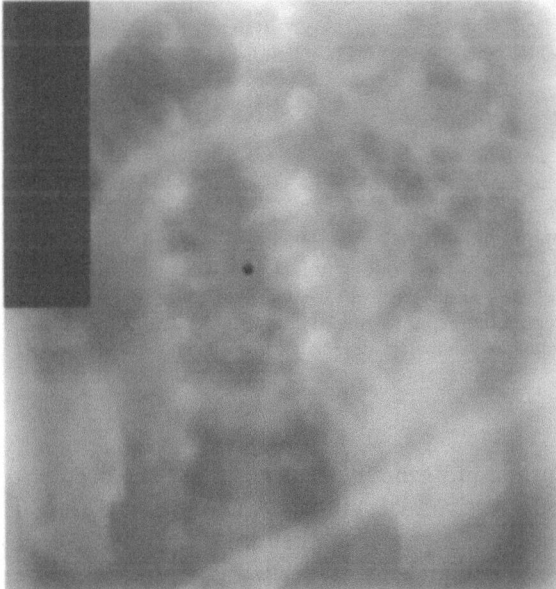

Fig. 9.35a, b. Vertebral hypoplasia. a Sagittal US of the spine of a 26-week-old fetus showing an absent ossification center at the fifth lumbar vertebra (*arrowhead*). Spinal curvature was normal and this anomaly was isolated. b Frontal view of the spine of the neonate showing the typical appearance of a butterfly fifth lumbar vertebra (*), explaining the US appearance observed in utero

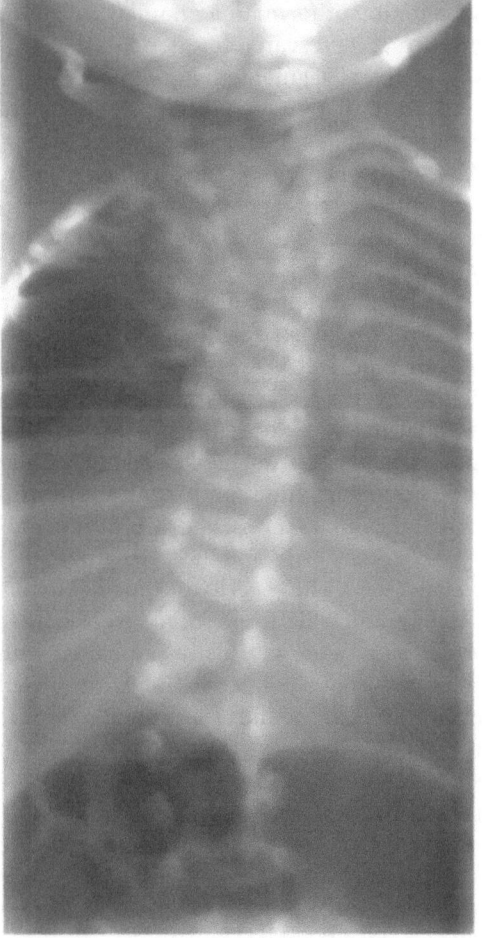

Fig. 9.36a, b. Segmentation anomalies. a Coronal US in this 28-week-old fetus shows abnormal distribution of the ossification centers of the lower thoracic vertebrae (*arrowhead*). b Corresponding radiograph of the spine of the neonate shows multiple levels of abnormal vertebral segmentation, including hemivertebrae, vertebral fusions and butterfly vertebrae. The ribs show abnormal morphology. These vertebral anomalies are associated with congenital scoliosis

liosis, lordosis or kyphosis. Their diagnosis relies upon the detection of abnormal fixed spinal curvature, associated with disruption of the normal alignment of the vertebral ossification centers, asymmetrical size of the ossification centers (in the case of hemivertebra and butterfly vertebra) and irregular positioning of the ribs when the malformation reaches the thoracic level (ABRAMS and FILLY 1985).

The malformation may be isolated, reaching one or several levels, may affect the whole spine (as in multiple vertebral segmentation disorders), or be part of a more complex malformation including neural tube defect, VATER association, limb body wall complex, amniotic band sequence, etc. (TORTORI-DONATI et al. 1999). The discovery of a vertebral segmentation or formation anomaly in a fetus must induce a careful search for associated anomalies. Any vertebral segmentation anomaly can be associated with diastematomyelia, which would appear as a bony spur splitting the spinal cord (Fig. 9.37). Also malformations of any system can be associated with vertebral malformations, particularly those of the central nervous system and the urinary tract.

When isolated, vertebral malformations have a relatively good prognosis for the neonate and the likelihood of a normal karyotype is high (ZELOP et al. 1993). Nevertheless, a postnatal survey must be performed in order to detect possible associated anomalies missed during pregnancy. Close follow-up is important due to a risk of rapid progression of congenital scoliosis (25% progress rapidly, 50% progress slowly and 25% remain stable) (ZELOP et al. 1993). The severity of the final deformation is unpredictable in utero. A severe degree of deformation in utero is usually associated with other malformations such as in limb body wall complex or amniotic band syndrome, and has a poorer prognosis (HARRISON et al. 1992). In the case of oligohydramnios, survival is unlikely (ZELOP et al. 1993).

9.7.2
Caudal Regression Syndrome

Caudal regression syndrome represents a continuum of congenital malformations ranging from agenesis of the lumbosacral spine to more severe cases of sirenomelia with lower extremities fusion and major structural malformations (VALENZANO et al. 1999). Maternal diabetes, vascular hypoper-

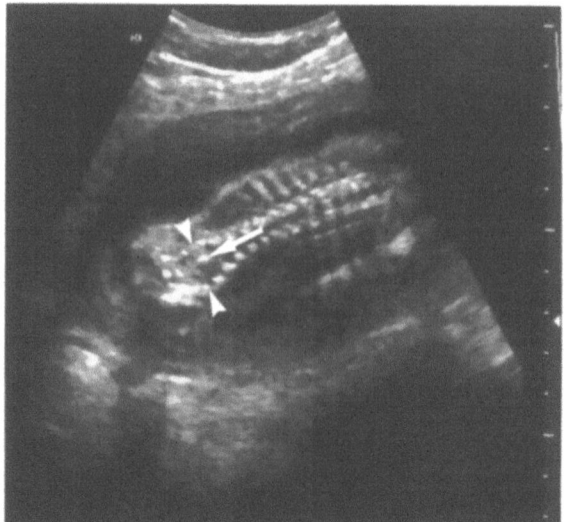

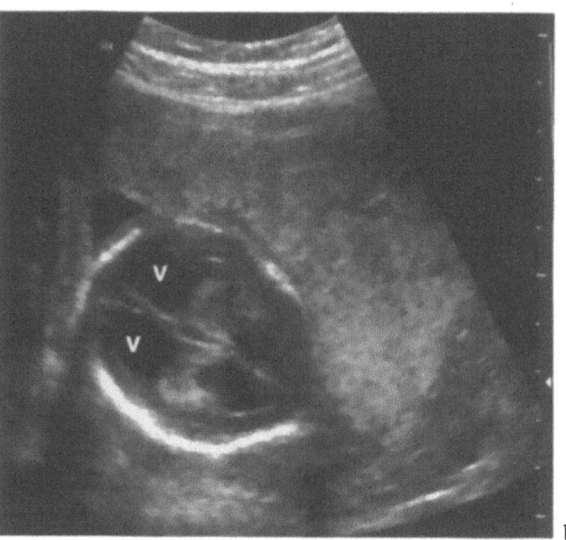

Fig. 9.37a, b. Diastematomyelia in a case of spina bifida. **a** Coronal US of the spine of this 19-week-old fetus shows focal splaying of the posterior ossification centers (*arrowheads*). A central bony spur (*arrow*) is also visible. **b** Axial US scan of the fetal head shows the associated hydrocephalus. *v* ventricles

fusion and genetic predisposition have been suggested as possible etiologies. Obstetrical US reveals the anomaly by demonstrating the absent distal vertebrae and the associated malformations after 16 weeks gestation (SUBTIL et al. 1998, HOUFFLIN et al. 1996, SONEK et al. 1990, BAXI et al. 1990). Prognosis is poor in terms of orthopedic capabilities and neurogenic bladder dysfunction. The prognosis also depends upon the associated structural anomalies (ADRA et al. 1994, CAMA et al. 1996) (Fig. 9.38).

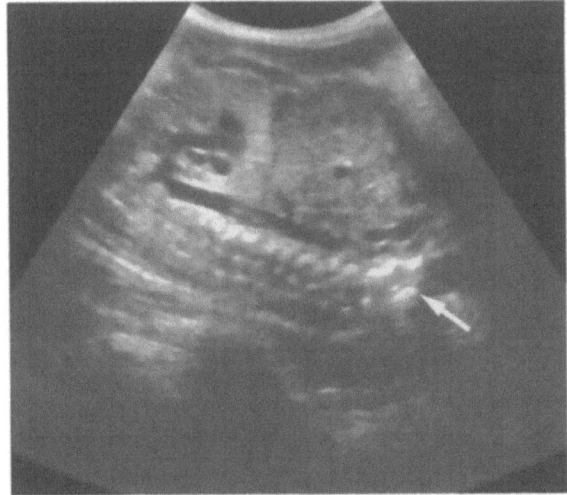

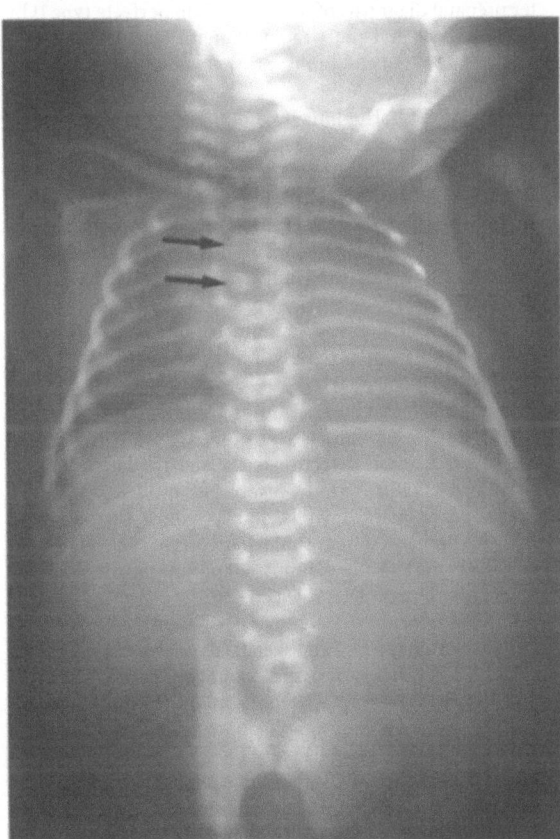

Fig. 9.38a, b. Caudal regression syndrome. **a** Sagittal US performed at 33 weeks gestation demonstrates no visible spine below the third lumbar vertebra (*arrow*), suggesting caudal regression sequence. (There was bilateral malpositioning of the feet, ventricular dilatation and abnormal segmentation of some thoracic vertebrae). **b** Frontal radiograph of the spine of the baby confirms abnormal segmentation of several thoracic vertebrae (*arrows*) and the absence of ossified vertebrae below the third lumbar level. Iliac wings are close one to another

9.7.3
Sacrococcygeal Teratoma

Although rare, sacrococcygeal teratoma (SCT) is the most common congenital neoplasm, occurring in 1 in 40,000 infants. Approximately 75% of affected infants are female. The tumor is derived from a pluripotential cell line originating in Hensen's node and contains components arising from all three germ layers.

Obstetrical US is very effective for the detection of the tumor. Early second trimester diagnosis is possible thanks to transvaginal US. US is helpful for characterizing the mass: this varies from purely cystic, through cystic with a few septa, to solid and calcified mass. US is less accurate than MRI in differentiating markedly septated cystic masses or hemorrhagic masses. MRI helps to determine the pelvic and/or abdominal extent of the mass, which is important for planning the postnatal management. Fetal SCT diagnosed in utero carries a high risk of preterm delivery (50%), a mortality of 15–35% and a morbidity of 12–68% according to various series (CHISHOLM et al. 1999, HOLTERMAN et al. 1998, WESTERBURG et al. 2000). The perinatal mortality and morbidity are high due to high-output cardiac failure, preterm delivery, anemia, dystocia and tumor rupture. Another important factor in the perinatal morbidity is the intrapelvic extent of the SCT and the effect on the urinary tract (CHISHOLM et al. 1999, BRACE et al. 2000). Prognosis seems to be related not to the size of the mass but rather to its content and extent. Solid hypervascularized masses carry a poorer prognosis than purely cystic masses. Fetal hydrops, hemorrhage or rupture of the SCT are the main complications associated with a high mortality. The degree of intrapelvic or abdominal extension of the mass affects the morbidity related to postnatal surgery. Compression of the fetal urinary tract may determine urological complications (42% in one series) (WESTERBURG et al. 2000). Therefore it is important to evaluate these tumors as precisely as possible. MRI is most helpful in determining the extent and content of the tumors (SHINMOTO et al. 2000, KIRKINEN et al. 1997) (see Chap. 13).

References

Abrams SL, Filly RA (1985) Congenital vertebral malformations: prenatal diagnosis using ultrasonography. Radiology 155:762–765

Adra A, Cordero D, MejidesA, Yasin S, Salman F, O'Sullivan MJ (1994) Caudal regression syndrome: etiopathogenesis, prenatal diagnosis, and perinatal management. Obstet Gynecol Surv 49:508–516

Anderson N, Boswell O, Duff G (1995) Prenatal sonography for the detection of fetal anomalies: results of a prospective study and comparison with prior series. AJR Am J Roentgenol 165:943–950

Avni EF, Rypens F, Zappa M, Donner C, Vanregemorter N, Cohen E (1996) Antenatal diagnosis of short limb-dwarfism: sonographic approach. Pediatr Radiol 26:171–178

Avni EF, Guibaud L, Robert Y, et al (2002) Fetal sacrococcygeal teratoma: diagnosis and assessment with MR imaging. AJR Am J Roentgenol (in press)

Azouz EM, Teebi AS, Eydoux P, Chen MF, Fassier F (1998) Bone dysplasias: an introduction. Can Assoc Radiol J 49:105–109

Baba K, Okai T, Kozuma S, Taketani Y (1999) Fetal abnormalities: evaluation with real-time processable three-dimensional US – preliminary report. Radiology 211:441–446

Baxi L, Warren W, Collins MH, Timor-Tritsch IE (1990) Early detection of caudal regression syndrome with transvaginal scanning. Obstet Gynecol 75:486–489

Benaceraff BR, Cnann A, Gelman R, Laboda LA, Frigoletto FD Jr (1989) Can sonographers reliably identify anatomic features associated with Down syndrome in fetuses? Radiology 173:377–380

Berge LN, Marton V, Tranebjaerg L, Kearny MS, Kiserud T, Oian P (1995) Prenatal diagnosis of osteogenesis imperfecta. Acta Obstet Gynecol Scand 74:321–323

Bowerman RA (1995) Anomalies of the fetal skeleton: sonographic findings. AJR Am J Roentgenol 164:973–979

Brace V, Grant SR, Brackley KJ, Kilby MD, Whittle MJ (2000) Prenatal diagnosis and outcome in sacrococcygeal teratomas: a review of cases between 1992 and 1998. Prenat Diagn 20:51–55

Bromley B, Benacerraf B (1995) Abnormalities of the hands and feet in the fetus: sonographic findings. AJR Am J Roentgenol 165:1239–1243

Brons JT, van der Harten HJ, Wladimiroff JW, et al (1988) Prenatal ultrasonographic diagnosis of osteogenesis imperfecta. Am J Obstet Gynecol 159:176–181

Brons JT, van Geijn HP, Bezemer PD, Nauta JP, Arts NF (1990) The fetal skeleton: ultrasonographic evaluation of the normal growth. Eur J Obstet Gynecol Reprod Biol 34:21–36

Bronshtein M, Keret D, Deutsch M, Liberson A, Bar Chava I (1993) Transvaginal sonographic detection of skeletal anomalies in the first and early second trimesters. Prenat Diagn 13:597–601

Brunelle F, Quere MP, Sonigo P et al (1999) Helical CT scanner in orthopedic malformation in fetus. Presented at the 36th Congress of the ESPR, Jerusalem, May 23–29

Budorick NE (2000) The fetal musculoskeletal system. In: Callen PW (ed) Ultrasonography in obstetrics and gynecology, 4th edn. Saunders, Philadelphia, pp 331–377

Budorick NE, Pretorius DH, Grafe MR, Lou KV (1991) Ossification of the fetal spine. Radiology 181:561–565

Bulas DI, Stern HJ, Rosenbaum KN, Fonda JA, Glass RB, Tifft C (1994) Variable prenatal appearance of osteogenesis imperfecta. J Ultrasound Med 13:419–427

Cama A, Palmieri A, Capra V, Piatelli GL, Ravergnani M, Fondelli P (1996) Multidisciplinary management of caudal regression syndrome (26 cases). Eur J Pediatr Surg 6[Suppl 1]:44–45

Camera G, Dodero D, Parodi M, Zucchinetti P, Camera A (1993) Antenatal ultrasonographic diagnosis of a proximal femoral focal deficiency. J Clin Ultrasound 21:475–479

Campbell J, Henderson A, Campbell S (1988) The fetal femur/foot length ratio: a new parameter to assess dysplastic limb reduction. Obstet Gynecol 72:181–184

Chervenak FA, Tortora M, Hobbins JC (1985) Antenatal sonographic diagnosis of clubfoot. J Ultrasound Med 4:49–50

Chisholm CA, Heider AL, Kuller JA, von Allmen D, McMahon MJ, Chescheir NC (1999) Prenatal diagnosis and perinatal management of fetal sacrococcygeal teratoma. Am J Perinatal 16:47–50

DiMaio MS, Barth R, Koprivnikar KE, et al (1993) First-trimester prenatal diagnosis of osteogenesis imperfecta type II by DNA analysis and sonography. Prenat Diagn 13:589–596

Driscoll DA (1991) Fetal limbs: normal and abnormal. Semin Roentgenol 26:12–20

Dugoff L, Coffin CT, Hobbins JC (1997) Sonographic measurement of the fetal rib cage perimeter to thoracic circumference ratio: application to prenatal diagnosis of skeletal dysplasias. Ultrasound Obstet Gynecol 10:269–271

Evans JA, Vitez M, Czeizel A (1994) Congenital abnormalities associated with limb deficiency defects: a population study based on cases from the Hungarian Congenital Malformation Registry (1975–1984). Am J Med Genet 49:52–66

Froster UG, Baird PA (1993) Amniotic band sequence and limb defects: data from a population-based study. Am J Med Genet 46:497–500

Gabrielli S, Falco P, Pilu G, Perolo A, Milano V, Bovicelli L (1999) Can transvaginal fetal biometry be considered a useful tool for early detection of skeletal dysplasias in high-risk patients? Ultrasound Obstet Gynecol 13:107–111

Gaffney G, Manning N, Boyd BA, Rai V, Gould S, Chamberland P (1998) Prenatal sonographic diagnosis of skeletal dysplasias – a report of the diagnostic and prognostic accuracy in 35 cases. Prenat Diagn 18:357–362

Garjian KV, Pretorius DH, Budorick NE, Cantrell CJ, Johnson DD, Nelson TR (2000) Fetal skeletal dysplasia: three-dimensional US – initial experience. Radiology 214:717–723

Geck MJ, Dorey P, Lawrence JF, Johnson MK (1999) Congenital radius deficiency: radiographic outcome and survivorship analysis. J Hand Surg 24:1132–1144

Gentili P, Trasimenti A, Giorlandino C (1984) Fetal ossification centers as predictors of gestational age in normal and abnormal pregnancies. J Ultrasound Med 3:193–197

Goncalves L, Jeanty P (1994) Fetal biometry of skeletal dysplasias: a multicentric study. J Ultrasound Med 13:977–985

Goto MP, Goldman AS (1994) Diabetic embryopathy. Curr Opin Pediatr 6:486–491

Hall JG (1986) Analysis of Pena Shokeir phenotype. Am J Med Genet 25:99–117

Harrison LA, Pretorius DH, Budorick NE (1992) Abnormal spinal curvature in the fetus. J Ultrasound Med 11:473–479

Hersh JH, Angle B, Pietrantoni M, et al (1998) Predictive value of fetal ultrasonography in the diagnosis of a lethal skeletal dysplasia. South Med J 91:1137–1142

Hill LM, Leary J (1998) Transvaginal sonographic diagnosis of short-rib polydactyly dysplasia at 13 weeks' gestation. Prenat Diagn 18:1198–1201

Ho NC (2000) Monozygotic twins with fetal akinesia: the importance of clinicopathological work-up in predicting risks of recurrence. Neuropediatrics 31:252–256

Hoffmann R, Lohner M, Bohm N, Leititis J, Helwig H (1993) Restrictive dermopathy: a lethal congenital skin disorder. Eur J Pediatr 152:95–98

Holterman AX, Filiatrault D, Lallier M, Youssef S (1998) The natural history of sacrococcygeal teratomas diagnosed through routine obstetric sonogram: a single institution experience. J Pediatr Surg 33:899–903

Houfflin V, Subtil D, Cosson M, et al (1996) Prenatal diagnosis of three caudal regression syndromes associated with maternal diabetes. J Gynecol Obstet Biol Reprod 25:389–395

James MA, McCarroll HR Jr, Manske PR (1999) The spectrum of radial longitudinal deficiency: a modified classification. J Hand Surg 24:1145–1155

Jeanty P, Romero R, d'Alton M, Venus I, Hobbins JC (1985) In utero sonographic detection of hand and foot deformities. J Ultrasound Med 4:595–601

Kirkinen P, Partanen K, Merikanto J, Ryynanen M, Haring P, Heinonen K (1997) Ultrasonic and magnetic resonance imaging of fetal sacrococcygeal teratoma. Acta Obstet Gynecol Scand 76:917–922

Kliewer MA, Hertzberg BS, Freed KS, et al (1996) Dysmorphic features of the fetal pelvis in Down syndrome: prenatal sonographic depiction and diagnostic implications of the iliac angle. Radiology 201:681–684

Koren G, Edwards MB, Miskin M (1987) Antenatal sonography of fetal malformations associated with drugs and chemicals: a guide. Am J Obstet Gynecol 156:79–85

Kurtz AB, Needleman L, Wapner RJ, et al (1990) Usefulness of a short femur in the in utero detection of skeletal dysplasias. Radiology 177:197–200

Lynch L, Berkowitz GS, Chitkara U, Wilkins IA, Mehalek KE, Berkowitz RL (1989) Ultrasound detection of Down syndrome: is it really possible? Obstet Gynecol 73:267–270

Mahony BS, Filly RA (1984a) High-resolution sonographic assessment of the fetal extremities. J Ultrasound Med 3:489–498

Mahony BS, Filly RA, Cooperberg PL (1984b) Antenatal sonographic diagnosis of achondrogenesis. J Ultrasound Med 3:333–335

Mahony BS, Callen PW, Filly RA (1985) The distal femoral epiphyseal ossification center in the assessment of third-trimester menstrual age: sonographic identification and measurement. Radiology 155:201–204

Malone FD, Marino T, Bianchi DW, Johnston K, D'Alton ME (2000) Isolated clubfoot diagnosed prenatally: is karyotyping indicated? Obstet Gynecol 95:437–440

Maroteaux P (1982) Maladies osseuses de l'enfant, 2nd edn. Flammarion Médecine Sciences, Paris

McCormick WF, Nichols MM (1981) Formation and maturation of the human sternum. I. Fetal period. Am J Forensic Med Pathol 2:323–328

Meizner I (1997) Fetal skeletal malformations revisited: steps in the diagnostic approach. Ultrasound Obstet Gynecol 10:303–306

Merz E, Kim-Kern MS, Pehl S (1987) Ultrasonic mensuration of fetal limb bones in the second and third trimesters. J Clin Ultrasound 15:175–183

Moerman P, Fryns JP, Vandenberghe K, Lauweryns JM (1992) Constrictive amniotic bands, amniotic adhesions and limb-body wall complex: discrete disruption sequences with pathogenetic overlap. Am J Med Genet 42:470–479

Moore KL, Persaud TVN (1993) The developing human: clinically oriented embryology, 5th edn. Saunders, Philadelphia

Munoz C, Filly RA, Golbus MS (1990) Osteogenesis imperfecta type II: prenatal sonographic diagnosis. Radiology 174:181–185

Odita JC, Okolo AA, Omene JA (1985) Sternal ossification in normal newborn infants. Pediatr Radiol 15:165–167

Pagnotta G, Maffulli N, Aureli S, Maggi E, Mariani M, Yip KM (1996) Antenatal sonographic diagnosis of clubfoot: a six-year experience. J Foot Ankle Surg 35:67–71

Pattarelli P, Pretorius DH, Edwards DK (1990) Intrauterine growth retardation mimicking skeletal dysplasia on antenatal sonography. J Ultrasound Med 9:737–739

Pretorius DH, Rumack CM, Manco-Johnson ML, et al (1986) Specific skeletal dysplasias in utero: sonographic diagnosis. Radiology 159:237–242

Ramus RM, Martin LB, Twickler DM (1998) Ultrasonographic prediction of fetal outcome in suspected skeletal dysplasias with use of the femur length-to-abdominal circumference ratio. Am J Obstet Gynecol 179:1348–1352

Reiss RE, Foy PM, Mendiratta V, Kelly M, Gabbe SG (1995) Ease and accuracy of evaluation of fetal hands during obstetrical ultrasonography: a prospective study. J Ultrasound Med 14:813–820

Romero R, Athanassiadis AP, Jeanty P (1990) Fetal skeletal anomalies. Radiol Clin North Am 28:75–99

Russ PD, Pretorius DH, Manco-Johnson ML, Rumack CM (1986) The fetal spine. Neuroradiology 28:398–407

Rypens F, Avni F (1994) Suivi échographique du développement squelettique fœtal normal. L'exemple de la colonne vertébrale et des membres inférieurs. J Cepur 14/2:31–37

Sanders RC, Blakemore K (1989) Lethal fetal anomalies: sonographic demonstration. Radiology 172:1–6

Sepulveda W, Weiner E, Bridger JE, Fisk NM (1994) Prenatal diagnosis of congenital absence of the fibula. J Ultrasound Med 13:655–657

Sharony R, Browne C, Lachman RS, Rimoin DL (1993) Prenatal diagnosis of skeletal dysplasias. Am J Obstet Gynecol 169:668–675

Shinmoto H, Kashima K, Yuasa Y, et al (2000) MR imaging of non-CNS fetal abnormalities: a pictorial essay. Radiographics 20:1227–1243

Shipp TD, Bromley B, Lieberman E, Benacerraf BR (1997) The iliac angle as a sonographic marker for Down syndrome in second-trimester fetuses. Obstet Gynecol 89:446–450

Skiptunas SM, Weiner S (1987) Early prenatal diagnosis of asphyxiating thoracic dysplasia (Jeune's syndrome). Value of fetal thoracic measurement. J Ultrasound Med 6:41–43

Sonek JD, Gabbe SG, Ladon MB, Stempel LE, Foley MR, Shubert-Moell K (1990) Antenatal diagnosis of sacral agenesis syndrome in a pregnancy complicated by diabetes mellitus. Am J Obstet Gynecol 162:806–808

Sorge G, Ardito S, Genuardi M, et al (1995) Proximal femoral focal deficiency (PFFD) and fibular A/hypoplasia (FA/H): a model of a developmental field defect. Am J Med Genet 55:427–432

Spirt BA, Oliphant M, Gottlieb RH, Gordon LP (1990) Prenatal sonographic evaluation of short-limbed dwarfism: an algorithmic approach. Radiographics 10:217–236

Stevens PM, Arms D (2000) Postaxial hypoplasia of the lower extremity. J Pediatr Orthop 20:166–172

Stoll C, Alembik Y, Dott B, Roth MP (1994) Evaluation of prenatal diagnosis of limb reduction defects by a registry of congenital anomalies. Prenat Diagn 14:781–786

Stoll C, Dott B, Alembik Y, Roth MP (1995) Evaluation of routine prenatal diagnosis by a registry of congenital anomalies. Prenat Diagn 15:791–800

Subtil S, Cosson M, Houfflin V, Vaast P, Valat A, Puech F (1998) Early detection of caudal regression syndrome: specific interest and findings in three cases. Eur J Obstet Gynecol 80:109–112

Tadmor OP, Kreisberg GA, Achiron R, Porat S, Yagel S (1997) Limb amputation in amniotic band syndrome: serial ultrasonographic and Doppler observations. Ultrasound Obstet Gynecol 10:312–315

Taybi H, Lachman RS (1996) Radiology of syndromes, metabolic disorders and skeletal dysplasia, 4th edn. Mosby, St Louis

Tillett RL, Fisk NM, Murphy K, Hunt DM (2000) Clinical outcome of congenital talipes equinovarus diagnosed antenatally by ultrasound. J Bone Joint Surg Br 82:876–880

Tortori-Donati P, Fondelli MP, Rossi A, Raybaud CA, Cama A, Capra V (1999) Segmental spinal dysgenesis: neuroradiologic findings with clinical and embryologic correlation. AJNR Am J Neuroradiol 20:445–456

Treadwell MC, Stanitski CL, King M (1999) Prenatal sonographic diagnosis of clubfoot: implications for patient counseling. J Pediatr Orthop 19:8–10

Valenzano M, Paoletti R, Rossi A, Farinini D, Garlaschi G, Fulcheri E (1999) Sirenomelia. Pathological features, antenatal ultrasonographic clues, and a review of current embryogenic theories. Hum Reprod Update 5:82–86

Van Allen MI, Siegel-Bartelt J, Dixon J, Zuker RM, Clarke HM, Toi A (1992) Constriction bands and limb reduction defects in two newborns with fetal ultrasound evidence for vascular disruption. Am J Med Genet 44:598–604

van Zalen-Sprock RM, Brons JT, van Vugt JM, van der Harten HJ, van Geijn HP (1997) Ultrasonographic and radiologic visualization of the developing embryonic skeleton. Ultrasound Obstet Gynecol 9:392–397

Weinblatt M, Petrikovsky B, Bialer M, Kochen J, Harper R (1994) Prenatal evaluation and in utero platelet transfusion from thrombocytopenia absent radii syndrome. Prenat Diagn 14:892–896

Weintroub S, Keret D, Bronshtein M (1999) Prenatal sonographic diagnosis of musculoskeletal disorders. J Pediatr Orthop 19:1–4

Westerburg B, Feldstein VA, Sandberg PL, Lopoo JB, Harrison MR, Albanese CT (2000) Sonographic prognostic factors in fetuses with sacrococcygeal teratoma. J Pediatr Surg 35:322–325

Winter RM, Sandin BM, Mitchell RA, Price AB (1984) The radiology of stillbirths and neonatal deaths. Br J Obstet Gynecol 91:762–765

Wolpert L (1999) Vertebrate limb development and malformations. Pediatr Res 46:247–254

Ylagan LR, Budorick NE (1994) Radial ray aplasia in utero: a prenatal finding associated with valproic acid exposure. J Ultrasound Med 13:408–411

Zalel Y, Lipitz S, Soriano D, Achiron R (1999) The development of the fetal sternum: a cross-sectional sonographic study. Ultrasound Obstet Gynecol 13:187–190

Zelop CM, Pretorius DH, Benacerraf BR (1993) Fetal hemivertebrae: associated anomalies, significance, and outcome. Obstet Gynecol 81:412–416

Zimmer EZ, Divon MY (1992) Sonographic diagnosis of IUGR – macrosomia. Clin Obstet Gynecol 35:172–184

Zimmer EZ, Bronshtein M (2000) Fetal polydactyly diagnosis during early pregnancy: clinical applications. Am J Obstet Gynecol 183:755–758

10 The Evaluation of Twin Pregnancy

Andrée Grignon and Josée Dubois

CONTENTS

10.1   Introduction   227
10.2   Embryological Reminder   227
10.3   General Considerations   228
10.3.1   Maternal Complications: Preterm Delivery   229
10.3.2   About the Perinatal Morbidity and Mortality   229
10.3.3   Fetal Demise   229
10.3.4   Vanishing Twin   229
10.3.5   Associated Malformations   229
10.3.6   About Normal Growth
         in Multifetal Gestations   230
10.3.6.1 Biometry   230
10.3.6.2 Normal Growth   230
10.3.7   About Amniotic Fluid   230
10.3.8   Doppler   231
10.4   How to Determine by US the Type
         of Twinning   231
10.4.1   The First Trimester   231
10.4.2   The Second Trimester   232
10.5   General Complications   234
10.5.1   Discordance Between Twins   234
10.5.2   Intrauterine Growth Restriction   235
10.5.3   Our Series: Abnormal Growth   235
10.5.3.1 Diamniotic Dichorionic Twins   236
10.6   Specific Complications   236
10.6.1   General Considerations   236
10.6.2   Stuck-Twin Syndrome   236
10.6.3   Twin Oligohydramnios-Polyhydramnios
         Sequence   237
10.6.4   Twin-Twin Transfusion Syndrome   238
10.6.5   Twin Embolization Syndrome   239
10.6.6   Acardius or Twin Reversal Arterial Perfusion   240
10.6.7   Monochorionic Monoamniotic Twins   240
10.6.8   Conjoined Twins   241
10.7   Conclusion   241
         References   241

A. Grignon, MD; J. Dubois, MD
Department of Medical Imaging, Sainte-Justine Hospital, 3175
Côte-Sainte-Catherine, Montréal, Québec H3T 1C5, Canada

pregnancies in the United States (Sepulveda 1997). This is mainly related to treatment of infertility and to an aging maternal population (Divon and Weiner 1995, Edwards et al. 1995).

Twin births occur in 1 of 90 pregnancies but account for almost 10% of all perinatal morbidity and mortality (Sepulveda 1997, Luke 1994, Ghai and Vidyasagar 1988). The mortality is 4–6 times as high as in singleton pregnancy and the morbidity is twice as high (Ghai and Vidyasagar 1988, Naeye et al. 1978). Multifetal gestations are also high-risk pregnancies for the mother, with a higher rate of preterm labor, premature rupture of membrane, pre-eclampsia, hypertension, abruptio placentae, placenta previa and pre- and postpartum hemorrhage. Also, they have a higher rate of perinatal complications such as prematurity, fetal anomalies, fetal demise, intrauterine growth retardation (IUGR), polyhydramnios, oligohydramnios, twin-twin transfusion syndrome, polyhydramnios, oligohydramnios, conjoined twin, acardiac twinning and traumatic delivery (Benirschke 1961).

Considering the impact of these complications, sonography is of great value in assessing the relative risk for morbidity and mortality by determining the type of twinning. Also, US allows the diagnosis of fetal anomalies and complications, and has a crucial impact on the medical management.

In this chapter, we will review from a practical approach the most important concepts that the sonographer has to know in order to diagnose the type of the twin pregnancy, and to recognize the anomalies and specific complications.

10.1
Introduction

The number of multifetal gestations has increased significantly since 1980, accounting for 1.5% of all

10.2
Embryological Reminder

There are two major classes of twins:

Dizygotic or non-identical twins result from two ova fertilized separately. The ova, therefore, reach in the uterus in the form of two cells or blastocysts, and

will always be, by definition, dichorionic (two placentas) and diamniotic (two amnions). This class of
twins represents the majority of twin pregnancies,
that is to say, 66%. The incidence of dizygote pregnancies varies from 1 in 20 to 1 in 500 live births
(GALL 1996). Generally, there is a maternal history of
twins in the family. Other predisposing factors are:
race (more frequent among black people), nutritional
status (well-nourished and strong women have more
chance of being pregnant with twins), and repeated
and close pregnancies.

Monozygotic or identical twins result from a single
fertilized egg but the types vary according to the time
of division of the morula (fertilized egg) (AISENBREY
et al. 1995, BENIRSCHKE and KIM 1973a,b):

1. If the division occurs early, during the first 3 days,
   the result is dichorionic, diamniotic monozygotes
   of the same sex. These represent 14–36% of monozygotes.
2. If the division occurs later, between 4 and 8 days,
   the result is monochorionic (a single placenta),
   diamniotic (two amnions) monozygotes. These
   represent about 70% of monozygotes.
3. If the division occurs between 8 and 13 days, the
   result is monochorionic (a single placenta), monoamniotic (a single amnion) monozygotes. These
   account for less than 1–4% of monozygotes;.
4. Finally, if division does not occur, the result is
   Siamese twins. The incidence is 1 in 200,000 births
   (<1%) (Sherer 1998).

The incidence of monozygotic twin pregnancies is
approximately 1 in 250 live births and is independent
of maternal history, age or race (BENIRSCHKE and
KIM 1973b, MACGILLIVRAY 1986).

It should be recalled that the majority of twin
pregnancies induced by medication are multizygotic
twin pregnancies. On the other hand, WENSTROM et
al. (1993) and CALLEN (2000) reported an incidence
of monozygotes 8 times higher in women treated for
infertility than in non-treated women.

Two important points should be remembered:
monochorionic twins are always monozygotic or
identical twins, but monozygotic twins may have different types of chorionicity and amniocity.

The different types of twin pregnancies studied by
ultrasonography are thus (Diagram 10.1):

- Dichorionic diamniotic dizygotes (di-di DZ): A.
- Dichorionic diamniotic monozygotes (di-di MZ):
  A.
- Monochorionic diamniotic monozygotes
  (mono-di MZ): B.
- Monochorionic monoamniotic monozygotes
  (mono-mono MZ): C.
- Siamese: D.
- Acardius. Rare monozygotic monochorionic twins
  where one of the fetuses (the parasite), without
  a normal cardiac structure, feeds passively at the
  expense of its twin, thanks to vascular connections (Fouron et al. 1994).

10.3
General Considerations

The following must be known before starting the US
examination.

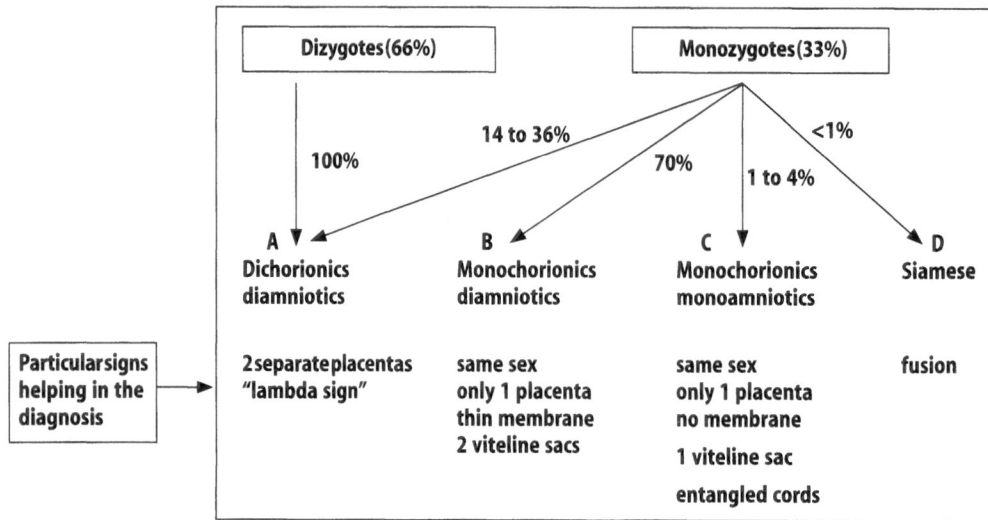

Diagram 10.1.
The different
types of twin
pregnancies

10.3.1
Maternal Complications: Preterm Delivery

The frequency of delivery <37 weeks in twin pregnancies is 25–55% (DIVON and WEINER 1995). At Sainte-Justine Hospital, 43% of preterm deliveries involve twins. It is mandatory to measure the cervical length at sonography, as this can predict the preterm delivery.

Cervical length can be measured by the endovaginal (WINN et al. 1989, KURTZ et al. 1992), transperineal (BROMLEY and BENACERRAF 1995), translabial (FINBERG 1992) or transabdominal route, with sensitivity varying according to the series (SAADE et al. 1998).

Cervical length less than 25 mm before the 26th week carries a 4-fold greater risk of preterm labor, according to a study presented by SEIS et al. at the Society of Perinatal Obstetricians (SPO) Meeting in January 1997. KUSHNIR et al. (1995) demonstrated well using US that cervical shortening is more pronounced in twin pregnancies than in single pregnancies after the 19th week of gestation. It is important to remember that cervical measurement must be done systematically at every US examination during a twin pregnancy. The presence of an anomalous fetus in twins increases the risk of preterm delivery (ALEXANDER et al. 1997).

10.3.2
About the Perinatal Morbidity and Mortality

The perinatal mortality rate in dichorionic twins is 10% compared with 25% in monochorionic diamniotic and 50% in monochorionic monoamniotic pregnancies. Even in cases of monoamniotic twinning, a perinatal mortality of 30–70% has been reported (BENIRSCHKE and KAUFMANN 1990). The higher complication rate in cases of monochorionic twin is related to the sharing of the same placenta between two fetuses. US is essential for the diagnosis of twinning in order to establish the chorionicity and amniocity and in the management of the perinatal complications. In preterm twin gestations, a birth weight discordance of >20% is associated with a high adverse perinatal and neonatal outcome (CHEUNG et al. 1994).

10.3.3
Fetal Demise

The frequency of co-twin demise (second and third trimesters) is 5–7% (DIVON and WEINER 1995).

10.3.4
Vanishing Twin

The only criterion for the diagnosis of vanishing twin is as follows: after a previous scan showing two living fetuses with documented heart pulsation, a follow-up sonogram demonstrates only one fetus with a heart beat.

In this circumstance, the twin pregnancy ends up as singleton. The frequency is between 20% and 50% (DIVON and WEINER 1995) but the diagnosis is often overestimated when, in retrospect, the so-called vanishing twin actually represents a hemorrhagic zone in the chorion.

10.3.5
Associated Malformations

Chromosomal Anomalies: The percentage of aneuploidy in twin pregnancies corresponds to 2 times the maternal age (SHERER 1998). It is rare for the chromosomal make-up to be abnormal in dichorionic diamniotic fetuses (SHERER 1998). With the exception of the very rare incidence of a mitotic disjunction in monozygotes, monozygotic twins share the same genetic make-up. Accordingly, during diagnostic amniocentesis, generally only one sac should be punctured (BALDWIN 1993).

Structural Anomalies: Structural anomalies are 1.2–2 times more frequent in twin pregnancies than in single pregnancies (ZALAR 1996) and 16 times higher in monozygotes (WINN et al. 1989). Certain types of malformations are more frequent. KOHL and CASEY (1975) reported a major malformation rate of 2.12% for twins compared with 1.05% for singletons. Twins are at increased risk for specific malformations involving the gastrointestinal tract, heart and skeleton. HOLLIER et al. (1997) reported the odd ratios for twins versus singletons for cardiac anomalies (2.42), tracheoesophageal fistula (11.38), esophageal atresia (15.62), syndactyly (9.85) and omphalocele (13.44). Upper neural tube anomalies are more frequent in twins whereas spina bifida (lower neural tube) is more frequent in singletons. According to BALDWIN (1993), the most frequent anomalies to look for are cardiac anomalies, neural tube anomalies, cerebral anomalies, labiopalatine clefts, gastrointestinal anomalies and abdominal wall defects.

Screening of these anomalies with antenatal sonography is mandatory, because the findings have important implications for the counseling, antepartum management, delivery and neonatal and infant outcome. Regarding the issue of selective termination, EVANS et al. (1999) have reported that in cases of dichorionic diamniotic twins the termination is safe when it is performed with potassium chloride with 83% of deliveries after 33 weeks and only 4.3% of deliveries between 25 and 28 weeks. All monoamniotic and monochorionic twins die after selective feticide.

10.3.6
About Normal Growth in Multifetal Gestations

10.3.6.1
Biometry

First Trimester: The rate of growth of crown-rump length (CRL) in early multifetal pregnancy is identical for twins and singleton pregnancies. Gestational age can be determined most accurately by averaging the CRLs of all embryos and estimating the gestational age from the mean CRL (SAADE et al. 1998) (Fig. 10.1).

Second and Third Trimester: The basic fetal measurements used to estimate the gestational age are the biparietal diameter (BPD), head circumference (HC), abdominal circumference (AC) and femur length (FL). We use the same singleton tables for the biometry of all types of twins except for the estimation of weight; ARBUCKLE et al. (1993) have published a

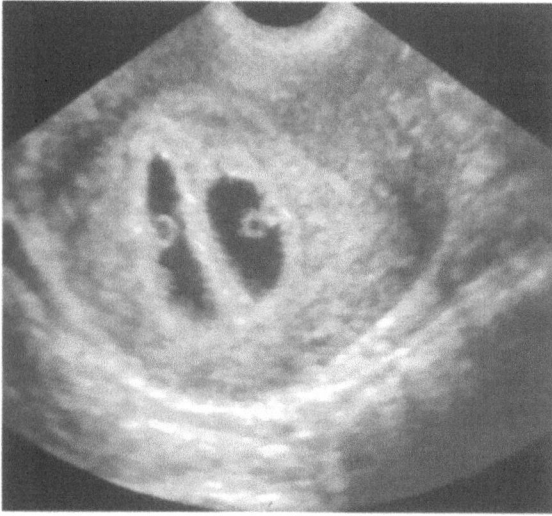

Fig. 10.1. Nine weeks of gestation. Two chorionic rings with their own vitelline sac

specific Canadian table for twin pregnancies taking into account the fetal gender.

10.3.6.2
Normal Growth

First Trimester

The normal growth between twins must be evaluated by the CRL. The difference between the two CRLs should be ≤3 mm.

Second Trimester

To evaluate the symmetry of growth between the twins:

$$\frac{\text{Abdominal circumference (AC) of the small fetus}}{\text{Abdominal circumference of the 'large' fetus}} \times 100 > 0{,}93 \quad \text{(normal)}$$

Third Trimester

Twins grow at the same speed as singletons until 28 weeks of gestation, independently of the type of twins. After this time, twins gain weight more slowly than singletons. ANANTH et al. (1998), who created a twin birth weight normogram, found that the growth table for singletons well approximates twin growth between 32 and 34 weeks of gestation and overestimates twin growth beyond 34 weeks.

To evaluate the symmetry of growth between the twins:

Third trimester:

AC large–AC small/AC large×100<20% (concordant normal)

The weight is estimated by the abdominal circumference and the femur length (HADLOCK et al. 1984).

Like singletons, during the late second trimester and the third trimester twins have to gain around 50–150 g/week.

10.3.7
About Amniotic Fluid

Evaluation of amniotic fluid in twin pregnancies can be done in different ways:
a) As suggested by PORTER et al. (1996), by summing the deeper amniotic pouches in the four uterine quadrants.
b) As CHAU et al. (1996) recommended, by measuring the deepest and largest of the amniotic

pouches of each sac (method used at Sainte-Jus-tine Hospital).

c) As WATSON et al. (1995) proposed, by doing both.

10.3.8
Doppler

The role of Doppler is of the utmost importance in determining the presence or absence of uteroplacental insufficiency in the fetus. Doppler sonography will establish specific criteria to confirm the diagnosis of twin-twin transfusion syndrome during the second and third trimesters.

10.4
How to Determine by US the Type of Twinning

Reminder:
   Chorionicity = Placentation
   Amniocity = Amniotic cavity

10.4.1
The First Trimester

The number of rings of chorion has to be determined. The sonographer must clearly determine, by the endovaginal or transvesical route, whether there are one or two decidual chorionic rings (i.e., one or two gestational sacs).

Scenario I (Fig. 10.2)

Two rings indicates a dichorionic twin pregnancy. The diagnosis can be made at over 5.5 weeks of gestation. At this stage it is impossible to establish precisely whether it will be a dichorionic, monozygotic or dizygotic twin pregnancy. Later, the only way will be to diagnose two fetuses of different gender. In any case, it will be a less risky twin pregnancy because each fetus will evolve with its own placenta and amniotic cavity.

Scenario II

One ring indicates a monochorionic twin pregnancy. The second step is then to find: a membrane (diamniotic) (Fig. 10.2) and/or two vitelline sacs (Fig. 10.3). The best time to visualize a membrane is at 8–9 weeks

of gestation. By a transvaginal approach the membrane can be identified after 7 weeks of gestation (HILL et al. 1996).

One yolk sac and/or no membrane corresponds to a monoamniotic monochorionic twin pregnancy.

Scenario III

The presence of one yolk sac implies a monoamniotic twin pregnancy, but it should be re-evaluated allowing a more confident confirmation or exclusion of monoamniocity (BROMLEY and BENACERRAF 1995).

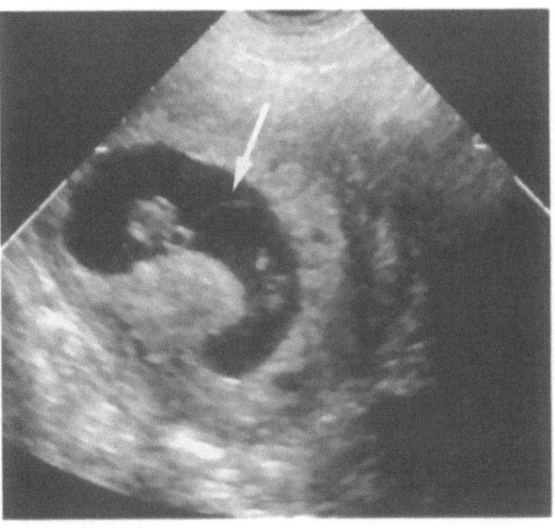

Fig. 10.2. Nine weeks of gestation. One chorionic ring, two embryos and one thin membrane between (*arrow*) = monochorionic diamniotic twins

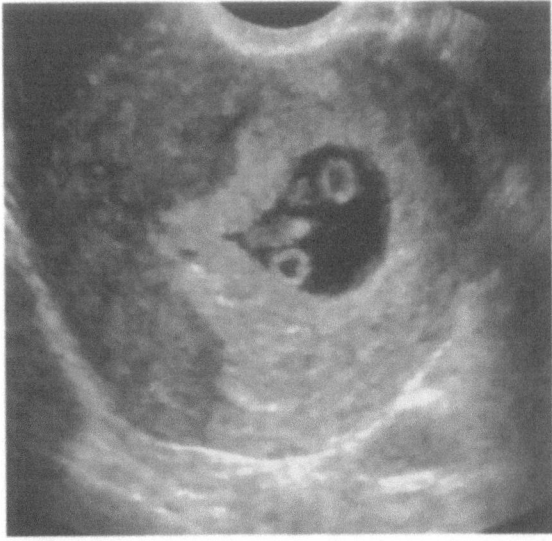

Fig. 10.3. Nine weeks of gestation. One chorionic ring and two vitelline sacs can be seen = monochorionic diamniotic twins

Pitfall

Contrary to the central position of the membrane, the chorioamniotic separation is seen in the peripheral area of the gestational sac (Figs. 10.4, 10.5).

Beware: if a dividing membrane cannot be visualized during the first trimester, US is necessary in the second trimester to clarify the type of twins. Such information is important because fetal risk assessment and subsequent management decisions can be affected.

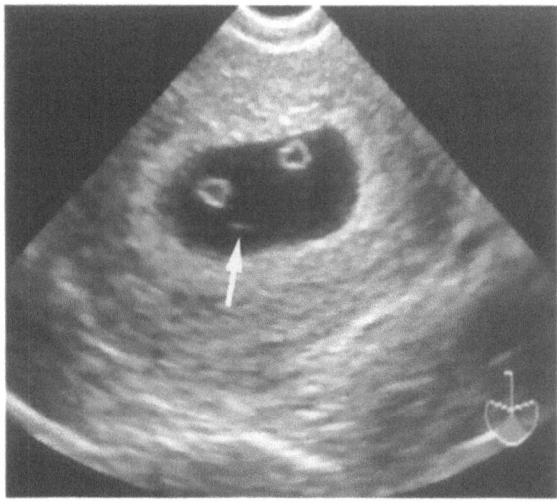

Fig. 10.4. Nine weeks of gestation. One chorionic ring, no membrane identified, two vitelline sacs = monochorionic diamniotic twins. Normal amniotic separation (*arrow*)

10.4.2
The Second Trimester

Fetal Gender: The identification of a male and female fetus indicates dichorionic diamniotic dizygotes with 100% reliability (Figs. 10.6, 10.7). This sign is found in 35% of twin pregnancies (HENDRIX and CHAUHAN 1998).

Number of Placentas The sonographic finding of two separate placentas (Fig. 10.8) is the only reliable sign to prove a dichorionic twin pregnancy in 100% of twin pregnancies (DZ or MZ) (HENDRIX and CHAUHAN 1998). The sonographic finding of one placenta is not reliable to determine the chorionicity because placental separation is not always visible at US. The two placentas may appear to be fused at US but will be separate at pathology. This pseudofusion is found in 66% of cases.

The Amniotic Membrane: Thick or Thin

Scenarios

a) The membrane is present and the sonographer needs to determine whether it is thick (dichorionic diamniotic) or thin (monochorionic diamniotic).
b) The membrane is absent, leading to the diagnosis of a monochorionic monoamniotic twin pregnancy. Cord entanglement is the only echographic sign that confirms it.

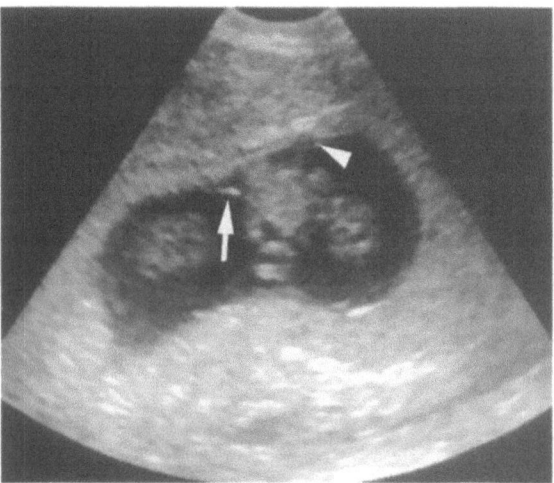

Fig. 10.5. Nine weeks of gestation. One chorionic ring, two embryos and one thin membrane (*arrow*). Note the normal amniotic separation (*arrowhead*)

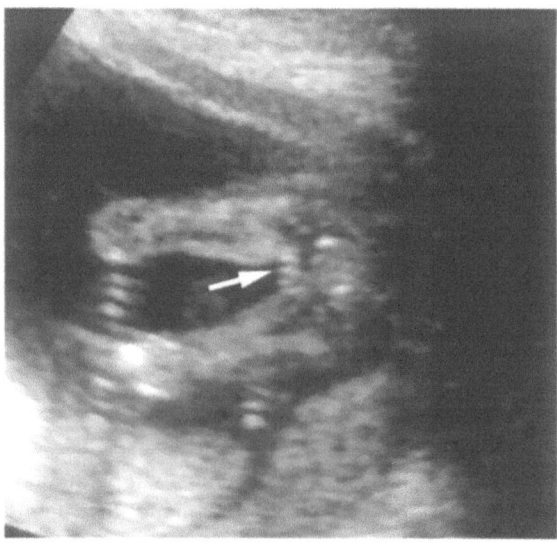

Fig. 10.6. Eighteen weeks of gestation. Female fetus (*arrow*)

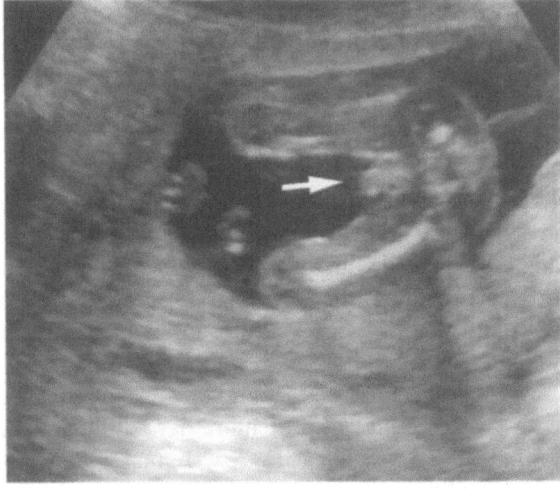

Fig. 10.7. Eighteen weeks of gestation. Male fetus (*arrow*)

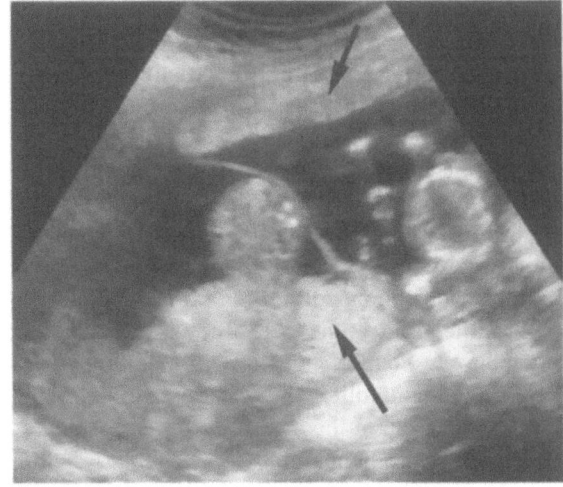

Fig. 10.8. Fifteen weeks of gestation. Two placentas (*arrows*) in a dichorionic diamniotic twin pregnancy

Qualifying the Membrane

Thick:	Dichorionic diamniotic >2 mm	*Thin*:	Monochorionic diamniotic Not measurable, <1 mm
	Four layers: two amnions, two chorions		Two layers: two amnions
	Hyperechoic Twin peak sign[a]		Faintly seen, wispy T-sign[b]

[a] Twin peak sign or lambda sign: The extension of placental tissue into the base of the intertwin membrane (FINBERG 1992) or the area between the uterine wall and the chorionic membrane will form a triangular villus-filled space. The accuracy of the twin peak or lambda sign is 100% for determining dichorionic twinning (Fig. 10.9).

[b] T-sign: No extension of the placental tissue is seen within the triangular villus-filled space (Fig. 10.10).

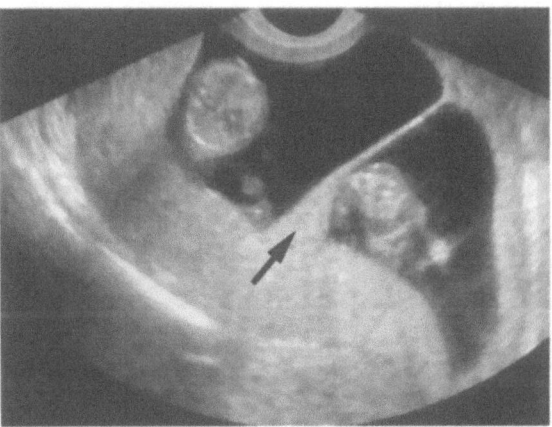

Fig. 10.9. Fourteen weeks of gestation. Twin peak sign (*arrow*) in dichorionic diamniotic twins with one fused placenta

Using the cut-off point of 2 mm for the thickness of the membrane, accuracy for monochorionic diamniotic pregnancies is 82% and 95% for dichorionic diamniotic (WINN et al. 1989). TOWNSEND et al. (1988) reported that a thick membrane 2 mm can be diagnosed in 89–90% of cases.

The evaluation of membrane thickness is always done more accurately earlier in pregnancy. With increasing gestational age, a thick membrane becomes progressively thinner in appearance.

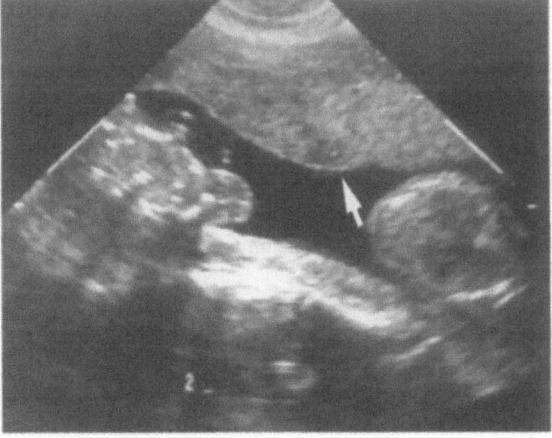

Fig. 10.10. Sixteen weeks of gestation. "T" sign (*arrow*) in monochorionic diamniotic twins

Pitfalls

A thin membrane appears artifactually thick when the ultrasound beam strikes the membrane perpendicularly. To avoid this artifactual thickening, the sonographer has to image the membrane in a plane not directly perpendicular to the sound beam.

The most frequent error is to report that the membrane is absent and identify a twin pregnancy as monochorionic monoamniotic. A practical US hint is to place the probe at the level of the limbs and wait. The failure to identify an intertwin membrane suggests a monoamniotic twin gestation. However, the non-visualization of the membrane does not definitively confirm the monoamniocity, particularly before 8 weeks or after 20 weeks of gestation because the membrane is often difficult to identify. The most reliable sign of monoamniocity is the demonstration of entanglement of the twin umbilical cords (Fig. 10.11).

With all these echographic criteria, the percentage error of twin subtypes is 2.7% in a Sainte-Justine Hospital series of 317 twin pregnancies, with 217 dichorionic diamniotic pregnancies and 110 monochorionic diamniotic twin pregnancies.

10.5
General Complications

10.5.1
Discordance Between Twins

First Trimester: Disparity of 3 mm in CRL (Fig. 10.12) raises the possibility of chromosomal abnormalities and is associated with an embryo loss rate of 50%. In early pregnancies, the differences of gestational sac (GS) and CRL are unrelated to differences in birth weight, length or fetal sex (SHERER 1998).

WEISSMAN et al. (1994) found that in all such pairs with a discordance of 5 or more days difference in estimated gestational age there were major congenital anomalies in the smaller twin.

Second Trimester: A study performed at Sainte-Justine Hospital indicated that the ratio of abdominal circumference of the smaller twin to the abdominal circumference of the larger twin multiplied by 100

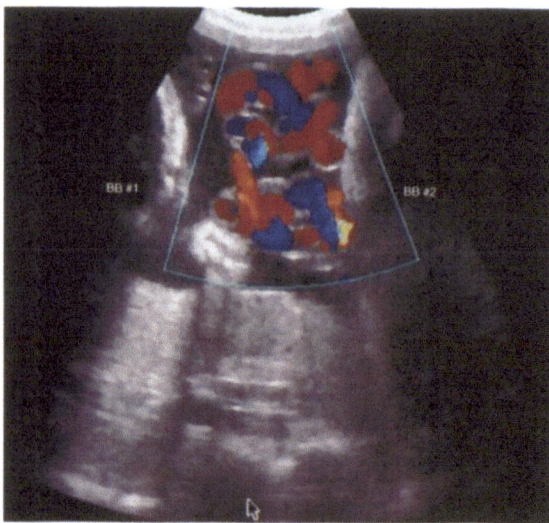

Fig. 10.11. Twenty-two weeks of gestation. Entanglement of the cords in monochorionic monoamniotic twins well illustrated by color Doppler

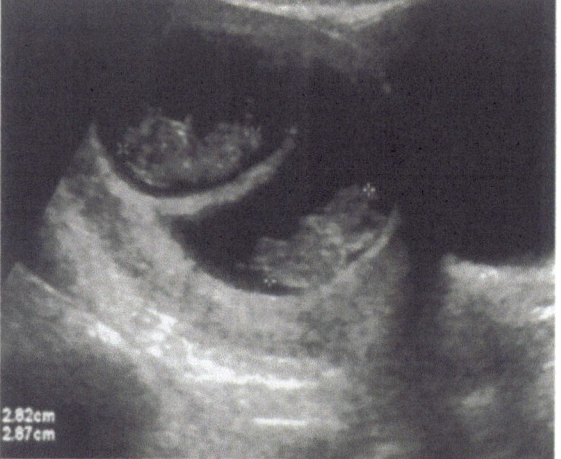

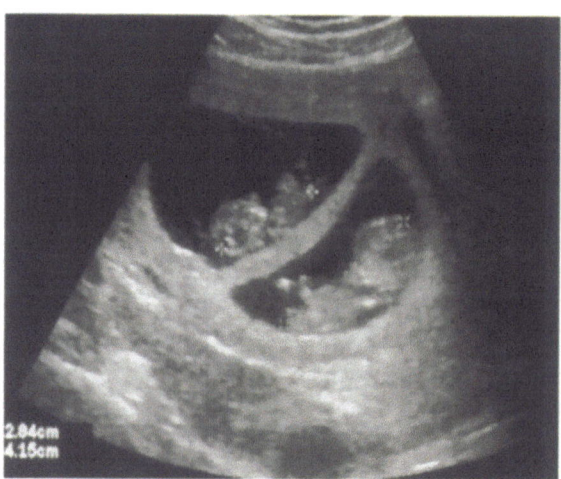

Fig. 10.12a, b. a Nine and a half weeks of gestation. Dichorionic diamniotic twins, symmetrical crown-rump length (CRL). **b** Eleven weeks of gestation. Dichorionic diamniotic twins, asymmetrical CRL

must be higher than or equal to 0.93 (Fig. 10.13). A ratio lower than 0.93 has a sensitivity of 78%, a specificity of 92%, a positive predictive value (PPV) of 70% and a negative predictive value (NPV) of 94% for detecting a population at risk, that is to say, growth restriction, twin-twin transfusion syndrome, chromosomal anomalies, etc. For a greater sensitivity, a ratio value of 0.89 may be used.

*Third Trimester: T*here are several definitions of discordance in the literature.

The weight difference is calculated as a percentage: The weight of the larger twin minus the weight of the smaller twin/the weight of the larger twin multiplied by 100. A difference between twins >20% (weights evaluated by abdominal circumference and femur length) is the definition of discordance found most frequently in the literature. However, STORLAZZI et al. (1987) found that an abdominal circumference difference of 20 mm or greater or a difference in estimated fetal weight (EFW) of 20% or more based on the weight of the heavier twin was the most sensitive indication of significant discordance. A difference in birth weight of 20% or more is reported to occur in as up to 23% of twin pairs and leads to significantly increased morbidity and mortality in the discordant twins (SONNTAG et al. 1996) (Fig. 10.14).

A weight difference of 20% or more is most frequently reported in the literature to define discordant twins and is used at Sainte-Justine Hospital.

In our series of 217 dichorionic diamniotic twin pregnancies, 19% were discordant. The percentage of discordance rises in the monochorionic diamniotic population to 29%.

10.5.2
Intrauterine Growth Restriction

The most common definition of IUGR, and the one we advocate, is that growth of a fetus is restricted if its weight is below the 10th percentile of gestational age (DOUBILET and BENSON 1990).

IUGR occurs in 10% of singleton pregnancies and rises to 15–47% in twin pregnancies, depending on the series (DIVON and WEINER 1995). In our institution we found 7% IUGR out of 217 dichorionic diamniotic twin pregnancies compared with 15.4% out of 110 monochorionic diamniotic twin pregnancies.

In the presence of IUGR we apply the same standards and protocol as for singleton follow-up regarding the frequency of sonography examinations and Doppler velocimetry.

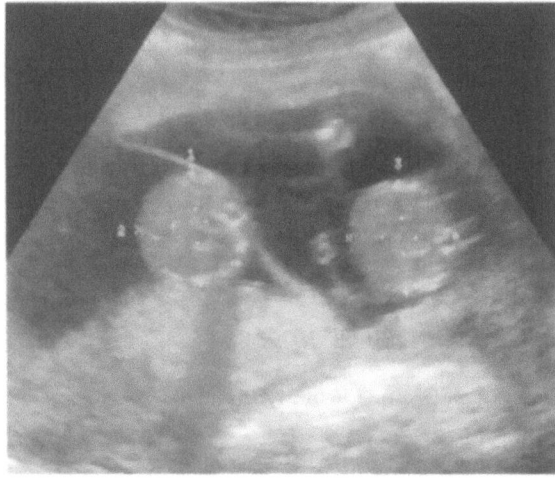

Fig. 10.13. Fifteen weeks of gestation. Symmetrical dichorionic diamniotic twins

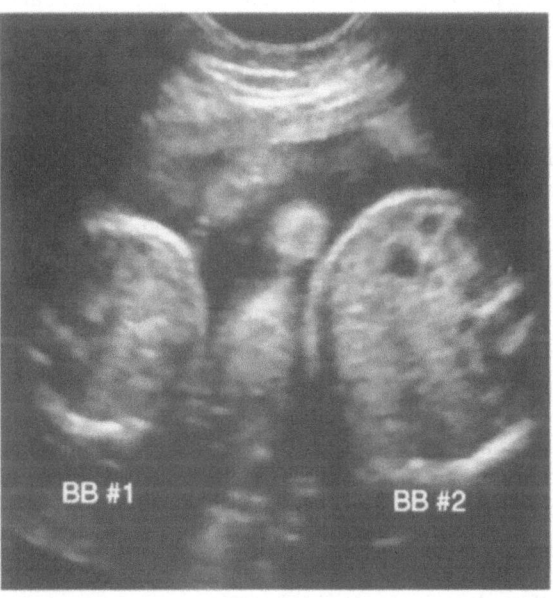

Fig. 10.14. Twenty-nine weeks of gestation. Discordant diamniotic dichorionic twins

10.5.3
Our Series: Abnormal Growth

Twin pregnancies carry a higher risk than single pregnancies. The role of the sonographer is pre-eminent for the detection of complications, and for providing information to the physician in charge. It is important to remember that the complications of monochorionic twin pregnancies are more numerous and more serious due to the fact that these fetuses share the same placenta (possibility of vascular communication) and the same amniotic sac (cord entanglement).

At Sainte-Justine Hospital, we reviewed our cases of twin pregnancy. In order to evaluate their complications and natural evolution, we compared the weight of the two fetuses (concordant or discordant), and reported the estimated weight in relation to the standard charts (normal growth or IUGR).

10.5.3.1
Diamniotic Dichorionic Twins

Concordant Group: 176 of 217 (81%)

A) With normal growth: 144 of 176 (81%).
Ultrasonography follow-up: should be performed every 3–4 weeks to assess fetal growth.

Outcome: in our series of 144 of 176 concordant twin pairs, 43% had a preterm labor between 34 and 35 weeks of gestation and the neonatal outcome was 100% normal.

B) With IUGR: 32 of 176 (19%)
The Doppler evaluation has an important role to play in the diagnosis and follow-up. In our series of 32 twin pairs, 17 had normal Doppler findings, 13 had abnormal Doppler findings and there were two deaths secondary to infection.

Ultrasonography follow-up should be performed every 2 weeks or, if the Doppler findings are abnormal, twice a week.

Outcome: The concordant twins with IUGR with normal Doppler findings (17/32, 53.1%) had no mortality or morbidity. In the group of concordant twin pairs with abnormal Doppler findings (13/32, 40.6%), the mortality was 37.5% and morbidity 40%.

Discordant Group: 41 of 217 (19%)

The etiology of the discordant growth in twins can result from biological variability, placental crowding (dysfunction?), poor placental implantation, chromosomal abnormality, fetal infection or other causes of IUGR.

A) With normal growth: 30 of 41 (73%)
Complications: preterm delivery, median 33 weeks.
Ultrasonography follow-up: Doppler analysis has to be included in the ultrasonography examination. If the Doppler findings are normal, the examination has to be repeated every 4 weeks, whereas the examination has to be done every week in the case of abnormal Doppler findings.

Outcome: The mortality and morbidity was 0 in 16 of 41 twin pairs. The hospitalization duration was 6 days.

B) With IUGR: 11 of 41 (27%)

Complications: preterm delivery, median 34.2 weeks.
Outcome: No mortality. The morbidity was 18%, including a hospitalization duration of more than 3 weeks, and the complications of prematurity such as pulmonary bronchodysplasia.

10.6
Specific Complications

10.6.1
General Considerations

The hemodynamic balance of the vascularization in the placenta is sometimes disturbed and can affect the other twin. Monochorionic twins share the same placenta.

There are four important heterogeneous groups of disorders concerning the complications of monochorionic twins:
1) Stuck-twin syndrome (STS), almost always monochorionic.
2) Twin oligohydramnios-polyhydramnios sequence (TOPS).
3) Twin-twin transfusion syndrome (TTTS).
4) Twin embolization syndrome (TES).

The mechanisms of these complications are not well established. They comprise a spectrum of complications with possible progression of STS to TOPS or TOPS to TTTS and TES.

10.6.2
Stuck-Twin Syndrome

Definition: A fetus trapped against the uterine wall, always by a retaining membrane. A trapped fetus necessarily implies a diamniotic twin pregnancy.

General Considerations: STS complicates up to 8% of twin pregnancies and 35% of monochorionic diamniotic gestations. Rarely it can occur in dichorionic and even dizygotic pregnancies. The etiologies in cases of dichorionic diamniotic pregnancies are placental insufficiency, kidney anomalies, chromosomal anomalies and premature membrane rupture in one sac.

Normal growth or growth restriction can be observed. Growth restriction is due to asymmetrical placental insufficiency, confirmed by Doppler.

US Findings

a) Type of twin: STS is far more common in monochorionic diamniotic than in dichorionic diamniotic pregnancies. Fetuses are mostly of the same sex or rarely of different sex (dichorionic diamniotic). There is one placenta in most cases.
b) Significant disparity in size of the fetuses.
c) Asymmetry of amniotic fluid: oligohydramnios of the stuck twin, the other twin in normal amniotic fluid or polyhydramnios (most frequently).
d) The membrane that holds the fetus in a fixed position also presses the umbilical cord against the trunk of the fetus. The fetus is held in place, adjacent to the lateral or anterior uterine wall.
e) Sometimes there is velamentous or peripheral insertion of the cord for the stuck twin.

10.6.3
Twin Oligohydramnios-Polyhydramnios Sequence

Definition: One fetus with an oligohydramnios ≥2 cm (STS), one fetus with a polyhydramnios 8 cm (Fig. 10.15).

The twins are always monochorionic and diamniotic. Outcome is sometimes a TTTS, but TOPS is not synonymous with TTTS.

US Findings

a) Fetuses of the same sex.
b) One placenta.
c) Asymmetry of amniotic fluid: oligo- and polyhydramnios (**>8 cm).
d) Growth: concordant or discordant with or without growth restriction.
e) Doppler velocimetry: with or without placental insufficiency: abnormal Doppler findings are seen frequently with the smaller fetus.
f) Peripheral insertion of the cord in some cases (velamentous insertion).
g) Cord edema in the polyhydramniotic fetus (Fig. 10.16a).
h) Bladder distention in the polyhydramniotic fetus (Fig. 10.16b).

Signs (a) to (c) are essential to establish the diagnosis.

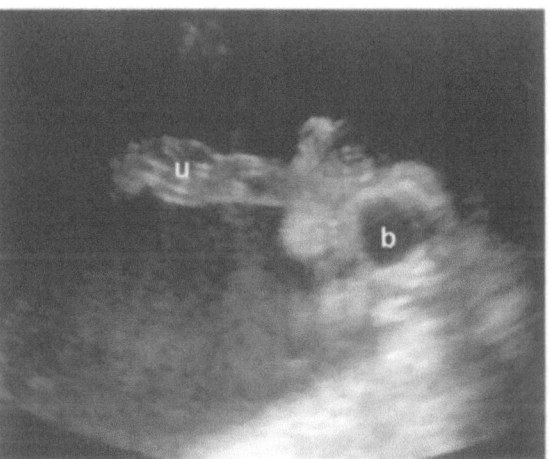

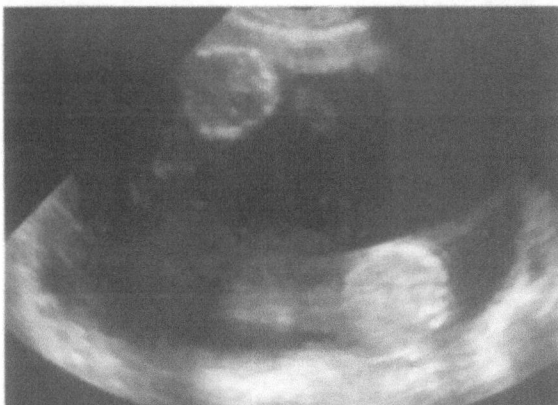

Fig. 10.15. Eighteen weeks of gestation. Twin oligohydramnios-polyhydramnios sequence (TOPS) in monochorionic diamniotic twins. The upper left embryo is a stuck twin. The lower-right embryo is in a polyhydramniotic sac

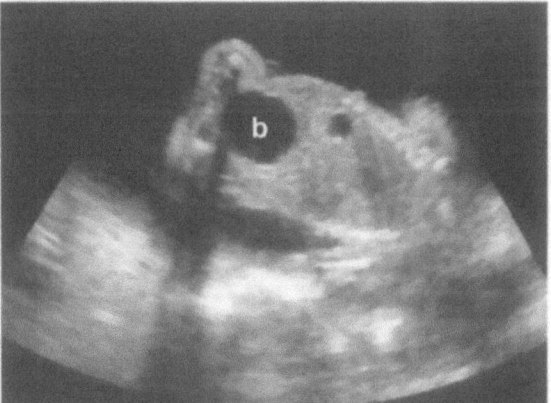

Fig. 10.16a, b. Eighteen weeks of gestation. TOPS in monochorionic diamniotic twins. a Umbilical cord edema (*u*) in the embryo that lies in the polyhydramniotic sac. b Huge bladder (*b*)

10.6.4
Twin-Twin Transfusion Syndrome

Definition (VILLE 1997): One or more vascular communication(s) (vein-vein, artery-vein, etc.) exist between the two twins. These vascular communications are deep in 80% of cases (BAJORIA et al. 1995). They are established between the donor, namely the transfuser, and the recipient, namely the transfusee. The process appears to start when an imbalance in anastomoses results in shunting of blood from the donor to the recipient twin. It complicates 4–35% of monochorionic twin pregnancies with 17% perinatal mortality and 20.4% of deaths after the neonatal period (SHERER 1998, VILLE 1997). The mortality rate is high, being from 40% to 70%. However, when TTTS is fully manifested by the ST phenomenon, it is a highly lethal entity. The perinatal morbidity was 100% for all twin pairs and prematurity occurred in all cases. Perinatal mortality was 88% for the larger twin and 96% for the smaller twin. Neurodevelopmental abnormalities in the survivors are 6–8 times more frequent than in any other type of pregnancy.

The donor is affected by anemia, hypovolemia, hypotension, reduced renal blood, oligohydramnios and loss of fetal weight. The recipient compensates for the additional volume received by high-output cardiac failure and increased urine output (ROSEN et al. 1990), followed by polyhydramnios and a preterm labor.

This hyperosmolarity state requires through the mother a larger quantity of circulating fluid. This condition results in polyhydramnios, secondary cardiac insufficiency, large liver, pancreas, adrenal cortex and hydrops. The dilated and hypertrophied heart secretes more atriopeptin, which increases its vascular exchange (NAGEOTTE et al. 1989).

In the first trimester there is asymmetry of nuchal lucencies (Fig. 10.17).

US Findings

a) Same sex: more frequent in females (63–89%).
b) One placenta.
c) Disparity in the amount of amniotic liquid.
d) Size disparity is a universal feature in this syndrome. The smaller twin may not be less than the 10th percentile for gestational age but may be discordantly small (20% smaller than the larger twin).

1. Small Fetus (Donor)

– Oligohydramnios.
– Intrauterine growth restriction.
– Doppler: high resistance at placenta blood flow.
– Velamentous cord insertion: 63% prevalence for this type of umbilical cord is found in monochorionic diamniotic fetuses with the transfuser-transfusee syndrome (Fig. 10.18).

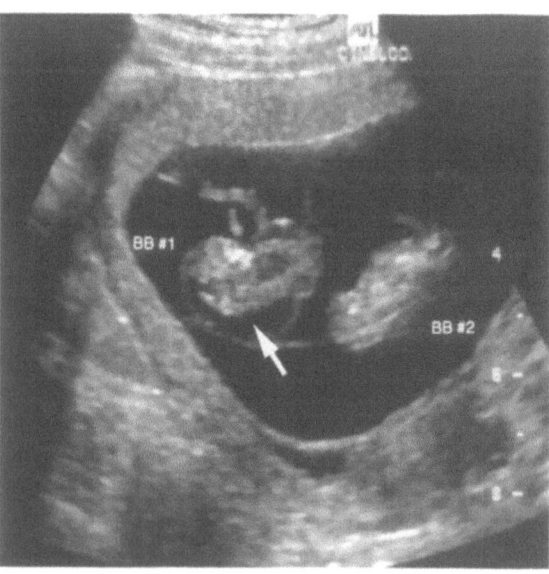 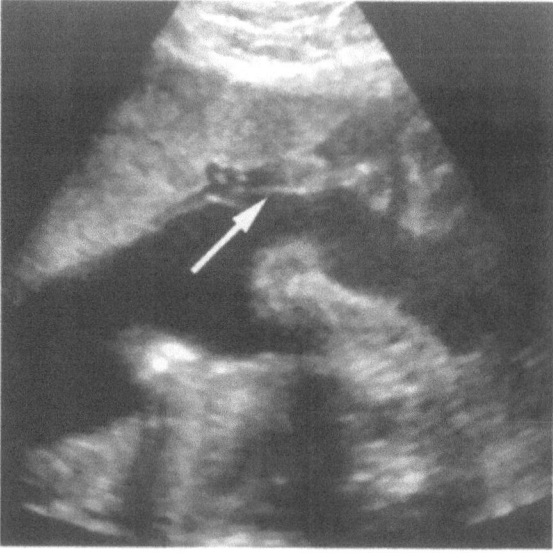

Fig. 10.17. Eleven weeks of gestation. Monochorionic diamniotic twins. BB #1 with abnormal nuchal lucency (*arrow*). Outcome: twin-twin transfusion syndrome (TTTS)

Fig. 10.18. Seventeen weeks of gestation. Monochorionic diamniotic twins with a proven velamentous cord insertion (*arrow*)

- Placenta: white (Fig. 10.19).
- Morphological signs: hyperdynamic heart with a thin wall (Fig. 10.20a), small bladder.

2. Large Fetus (Recipient)

- Polyhydramnios.
- Intrauterine growth restriction: rare but can be seen.
- Doppler: Normal low resistance to blood flow.
- Cord: central insertion, cord edema.
- Placenta: dark.
- Morphological signs: cardiomegaly with a thickened wall (Fig. 10.20b), large bladder, hydrops in cases of cardiac failure.

A Word of Caution: In cases of TTTS, an inversion of the process can be seen during evolution (BROMLEY and BENACERRAF 1996). TTTS may also occur with weight discordance of less than 20–25% and without development of polyhydramnios and oligohydramnios (SEPULVEDA 1997).

10.6.5
Twin Embolization Syndrome

Twin embolization syndrome is a rare complication of monochorionic twins that follows the in utero demise of one twin.

Etiopathology: The infarcted organs in the surviving twin result from the transfusion of thromboplas-

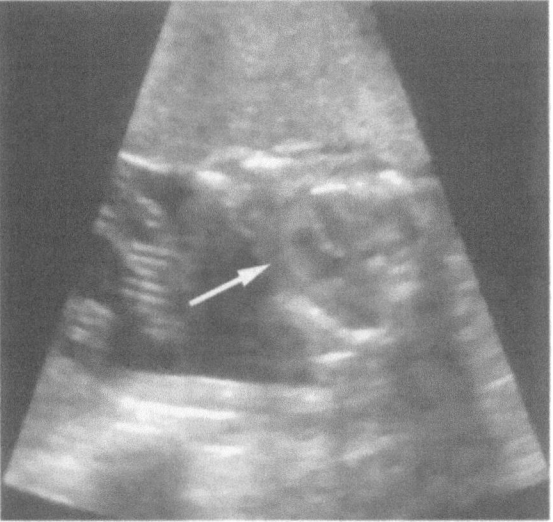

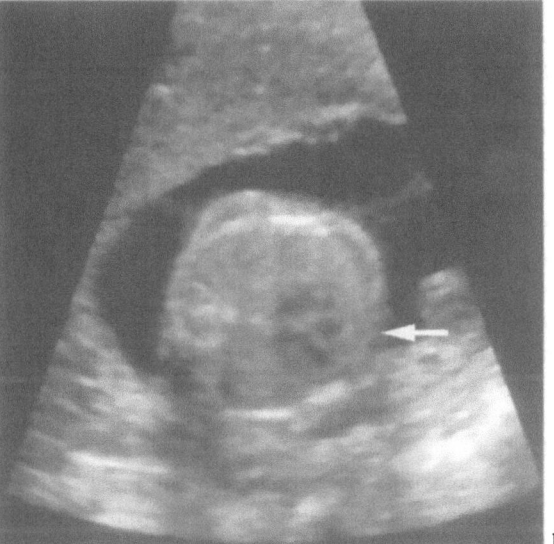

Fig. 10.20a, b. The twins of a TTTS. **a** The smaller fetus with normal myocardial wall (*arrow*). **b** The larger fetus with myocardial wall thickening (*arrow*)

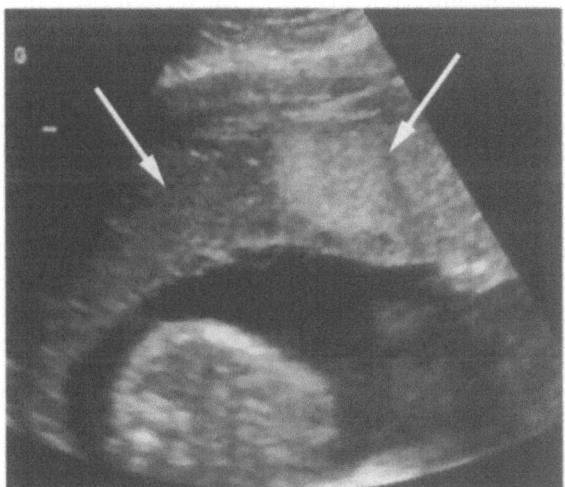

Fig. 10.19. Twenty-two weeks of gestation. Monochorionic diamniotic twins. There are two types of density in this unique placenta (*arrows*)

tin-rich blood from the dead twin to the live twin through vascular communications and/or sudden hemodynamic changes and/or ischemic modifications (FILLY et al. 1990, OKAMURA et al. 1994).

The prevalence of TES in the setting of antepartum demise of one twin is not firmly established. The recognition of TES has an important potential therapeutic implication. Theoretically the delivery of the affected surviving twin can reduce the organ damage but the benefit must be balanced against the inherent risks of preterm delivery.

The death of one of the monochorionic twins can cause the death of the other twin in 25% of cases. If the second twin survives, there is 25% chance of it developing neurological handicaps (YOSHIDA and MATAYOSHI 1990).

The intracranial changes that the ultrasonographer has to look for are: ventriculomegaly (the most commonly identified abnormality), porencephalic cyst formation, diffuse cerebral atrophy and microcephaly (FUSI et al. 1991). Other anomalies to search for are digestive atresias, renal cortical necrosis and liver embolism. These signs can be found from day 6 after the death of the first twin.

10.6.6
Acardius or Twin Reversal Arterial Perfusion

Acardius twin, known in the past as chorioangiopagus parasiticus, is the most extreme manifestation of multifetal pregnancy, with an incidence of 1% of monochorionic twin pregnancies (1 in 35,000 pregnancies).

The acardius has no functional heart. The normal twin (donor) circulates the acardiac twin (recipient), which is kept alive through vascular anastomoses. The blood flow in the acardiac twin is pumped directly from the umbilical cord of the co-twin into the umbilical artery of the acardiac twin. It is characterized by a twin reversed arterial perfusion syndrome (TRAP) with hypoxia of the upper part of the body.

Chromosomal disorder is found in 50% (VAN ALLEN et al. 1983) and there is a high incidence (10%) of major malformations: hydrocephalus, major heart or vascular malformation (SOGAARD et al. 1999).

US Findings and Follow-up

- The dead fetus seems to be growing, particularly during the first trimester.
- Monstrous appearance of the edematous acardius: solid mass with a cystic component (Fig. 10.21).
- Upper extremities are absent or rudimentary.
- Lower extremities are better formed.
- Absence of any visible cardiac pulsation.
- Umbilical cord of the acardius sometimes has a velamentous insertion.
- On Doppler examination there is a retrograde pattern of fetal perfusion throughout the umbilical and iliac arteries.

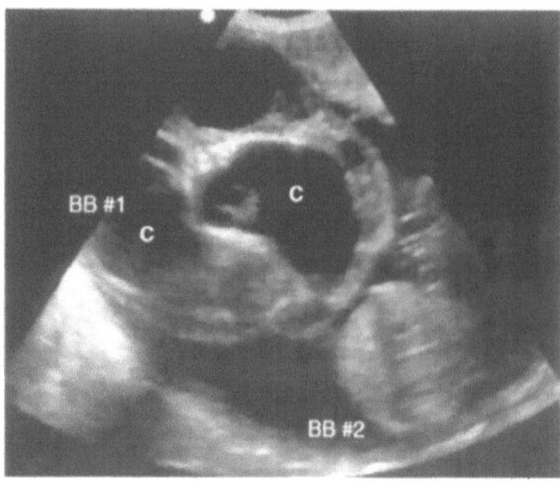

Fig. 10.21. Eighteen weeks of gestation. Monochorionic diamniotic twins with a cystic (c) acardius. Abdominal transverse section of both fetuses

- Ultrasonography has to be performed every week.

Outcome is influenced by the congenital abnormalities. The mortality is 50–75%.

10.6.7
Monochorionic Monoamniotic Twins

Monoamniotic twin pregnancies are important to recognize, especially for the prognosis and the obstetrical management. They comprise approximately 1% of monozygotic twin pregnancies and carry the highest mortality. The twins share the same amniotic fluid. No dividing membrane exists. Knotted cords may be seen with a good outcome for both twins, however, knotted cords may cut off the circulation resulting in sudden death, and account for the high fetal loss rate. The specific important complication is the cord entanglement. This event is unpredictable. Cesarean delivery can be safer than vaginal delivery (BEASLEY et al. 1999).

US Findings

- Lack of membrane.
- Contact of the two umbilical cords: it is important to trace both fetal cords to evaluate the possibility of entanglement.

10.6.8
Conjoined Twins

Conjoined twins are rare. The incidence is 1 in 50,000 to 1 in 100,000 births.

General Considerations

The precise diagnosis concerning the conjoining is important to determine the postnatal viability, separability and mode of delivery. Thoracopagus, omphalopagus and thoraco-omphalopagus twins account for more than 70% of cases. Seventy-five percent are stillborn or die within 24 h.

US Findings

- No membrane.
- Twin fusion: most are usually anterior-anterior. Involve one body region or more:
  - Head to head: craniopagus
  - Chest to chest: thoracopagus (Fig. 10.22)
  - Abdomen to abdomen: omphalopagus
  - Side to side – more extensive: inability to detect separate skin contours, joined fetal parts; shared heart, liver, brain or other organs; single umbilical cord with more than three vessels.

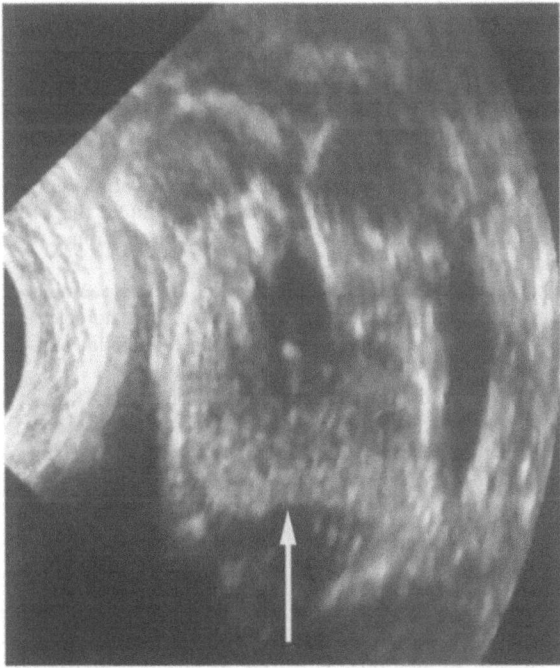

Fig. 10.22. Seventeen weeks of gestation. Omphalopagus (*arrow*) conjoined twins

10.7
Conclusion

All twin pregnancies are at high risk for perinatal morbidity and mortality compared with singleton gestation. Ultrasonography has a major impact concerning the obstetrical management. It permits the determination of the type of twin, can exclude syndromes or assess the complications of twinning. Despite the rarity of some entities, it is crucial to be familiar with problems related to chorionicity and amniocity and their sonographic evaluation, diagnosis and sometimes therapeutic implications.

References

Aisenbrey GA, Catanzrite VA, Hurley TJ, Spiegel JH, Schrimmer DB, Mendoza A (1995) Monoamniotic and pseudomonoamniotic twins: sonographic diagnosis, detection of cord entanglement, and obstetric management. Obstet Gynecol 86:218–222

Alexander JM, Ramus R, Cox SM, Gilstrap LC (1997) Outcome of twin gestations with a single anomalous fetus. Am J Obstet Gynecol 176:S75

Ananth CV, Vintzileos AM, Shen-Schwarz S, Smulian JC, Lai YL (1998) Standards of birth weight in twin gestations stratified by placental chorionicity. Obstet Gynecol 91:917–924

Arbuckle TE, Wilkins R, Sherman GJ (1993) Birth weight percentiles by gestational age in Canada. Obstet Gynecol 81:39–48

Bajoria R, Wigglesworth J, Fisk NM (1995) Angioarchitecture of monochorionic placentas in relation to the twin-twin transfusion syndrome. Am J Obstet Gynecol 172:856–863

Baldwin VJ (1993) Pathology of multiple pregnancy. Springer, Berlin Heidelberg New York

Beasley E, Megerian G, Gerson A, Roberts NS (1999) Monoamniotic twins: case series and proposal for antenatal management. Obstet Gynecol 93:130–134

Bebbington MW, Wittmann BK (1989) Fetal transfusion syndrome: antenatal factors predicting outcome. Am J Obstet Gynecol 160:913–915

Benirschke K (1961) Twin placenta in perinatal mortality. NY State J Med 61:1499

Benirschke K, Kim CK (1973a) Multiple pregnancy: 1. N Engl J Med 288:1276–1284

Benirschke K, Kim CK (1973b) Multiple pregnancy: 2. N Engl J Med 288:1329–1336

Benirschke K, Kaufmann P (1990) Pathology of the human placenta, 2nd edn. Springer, Berlin Heidelberg New York

Brennan JN, Diwan RV, Rosen MG, Bellon EM (1982) Fetofetal transfusion syndrome: prenatal ultrasonographic diagnosis. Radiology 143:535–536

Bromley B, Benacerraf B (1995) Using the number of yolk sacs to determine amnionicity in early first trimester monochorionic twins. J Ultrasound Med 14:415–419

Bromley B, Benacerraf BR (1996) Acute reversal of oligohydramnios-polyhydramnios sequence in monochorionic twins. Int J Obstet Gynecol 55:281–283

Bruner JP, Anderson TL, Rosemond RL (1998) Placental patho-physiology of the twin oligohydramnios-polyhydramnios sequence and the twin-twin transfusion syndrome. Placenta 19:8–86

Callen PW (2000) Ultrasonography in obstetrics and gynecology, 4th edn. Saunders, Philadelphia

Chau AC, Kjos SL, Kovacs BW (1996) Ultrasonographic measurement of amniotic fluid volume in normal diamniotic twin pregnancies. Am J Obstet Gynecol 174:1003–1007

Cheung VYT, Bocking AD, DaSilva OP (1994) Preterm discordant twins: what birthweight difference is significant ? Am J Obstet Gynecol 170:345

Di Salvo DN, Benson CB, Laing FC, Brown DL, Frates MC, Doubilet PM (1998) Sonographic evaluation of the placental cord insertion site. AJR Am J Roentgenol 170:1295–1298

Divon MY, Weiner Z (1995) Ultrasound in twin pregnancy. Semin Perinatol 15:404–412

Doubilet PM, Benson CB (1990) Fetal growth disturbances. Semin Roentgenol 25:309–316

Edwards MS, Ellings JM, Newman RB, Ménard MK (1995) Predictive value of antepartum ultrasound examination for anomalies in twin gestations. Ultrasound Obstet Gynecol 6:43–49

Evans MI, Goldberg JD, Horenstein J, et al (1999) Selective termination for structural, chromosomal, and mendelian anomalies: international experience. Am J Obstet Gynecol 18:893–897

Filly RA, Goldstein RB, Callen PW (1990) Monochorionic twinning: sonographic assessment. AJR Am J Roentgenol 154:459–469

Finberg HJ (1992) The „twin peak" sign: reliable evidence of dichorionic twinning. J Ultrasound Med 11:571–577

Fouron JC, Leduc L, Grignon A, Maragnes P, Lessard M, Drblik SP (1994) Importance of meticulous ultrasonographic investigation of the acardiac twin. J Ultrasound Med 13:1001–1004

Fries MH, Goldstein RB, Kilpatrick SJ, Golbus MS, Callen PW, Filly RA (1993) The role of velamentous cord insertion in the etiology of twin-twin transfusion syndrome. Obstet Gynecol 81:569–574

Frisch L, Arava J, David H, Jaschevatzky OE, Ballas S (1997) Severe twin-to-twin transfusion syndrome: a new sonographic feature of the placenta. Ultrasound Obstet Gynecol 10:145–146

Fusi L, McParland P, Fisk N, Nicolini U, Wigglesworth J (1991) Acute twin-twin transfusion: a possible mechanism for brain-damaged survivors after intrauterine death of a monochorionic twin. Obstet Gynecol 78:51–520

Gall S (1996) Multiple pregnancy and delivery. Mosby, St Louis

Ghai V, Vidyasagar D (1988) Morbidity and mortality factors in twins. An epidemiologic approach. Clin Perinatol 15:123–140

Hadlock FP, Harrist RB, Carpenter RJ, Deter RL, Park SK (1984) Sonographic estimation of fetal weight. The value of femur length in addition to head and abdomen measurements. Radiology 150:535–540

Hendrix NW, Chauhan SP (1998) Sonographic examination of twins. From first trimester to delivery of second fetus. Obstet Gynecol Clin North Am 25:609–621

Hill LM, Chenevey P, Hecker J, Martin JG (1996) Sonographic determination of first trimester twin chorionicity and amnionicity. J Clin Ultrasound 24:305–308

Hollier L, Leveno K, Kelly M, Cunningham FG (1997) A comparison of malformation rates in twin versus singleton gestations. Am J Obstet Gynecol 176:S75

Hrubec Z, Robinette CD (1984) The study of human twins in medical research. N Engl J Med 310:435–441

Kohl SG, Casey G (1975) Twin gestation. Mt Sinai J Med 42:523–539

Kurtz AB, Wapner RJ, Mata J, Johnson A, Morgan P (1992) Twin pregnancies: accuracy of first-trimester abdominal US in predicting chorionicity and amnionicity. Radiology 185:759–762

Kushnir O, Vigil DA, Izquierdo L, Schiff M, Curet LB (1990) Vaginal ultrasonographic assessment of cervical length changes during normal pregnancy. Am J Obstet Gynecol 162:991–993

Kushnir O, Izquierdo LA, Smith JF, Blankstein J, Curet LB (1995) Transvaginal sonographic measurement of cervical length: evaluation of twin pregnancies. J Reprod Med 40:380–382

Lipitz S, Meizner I, Yagel S, Shapiro I, Achiron R, Schiff E (1995) Expectant management of twin pregnancies discordant for anencephaly. Obstet Gynecol 86:969–972

Luke B (1994) The changing pattern of multiple births in the United States: maternal and infant characteristics, 1973 and 1990. Obstet Gynecol 84:101–110

MacGillivray I (1986) Epidemiology of twin pregnancy. Semin Perinatol 10:4–8

Mahony BS, Nyberg DA, Luthy DS, Hirsch JH, Hickok DE, Petty CN (1990a) Translabial ultrasound of the third-trimester uterine cervix. Correlation with digital examination. J Ultrasound Med 9:717–723

Mahony BS, Petty CN, Nyberg DA, Luthy DA, Hickok DE, Hirsch JH (1990b) The "stuck twin" phenomenon: ultrasonographic findings, pregnancy outcome, and management with serial amniocenteses. Am J Obstet Gynecol 163:1513–1522

Naeye RL, Tafari N, Judge D, Marboe CC (1978) Twins: causes of perinatal death in 12 United States cities and one African city. Am J Obstet Gynecol 131:267–272

Nageotte MP, Hurwitz SR, Kaupke CJ, Vaziri ND, Pandian MR (1989) Atriopeptin in the twin transfusion syndrome. Obstet Gynecol 73:867–870

Ohno Y, Ando H, Tanamura A, Kurauchi O, Mizutani S, Tomoda Y (1994) The value of Doppler ultrasound in the diagnosis and management of twin-twin transfusion syndrome. Arch Gynecol Obstet 255:37–42

Okamura K, Murotsuki J, Tanigawara S, Uehara S, Yajima A (1994) Funipuncture for evaluation of hematologic and coagulation indices in the surviving twin following co-twin's death. Obstet Gynecol 83:975–978

Porter TF, Dildy GA, Blanchard JR, Kochenour NK, Clark SL (1996) Normal values for amniotic fluid index during uncomplicated twin pregnancy. Obstet Gynecol 87:699–702

Raga F, Simon C, Strasser J, Bonilla-Musoles F (1992) Abdominal, perineal and vaginal sonographic diagnosis of cervix insufficiency. Ultraschall Med 13:24–27

Richey SD, Ramin KD, Roberts SW, Ramin SM, Cox SM, Twickler DM (1995) The correlation between transperineal sonography and digital examination in the evaluation of the third-trimester cervix. Obstet Gynecol 85:745–748

Rosen DJ, Rabinowitz R, Beyth Y, Fejgin MD, Nicolaides KH

(1990) Fetal urine production in normal twins and in twins with acute polyhydramnios. Fetal Diagn Ther 5:57–60

Saade GR, Gray G, Belfort MA, Carpenter RJ Jr, Moise KJ Jr (1998) Ultrasonographic measurement of crown-rump length in high-order multifetal pregnancies. Ultrasound Obstet Gynecol 11:438–444

Sepulveda W (1997) Chorionicity determination in twin pregnancies: double trouble. Ultrasound Obstet Gynecol 10:79–81

Sharma S, Gray S, Guzman ER, Rosenberg JC, Shen-Schwarz S (1995) Detection of twin-twin transfusion syndrome by first trimester ultrasonography. J Ultrasound Med 14:635–637

Sherer DM (1998) First trimester ultrasonography of multiple gestations: a review. Obstet Gynecol Surv 53:715–726

Sogaard K, Skibsted L, Brocks V (1999) Acardia twins: pathophysiology, diagnosis, outcome and treatment. Six cases and review of the literature. Fetal Diagn Ther 14:53–59

Sonntag J, Waltz S, Schollmeyer T, Schuppler U, Schroder H, Weisner D (1996) Morbidity and mortality of discordant twins up to 34 weeks of gestational age. Eur J Pediatr 155:224–229

Storlazzi E, Vintzileos AM, Campbell WA, Nochimson DJ, Weinbaum PJ (1987) Ultrasonic diagnosis of discordant fetal growth in twin gestations. Obstet Gynecol 69:363–367

Townsend R, Simpson GF, Filly RA (1988) Membrane thickness in ultrasound prediction of chorionicity of twin gestations. J Ultrasound Med 7:327–332

Van Allen MI, Smith DW, Shepart TH (1983) Twin reversed arterial perfusion (TRAP) sequence: a study of 14 twin pregnancies with acardius. Semin Perinatol 7:285–293

Ville Y (1997) Monochorionic twin pregnancies: «les liaisons dangereuses». Ultrasound Obstet Gynecol 10:82–85

Watson WJ, Harlass FE, Menard MK, McCurdy CM, Brady K, Miller RC (1995) Sonographic assessment of amniotic fluid in normal twin pregnancy. Am J Perinatol 12:122–124

Weissman A, Achiron R, Lipitz S, Blickstein I, Mashiach S (1994) The first-trimester growth-discordant twin: an ominous prenatal finding. Obstet Gynecol 84:110–114

Wenstrom KD, Syrop CH, Hammit DG, Van Voorhis BJ (1993) Increased risk of monochorionic twinning associated with assisted reproduction. Fertil Steril 60:510–514

Winn HN, Gabrielli S, Reece EA, Roberts JA, Salafia C, Hobbins JC (1989) Ultrasonographic criteria for the prenatal diagnosis of placenta chorionicity in twin gestations. Am J Obstet Gynecol 161:1540–1542

Yoshida K, Matayoshi K (1990) A study on prognosis of surviving cotwin. Acta Genet Med Gemellol 39:383–388

Zalar RW Jr (1996) Transvaginal ultrasound and preterm prelabor: a nonrandomized intervention study. Obstet Gynecol 88:20–23

11 Ultrasound and Perinatal Infection

CATHERINE DONNER, FRANÇOISE RYPENS, FRED E. AVNI

CONTENTS

11.1 Introduction 245
11.2 Sonographic Findings 246
11.2.1 CNS Findings 246
11.2.1.1 Ventriculomegaly
11.2.1.2 Intracranial Calcifications 246
11.2.1.3 Microcephaly 246
11.2.1.4 Gyration Anomalies 247
11.2.2 Visceral Signs 247
11.2.2.1 Cardiac Abnormalities 247
11.2.2.2 Hepatomegaly and Splenomegaly 247
11.2.2.3 Effusions and Hydrops 248
11.2.2.4 Intra-abdominal Calcifications
 and Hyperechoic Bowel 248
11.2.3 Placental Anomalies 249
11.2.4 Abnormalities of Amniotic Fluid Volume 249
11.2.5 Intrauterine Growth Restriction 249
11.3 Specific Congenital Infections
 and Sonographic Evaluation 250
11.3.1 Rubella 250
11.3.2 Toxoplasmosis 251
11.3.3 Cytomegalovirus 251
11.3.4 Parvovirus B19 252
11.3.5 Varicella zoster Virus 253
11.4 Antenatal Diagnosis and Fetal Sampling 253
11.5 Conclusion 254
 References 254

C. DONNER, MD, PhD
Department of Obstetrics and Gynecology, Erasme Hospital, Route de Lennick 808, 1070 Brussels, Belgium
F. RYPENS, MD
Department of Medical Imaging, Sainte Justine Hospital, 3175 Côte Sainte Catherine, Montréal, Québec H3T 1C5, Canada
F.E. AVNI, MD, PhD
Department of Pediatric Imaging, University Children's Hospital Queen Fabiola, Avenue J. J. Crocq 15, 1020 Brussels, Belgium

11.1
Introduction

The management of the patient at risk for fetal infection is still challenging and often controversial.

The diagnosis of fetal infection was historically made at birth in the presence of an association of neonatal sequelae and maternal disease. Rubella was the first observed congenital infection diagnosed by culture and IgM detection in the blood of the neonate. This evaluation was not entirely reliable as IgM is not always present in congenital infection, neonates are not always symptomatic at birth and maternal disease in usually asymptomatic. In the majority of cases, fetal infection is due to a virus but bacteria, protozoans, helminths and fungi can also be responsible.

The fetus can become infected via ascending or transcervical and transplacental routes. Infection via the ascending route results in chorioamnionitis and the causal agents are usually bacteria. Infection via the placental route, however is habitually viral, from infectious agents present in the maternal blood. Fetal vulnerability varies with gestational age and maturation of the organ systems. The effects of viral infections on the fetus include abortion, stillbirth, physical defects, growth deficit and physiological dysfunction. The intrauterine infection may result in continuing postnatal damage because of persistence of the virus in infants organs. Nowadays, viruses can be detected by polymerase chain reaction (PCR). This method is usually more sensitive than culture or IgM detection.

Advanced ultrasound technology has added to clinical ability in the diagnosis of fetal infection by permitting the observation of signs associated with infection and fetal sampling (amniotic fluid, fetal blood) under ultrasound guidance. In cases of known fetal infection, the observation of sonographic signs can give important information about its severity. Conversely, ultrasound can suggest fetal infection still unknown.

This chapter reviews the sonographic signs and prenatal management of prenatal infection.

11.2
Sonographic Findings

Several sonographic (US) findings can indicate fetal
infection. The most frequent observations are associated with central nervous system (CNS) lesions,
cardiac abnormalities, effusions, parenchymal calcifications, abnormalities in amniotic fluid volume, placental enlargement and intrauterine growth restriction (IUGR).

In a recent work (WEINER 1997) the authors systematically searched for infection in fetuses with
sonographic abnormalities on PCR. Viral DNA was
found in 40% of cases (301 fetuses) and in half of
them adenovirus was identified. These results indicate that any US finding could be associated with fetal
infection and that the incidence of viral fetal infection has been underestimated.

11.2.1
CNS Findings

11.2.1.1
Ventriculomegaly

The lateral ventricular measurement is obtained
in an axial plane just above the one used for biparietal diameter at the posterior aspect of the choroid
plexus. This measurement remains nearly constant
at 4–8 mm from 15 weeks to term. The upper limit is
10 mm. Neural tube defect is the most frequent cause
of ventriculomegaly (36%).

In 5% of cases the enlargement is related to fetal
infection, and the figure reaches 10% when ventriculomegaly is isolated (Fig. 11.1a) (VALAT et al. 1998).
This cerebral lesion can result from different mechanisms including cellular death, mitosis inhibition
and inflammatory responses, and can progress to
hydrocephaly or hydranencephaly. Ventriculomegaly
is almost always symmetrical but has been observed
unilaterally in cases of cytomegalovirus (CMV) and
toxoplasmosis infection.

11.2.1.2
Intracranial Calcifications

Fetal intracranial calcifications are consistent with
local cerebral necrosis with secondary calcification.
The lesions are not specific to fetal infections. Periventricular hyperechoic foci are characteristic of fetal
intracranial calcifications. These are small, isolated
or grouped together (Fig. 11.1b) and do not exhibit

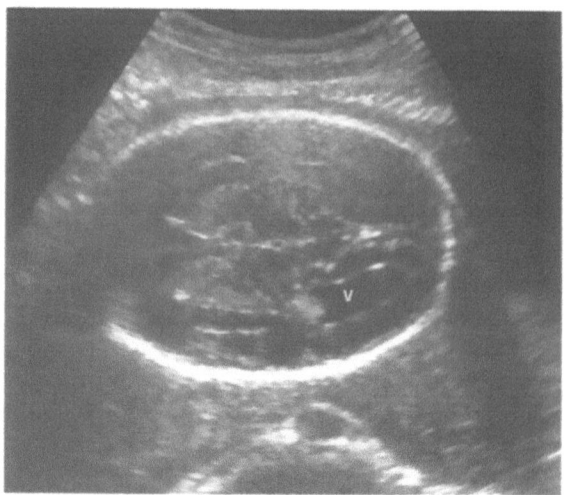

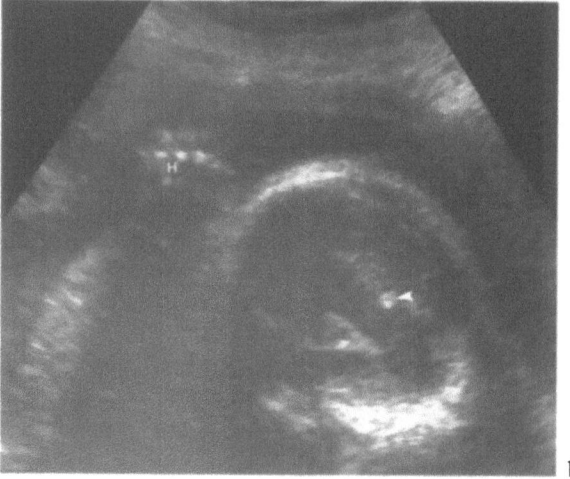

Fig. 11.1a, b. Toxoplasmosis. End of second trimester. **a** Ventriculomegaly. Transverse scan of the fetal head. The width of
the lateral ventricle (*v*) is 15 mm. **b** Intracranial calcification.
Oblique sagittal view of the fetal brain. A hyperechoic focus is
visible (*arrowhead*) in the parieto-occipital area. *h* hand

acoustic shadowing. They are difficult to demonstrate
during the antenatal period but are easier to visualize postnatally (Fig. 11.2). In a 1995 review on US
signs and congenital toxoplasmosis, intracranial calcifications were seen antenatally in only 44% of cases
diagnosed during the neonatal period (ABBOUD et al.
1995). The main differential diagnosis includes periventricular hamartoma in cases of tuberous sclerosis.

11.2.1.3
Microcephaly

Microcephaly corresponds to a cerebral circumference below the 3rd centile for gestational age. The

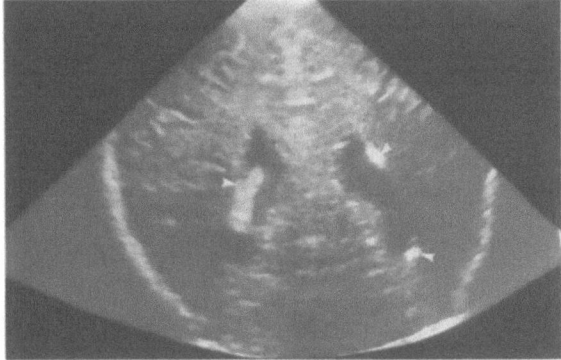

Fig. 11.2. Toxoplasmosis. Periventricular calcifications. Postnatal transfontanellar ultrasound. Coronal view. Several hyperechoic foci (*arrowheads*) are visible in the periventricular areas

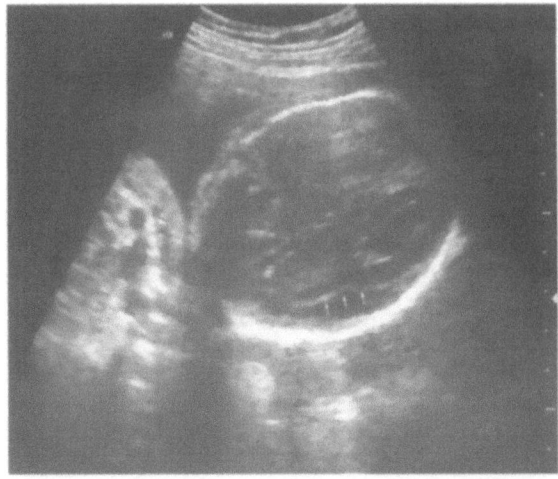

a

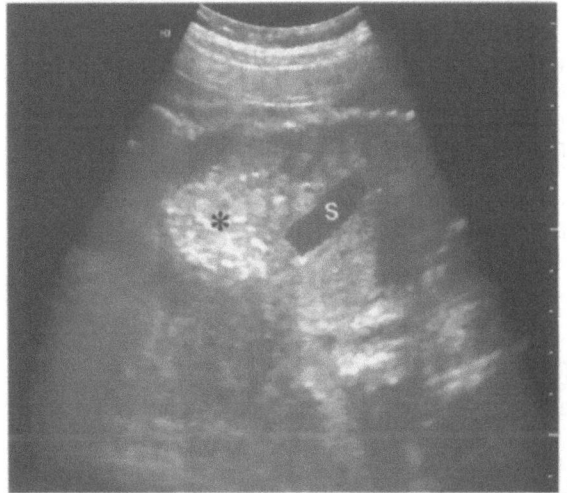

b

Fig. 11.3a, b. CMV. End of second trimester. **a** Gyration anomalies. Transverse scan of the fetal head. Abnormal operculation of the sylvian fissure (*arrows*). **b** Hyperechoic intestinal loops (***). Sagittal scan of the fetal trunk. *S* stomach

biparietal diameter is a less reliable measurement as variations may depend on the skull shape. It can result from a significant reduction of the brain mass as has been reported in CMV, rubella, herpes simplex congenital infection and, less frequently, in toxoplasmosis. Viral infection clearly affects the growth of brain and cerebellum.

11.2.1.4
Gyration Anomalies

Gyration anomalies can result from an infection occurring during the early second trimester. The cardinal sign is lack of operculization of the sylvian fissure (Fig. 11.3a). Anomalies can be confirmed by fetal MR imaging (Fig. 11.4a).

11.2.2
Visceral Signs

11.2.2.1
Cardiac Abnormalities

Cardiomegaly is the most frequent cardiac anomaly encountered in congenital infection, especially in CMV fetal infection (Fig. 11.5). It can be quantified by measuring the cardiothoracic ratio (CTR). The CTR, which is the cardiac circumference divided by the chest circumference, can be obtained at the level of the four-chamber view. This ratio is fairly constant throughout pregnancy, from 0.45 at 17 weeks' gestation to 0.5 at term.

Myocarditis and pericardial effusion can be observed in parvovirus B19 infection (Fig. 11.6a). In congenital rubella infection, structural cardiac anomalies such as ventricular and atrial septal defects, pulmonary artery stenosis and coarctation of the aorta are common findings when maternal infection occurs during the first trimester of pregnancy.

11.2.2.2
Hepatomegaly and Splenomegaly

Hepatomegaly can be recognized by a shift to the left of the umbilical vein in its intra-abdominal portion or from a longitudinal measurement of the liver from the dome of the right hemidiaphragm to the tip of the right lobe (VINTZILEOS et al. 1985).

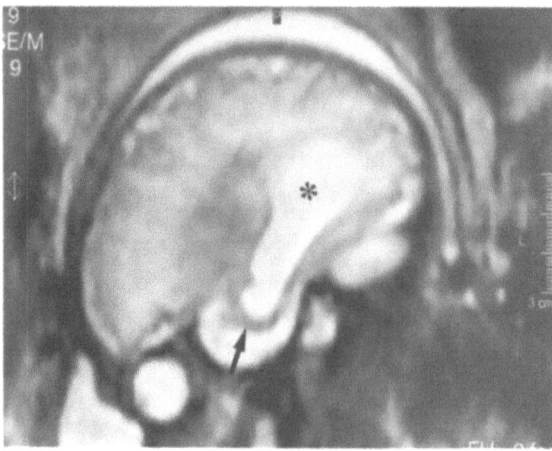

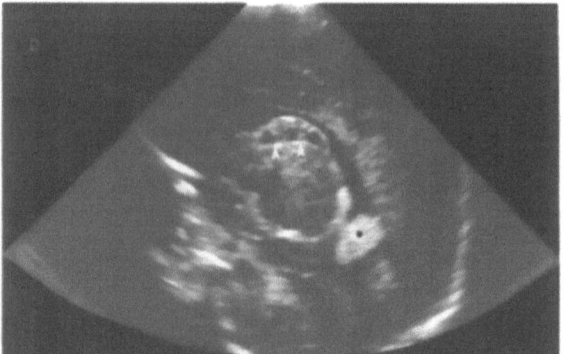

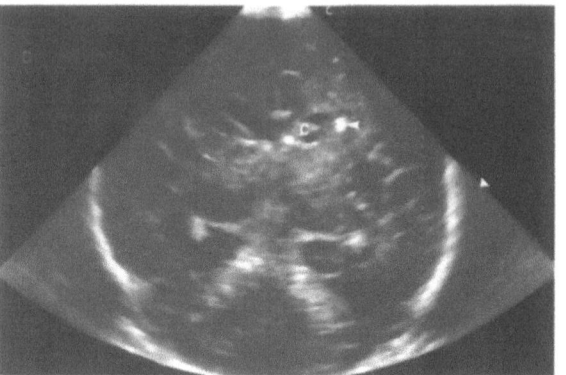

Fig. 11.4a–c. CMV. Third trimester. **a** In utero. Fetal MR imaging, T2-weighted sequence. Parasagittal scan. The ventriculomegaly (*) is associated with gyration anomalies of the temporal lobe surface (*arrow*). **b** Postnatal head US. Sagittal view. Subependymal necrotic cysts (*arrowheads*). *Asterisk* indicates the choroid plexus. **c** Postnatal head US. Coronal view. A left periventricular calcification is visible (*arrowhead*). *c* subependymal cysts

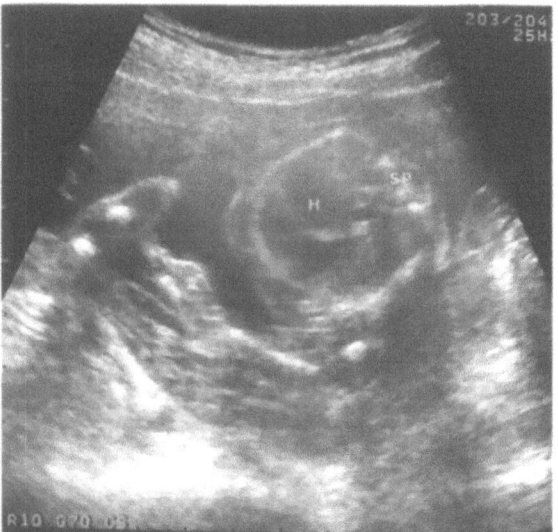

Fig. 11.5. CMV. Second trimester. Cardiomegaly. Transverse scan of the fetal chest. The heart (*H*) is markedly enlarged and occupies more than two thirds of the chest. *SP* spine

The splenic circumference is measured behind the stomach at the level of the transverse abdominal section (OEPKES et al. 1993). Hepatosplenomegaly has been reported in all congenital infections but is often a transient finding (Fig. 11.7).

11.2.2.3
Effusions and Hydrops

Ascites may also be present, pleural and pericardial effusions have been observed and evolution to fetal hydrops is possible (Fig. 11.6b, c). All these visceral signs can regress spontaneously (ABBOUD et al. 1995).

11.2.2.4
Intra-abdominal Calcifications and Hyperechoic Bowel

Intrahepatic calcifications are a classical but non-specific sign of fetal infection. Intra-abdominal fetal calcifications can be found in various locations, including the peritoneal surface, intestinal lumen and organ parenchyma. Hyperechoic bowel appears in the inferior part of the fetal abdomen with an echogenicity similar to that of bone (Fig. 11.3b). This image has been associated with chromosomal anomalies, cystic fibrosis, IUGR, fetal infection and may also correspond to a normal variant. Among 182 cases of hyperechoic bowel during the second and third trimester studied recently, seven congenital infections were diagnosed (3.8%). This result could, however, have been an underestimate as viral DNA was not searched

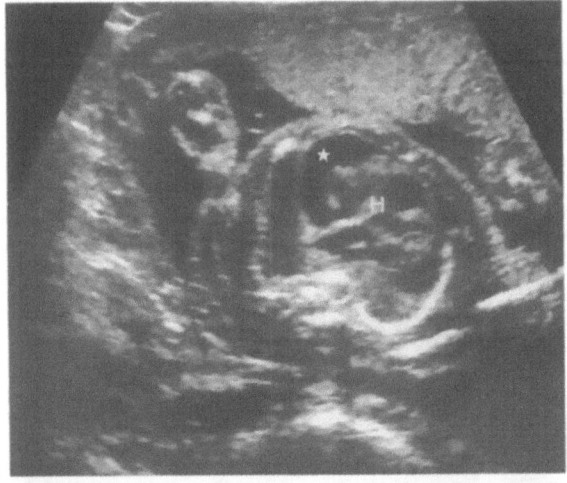

a

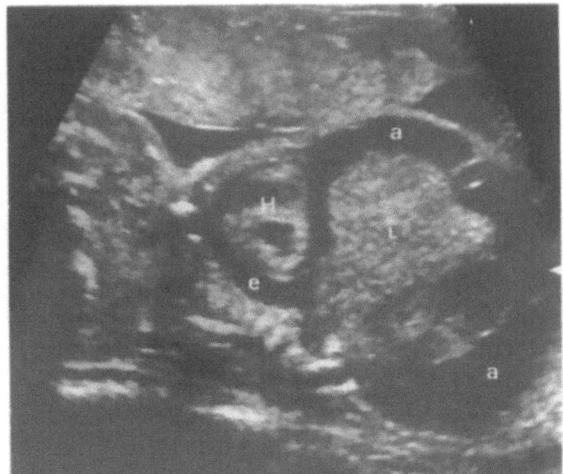

b

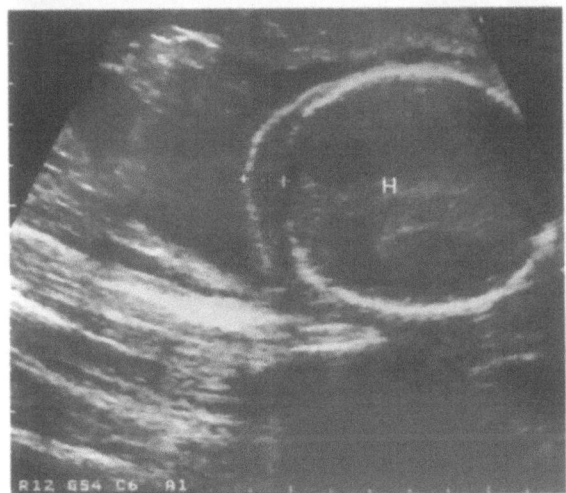

c

Fig. 11.6a–c. CMV. Second trimester. Fetal hydrops and effusions. **a** Massive pericardial effusion (*) seen on a transverse scan of the fetal chest. *H* heart. **b** Pleural effusions (*e*) and abdominal ascites (*a*). Sagittal scan of the fetal trunk. *H* heart, *L* liver. **c** Nuchal soft tissue thickening (7 mm between crosses). Transverse scan of the fetal head (*H*)

for systematically (MULLER et al. 1995). Among the infected fetuses, CMV was the most frequent virus.

11.2.3
Placental Anomalies

Maternal infection and viremia can cause placentitis. Among placental lesions necrosis, edema and thrombosis are common. Abnormally large and abnormally small placentae have both been observed in intrauterine infections. The placenta appears thicker and more echogenic (Fig. 11.8). Placental "size" is assessed subjectively; measurement standardization has been attempted without success (CRINO 1999). Fetal lesions can be the consequence of an infectious agent in fetal tissue but also of placental insufficiency. Fetal vulnerability depends on gestational age but the presence of placental infection does not result in fetal sequelae in all cases.

11.2.4
Abnormalities of Amniotic Fluid Volume

Polyhydramnios and oligohydramnios have been associated with congenital infection. The amniotic fluid index (AFI) is the most commonly criterion to assess the quantity of amniotic fluid. The AFI is defined as the sum of the measurements of the largest fluid pocket in each of the four quadrants of the uterus (PHELAN et al. 1987). The nomogram for each gestational age has been published (MOORE and CAYLE 1990).

11.2.5
Intrauterine Growth Restriction

IUGR has been defined as a birth weight less than the 10th centile. During the antenatal period, the criterion most often used is abdominal circumference

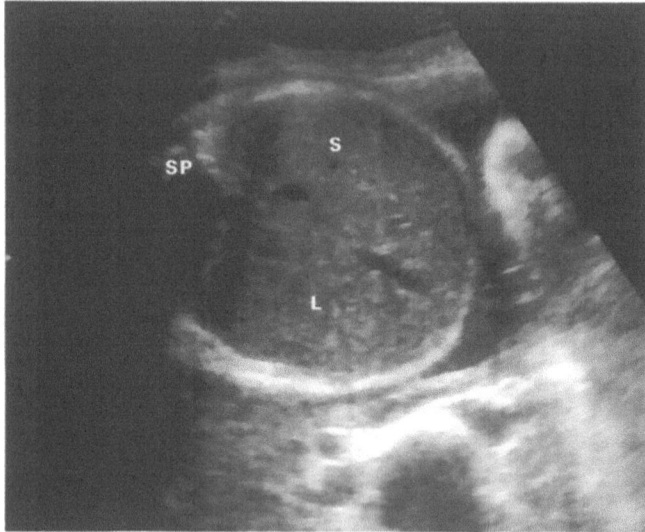

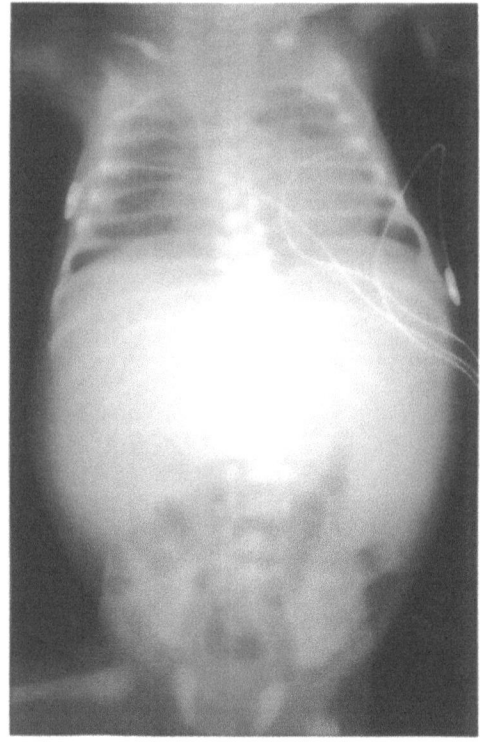

Fig. 11.7a, b. CMV. Hepatosplenomegaly. **a** In utero third trimester. Transverse scan of the fetal abdomen. Enlarged liver (*L*) and spleen (*S*). *SP* spine. **b** At birth. The babygram confirms the hepatosplenomegaly

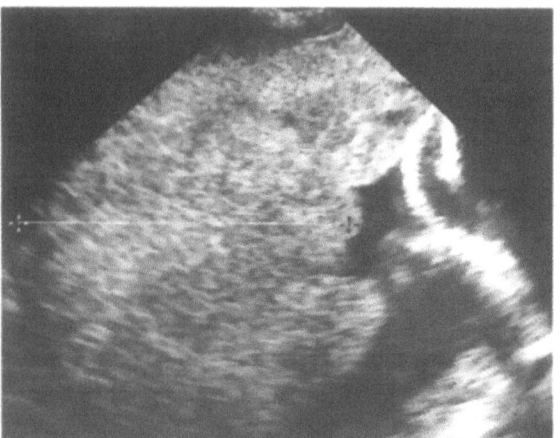

Fig. 11.8. Placentomegaly. Case of varicella. Third trimester. Thickened (6 cm between *crosses*) and hyperechoic placenta. Fetal hydrops (not shown) was also present

less than the 5th centile. Severe IUGR in cases of fetal infection is due to a reduction of the growth potential (cell death, mitosis inhibition, etc.), multisystemic involvement and/or placental insufficiency. In some cases, the Doppler flow measurement can be abnormal, showing increased vascular resistance which can result in fetal hypoxia and acidosis. Peri-

natal infections may affect any organ but the CNS is particularly vulnerable.

11.3
Specific Congenital Infections and Sonographic Evaluation

Although infection semiology in fetal infection is highly variable, certain specific signs can suggest one or another infectious agent.

11.3.1
Rubella

In 1941, maternal rubella infection was for the first time associated with congenital cataract. Vaccination was introduced in 1969. Congenital rubella is thus rare in modern obstetrics, with an incidence of less than 1/100,000 live births in the USA (COOPER et al. 1995). Few cases diagnosed antenatally by US have been reported, though specific signs associated with rubella such as microcephaly, cardiac malformation, cataract and ventriculomegaly would be detectable by obstetrical US.

11.3.2
Toxoplasmosis

The risk of congenital infection increases with gestational age, being the lowest during the first trimester of pregnancy (1–10%), higher during the second trimester (10–25%) and highest when maternal infection occurs during the third trimester (60–90%) (JEFFREY et al. 2001). However, the severity of the fetal disease is worse when infection is acquired in the first trimester.

The most frequent manifestations of congenital toxoplasmosis are hydrocephaly, chorioretinitis and intracranial calcifications (Fig. 11.1). The timing of the appearance of ventriculomegaly after maternal seroconversion is variable and may be rapidly progressive. Inflammatory lesions may develop in the brain parenchyma and areas of necrosis develop. This type of lesion is best assessed by fetal MR imaging (Fig. 11.10). Hydrocephaly is far more frequent than other lesions, being present in 78% of fetuses with one or more sonographic abnormality. Inflammatory changes can be associated with the ventriculomegaly and produce a thick hyperechoic ependyma (Fig. 11.9).

In our center, the following data were obtained: in 185 pregnancies with maternal seroconversion, 17 fetuses were infected (9.2%). Among these, seven (41%) had sonographic signs, of which six (85%) presented ventriculomegaly or hydrocephaly.

The frequency of abnormal US signs diminishes with gestational age at the time of maternal seroconversion (58% in the first trimester, 22% in the second trimester,

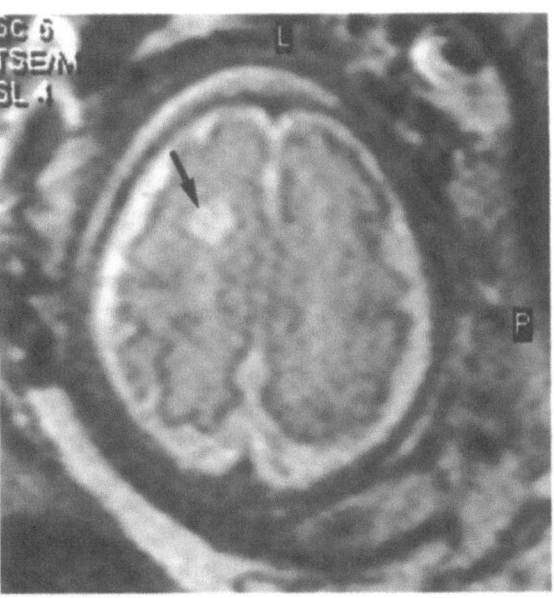

Fig. 11.10. Toxoplasmosis. Porencephalic cavity. Third trimester. Fetal MR imaging, T2-weighted sequence. A hyperintense porencephalic cavity is visualized within the frontal lobe parenchyma (*arrow*)

6% in the third trimester) (ABBOUD et al. 1995). The appearance of cerebral sequelae provides evidence of severe and irreversible fetal disease. Moreover normal cerebral sonographic findings do not guarantee the integrity of cerebral tissue (HOHLFELD et al.1991).

Ventriculomegaly and brain calcifications are the most common signs in cases of toxoplasmosis.

11.3.3
Cytomegalovirus

With an incidence of 0.2–2.2% of live births, CMV infection is the most frequent congenital infection worldwide (ENDERS et al. 2001). It is a common cause of deafness and intellectual function impairment. Ninety percent of congenitally infected newborns are asymptomatic at birth, but 5–17% will develop symptoms, usually during the first 2 years of life. Among the 10% of symptomatic newborns, 20% will die and 90% of the survivors will develop severe sequelae.

The most frequent sonographic anomalies encountered are ventriculomegaly (Fig. 11.4), IUGR, intracranial calcifications, oligohydramnios, hyperechoic bowel (Fig. 11.3b), hepatosplenomegaly (Fig. 11.7), cardiomegaly (Fig. 11.5), ascites and hydrops. Intracranial calcifications affect particularly the thalamostriated vessels – producing the so-called candlestick appearance on US (Fig. 11.11a) – and the pericallosal

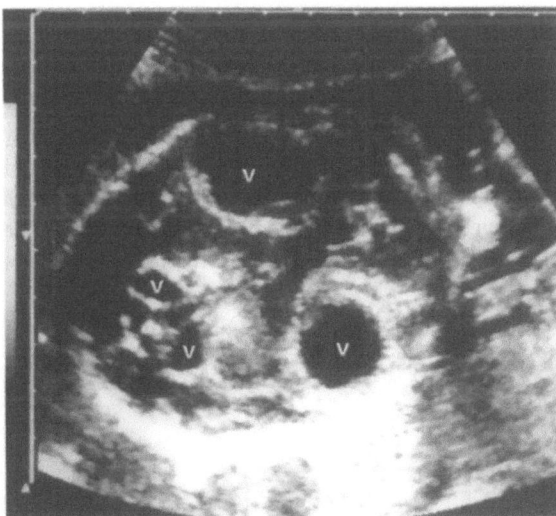

Fig. 11.9. Toxoplasmosis-related ventriculitis Third trimester. Transverse scan of the fetal head. Dilated ventricles (*v*) with hyperechoic thick ventricular walls

artery (Fig. 11.11b). Rapidly evolving subependymal necrosis is also typical, though it might be difficult to visualize in utero (Fig. 11.11a). Calcifications and subependymal cysts are easier to demonstrate after birth (Fig. 11.4b, c). Very rarely, the kidneys may be affected ; they will appear with a cortical hyperechogenicity. Moderate renal failure developing after birth may ensue (Fig. 11.12).

Since 1986 in our center, 237 pregnancies at risk for congenital CMV infection have been investigated, and 55 fetuses were found to be infected. Among them 14 (25%) had sonographic signs (3 hydrocephaly, 2 microcephaly, 4 IUGR, 5 hyperechogenic bowel) (Liesnard et al.2000). Major cerebral abnormalities were found in five of 55 infected fetuses (9%). All abnormal cerebral signs appeared when maternal seroconversion occurred before 20 weeks gestation. Abnormal US findings in combination with a positive

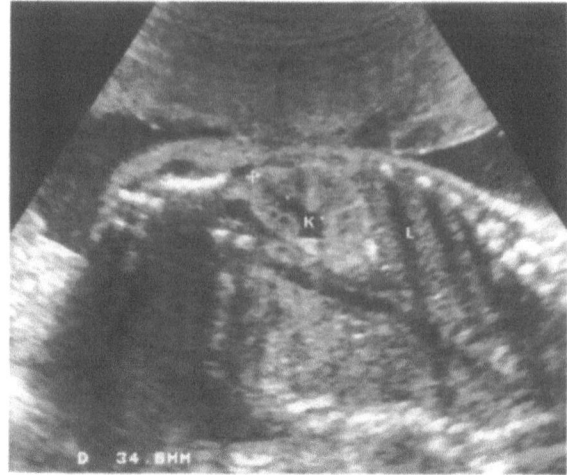

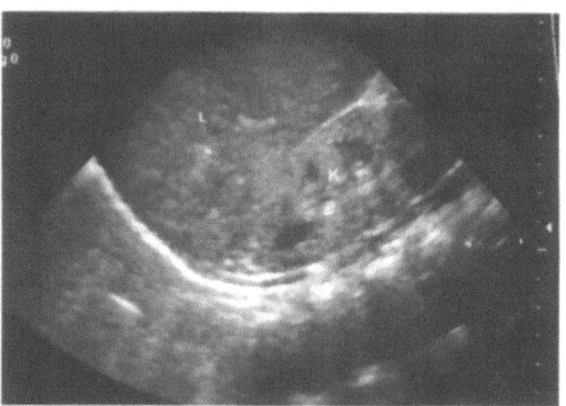

Fig. 11.12a, b. CMV. Kidney involvement. a In utero, Third trimester. Sagittal scan of fetal abdomen. Hyperechogenicity of the renal cortex. *L* liver, *K* kidney (between *crosses*). b Postnatally (moderate renal failure was present). Persistently hyperechoic renal cortex. *L* liver, *K* kidney

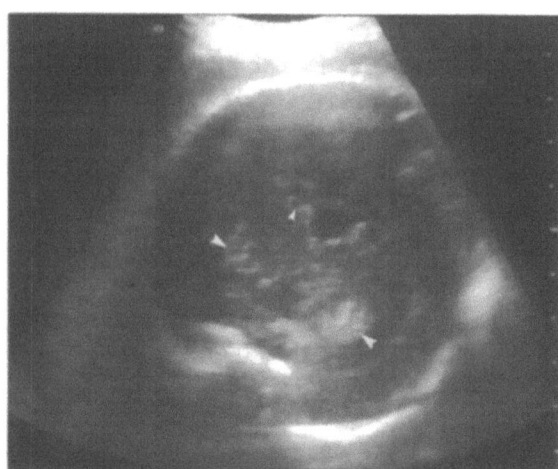

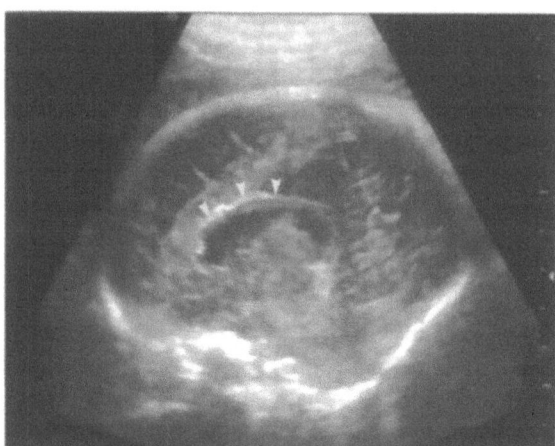

Fig. 11.11a, b. CMV. Cranial lesions. a Frontal view of the fetal head. Bilateral calcified thalamo-striated vessels ("candlestick appearance") (*large arrowheads*) and subependymal necrotic cysts (*small arrowhead*). b Midsagittal scan demonstrating calcification of the pericallosal artery (*arrowheads*)

antenatal diagnosis of congenital CMV infection by amniotic fluid and fetal blood sampling is a marker of poor fetal prognosis. However, fetal lesions may appear very late during pregnancy, and thus serial examinations are recommended (Enders et al. 2001). Moreover, as for toxoplasmosis, not all sequelae of congenital infection are detectable by antenatal sonography.

CMV affects every organ; CNS lesions are predictive of outcome; some lesions are easier to visualize after birth.

11.3.4
Parvovirus B19

Parvovirus B19 is known as the "fifth disease" in children (producing erythema, arthralgia) and can cause anemia in adults. Classically, this infection is not associated with congenital malformations. Fetal infection can lead to no consequences, miscarriage during the first half of pregnancy or severe fetal anemia with possible hydrops (Fig. 11.6) and fetal death (3–6% of pregnancies with maternal infection) (LEVY et al. 1997). Eight to ten percent of cases of non-immune hydrops are due to parvovirus fetal infection. The appearance of hydrops is the result of both anemia and some degree of fetal myocarditis. In the majority of cases, the fetus heals spontaneously. Follow-up should be continued for 12 weeks after diagnosis of maternal infection. In cases of mild hydrops, a conservative approach should be adopted; at any signs of worsening and fetal distress, cordocentesis should be proposed after 20 weeks of gestation. Eighty cases of intrauterine fetal transfusion have been reported in the literature (LEVY et al.1997) with a survival rate of 77%. In all cases the hemoglobin level was less than 8 g/100 ml. Additional cases of intrauterine transfusion have been reported more recently with a successful outcome in 83.8% (SCHILD et al. 1999, KAILASAM et al. 2001).

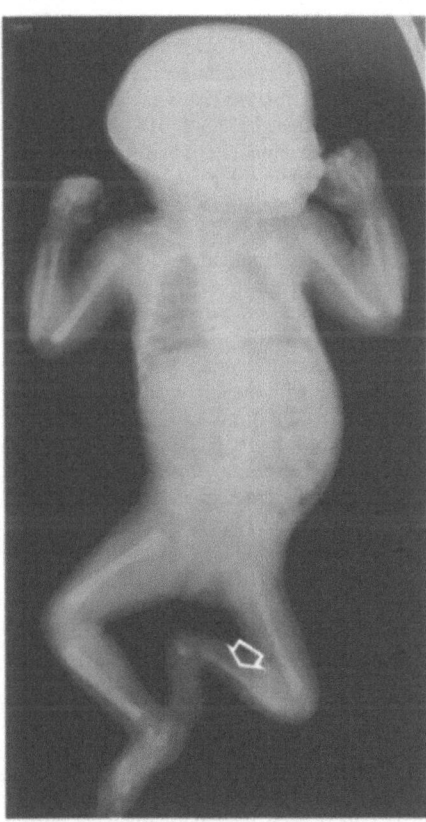

Fig. 11.13. Varicella zoster infection. Babygram at birth demonstrates lytic destruction of the left fibula and tibia. (The baby was covered with typical vesicles. The mother had developed hepatitis of unknown origin during pregnancy)

11.3.5
Varicella zoster Virus

The incidence of varicella is estimated to be from 1 to 7/10,000 pregnancies and the rate of fetal transmission around 25%. Fetal infection can cause miscarriage, in utero death or severe embryopathy. The risk of fetal disease before 20 weeks' gestation is estimated at 2% (ENDERS et al. 1994). Antenatal diagnosis is possible by amniocentesis and subsequent search for viral infection by PCR. Cordocentesis can also be proposed and the presence of specific IgM antibodies revealed (PETIGNAT et al. 2001). However, US is the best indicator of severe fetal disease. In 1992 (PRETORIUS et al. 1992), 37 cases of maternal varicella before 20 weeks gestation were reviewed. Five fetuses had abnormal sonographic findings (limb deformities (Fig. 11.13), cerebral ventriculomegaly, parenchymal liver calcifications, hydrops, hepatomegaly, hydramnios). None of the 32 other infants had any sequelae. US examination efficacy has, however, to be viewed with caution as in some cases the lesions are solely ocular, skin scarring or even neurological.

11.4
Antenatal Diagnosis and Fetal Sampling

Antenatal sampling can be proposed when there is US evidence suggesting fetal infection or when maternal serological tests show seroconversion during pregnancy. Present procedures available are amniocentesis and cordocentesis under US guidance. Amniotic fluid and blood sampling permit the search for specific and non-specific signs of fetal infection (DAFFOS et al. 1988). Non-specific signs include an increase in leukocytes, thrombopenia and abnormal hepatic tests. Specific signs are the presence of IgM, IgA, DNA seen on PCR and virus found by culture. The sensitivity of antenatal diagnosis is variable depending on the technique and from one team to another (PRALONG et al. 1998). This factor, the absence of fetal therapy or not and the inherent risk of invasive procedures, make the management of pregnancies at risk for congenital infection difficult and controversial. In our experience and that of others (DAFFOS et al. 1988, DONNER et al. 1994) the risk of fetal loss after cordocentesis in these pregnancies is 0.2–0.5%.

11.5
Conclusion

The utility of sonography for investigating pregnancies at risk for fetal infection has been demonstrated, although limiting factors have to be taken into account. A normal US examination in an infected fetus does not guarantee absence of fetal lesions. Some lesions can be seen only months or even years after birth. Some lesions diagnosed by US can have a pejorative evolution or on the contrary can regress spontaneously, emphasizing the need for repeat US. The high rate of therapeutic abortion after diagnosis of fetal infection restricts the correlation between sonographic signs and the severity of the disease. More cases must be studied to improve knowledge of the natural history of congenital diseases. The need for antiviral therapy in congenitally infected fetuses is obvious. Further studies on antiviral agents in congenitally infected infants are needed to determine the potential benefit of drugs such as ganciclovir for CMV. Prenatal therapy with nontoxic antiviral drugs or immunoglobulins should be considered and studied.

References

Abboud A, Horika G, Saniez D, Gabriel R, Bednarezyk F, Chemk C, Quereux C (1995) Signes échographiques de la foetopathie toxoplasmique. J Gynecol Biol Reprod 24:733–738

Achiron R, Yagel S, Rotstein Z, Inbar O, Mashiach S, Lipitz S (1997) Cerebral lateral ventricular asymmetry: is this a normal ultrasonographic finding in the fetal brain? Obstet Gynecol 89:233–237

Cazenave J, Forestier F, Bessières M, Broussin B, Begueret J (1992) Contribution of a new PCR assay to the prenatal diagnosis of congenital toxoplasmosis. Prenat Diagn 12:119–127

Cooper LZ (2001) Current lessons from 20th century serosurveillance data on rubella. Clin Infect Dis 33:1287

Crino JP (1999) Ultrasound and fetal diagnosis of prenatal infection. Clinical Obstet Gynecol 42:71–80

Daffos F, Forestier F, Cappella-Pavlovsky M, Thulliez P, Aufrant C, Valenti C, Cox W (1988) Prenatal management of 746 pregnancies at risk for congenital toxoplasmosis. N Engl J Med 318:217–225

Donner C, Liesnard C, Content J, Busine A, Aderca J, Rodesch F (1993) Prenatal diagnosis of 52 pregnancies at risk for congenital cytomegalovirus infection. Obstet Gynecol 82:481–486

Donner C, Liesnard C, Brancart F, Rodesch F (1994) Accuracy of amniotic fluid testing before 21 weeks' gestation in perinatal diagnosis of congenital cytomegalovirus infection. Prenat Diagn 14:1055–1059

Enders G, Miller E, Cradock-Watson J, Bolley I, Ridehaigh M (1994) Consequences of varicella and herpes zoster in pregnancy: prospective study of 1739 cases. Lancet 343:1548–1551

Enders G, Bader U, Lindeman L, Schalasta G, Daiminger A (2001) Prenatal diagnosis of congenital cytomegalovirus infection in 189 pregnancies with known outcome. Prenat Diagn 21:362–377

Hohlfeld P, Aleese D, Cappella-Pavlovsky M, Giovangrandi Y, Thulliez P, Forestier F, et al (1991) Fetal toxoplasmosis: ultrasonographic signs. Ultrasound Obstet Gynecol 1:241–244

Jeffrey L, Lopez A, Wilson M, Schulkin J, Gibbs R (2001) Congenital toxoplasmosis: a review. Obstet Gynecol Surv 56:296–305

Jones J, Lopez A, Wilson M, Schulkin J, Gibbs R (2001) Congenital toxoplasmosis: a review. Obstet Gynecol Surv 56:296–305

Kailasam C, Brennand J, Cameron A (2001) Congenital parvovirus B19 infection: experience of a recent epidemic. Fetal Diagn Ther 16:18–22

Levy R, Weissman A, Blombery G, Hagay Z (1997) Infection by parvovirus B19 during pregnancy: a review. Obstet Gynecol Surv 52:254–259

Liesnard C, Donner C, Brancart F, Gosselin F, Delforge ML (2000) Prenatal diagnosis of congenital cytomegalovirus infection: prospective study of 237 pregnancies at risk. Obstet Gynecol 95: 881–888

Moore TR, Cayle JE (1990) The amniotic fluid index in normal human pregnancy. Am J Obstet Gynecol 162:1168–1173

Muller F, Dommergues M, Aubry MC, Simon-Bouy B, Gautier E, Oury J, Narcy, F. (1995) Hyperechogenic fetal bowel: an ultrasonographic marker for adverse fetal and neonatal outcome. Am J Obstet Gynecol 173:508–513

Oepkes D, Meerman R, Vandenbussche F, Van Kamp I, Kok F, Kanhai H (1993) Ultrasonographic fetal spleen measurements in red blood cell-alloimmunized pregnancies. Am J Obstet Gynecol 169:121–128

Petignat P, Vial Y, Laurini R, Hohlfeld P (2001) Fetal varicella-herpes zoster syndrome in early pregnancy: ultrasonographic and morphological correlation. Prenat Diagn 21:121–124

Phelan JP, Smith CV, Broussard P, Small M (1987) Amniotic fluid volume assessment with the four-quadrant technique at 36–42 weeks' gestation. J Reprod Med 32:540–542

Pralong F, Boulot P, Villena I, Issert E, Tamby I, et al (1998) Antenatal diagnosis of congenital toxoplasmosis: evaluation of the biological parameters in a cohort of 286 patients. Br J Obstet Gynaecol 130:552–557

Pretorius D, Hayward I, Jones K, et al (1992) Sonographic evaluation of pregnancies with maternal varicella infection. J Ultrasound Med 11:459–463

Schild RL, Bald R, Eis-Hubinger AM, Enders G, Hansmann M (1999) Intrauterine management of fetal parvovirus B19 infection. Ultrasound Obstet Gynecol 13: 161–166

Valat A, Dehouck M, Dufour P, Dubos J, Djebara A, Dewisma L, Robert Y, Puech F (1998) Ventriculomégalie cérébrale foetale. J Gynecol Obstet Biol Reprod 27:782–789

Vintzileos A, Neckles S, Campbell W, Andreoli J, Kaplan B, Nochinson D (1985) Fetal liver measurements during normal pregnancy. Obstet Gynecol 66:477–480

Weiner C (1997) The elusive search for fetal infection. Obstet Gynecol Clin North Am 24:19–32

12 Fetal Chromosomal Anomalies

Fred E. Avni, Judy Estroff, Anne Massez, Nicole Vanregemorter

CONTENTS

12.1	Indications and Techniques	255
12.2	Chromosomal Anomalies	255
12.2.1	First Trimester	255
12.2.2	Trisomy 21 (Down's Syndrome)	256
12.2.2.1	Major Structural Anomalies	257
12.2.2.2	Minor Structural Anomalies	257
12.2.3	Trisomy 18 (Edwards' Syndrome)	261
12.2.3.1	Craniofacial Anomaly	262
12.2.3.2	Cardiovascular System	262
12.2.3.3	Abdomen	262
12.2.3.4	Skeletal System	262
12.2.3.5	Umbilical Cord	262
12.2.4	Trisomy 13 (Patau's Syndrome)	262
12.2.5	Sex Chromosomes	262
12.2.6	Other Chromosome Anomalies	263
12.3	Conclusion	265
	References	265

12.1
Indications and Techniques

A chromosomal anomaly is estimated to occur in 1/156 pregnancies. Generally it is considered that women above the age of 36 years are at increased risk and should be offered the possibility of a chromosomal analysis. For the others, US plays an important role in the detection of pregnancies at risk (NICO-

LAIDES et al. 1992, SNIJDERS et al. 1995). For instance, the detection during obstetrical US of any major structural anomaly is potentially associated with abnormal chromosomes. This is even more the case in the presence of multiple anomalies. More problematic and controversial is the presence at the US examination of minor structural anomalies; this has prompted the development of scoring systems in order to optimize the obstetrical US conclusions. Other clinical and biological data may help in the decision (see below) (GONEN et al. 1995, SHOHAT et al. 1995).

The technique utilized for the karyotype analysis depends upon the age of the pregnancy. During the first trimester, the karyotype is obtained through a chorionic villous biopsy, during early second trimester through amniotic fluid puncture and during the third trimester through cordocentesis or amniotic fluid puncture (SHERER et al. 1997).

12.2
Chromosomal Anomalies

Trisomy 13, 18 and 21 account for over 65% of all fetuses born with a karyotype anomaly. Anomalies of all other chromosomes have been reported (GONEN et al. 1995).

12.2.1
First Trimester

Measurement of the nuchal translucency in the fetus is now part of the systematic evaluation of first trimester pregnancies. This measurement is best performed on a sagittal view of the fetus. Normally the thickness must be below 3 mm.

There is a strong association between chromosomal anomalies and nuchal thickness equal to or exceeding 3 mm (Fig. 12.1). At 3 mm, there is a 4-fold increase and above 3 mm there is a 29-fold increase in

F. E. Avni, MD, PhD
Department of Pediatric Imaging, University Children's Hospital Queen Fabiola, Avenue J. J. Crocq 15, 1020 Brussels Belgium
J. Estroff, MD
Department of Pediatric Radiology, Children Hospital Medical Center, 300 Longwood Avenue, Boston, MA 02115, USA
A. Massez, MD
Department of Pediatric Imaging, University Clinics of Brussels, Erasme Hospital, Route de Lennick 808, 1070 Brussels, Belgium
N. Vanregemorter, MD
Department of Medical Genetics, University Clinics of Brussels, Erasme Hospital, Route de Lennick 808, 1070 Brussels, Belgium

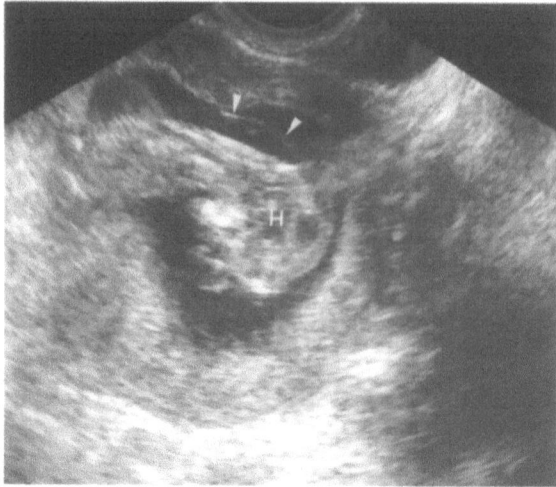 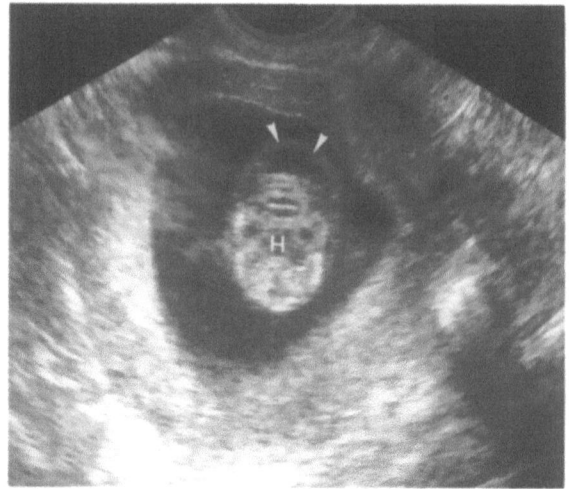

a   b

Fig. 12.1a, b. Nuchal thickening. First trimester. Case of trisomy 21. **a** Sagittal view of the fetus demonstrating abnormal 6 mm thickening of the soft tissues of the neck (*arrowheads*). *H* head. **b** Transverse scan showing the abnormal thickening (*arrowheads*) behind the head (*H*)

chromosomal anomalies. In these pregnancies, a chromosomal analysis should be proposed. The nuchal thickening may resolve spontaneously (Fig. 12.2), but this feature does not exclude chromosomal anomaly.

In fetuses with translucency of 4 mm and above and a normal karyotype there is a high incidence of other defects, especially cardiac anomalies, and poor outcome.

The prognosis can be considered more favorable only in patients in whom chromosomal or structural anomalies have been completely excluded (BRADY et al. 1998, SHERER et al. 1997, PANDYA et al. 1994, SNI-JDERS 2001).

12.2.2
Trisomy 21 (Down's Syndrome)

Trisomy 21 or Down's syndrome is the most frequent chromosomal anomaly observed at birth (1/800) in Western countries. The syndrome includes severe mental retardation and multisystem anomalies (mainly heart and digestive tract malformations). The aim of obstetrical US is to detect those pregnancies at highest risk for the syndrome and to optimize the use of methods allowing the evaluation of the karyotype. During the first trimester, screening is mainly based on the measurement of nuchal trans-

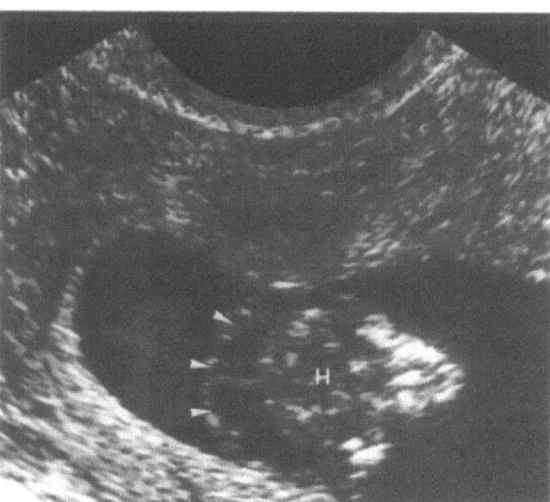 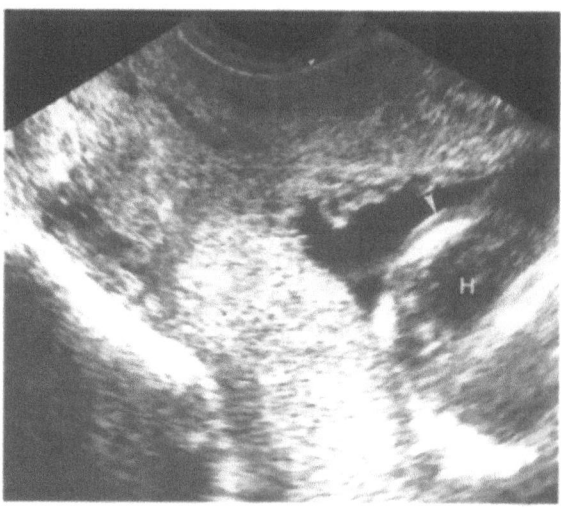

a   b

Fig. 12.2a, b. Spontaneously resolving nuchal thickening. First trimester. Normal karyotype. **a** At 10 weeks LMP there is marked and septated thickening (*arrowheads*). *H* head pole. **b** At 13 weeks the transverse scan shows normal soft tissues (*arrowhead*). *H* fetal head

lucency (see above). During the second trimester, screening is based on the demonstration of major and minor structural anomalies (WLADIMOROFF et al. 1995, RIZZO et al. 1996). Any circumstance (maternal age, triple screening test, etc.) that increases the risk of trisomy should prompt a complete and detailed US examination looking for major and mild anomalies; this analysis constitutes the so-called genetic US. A completely normal examination lowers the risk of chromosomal anomaly by 62–80% (DEVORE 2001, VINTZILEOS et al. 1996, VINTZILEOS et al. 1999).

12.2.2.1
Major Structural Anomalies

Any major structural anomaly should prompt a karyotype analysis; among the many malformations that may occur, fetal soft tissue, heart and digestive tract anomalies are more commonly associated with trisomy 21 (Table 12.1). Fetal hydrops, atrioventricular defects and duodenal atresia are the classical malformations that may be associated with the syndrome (Figs. 12.3, 12.4) (NYBERG et al. 1990, HILL 1996, ROTMENSCH et al. 1997, DICKE and CRANE 1991, GRAUPE et al. 2001).

Table 12.1. Major structural anomalies commonly associated with trisomy 21

| Cystic hygroma |
| Hydrops |
| Ventricular defect |
| Atrial defect |
| Duodenal atresia |
| (Intrauterine growth retardation) |

12.2.2.2
Minor Structural Anomalies

Various US signs have been reported as potential minor signs of trisomy 21 (Table 12.2). The most significant is nuchal thickening above 6 mm in the second trimester. For the others, it seems that when they appear as an isolated finding they are not associated with an increased risk, but when several are present the risk is increased. This has led to the description of a "trisomy scoring index", where any major structural anomaly or nuchal thickening determines a score of 2, any minor anomaly a score of 1; a total of 2 or more is required to indicate the need for a karyotype analysis (BENACERAFF et al. 1994, NYBERG

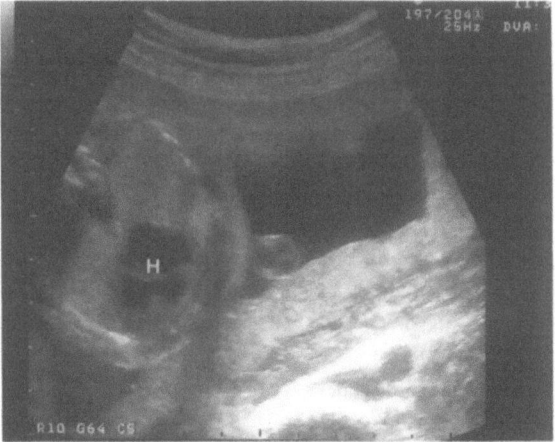
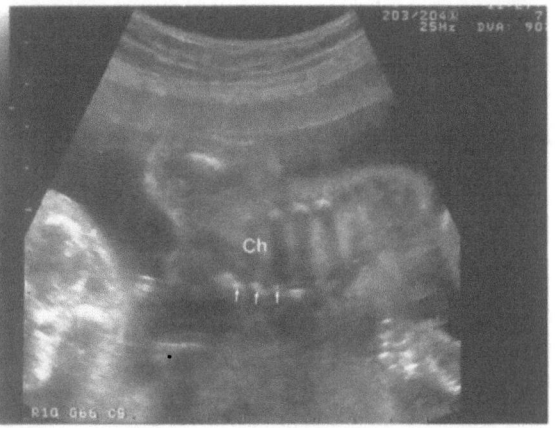

Fig. 12.3a, b. Trisomy 21: major structural defects. Second trimester. **a** Congenital heart disease. Transverse scan of the fetal chest, four-chamber view. Complex atrioventricular malformation. *H* heart. **b** Associated advanced and irregular sternal ossification. Frontal view of the ossified sternum (*arrows*). *Ch* chest

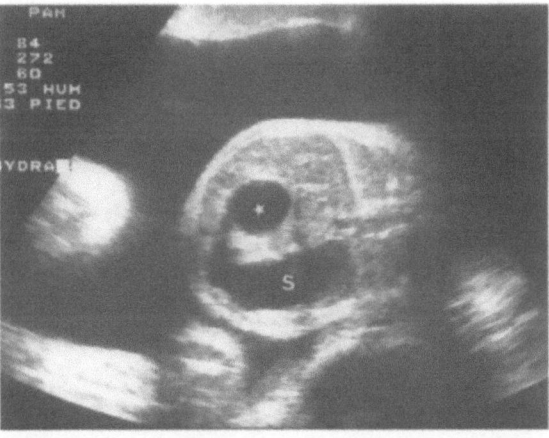

Fig. 12.4. Trisomy 21: major structural anomalies. Duodenal atresia. Third trimester. Transverse scan of the fetal abdomen showing the typical double bubble sign. *S* stomach, * distended duodenal bulb

Table 12.2. US minor signs for trisomy 21 during the second trimester

Nuchal thickening above 6 mm
Shortening of long bones
Pyelectasis
Widening of the iliac wing angle
Hypoplasia of the second phalanx of the fifth digit
"Sandal gap"
Shortening of the nasal bone
Biliary sludge
Echogenic bowel
Echogenic cardiac foci
Mild ventriculomegaly
Frontal lobe hypoplasia

et al. 1990, Vinzileos et al. 1997, Vautier-Rit et al. 2000, Wilkins 1994).

12.2.2.2.1
Nuchal Thickening

Nuchal thickening is measured during the second trimester on a transverse scan of the head that includes the thalami and the posterior fossa; it must be measured from the occipital bone to the margin of the skin. Thickening is significant above 6 mm (Fig. 12.5a). In a general population (risk of trisomy >1/800), nuchal thickening has a sensitivity of 37% and a positive predictive value of 14% (false positive 2.2%) (Grandjean and Saramon 1995, Watson et al. 1994).

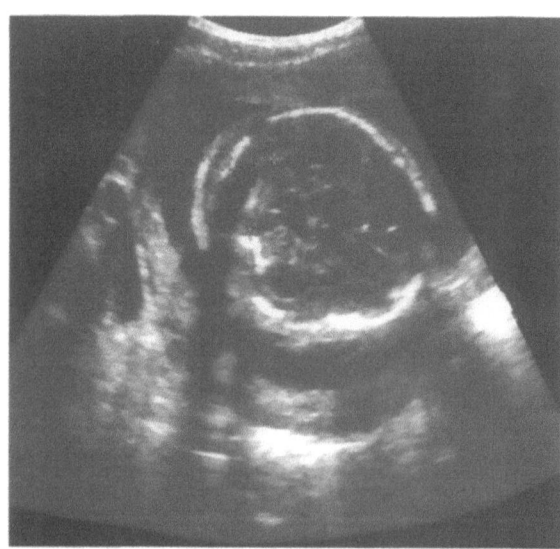

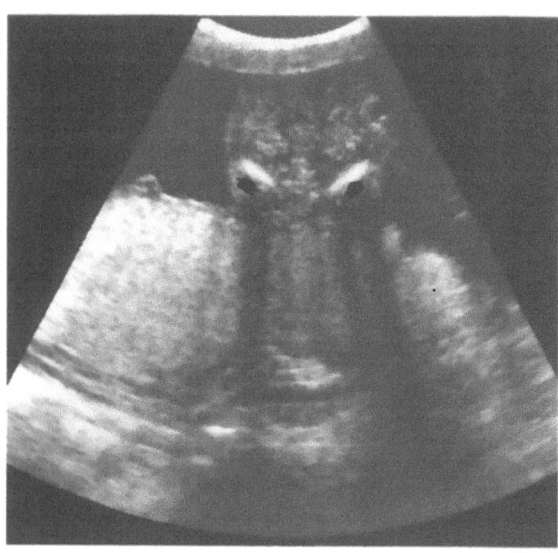

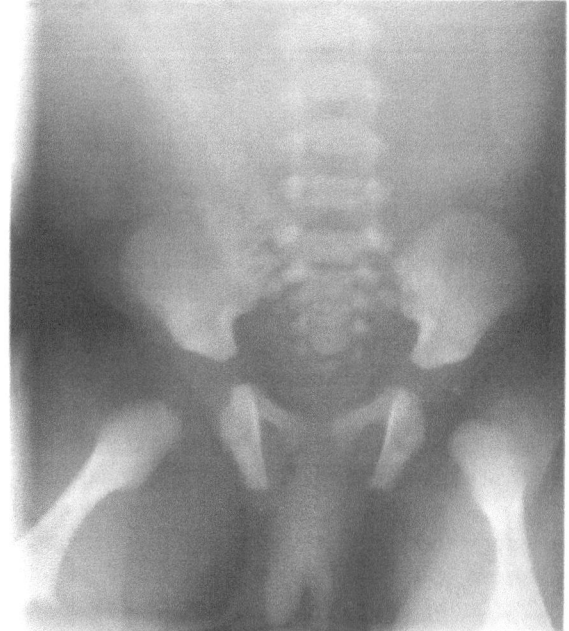

Fig. 12.5a–c. Trisomy 21: associated findings. Second trimester. **a** Transverse scan of the fetal head (*H*). Nuchal thickening at 6 mm (between *XX*). The cerebellum is measured as well (between *crosses*). **b** Transverse scan of the fetal pelvis, obtained at an upper level of the iliac bones (*arrows*). The iliac wing angle measures 105°. **c** Pelvic bone radiograph showing flattened and widened iliac wings

12.2.2.2.2
CNS and Facial Minor Markers

Mild ventriculomegaly and bilateral choroid plexus cysts (Fig. 12.6) have been reported as potentially associated with trisomy 21 (VERGANI et al. 1998, REINSCH 1997). Protruding tongue can be encountered in trisomy 21 patients. Hypoplasia of the nasal bones and relative flattening of the face can be encountered in trisomy 21 fetuses (Figs. 12.7, 12.8) (GUIS et al. 1995).

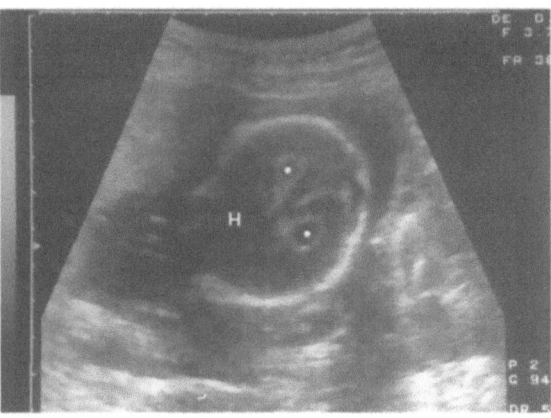

Fig. 12.6. Bilateral choroid plexus cysts (*); the karyotype was normal in this case. *H* head

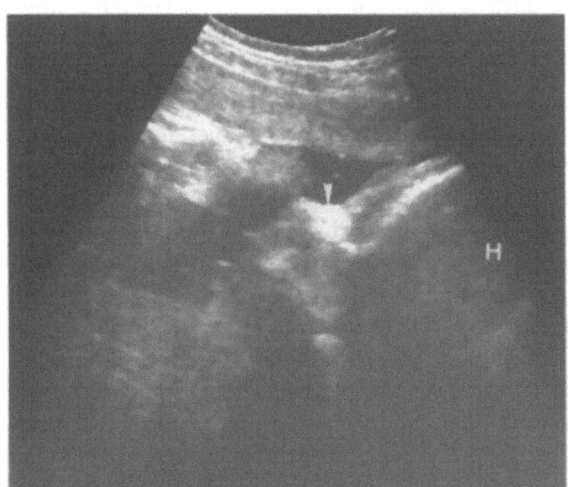

a

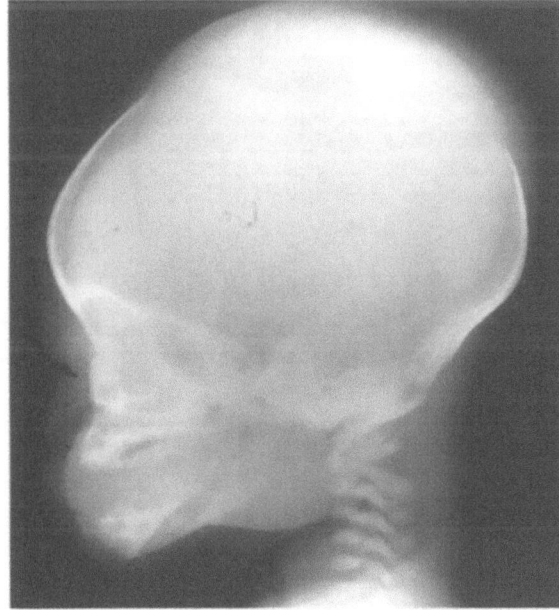

b

Fig. 12.7. Trisomy 21: minor findings. Nasal bone hypoplasia. Second trimester. **a** Profile view of the fetus showing thickened and shortened nasal bones (*arrowhead*). *H* head. **b** After termination of the pregnancy. Lateral skull radiograph shows hypodense and shortened nasal bones

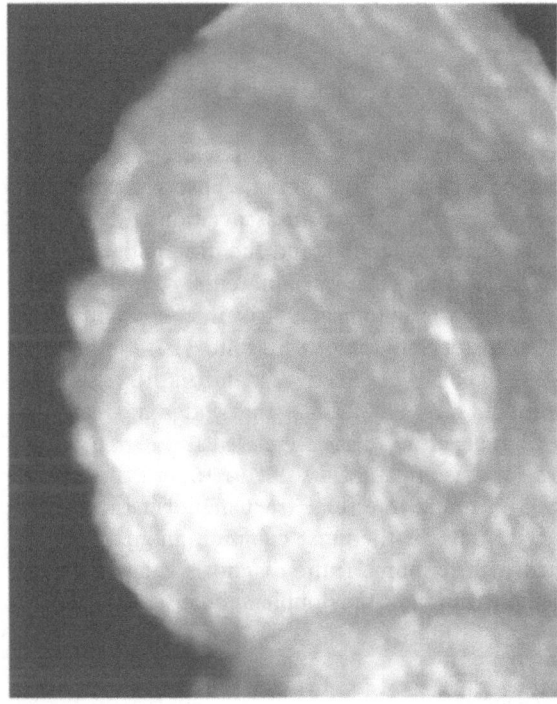

Fig. 12.8. Trisomy 21. Three-dimensional view of the face with obvious anteroposterior flattening

12.2.2.2.3
Intracardiac Echogenic Foci

Hyperechoic focus at the level of the cardiac tendinae chordis is associated, when combined with other anomalies, with an increased risk of trisomy 21 (Fig. 12.9) (BROMLEY et al. 1998, SOHL et al. 1999, SIMPSON 1999).

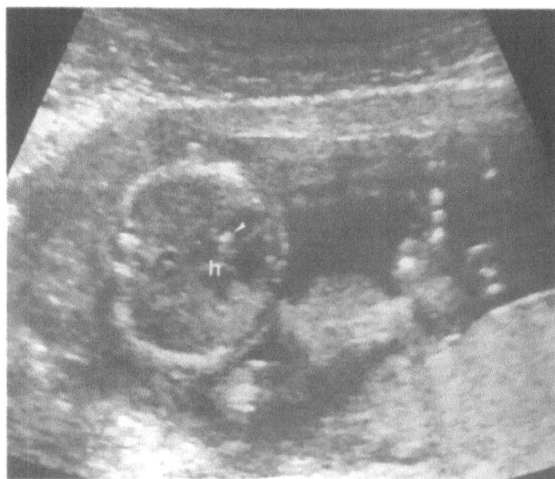

Fig. 12.9. Trisomy 21: minor signs. Cardiac hyperechoic focus. Second trimester. Four-chamber view of the heart (*h*) demonstrating a hyperechoic spot (*arrowhead*)

12.2.2.2.4
Hyperechoic Bowel and Digestive Tract

Hyperechoic bowel corresponds to an echogenicity of fetal bowel equal to that of bone, observed during the early second trimester. An association with trisomy 21 has been suggested, and the differential diagnosis includes normal variant (empty small bowel), cystic fibrosis, cytomegalovirus infection and a previous history of amniotic bleeding (HILL et al. 1994, NYBERG et al. 1993, SLOTNICK and ABUHAMAD 1996, SCIOSCIA et al. 1992). Echogenic sludge and fetal cholecystomegaly are also considered as potential markers for trisomy 21 (Fig. 12.10) (SEPULVEDA et al. 1995). Among intestinal tract malformations, duodenal atresia is the most common anomaly associated with trisomy 21; the diagnosis is based on the demonstration of the double bubble sign (Fig. 12.4).

12.2.2.2.5
Pyelectasis

A diameter of renal pelvis (uni- or bilateral) above 4 mm – on a transverse scan – during the second trimester is considered a minor sign for trisomy 21 (Fig. 12.11) (BENACERAFF 1990 et al., WICKSTROM et al. 1996a).

12.2.2.2.6
Skeletal System

Better than the *shortening of the long bones* (femur and humerus) itself, various ratios seem to indicate

a risk of trisomy 21: most frequently, a ratio of femur measured/femur expected <0.91 is considered suspicious (JOHNSON et al. 1995, NYBERG et al. 1993, BIAGIATTI 1994, BORRELL 1997). *Hypoplasia of the middle phalanx of the fifth digit* is present in 60% of neonates with trisomy 21 and can be evaluated in utero (Fig. 12.12); this digit may also show a radial deviation (clinodactyly) (BENACERAFF et al. 1990, GOLDSTEIN et al. 1995, KJAER 1998).

It has been known through neonatal radiographs that the iliac wings are flared and that the *iliac angle* is widened in trisomy 21. This has been studied and confirmed antenatally (Fig. 12.5b, c). The angle must be measured on a transverse scan of the fetal pelvis that includes the sacrum; the scan must be as symmetrical as possible. An angle below 90° apparently excludes trisomy 21; in most studies, this angle has a mean of 60–70° in normal fetuses and an angle above 100°in trisomy 21. It is noteworthy that the value of this angle depends upon the fetal position: it is wider in all fetuses in a prone or decubitus position as opposed to a lateral position (KLIEWER et al. 1996, SHIPP et al. 1997, BORK et al. 1997, KLIEWER et al. 2000).

Any major structural anomaly can be associated with trisomy 21 (especially anomalies of the heart and duodenum). Various minor signs have been described as markers for trisomy 21, their value becomes significant and justifies chromosomal analysis when more than two are found.

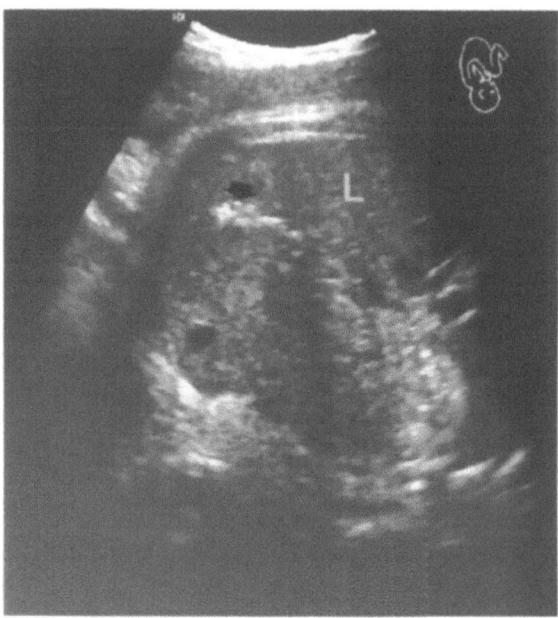

Fig. 12.10. Trisomy 21: minor signs. Biliary sludge. Third trimester. Transverse scan of the fetal abdomen demonstrating echogenic content within the gallbladder (*arrow*). *L* liver

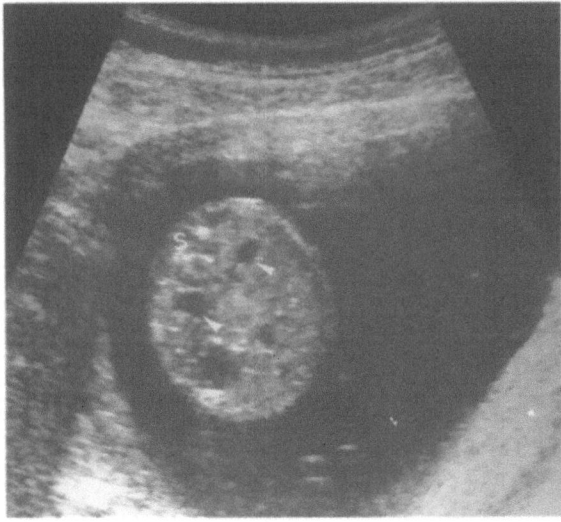

Fig. 12.11. Trisomy 21: minor signs. (Bilateral) pyelectasis. Second trimester. Transverse scan of the fetal abdomen demonstrating bilateral pyelectasis (*arrowheads*). *S* spine

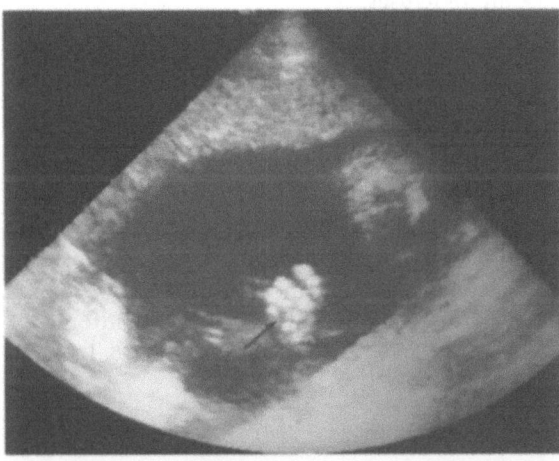

a

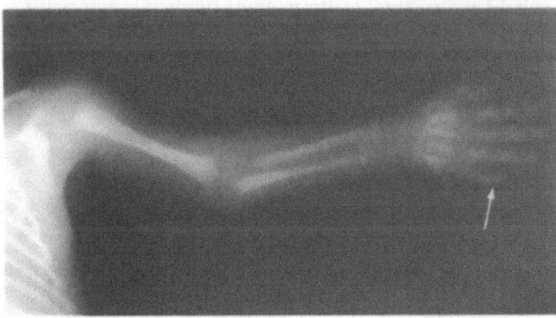

b

Fig. 12.12a, b. Trisomy 21: minor signs. Hypoplasia of the middle phalanx of the fifth finger. **a** In utero. Second trimester (the *arrow* points to the hypoplastic fifth digit). **b** After termination of pregnancy. Radiograph of the arm confirming the anomaly (*arrow*)

12.2.3
Trisomy 18 (Edwards' Syndrome)

After Down's syndrome, trisomy 18 is the most common autosomal trisomy, with an incidence of 1/5,000 births. The prevalence is even higher in first and second trimester pregnancies since many affected fetuses die in utero. The spectrum of associated congenital malformations is wide; the most common malformations are listed in Table 12.3. Intrauterine growth retardation is also associated with the syndrome, 30% of second trimester and 90% of third trimester fetuses with trisomy 18 being growth restricted. Polyhydramnios is another frequent finding (HILL 1996, DEVORE 2000, NYBERG et al. 1993).

Table 12.3. Structural anomalies commonly associated with trisomy 18

Bilateral choroid plexus cysts
Central nervous system malformations
Abnormal nuchal fold skin
Ventricular septal defect
Outflow tract anomalies of the heart
Right to left chamber disproportion of the heart
Omphalocele
Diaphragmatic hernia
Clubbed hands and feet (bilateral)

12.2.3.1
Craniofacial Anomaly

Hypoplasia of the frontal lobes and of the face determines a strawberry-like cranium. Patients with trisomy 18 present with micrognathia and low-set ears.

Microcephaly, and cerebellar hypoplasia with enlarged cisterna magna are typical anomalies that can be associated with the syndrome. Other CNS malformations can also be present (Fig. 12.13). Bilateral choroid plexus cysts are frequently found (YODER et al. 1999). The anomalies are rarely isolated.

12.2.3.2
Cardiovascular System

Cardiovascular anomalies are frequently encountered in trisomy 18. Ventricular septal defect, outflow tract abnormalities and right to left disproportion of the fetal heart are the most common anomalies encountered.

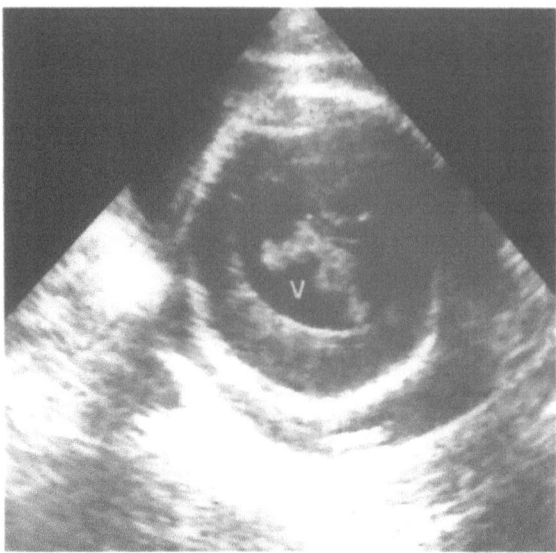

Fig. 12.13. Trisomy 18: CNS malformation. Holoprosencephaly. Third trimester. Transverse scan of the brain showing a single ventricle (*v*)

12.2.3.3
Abdomen

Small size omphalocele and diaphragmatic hernia as well as cystic kidneys are typical associated anomalies in trisomy 18 (Fig. 12.14).

12.2.3.4
Skeletal System

Clubfeet, clubhands, and overlapping fingers are typical findings in trisomy 18. (Fig. 12.15).

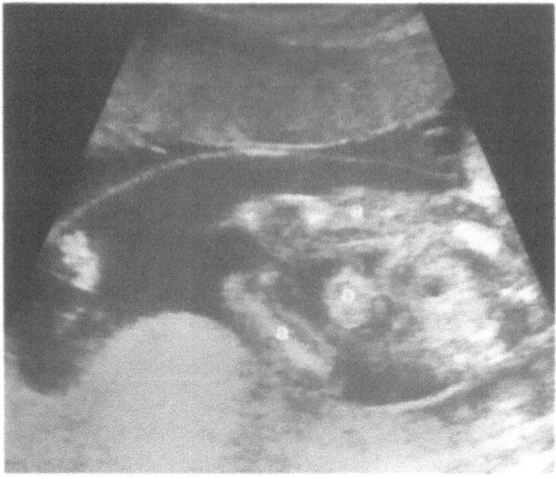

Fig. 12.14. Trisomy 18: digestive malformation. Second trimester. A small omphalocele is visible (*o*); it was associated with clubbed hands. *a* arms

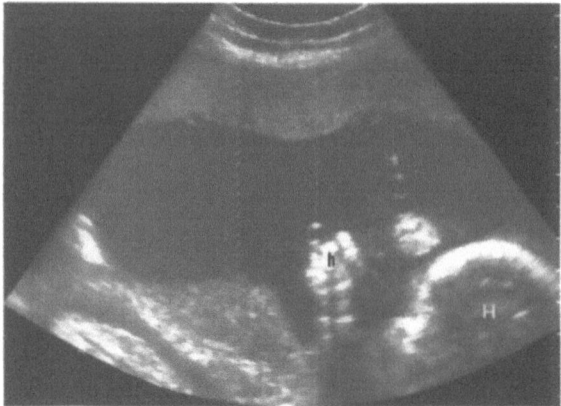

Fig. 12.15. Trisomy 18: skeletal malformation. Second trimester. Typical clenched hand (*h*). *H* head

12.2.3.5
Umbilical Cord

Umbilical cord cysts are a typical finding of trisomy 18. Major CNS and cardiac malformations, omphaloceles and clenched hands are typical findings in trisomy 18 fetuses.

12.2.4
Trisomy 13 (Patau's Syndrome)

Fetuses with trisomy 13 tend to have major brain and craniofacial malformations: median clefting, microphthalmos and holoprosencephaly. Postaxial polydactyly is present in 80% of affected fetuses. Cystic kidneys are usually part of the syndrome too (Table 12.4; Figs. 12.16–12.18) (HILL 1996, LEHMAN et al. 1995).

Table 12.4. Structural malformations commonly associated with trisomy 13

Nuchal thickening
Facial clefts
Microphthalmos
Holoprosencephaly
Meningo-cephalocele
Cardiac malformations
Omphalocele
Diaphragmatic hernia
Cystic kidneys
Polydactyly
Bilateral clubfeet

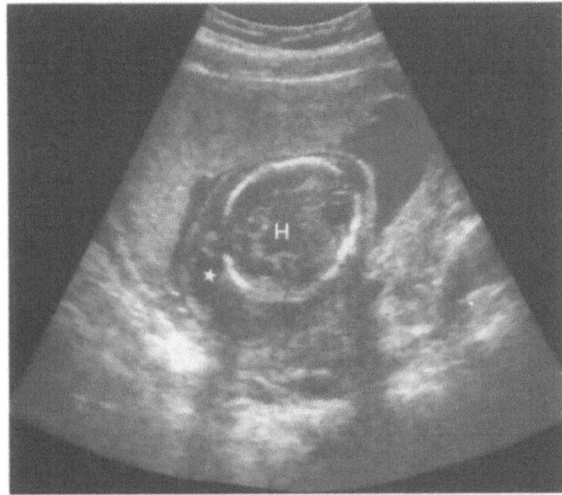

a

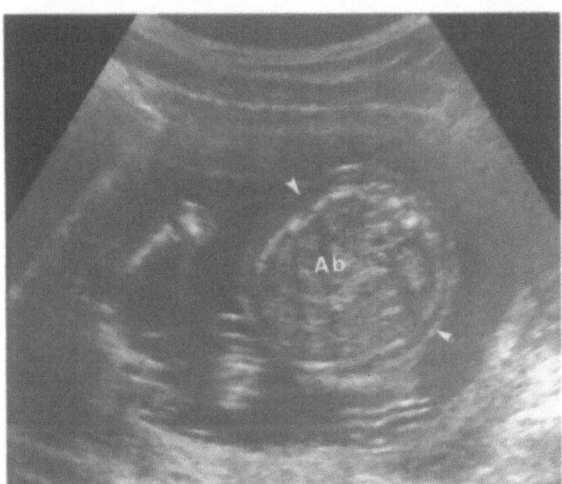

b

Fig. 12.16a, b. Trisomy 13: hydrops. Second trimester. **a** Transverse scan of the fetal head (*H*) with an obvious thickening of the soft tissues (*). **b** Transverse scan of the fetal abdomen (*Ab*) with thickening of the soft tissues (*arrowheads*)

12.2.5
Sex Chromosomes

Anomalies of sex chromosomes occur in about 3% fetuses at birth (ROBINSON et al. 1992). The prognosis is very variable and depends upon the type of anomaly and associated malformations. The most common anomalies are Turner (XO) and Klinefelter (XXY) syndromes, which represent 80% of cases detected (Figs. 12.19, 12.20). Detection can be based upon the demonstration of structural anomalies (i.e., cystic hygroma in the case of Turner (XO) syndrome) but many cases present without any or with minor US anomalies (i.e., Klinefelter (XXY) syndrome; Fig. 12.20) (PERROTIN et al. 2000) The anomalies encountered in Turner syndrome are variable and

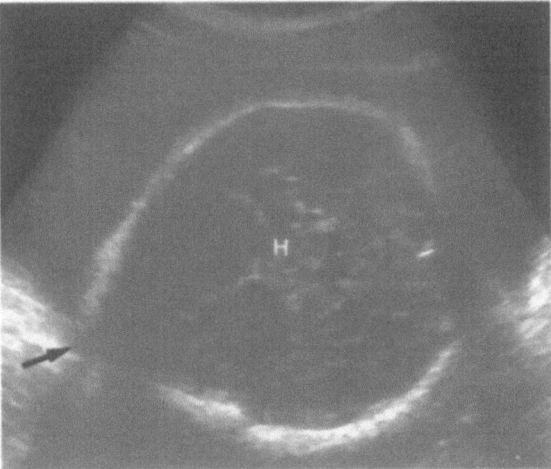

Fig. 12.17. Trisomy 13: CNS malformation. Third trimester. Hypoplasia of the frontal lobes. Transverse scan of the fetal head (*H*). The frontal bones point forward (*arrow*) due to the frontal lobe hypoplasia

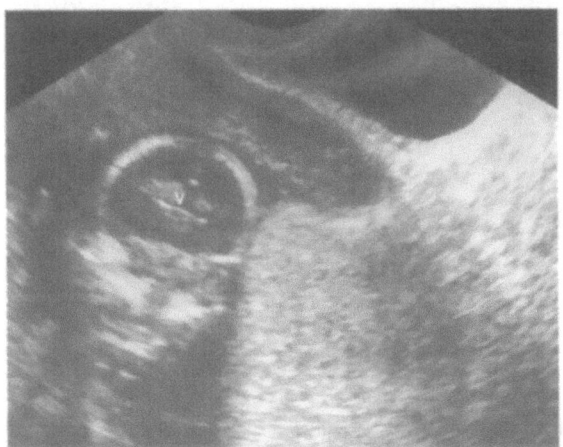

a

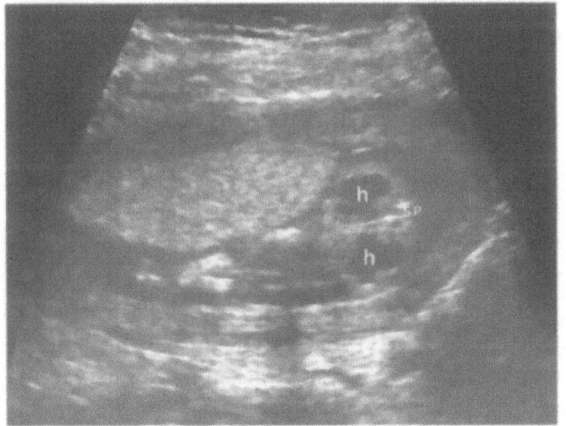

b

Fig. 12.18a, b. Trisomy 13: CNS and urinary malformations. Early second trimester. **a** Frontal view of the head demonstrating a holoprosencephaly variant with a single ventricle (*v*). **b** Transverse scan of the abdomen demonstrating bilateral hydronephrosis (*h*). *SP* spine

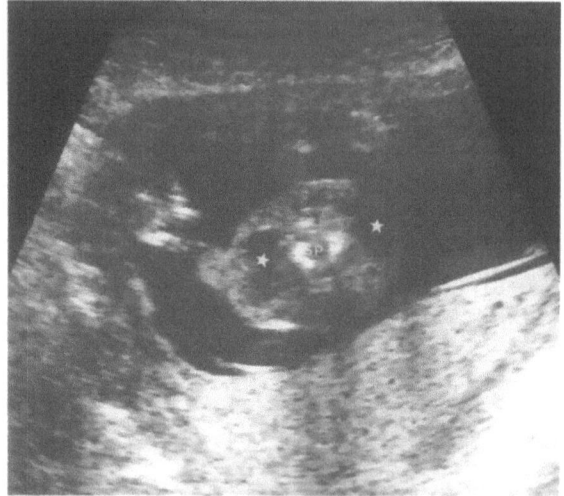

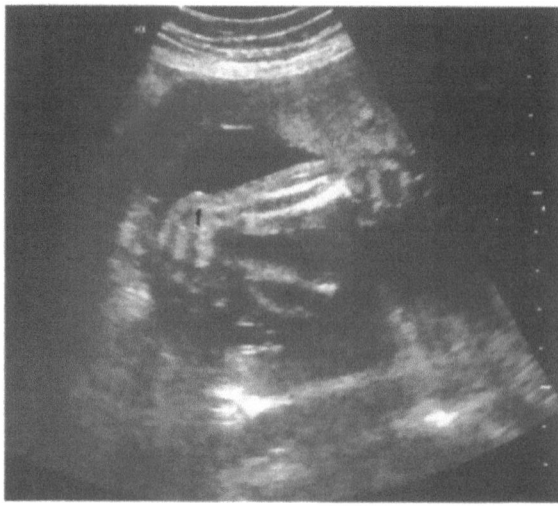

Fig. 12.20. Klinefelter syndrome (XXY). Third trimester. Bilateral clubfeet (*f*) was the only anomaly

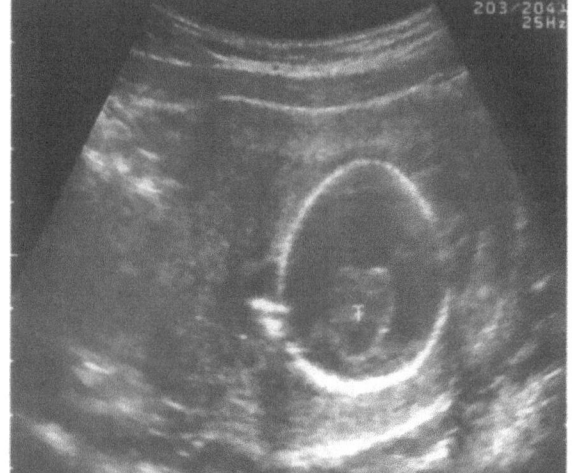

Fig. 12.19a, b. Turner syndrome (XO). Second trimester. a Cystic hygroma. Transverse scan at the level of the neck showing typical bilateral cystic hygroma (*). *SP* spine. b Clubfoot (*f*) deformity

most systems may be affected. Most commonly, nuchal translucency and cystic hygroma are encountered as US markers. Other characteristics include fetal hydrops, cystic kidneys or hydronephrosis and short-limb dwarfism (BOYD et al. 1996). Triploidy (XXX) (Fig. 12.21) may be diagnosed through the demonstration of a cystic thickening of the placenta and rarely by the detection of structural anomalies.

Fig. 12.21a, b. Triploidy syndrome (XXX). Second trimester. a Typical holoprosencephaly with fused thalami (*T*). Transverse scan of the fetal head. b Clubfoot (*f*)

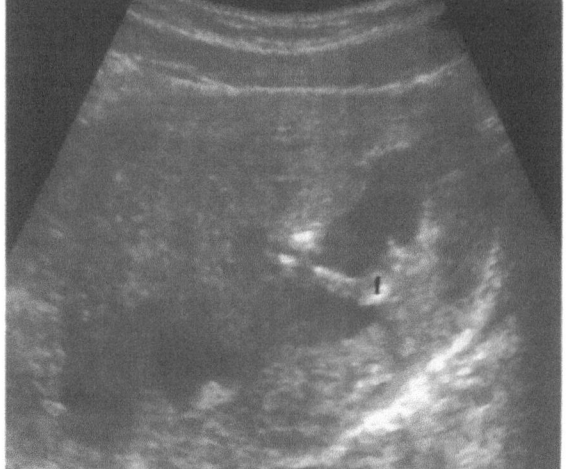

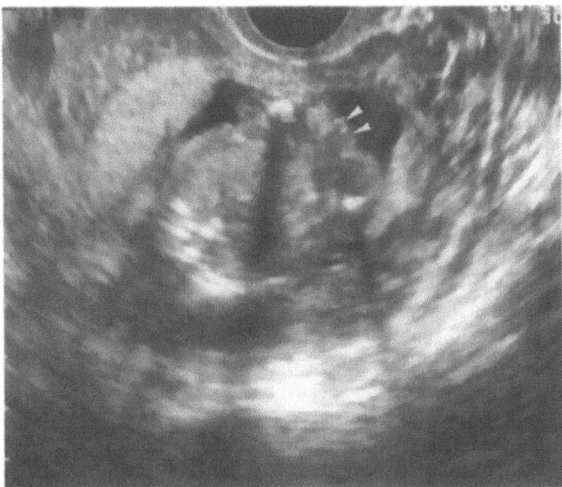

Fig. 12.22. Unbalanced translocation of chromosome 9: ambiguous genitalia. Second trimester. Transverse scan of the fetal perineum showing a female phenotype (*arrowheads*) while karyotype analysis revealed XY genotype. The anomaly was associated with anal atresia, mild ventriculomegaly and nuchal thickening

12.2.6
Other Chromosome Anomalies

As mentioned, anomalies have been detected for most chromosomes; the type and degree of malformations that are associated are very variable. It is of note that the development and improvements in the various techniques for high-resolution karyotype analysis have led to the detection of more and more chromosomal translocation with variable associated anomalies (SALIHU et al. 2001) (Fig. 12.22).

Among the anomalies presenting with monosomies, monosomy 22 is important since it is part of DiGeorge syndrome, which includes cardiac malformation and thymic agenesis (MERINO et al. 1995).

12.3
Conclusion

The detection of any major morphological anomaly justifies an analysis of the fetal chromosomes. The detection of more subtle or minor anomalies should prompt an in-depth analysis of the fetus in order to detect other anomalies. An extensive analysis of the heart is mandatory.

References

Benaceraff BR, Harlow BL, Frigopletto RL (1990) Hypoplasia of the middle phalanx of the 5th digit. J Ultrasound Med 9 :389–394

Benaceraff BR, Mandell, J Estroff JA, et al (1990) Fetal pyelectasis: a possible association with Down syndrome. Obstet Gynecol 76:56–60

Benaceraff BR, Nader A, Bromley B (1994) Identification of second trimester fetuses with autosomal trisomy by use of a sonographic scoring index, Radiology 193:135–140

Biagiatti R, Periti E, Cariati E (1994) Humerus and femoral length in fetuses with Down syndrome. Prenat Diagn 14:429–434

Bork MD, Egan JF, Cusick W, et al (1997) Iliac wing angle as a marker for Down syndrome in the second trimester, Obstet Gynecol 89:734–737

Borrell A, Costa D, Ojuel J, et al (1997) Limited effectiveness of humerus and femur shortening as markers of Down syndrome in early midtrimester fetuses. Fetal Diagn Ther 12:156–162

Boyd PA, Anthony MY, Manning M, et al (1996) Antenatal diagnosis of cystic hygroma or nuchal pad, Arch Dis Child 74:F38–F42

Brady AF, Pandya PP, Yuksel B, et al (1998) Outcome of chromosomally normal fetuses with increased nuchal translucency. J. Med Genet 35:222–224

Bromley B, Lieberman E, Shipp TD, et al (1998) Significance of an echogenic intracardiac focus in fetuses at high and low risk for aneuploidy, J Ultrasound Med 17:127–131

Devine PC, Malone FD (1999) First trimester screening for structural fetal abnormalities: nuchal translucency. US Semin Perinatol 23:382–392

DeVore GR (2000) Second trimester US may identify 77–97% of fetuses with T18. J Ultrasound Med 19:565–576

DeVore GR (2001) The genetic sonogram. Prenat Diagn 21: 40–45

Dicke JM, Crane JP (1991) US recognition of major malformations and aberrant fetal growth in trisomic fetuses. J Ultrasound Med 10:433–438

Goldstein I, Gomes K, Copel JA (1995) Fifth digit measurement in normal pregnancies: a potential sign of Down's syndrome. Ultrasound Obstet Gynecol 5:34–37

Gonen R, Dar H, Degani S (1995) The karyotype of fetuses with anomalies detected by second trimester US. Eur J Obstet Gynecol 58:153–155

Grandjean H, Saramon MF, et al (1995) US measurement of nuchal skinfold thickness for detection of Down syndrome in the second trimester fetus. Obstet Gynecol 85:103–106

Graupe M, Naylor SC, Greene NH et al (2001) Trisomy 21. Clin Perinatol 28:303–332

Guis F, Ville Y Vincent Y, et al (1995) US evaluation of the length of the nasal bones throughout gestation. Ultrasound Obstet Gynecol 5:304–307

Hill LM, Fries J, Hecker J, et al (1994) Second trimester echogenic small bowel. Prenat Diagn 14:845–850

Hill LM (1996) The US detection of trisomies 13, 18 and 21. Clin Obstet Gynecol 39:831–850

Johnson MP, Michaelson JE, Barr M, et al (1995) Combining humerus and femur length for improved US identification of pregnancies at risk for trisomy 21. Am J Obstet Gynecol 172:1229–1235

Kjaer MS, Seeling JW, Andersen E, et al (1998) Hand development in T21. Am J Med Genet 79:337–342

Kliewer MA, Herzberg BS, Freed KS, et al (1996) Dysmorphologic features of fetal pelvis in Down syndrome. Radiology 201:681–684

Kliewer MA, Herzberg BS, Freed K, et al (2000) Normal fetal pelvis: important factors for morphometric characterization with US. Radiology 215:453–457

Lehman CD, Nyberg DA, Winter TC, et al (1995) Trisomy 13 syndrome: prenatal US findings in 33 cases. Radiology 194:217–222

Merino A, Deperdigo A, Nomballais F, et al (1995) DiGeorge syndrome with total monosomy 22 diagnosed prenatally. Prenat Diagn 15:189–192

Nicolaides KH, Snijders RJM, Goswen CM, et al (1992) US detectable markers of fetal chromosomal abnormalities. Lancet 340:704–707

Nyberg DA, Resta RG, Luthy DA (1990) Prenatal US findings of Down syndrome: review of 94 cases. Obstet Gynecol 76:360–377

Nyberg DA, Resta RG, Luthy DA, et al (1993) Humerus and femoral length shortening in the detection of Down's syndrome. Am J Obstet Gynecol 168:534–538

Nyberg DA, Resta RG, Mahonny BS, et al (1993) Fetal hyperechoic bowel and Down's syndrome. Ultrasound Obstet Gynecol 3:330–333

Nyberg DA, Kramer D, Resta RG, et al (1993) Prenatal US findings of T18: review of 47 cases. J Ultrasound Med 2:103–113

Pandya PP, Brizot ML, Kuhn P, et al (1994) First trimester nuchal translucency thickness and risks for trisomy. Obstet Gynecol 84:420–423

Perrotin F, Guichet A, Marret H, et al (2000) Devenir prenatal des anomalies des chromosomes sexuels diagnostiquées pendant la grossesse. J Gynecol Biol Reprod 29:668–676

Reinsch RC (1997) Choroid plexus cysts: an association with trisomy. Am J Obstet Gynecol 176:1381–1383

Rizzo N, Pittalis MC, Pilu G, et al (1996) Distribution of abnormal karyotypes among malformed fetuses detected through US, Prenat Diagn 16:159–163

Robinson A, Bender BG, Linden MG, et al (1992) Prognosis of prenatally diagnosed children with sex chromosome aneuploidy, Am J Med Genet 44:365–368

Rotmensch S, Liberati M, Bronshtein M, et al (1997) Prenatal US findings in fetuses with Down syndrome. Prenat Diagn 1997 17:1001–1009

Salihu HM, Boos R, Tchuinghem G, et al (2001) Prenatal diagnosis of translocation and a single pericentric inversion 9: the value of fetal US. J Obstet Gynecol 21:474–477

Scioscia AJ, Pretorius DH, Budorick NE, et al (1992) Second trimester echogenic bowel. Am J Obstet Gynecol 167:889–894

Sepumlveda W, Nicolaidis P, Hollingsworth J, et al (1995) Fetal cholecystomegaly: a prenatal marker of aneuploidy. Prenat Diagn 15:193–197

Simpson J (1999) The echogenic intracardiac focus. Prenat Diagn 19:972–975

Sherer DM, Bombard AT, Kellner LH, et al (1997) Noninvasive first trimester screening for fetal aneuploidy. Obstet Gynecol Surv 52:123–129

Shipp TD, Bromley B, Lieberman E, Benaceraff BR (1997) The iliac angle as a sonographic marker for Down syndrome in second trimester fetuses. Obstet Gynecol 89:446–450

Shohat M, Legum C, Romem Y, et al (1995) Down syndrome prevention program in a population with an older maternal age. Obstet Gynecol 85:368–373

Slotnick RN, Abuhamad AZ (1996) Prognostic implications of fetal echogenic bowel. Lancet 347:85–87

Snijders RJM, Sebire NJ, Nicolaides KH (1995) Maternal age and gestational age-specific risk for chromosomal defects. Fetal Diagn Ther 10:356–367

Snijders R (2001) First trimester US. Clin Perinatol 28:333–352

Sohl BD, Scioscia AL, Budorick NE, et al (1999) Utility of minor US markers in the prediction of abnormal fetal karyotype. Am J Obstet Gynecol 181:898–903

Vautier-Rit S, Subtil D, Vaast P, et al (2000) Signes échographiques de trisomie 21 au 2ème trimestre de la grossesse. J Gynecol Biol Reprod 29:445–453

Vergani P, Locatelli A, Strobelt N, et al (1998) Clinical outcome of mild ventriculomegaly. Am J Obstet Gynecol 178:218–222

Vintzielos AM, Campbell WA, Rodis JF, et al (1996) The use of second trimester genetic sonogram in guiding clinical management of patients at increased risk for trisomy 21. Obstet Gynecol 87:948–952

Vintzielos AM, Campbell WA, Guzman ER, et al (1997) Second trimester US markers for detection of trisomy 21. Obstet Gynecol 89:941–944

Vintzileos AM, Guzman ER, Smyulian JC, et al (1999) Indication specific accuracy of second trimester genetic US for the detection of trisomy 21. Am J Obstet Gynecol 181:1045–1048

Watson WJ, Miller RC, Menard MR (1994) US measurement of fetal nuchal skin to screen for fetal chromosomal abnormalities. Am J Obstet Gynecol 170:583–586

Wickstrom E, Maizels M, Sabbagha RE, et al (1996a) Isolated fetal pyelactasis. Ultrasound Obstet Gynecol 8:236–240

Wickstrom EA, Thangavelu M, Barilla BV, et al (1996b) A prospective study of the association between isolated fetal pyelectasis and chromosomal abnormality. Obstet Gynecol 88:379–382

Wilkins I (1994) The separation of the great toe in fetuses with Down syndrome. J Ultrasound Med 13:229–231

Wladimoroff JW, Bhaggoe WR, Kristelijn M, et al (1995) US determined anomalies and outcome in 170 chromosomally abnormal fetuses. Prenat Diagn 15:431–438

Yoder PR, Sabbagha RE, Gross SJ, et al (1999) The second trimester fetus with isolated choroid plexus cysts. Obstet Gynecol 93:869–872

13 Fetal Tumors and Pseudotumors

Fred E. Avni, Marie Cassart, Christine Devalck, Danièle Eurin

CONTENTS

13.1   Introduction   267
13.2   Central Nervous System   268
13.3   Face and Neck   272
13.3.1   Facial Tumors   272
13.3.2   Neck Masses   272
13.4   Chest   273
13.4.1   Lungs and Chest Wall   273
13.4.2   Mediastinum   273
13.4.3   Heart   274
13.5   Abdomen   274
13.5.1   Peritoneum   274
13.5.1.1 Liver   274
13.5.1.2 Peritoneal Cavity   275
13.5.2   Retroperitoneum   276
13.5.2.1 Kidney   276
13.5.2.2 Adrenal   276
13.5.2.3 Other   276
13.6   Ovary and Testis   278
13.7   Soft Tissues   279
13.8   Sacro-coccygeal Teratoma   279
13.10   Conclusion   281
          References   281

F. E. Avni, MD, PhD
Department of Pediatric Imaging, University Children's
Hospital Queen Fabiola, Avenue J. J. Crocq 15, 1020 Brussels,
Belgium
M. Cassart, MD
Division of Perinatal Imaging, University Clinics of Brussels,
Erasme Hospital, Route de Lennick 808, 1070 Brussels
C. Devalck, MD
Department of Pediatric Oncology, University Children's
Hospital Queen Fabiola, Avenue J. J. Crocq 15, 1020 Brussels,
Belgium
D. Eurin, MD
Department of Pediatric Imaging, Charles Nicolle Hospital,
rue de Germont 1, 76031 Rouen Cedex, France

13.1 Introduction

Less than 3% of all childhood neoplasms are diagnosed within the first month of life. Their overall incidence is estimated to be 1/100,000 live births (0.89/100,000 for solid-type tumors). Although rare, tumors develop during fetal life and even metastasize. Any organ can be involved but some sites and tumors types are more frequent (Table 13.1) (Salloum et al. 1990, Teinturier et al. 1992, Parkes et al. 1994, Grundy et al. 2001). The prognosis depends upon the tumoral type and extent at diagnosis. Therefore, it is mandatory to detect and assess the anomaly as early as possible ,especially during fetal life, so that postnatal management can be optimized (Meizner 2000).

Table 13.1. Perinatal tumors

Teratoma	29%
Neuroblastoma	18%
Leukemias	12%
Soft tissue tumors	10%
Brain and CNS	8%
Retinoblastoma	8%
Kidney tumors	5%
Liver tumors	5%
Other	5%

In most instances, the sonographic diagnosis is straightforward, demonstrating a well-circumscribed mass; US is usually accurate enough in defining the content of the mass and its location. However, in some cases the diagnosis is less easy and true tumors have to be differentiated from pseudo-tumors or even from simple organomegaly. Furthermore, some tumors correspond to a true neoplasm while others constitute a congenital malformation determining a mass effect. In many instances, MR imaging will provide additional information in terms of tissue content and tumoral extent.

13.2
Central Nervous System

Central nervous system (CNS) tumors are rare during fetal life (0.5/1000000 life births). *Cystic masses* in the CNS most commonly represent arachnoid cysts; they may develop in any space and their size is variable (Fig. 13.1). Cysts may also develop in the choroid plexus (see Chap. 4).

Various *non-cystic tumors* have been diagnosed in utero and over 50% have been teratomas (benign or malignant) (Fig. 13.2); other lesions included astrocytoma, ependymoma, glioblastoma, medulloblastoma, choroid plexus papilloma, craniopharyngioma, hemangioendothelioma, sarcoma, lipoma and hamartomatous tubers (in patients with tuberous sclerosis). The tumors are most frequently associated with hydrocephalus and diagnosed during the third trimester. Fetal tumors are usually supratentorial but all locations have been described (SCHLEMBACH et al. 1999, PINTO et al. 1999, LEE et al. 1999, ADRA et al. 1994, VANLIEFERINGHEN et al. 1993). A rare case of cerebellar hemangioendothelioma has been reported (Fig. 13.3) (SHARONY et al. 1999).

Sonographically, the tumors are usually completely echogenic or appear in a more complex cystic and solid-type pattern. At diagnosis, except for tubers and some lipomas, CNS tumors are large and/or enlarge rapidly producing secondary hydrocephalus and increasing biparietal diameter. Their prognosis is poor, mainly because of the mass effect upon the developing brain; very few affected fetuses survive (SCHLEMBACH et al. 1999). Lipoma and tubers have a much better prognosis; in fact the prognosis will be that of the associated anomalies. Lipomas are usually highly echogenic tumors that develop in any cisternal space and correspond to a deficient reabsorption of the primitive pia. They are most frequently located in the pericallosal cisterna and are associated with partial or complete agenesis of the corpus callosum. Two types can be demonstrated: a nodular and a tubular pattern (Figs. 13.4–13.6) (TRUWIT and BARCHOVITZ 1990, ICKOWITZ et al. 2001).

Tubers affecting the CNS are difficult to diagnose by obstetrical US and are mainly demonstrated by MR imaging (Fig. 13.7). They are usually detected after cardiac rhabdomyoma has been found at obstetrical US or in patients with a positive family history

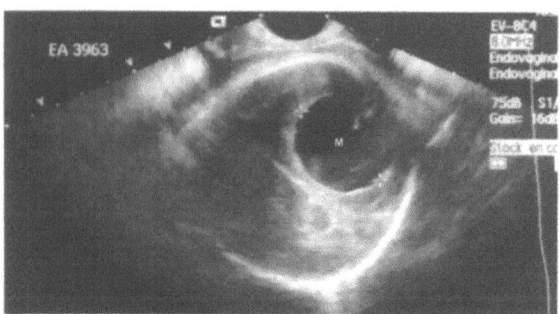

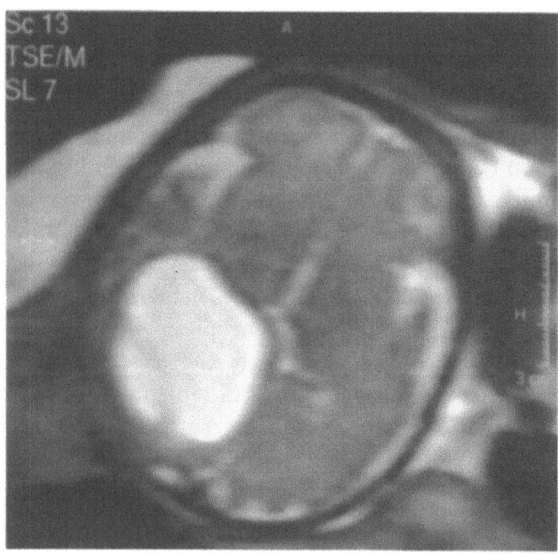

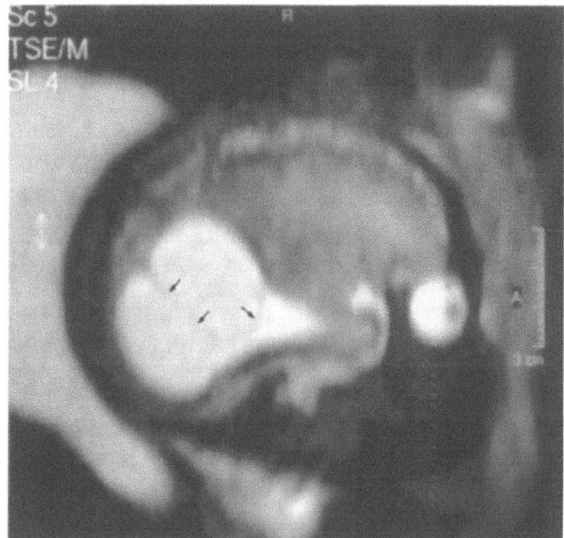

Fig. 13.1a–c. Glio-ependymal cyst. Third trimester. **a** US. Transverse scan of the fetal head (endovaginal). A hypoechoic cystic mass (*M*, limited by *crosses*) is visible in the right occipital area. **b** Fetal MR imaging, T2-weighted sequence. Transverse scan demonstrating the cyst close to the ventricle but without mass effect. **c** Fetal MR imaging. Sagittal scan. There are septations (*arrows*) within the cyst. (It was removed after birth)

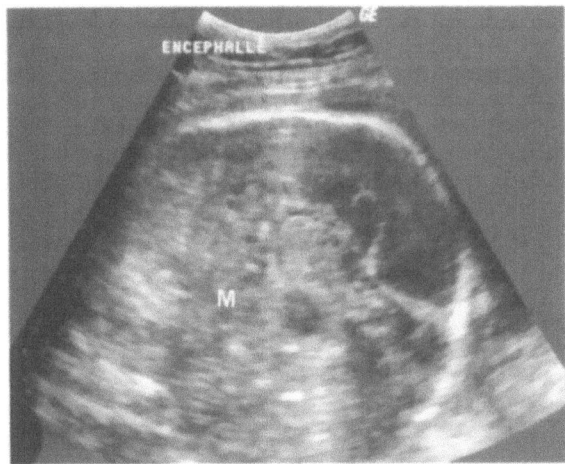

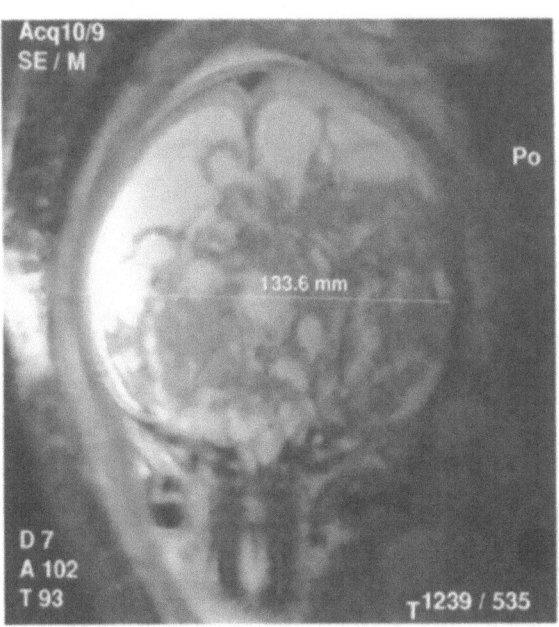

Fig. 13.2a, b. Cystic teratoma. Third trimester. **a** US. Transverse scan. A huge heterogeneous mass (*M*) has replaced the normal brain parenchyma. **b** Fetal MR imaging, T2-weighted sequence. Coronal view. Confirmation of the complete destruction of the brain by the mixed-type mass

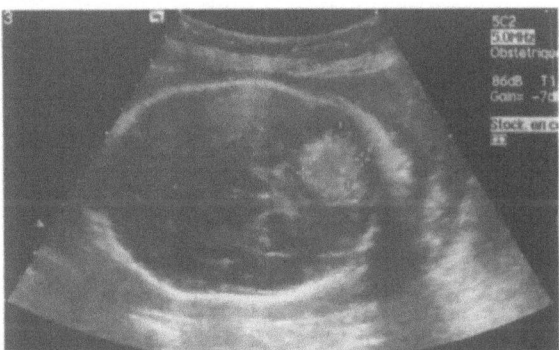

Fig. 13.3a–c. Pericerebellar hemangioma. Third trimester. **a** US. Transverse scan of the fetal head demonstrating a hyperechoic mass (3×4 cm between *crosses*) within the posterior fossa. **b** Fetal MR imaging, T2-weighted sequence. Axial scan. A slightly hyperintense and heterogeneous mass (*M*) displaces the cerebellum and produces ventricular dilatation. **c** Fetal MR imaging, T2-weighted sagittal sequence. The mass (*M*) and the ventricular dilatation are seen

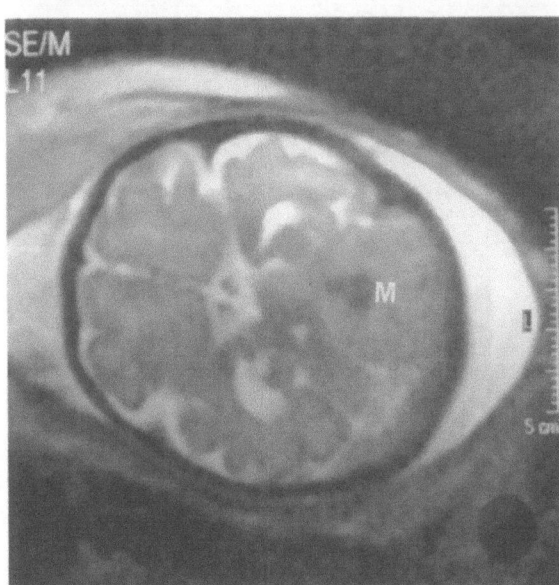

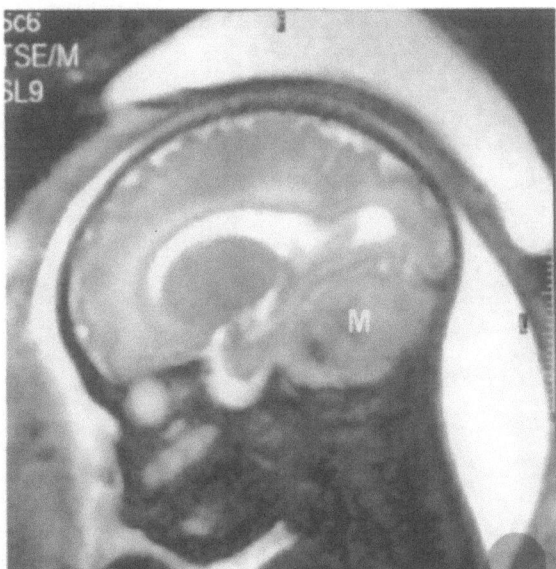

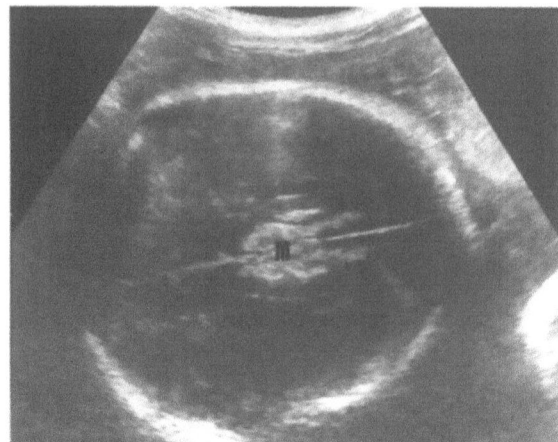

Fig. 13.4a–c. Pericallosal lipoma, tubular type with partial agenesis of the corpus callosum. a US in utero. Third trimester. Biparietal view. A hyperechoic mass (*M*) is visible on both sides of the interhemispheric falx. It has frontal extensions (*arrows*). b MR imaging at birth, TSE T1-weighted sequence. Sagittal scan. Hyperintense mass in the pericallosal cistern; only the anterior part of the corpus callosum has developed (*arrow*). c MR imaging at age 3 years. Sagittal scan. The lipoma has grown. The child was still asymptomatic

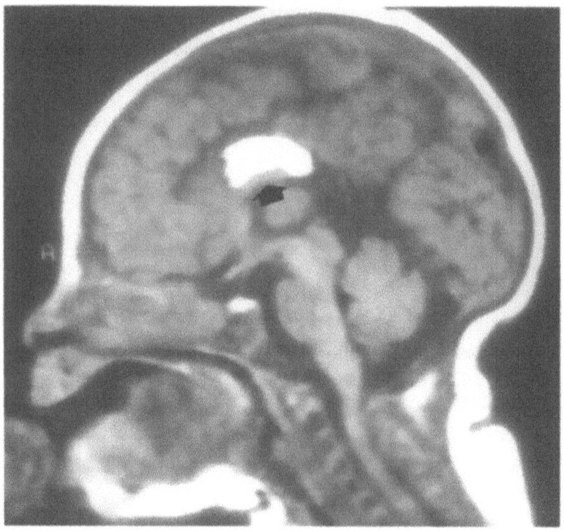

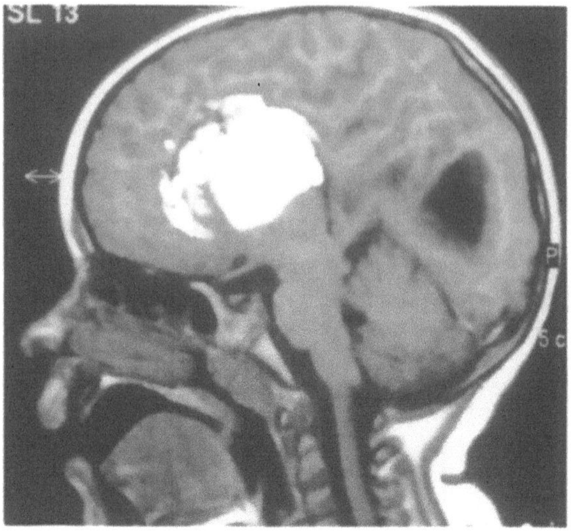

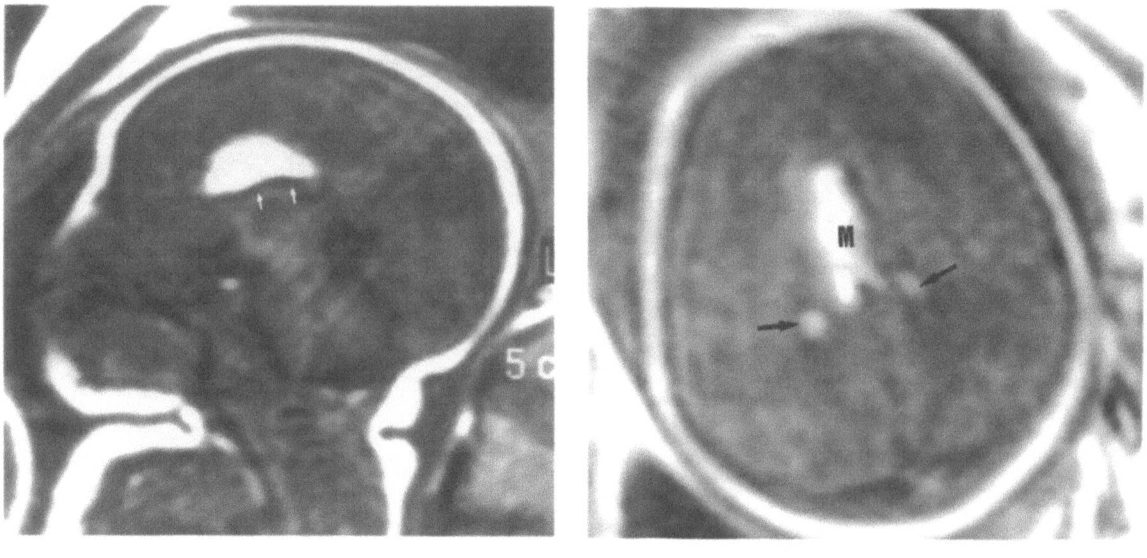

Fig. 13.5a, b. Fetal pericallosal lipoma, tubular type with normal corpus callosum. Fetal MR imaging, T1-weighted sequences. a Sagittal scan. The lipoma is seen as well as the corpus callosum (*arrows*). b Transverse view. The lipomatous mass (*M*) has extensions into the choroidal fissures (*arrows*)

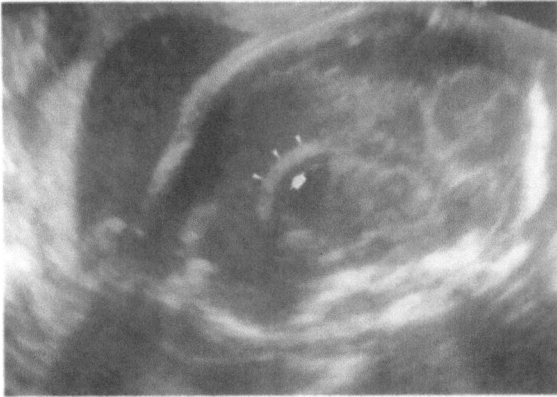

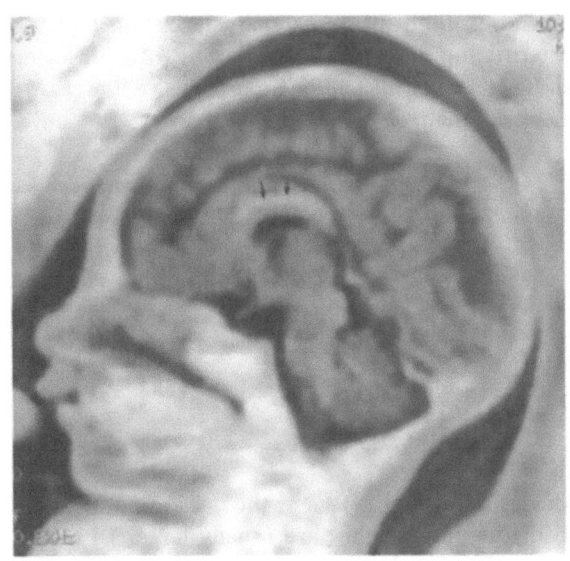

Fig. 13.6a, b. Pericallosal lipoma, curvilinear type. Second trimester. **a** US in utero. Sagittal view. The hyperechoic lipoma (*arrowheads*) parallels the normal corpus callosum (*arrow*). **b** Fetal MR imaging, T1-weighted sequence. The hyperintense lipoma and the normal corpus callosum are seen

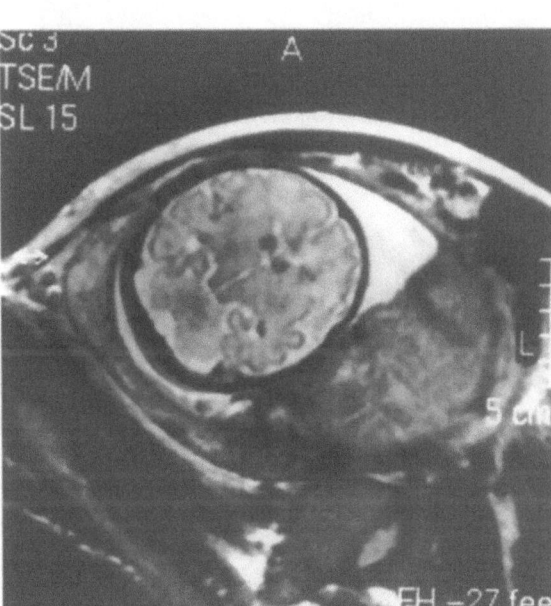

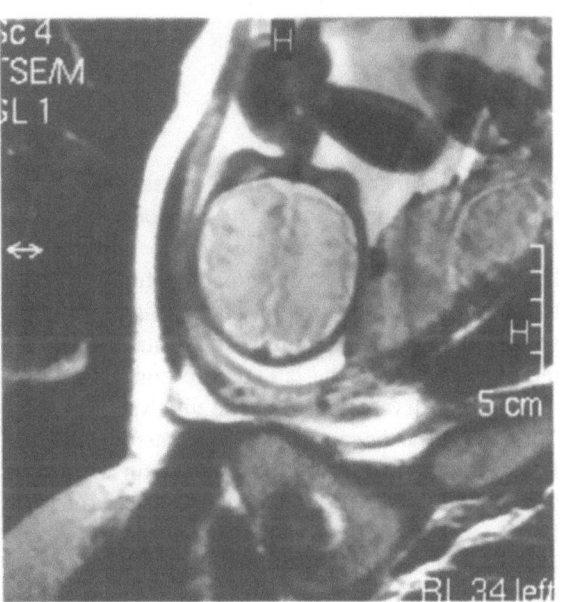

Fig. 13.7a, b. CNS involvement of tuberous sclerosis. Fetal MR imaging, T2-weighted sequences. **a** Transverse scan demonstrating the hypointense tubers (*arrows*). **b** Transverse scan somewhat higher than **a** showing diffuse areas of abnormal signal in the fetal brain

for tuberous sclerosis. CNS tubers are mainly located in the subependymal area (Fig. 13.7) (LEVINE et al. 2000, MITRA 2000, SONIGO et al. 1998).

CNS tumors may be associated with other anomalies of other systems that should be searched for (face, kidneys, skeletal, heart, etc.) and more rarely with chromosomal anomalies. Associated anomalies may alter the prognosis and the postnatal management.

Differential diagnosis of CNS tumors includes vascular malformations such as cavernous hemangioma

(particularly those that are thrombosed), for which Doppler analysis can be helpful and can demonstrate the vascular nature of the anomaly (LEE et al. 2000, HELLING et al. 2000, PILU et al. 1997, SHARONY et al. 1999). Another important differential diagnosis is hemorrhagic foci, which may occur at any level of the CNS and at any time during gestation. They also appear as hyperechoic areas with, eventually, a mass effect (VERGANI et al. 1996, REISS et al. 1996, RANZINI et al. 1998). MR imaging is an important complementary technique for all these differential diagnoses, both for tissue characterization and for determining the extent of the lesion (KURIHARA et al. 2001, BAILEY et al. 1990, KUELTUERSAY et al. 1995) (see also Chap. 4).

> CNS tumors are rare. Both cystic and solid tumors can be encountered. Teratoma is the most common solid tumor. Fetal MR imaging is essential in order to assess CNS tumors.

13.3
Face and Neck

Masses affecting the face or the neck are important to detect because they are usually large. This may induce dystocia during delivery and neonatal distress after birth due to compression.

13.3.1
Facial Tumors

Facial tumors are rare in the fetus. Masses involving the nose, mouth pharynx and orbits have been reported. Nasal teratoma and facial hemangioendothelioma have been described as mixed-pattern tumors. Other facial tumors include oropharyngeal masses that may protrude through the mouth. These masses may be teratoma or epulis; the latter corresponds to a soft tissue mass developing from the gingiva (Fig. 13.8). The differential diagnosis includes a macroglossia that is associated with Beckwith-Wiedemann syndrome and Down's syndrome (SHIPP et al. 1995, LOPEZ DE LACALLE et al. 2001). Ocular retinoblastoma is a classical neonatal tumor, often bilateral, but it has rarely been reported in utero. The intraocular calcified mass has to be differentiated from benign dacryocystoceles that develop in the internal part of the orbit but outside the eyeball (SALIM et al. 1998) (see Chap. 4).

13.3.2
Neck Masses

Masses that develop in the neck must be separated into anterior and posterior masses (MERNAGH et al. 1999, SUCHET 1995). Teratoma occurs more typically in the anterior compartment, and presents a mixed-type pattern (KERNER et al. 1998). It must be differentiated from enlarged thyroid, thyroglossal or branchial cleft cysts (AVNI et al. 1992, BROMLEY

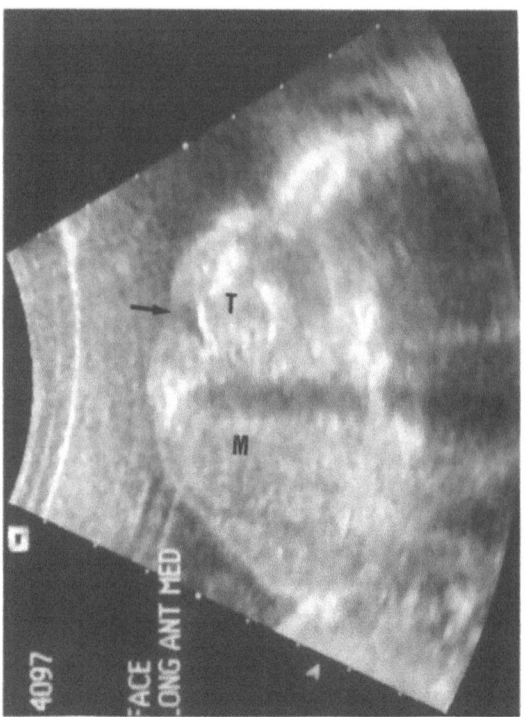

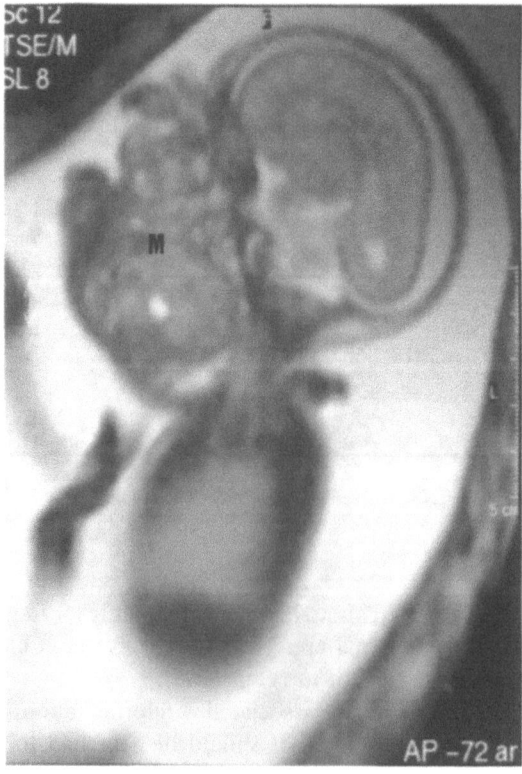

Fig. 13.8a, b. Gingival epulis tumor. Third trimester. **a** US. Sagittal view of fetal neck. The mass (*M*) extends downwards and upwards, and displaces the tongue (*T*) upwards. The *arrow* points to the mouth opening. **b** Fetal MR imaging, T2-weighted sequence. This demonstrates and delineates the extent of the mass (*M*) better than US

et al. 1992). Rarely but classically, neuroblastoma may develop in the posterior compartment of the neck, associated or not with a mediastinal extension (ABRAMSON et al. 1993). Posterior masses must be differentiated from cephalocele, vascular malformations and scalp cysts (OGDE and JAUNIAUX 1999).

Cystic lymphangiomas develop in both anterior and posterior compartments. Sonographically the mass appears mainly cystic with multiple septa. The mass may invade the pharynx and the mediastinum. An important differential diagnosis is rhabdomyosarcoma, which also may develop in any compartment and has a poorer prognosis. Also important for the differential diagnosis is neonatal myofibromatosis, as about 50% of cases arise in the head and neck and may involve the superficial and deep soft tissues. They appear as solid-type tissue (BECK 1999). It can be difficult to differentiate all these tumors from hemangioendothelioma, which has a similar US appearance; in markedly vascularized tumors, color Doppler may help in the differentiation (SHIRAISHI et al. 2000, GONCALVES et al. 2000, YANCEY et al. 1993).

MR imaging may provide essential information regarding tissue content and the extent of the mass in order to optimize postnatal management (LIECHTEY and CROMBLEHOLME 1999, POUTAMO et al. 1999) (see Chap. 4).

> Cystic lymphangioma is the commonest mass developing in the neck region.

13.4
Chest

13.4.1
Lungs and Chest Wall

True lung tumors in the fetus are exceedingly rare; few reports exist of embryonic rhabdomyosarcoma (ONDEROGLU et al. 1999, LEVINE et al. 2001). Hamartoma, teratoma, and mesenchymal tumors with leiomyomatous, blastomatous and fibrosarcomatous features have been described in the neonatal period. Due to their volume, bronchopulmonary malformations produce a mass effect on adjacent structures (LEVINE et al. 2001) and should not be misinterpreted as true neoplasms. Masses can develop in the soft tissues of the chest. Cystic lymphangioma is the main diagnosis to consider (Fig. 13.9).

Bronchopulmonary malformations are the main cause of space-occupying lesions in the lungs.

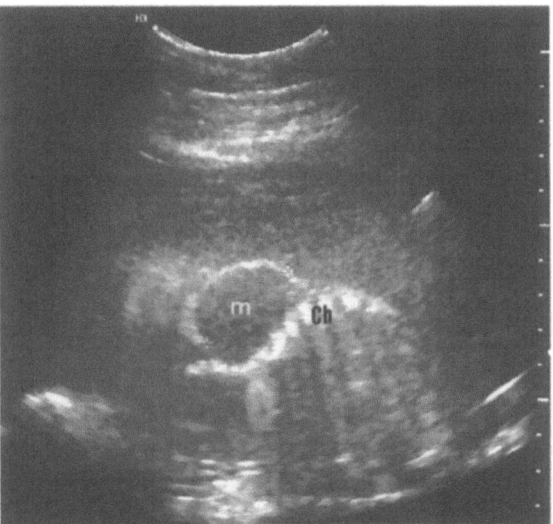

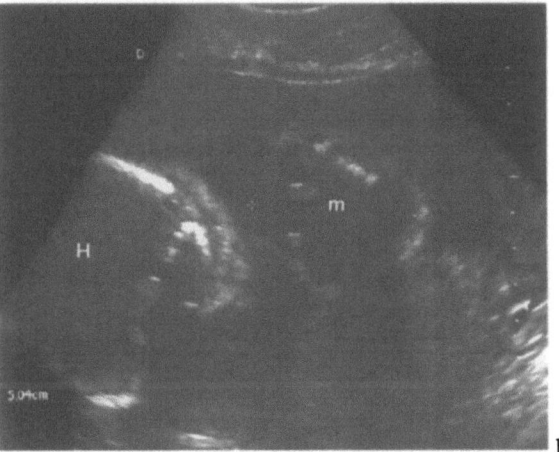

Fig. 13.9a, b. Chest wall soft tissue cystic lymphangioma. a Second trimester. A cystic mass (*m*, 3 cm between the *crosses*) is depressing the chest wall (*Ch*). b Third trimester: The mass (*m*) has grown and measures 5 cm. It was removed after birth. *H* head

13.4.2
Mediastinum

The differential diagnosis of a mediastinal tumor includes cystic lymphangioma, teratoma, thoracic neuroblastoma and mediastinal sequestration (JUNG et al. 2000, WANG et al. 2000). All may present a solid or a mixed-type pattern; neuroblastoma and teratoma may present calcifications. Solid-type tumors usually escape the US diagnosis, probably because they cannot be differentiated from surrounding structures. The tumors are usually detected during the end of the second or third trimester when they tend to enlarge (sometimes rapidly) and compress the upper airways, the esophagus and the vena cava. Hydrops and poly-hydramnios may develop. The effect on the upper airways is best assessed by MR imaging.

Masses that develop at the thoraco-abdominal limit usually represent foregut duplication cysts that typically develop both in the posterior mediastinum and in the upper abdomen; they may consist of a cystic part and an echogenic part. Their differential diagnosis includes sequestration (feeding vessel) and diaphragmatic hernia (herniated digestive loops) (MARKERT et al. 1996, CURROS and BRUNELLE 2001) (see Chap. 5).

> Teratoma and mediastinal neuroblastoma should be considered in cases of solid-type mediastinal tumors.

13.4.3
Heart

Rhabdomyomas appear typically as unique or multiple rounded echogenic intracardiac tumors; they grow within the myocardium (Fig. 13.10). They represent a marker for tuberous sclerosis and should prompt a search for typical CNS anomalies that are best assessed by fetal MR imaging. Rhabdomyomas may resolve progressively after birth. Other tumors such as teratoma and hemangioma may develop, usually within the cardiac chambers (TSENG et al. 1999, GEIPEL et al. 2001, CHOI et al. 2000, GROVES et al. 1992). Teratoma and angioma may develop in the pericardium and some pericardial effusion may be associated (DE BUSTAMENTE 2000, SEPULVEDA et al. 2000).

13.5
Abdomen

13.5.1
Peritoneum

13.5.1.1
Liver

Cystic masses in the liver usually correspond to simple hepatic cysts (HACKMON-RAM et al. 2000, MACKEN et al. 2000). The differential diagnosis includes choledochal cyst (next to the gallbladder), intrahepatic vascular malformations and other abdominal cavity cysts (MEJIDES et al. 1995, GALLAGHER et al. 1993). Rarely, they may correspond to a cystic hamartoma.

The differential diagnosis of intrahepatic solid or mixed-type tumors includes primary tumors and metastases. Hepatoblastoma and liver hamartoma appear as large, usually well-circumscribed echogenic masses (SHIH et al. 2000, BESSHO et al. 1996, DICKINSON et al. 1999). Liver hemangioma, the most common benign hepatic tumor in infants, may appear as an isolated large mass (Fig. 13.11) or multiple small hypoechoic masses. Color Doppler analysis may show hypervascularization and confirm the enlargement of the aorta at the level of the liver (MEIROWITZ et al. 2000, ABUHAMAD et al. 1993, SEPULVEDA et al. 1993, DE BIEVRE et al. 1994, DREYFUS et al. 1996).The masses may grow rapidly in utero during the third trimester or directly after birth. Heart failure may occur and, if necessary, cor-

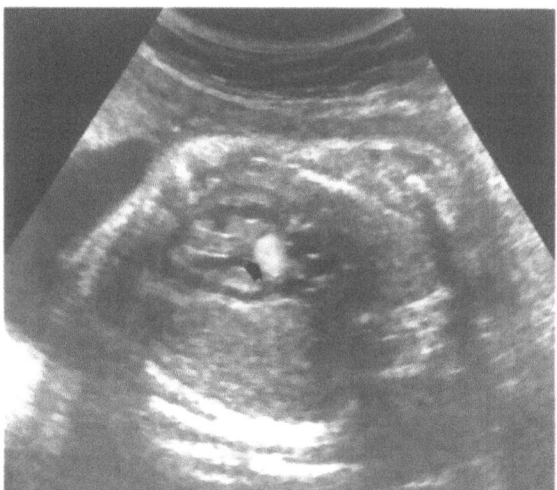
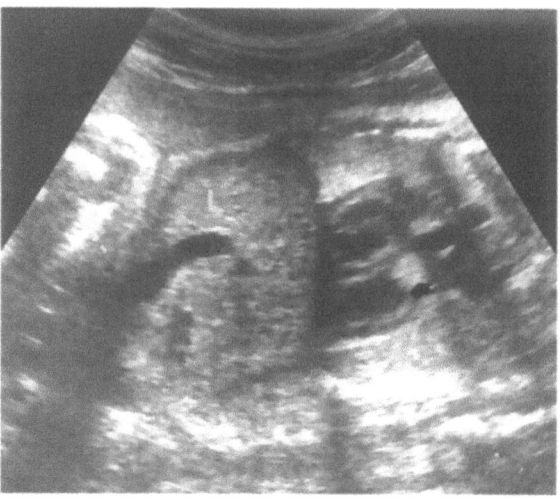

a   b

Fig. 13.10a, b. Cardiac rhabdomyoma. Third trimester. Case of tuberous sclerosis.. **a** Transverse US scan of the chest, four-chamber view showing a hyperechoic mass (*arrow*) centrally located within the heart. **b** Sagittal US scan The mass (*arrow*) is visible at the atrioventricular junction. *L* liver

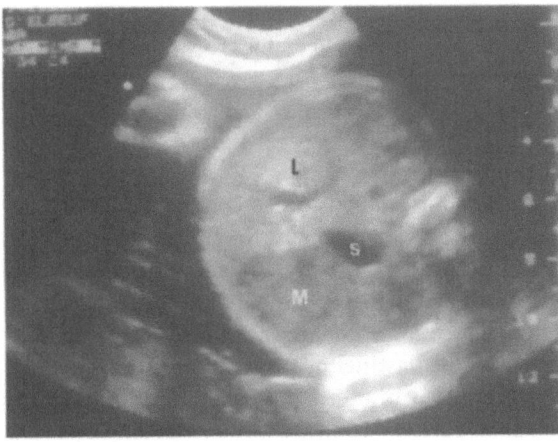
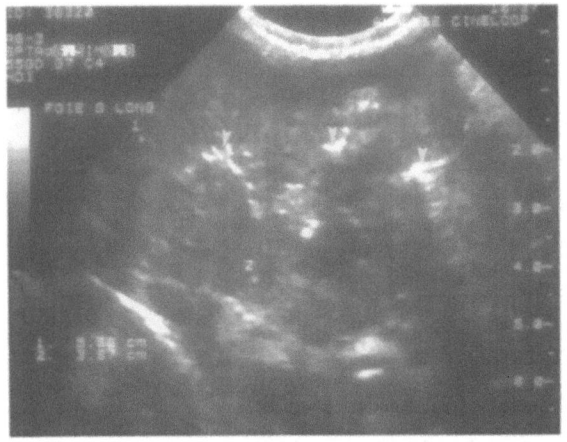

a

b

Fig. 13.11a, b. Hepatic hemangioendothelioma. **a** US in utero, Third trimester. Transverse scan of the fetal liver (*L*). A large hypoechoic mass (*M*) (4×5 cm) occupies the left lobe. *S* stomach. **b** US after birth. Sagittal scan of the left lobe of the liver demonstrates diffuse multiple areas of calcification (*arrowheads*) within the mass. The mass resolved spontaneously after birth

ticosteroid therapy may be started in utero (MORRIS et al. 1999). Liver metastasis may develop in utero secondary to neuroblastoma or to maternal cancer (melanoma, choriocarcinoma) (JAFFA et al. 1993, LIYANAGE and KATOCH 1992, TOMA et al. 1994). Metastases may appear as single or multiple masses. Calcification within liver masses should suggest a calcified metastasis, resolving hemangioendothelioma (Fig. 13.11b) or intrahepatic teratoma (MAGNUS et al. 1999). MR imaging may provide additional information in terms of tumoral content and extent of liver involvement.

> Solid-type liver tumors can correspond to primary (hamartoma, hemangioendothelioma) or secondary tumor (metastasis of neuroblastoma).

13.5.1.2
Peritoneal Cavity

Solid-type masses are extremely rare and may correspond to mesenchymal hamartoma or teratoma (HIRATA et al. 1990, SHIH et al. 1997).

Cystic lymphangioma and hemangioendothelioma may also extend into the peritoneal cavity. They appear as mixed, cystic or solid-type masses; color Doppler may demonstrate the vascular pedicle and eventual hypervascularization (DEVESA et al. 1997, DESHPANDE et al. 2001, SUZUKI et al. 1998). These tumors are usually large and displace the intra-abdominal structures. The differential diagnosis includes in utero ovarian torsion cysts and meconium pseudocysts. which may appear as echogenic mixed-type masses (Fig. 13.12) (KATZ et al. 1996)

Duplication cyst, urachal cyst or hydrocolpos may appear as large masses but they are usually not septated (Tables 13.2–13.4) (BAKER 1988).

Table 13.2. Solid-type abdominal tumors

Hepatic hemangioma
Hepatoblastoma
Metastasis (from neuroblastoma)
Teratoma (fetus in fetu)
Neuroblastoma
Infradiaphragmatic sequestration
Mesoblastic nephroma

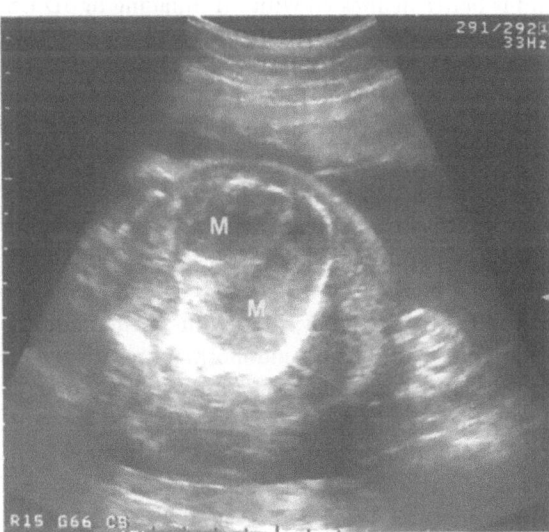

Fig. 13.12. Meconium pseudocyst. Third trimester. Transverse US scan of the fetal abdomen demonstrating a large echogenic mass (*M*) with a calcified rim. It was associated with an intestinal obstruction

Table 13.3. Abdominal cystic tumors

Choledochal cyst
Liver cyst
Splenic cyst
Pancreatic cyst
Ovarian cyst
Duplications
Urachal cyst
Adrenal cyst
Renal cyst
Hydrocolpos
Wolffian duct remnant cyst

Table 13.4. Mixed pattern cystic/solid tumors

Cystic lymphangioma
Cystic teratoma
Hemolymphangioma
Ovarian torsion cyst
Meconium pseudocyst

13.5.2
Retroperitoneum

13.5.2.1
Kidney

More than half of all congenital abdominal masses found in the neonatal period originate in the kidney (Fig. 13.13). The most common renal tumor that can be diagnosed during fetal life is mesoblastic nephroma. It appears as a solid-type mass somewhat difficult to differentiate from the kidney parenchyma, and is better delineated with MR imaging or 3D US. The tumor may appear partially or completely cystic. Associated polyhydramnios is usual; hypertension may develop at birth and resolve after curative nephrectomy (Schild et al. 2000, Haddad et al. 1996, Irsutti et al. 2000, Campagnola et al. 1998). Rare cases of Wilms' tumor have been reported with good postnatal prognosis; fetal hydrops may be an associated finding (Applegate et al. 1999, Bove 1999, Suresh 1 et al. 997, Vadeyar et al. 2000). Patients with hemi-hypertrophy, Beckwith-Wiedemann or Perlmann syndrome, pseudohermaphroditism and aniridia are at risk of developing Wilms' tumor or nephroblastomatosis (Beckwith 1999). The latter may cause diffuse enlargement of the kidneys (that appear hyperechoic) or bilateral nodular tumoral development (Lonergan et al. 1998, Ambrosino et al. 1990).

The differential diagnosis of an unilateral renal tumor is multicystic dysplastic kidney in which the entire kidney is affected.

Mesoblastic nephroma is the most common solid-type tumor of the kidney in utero.

13.5.2.2
Adrenal

Neuroblastoma is the most common solid malignant tumor in the neonate. Several cases have been detected in utero, usually at the end of the second trimester or during the third trimester (Fig. 13.14). Adrenal location is the most commonly encountered. Cervical, mediastinal or pelvic locations have rarely been reported in utero and are more typical of the neonatal period (Acharya et al. 1997, Saylors et al. 1994, Kesrouani et al. 1999, Lin et al. 1999).

Fetal adrenal neuroblastoma may display various patterns – solid, mixed solid and cystic or completely cystic – raising a sometimes difficult differential diagnosis (Table 13.5). Among adrenal masses, the main differential diagnosis is with adrenal hemorrhage. This differential is quite difficult since neuroblastoma may bleed (Morgan 1995, Jennings et al. 1993, Dreyfus et al. 1994). Calcifications rarely develop in utero (Schwärzler et al. 1999, Burbige 1993, Vollersen et al. 1996, Morganti and Anderson 1991, McCauley et al. 1991, Patti et al. 1993, Srouse 1999).

The differential diagnosis with non-adrenal masses can be achieved by demonstrating normal-appearing adrenals clearly separated from the mass (that still can correspond to an extra-adrenal neuroblastoma) (Duncan et al. 1992, Rubenstein et al. 1995, Davies et al. 1989, Richards et al. 1996).

During gestation the neuroblastoma may grow and metastasize to the liver (see above) (Toma et al. 1994, Liyanage and Katoch 1992). Even so, the prognosis is mostly favorable since most cases represent stages I, II and IVS, with a favorable outcome in cases confirmed (by mIBG scan and urinary catecholamines) and treated at birth (Teinturier et al. 1992). It is noteworthy that the various types of masses affecting the adrenals have a potential for spontaneous involution, even neuroblastoma (Fig. 13.14) (Jennings et al. 1993, Daneman et al. 1997, Holgerson et al. 1996).

13.5.2.3
Other

Teratoma may develop within the retroperitoneal cavity and appear as a mixed-pattern mass with eventual calcifications. The differential diagnosis includes pancreatic masses (hamartoma, pancreatoblastoma) (Burt et al. 1983, Fremond et al. 1997, Hanquinet et al. 1997).

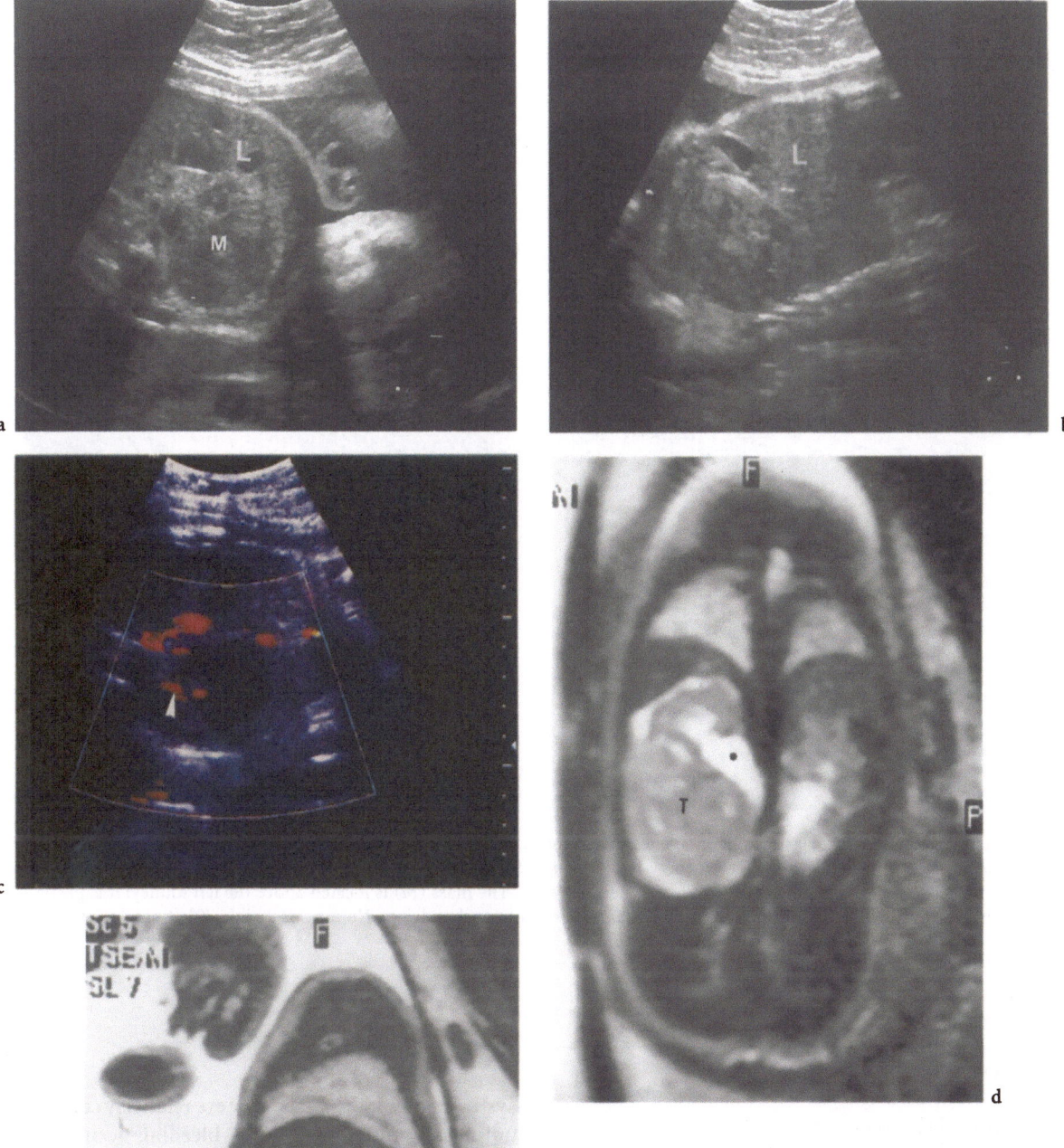

Fig. 13.13a–e. Mesoblastic nephroma. Third trimester. **a** US in utero. Transverse scan of the fetal abdomen. A mass (*M*) is hardly visible behind the left lobe of the liver (*L*). It measured 5 cm in diameter. **b** US in utero. Sagittal scan of the fetal trunk. The mass has an anteroposterior diameter of 5.35 cm (between *crosses*). Normal kidney is difficult to delineate from the mass. *L* liver. **c** Color Doppler demonstrates only one arterial branch entering the mass (*arrowhead*). **d** Fetal MR imaging. Frontal view. The tumor (*T*) invades the lower pole of the right kidney and produces some renal dilatation (***). **e** Fetal MR imaging. Sagittal view showing the normal upper pole (***) and the tumor (*T*) invading the lower pole. The tumor was removed at birth and this cured the neonatal hypertension

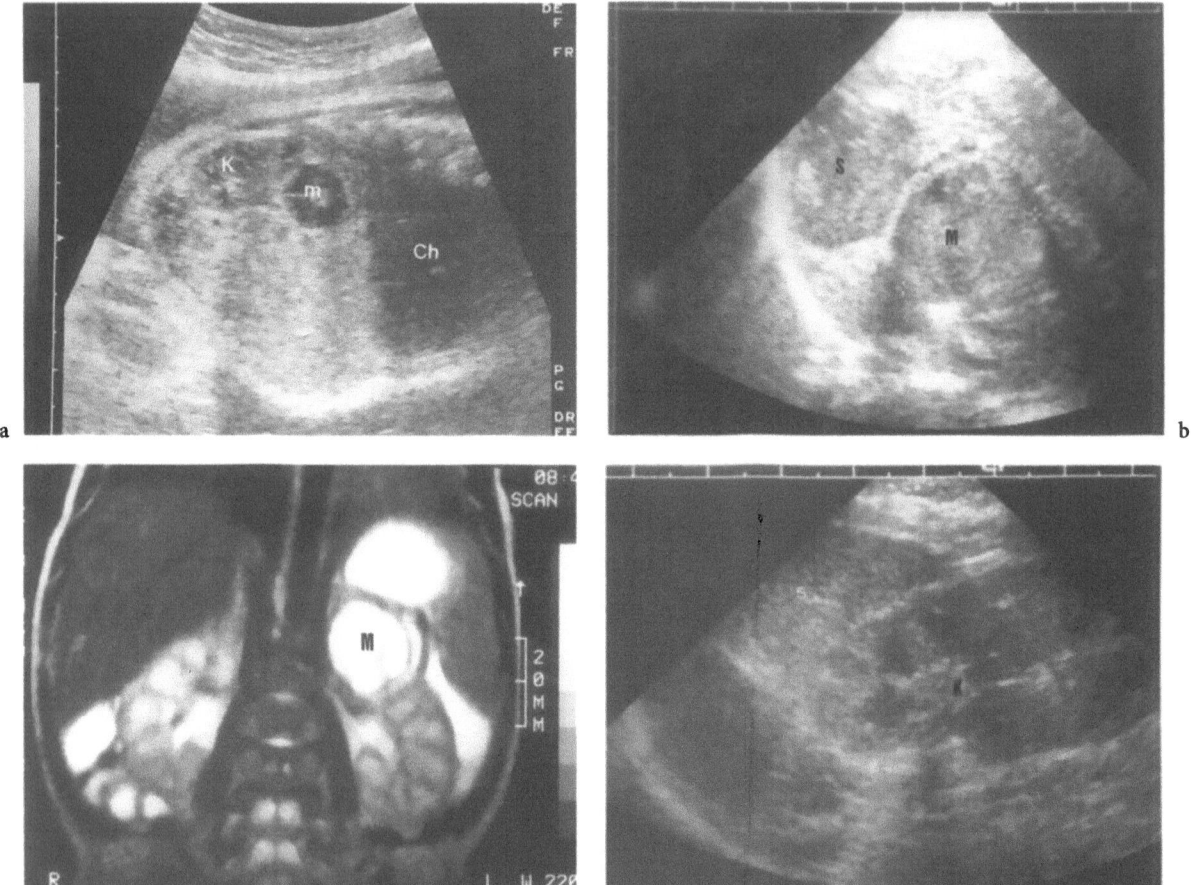

Fig. 13.14a–d. Adrenal neuroblastoma, spontaneous involution. **a** US in utero. Third trimester. A 3 cm heterogeneous mass (*m*) is visible in front of the left kidney (*K*). *Ch* chest. **b** US at birth. Sagittal scan of the left hypochondrium The mass (*M*) is still present. *s* stomach. **c** MR imaging at birth, T2-weighted sequence. The mass (*M*) is located above the left kidney; it is partially cystic (hemorrhagic?). **d** US at age 1 year. Sagittal scan of the left hypochondrium. No mass is visible. *K* left kidney, *s* spleen

Table 13.5. Differential diagnosis of an adrenal tumor

Neuroblastoma
Adrenal hemorrhage
Adrenal simple cyst
Cortical (hemorrhagic) cysts (associated with
    Beckwith-Wiedemann syndrome)
Renal cyst
Duplex kidney with dysplastic cystic upper pole
Mesoblastic nephroma
Wilms' tumor
Enteric duplication cyst
Infradiaphragmatic pulmonary sequestration
Teratoma

13.6
Ovary and Testis

Cystic lesions of the fetal ovary are relatively common and usually functional. When bleeding occurs with the cyst the mass appears hyperechoic and septated, but is still benign and may resolve spontaneously (Fig. 13.15) (see Chap. 8).

Testicular tumors may develop in the perinatal period and must be differentiated from testicular enlargement related to perinatal torsion. Yolk sac tumor, gonadal stromal tumors and juvenile granulosa cell tumors are the most common type. The prognosis is usually favorable. Note that teratoma may develop in the intra-abdominal undescended testis (LEVY et al. 1994). Rare inguino-scrotal hernia may develop in utero and have a pseudotumoral appearance (see Chap. 8).

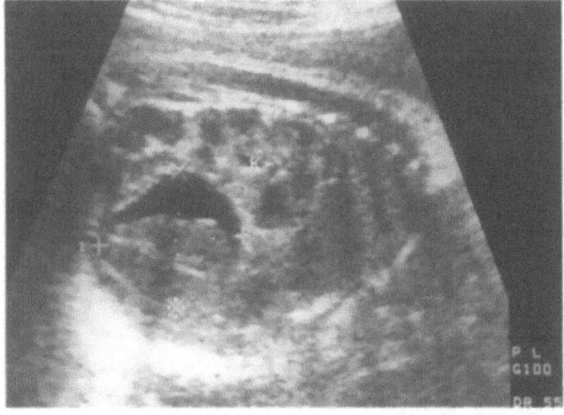

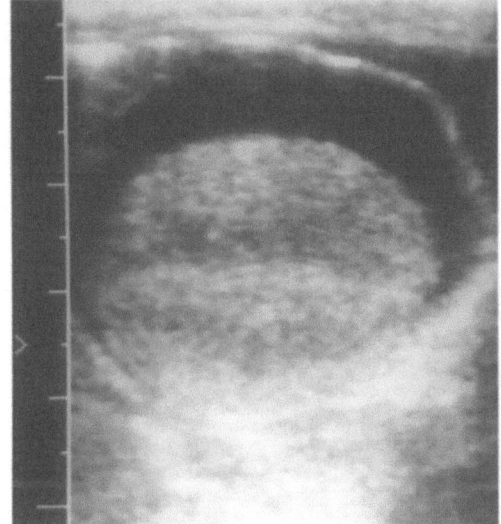

a

b

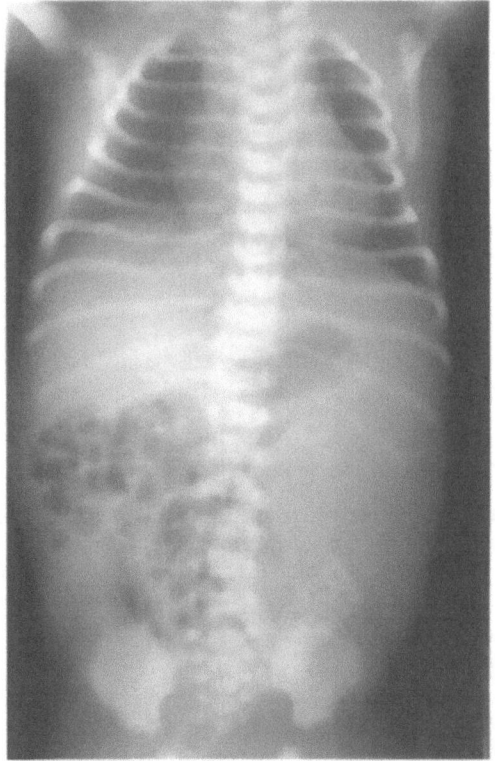

c

Fig. 13.15a–c. Ovarian cyst, pseudo-solid type. **a** US in utero. Third trimester. A mixed solid/cystic-type mass (3×2 cm between *crosses*) is visible in the fetal abdomen in front of the left kidney (*K*). **b** US at birth. The mass displays a similar appearance. **c** Plain film of the abdomen with a mass effect in the left flank (at surgery the ovarian cyst had bled and the content had coagulated)

13.7
Soft Tissues

Soft tissue neoplasms are an important category of tumors developing in the neonate and account for 10–25% of all congenital tumors. Some cases of rhabdomyosarcoma, lymphangioma, hemangiopericytoma and fibrous tumors have been reported in utero. They appeared as solid-type hypervascularized tumors. Malignant tumors have a poor postnatal prognosis and metastases are frequent (TEINTURIER et al. 1992, MEIZNER 2000, GRUNDY et al. 2001, SALLOUM et al. 1990, TADMOR et al.1998, PARKES et al. 1994, EICH et al. 1998, PATRICK et al. 1996). Lymphangioma and hemolymphangioma are relatively common; they present as very large tumors with a mixed solid and cystic pattern and may affect any part of the body (SENOH et al. 2001, GONCALVES et al. 2000, ROBERTS and SEPULVEDA 1997). MR imaging is helpful in demonstrating the extent of the tumor.

13.8
Sacro-coccygeal Teratoma

Sacro-coccygeal teratoma (SCT) represents the most common tumor in the neonate (1/35,000 births); fortunately only 2.5–10% are malignant in the neonatal period and therefore an early diagnosis and resection is mandatory. These tumors are associated with high incidence of prematurity (<50%), mortality 15–35% and morbidity 45–68%. Obstetrical US allows an early diagnosis around the early second trimester and helps to detect associated malformations (CNS, genitourinary or gastrointestinal). The tumor may be completely cystic, solid with calcifications or mixed solid and cystic (Figs. 13.16, 13.17). The size of SCT is variable at presentation; it is usually 3–4 cm diameter in the second trimester, but the tumor may grow rapidly and massively during the third trimester. The growth of the tumor may produce high-output cardiac failure and fetal hydrops. A large vascularized tumor is more

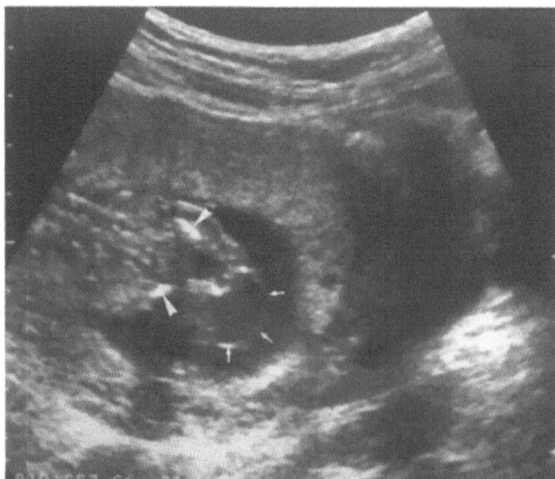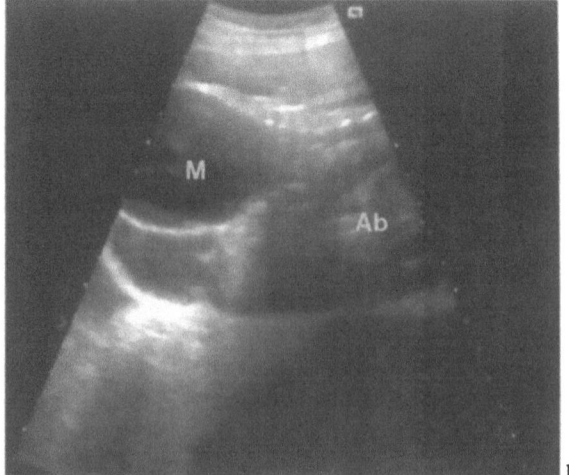

Fig. 13.16a, b. Sacrococcygeal teratoma, cystic type. **a** US in utero. Second trimester. Sagittal scan of the buttocks demonstrating a 1.5 cm mainly cystic mass (*arrows*). *Arrowheads* indicate the iliac wings. **b** Third trimester. A cystic septated 5×6 cm mass (*M*) is seen. The mass was limited to the perineum without intra-abdominal extension. *Ab* fetal abdomen

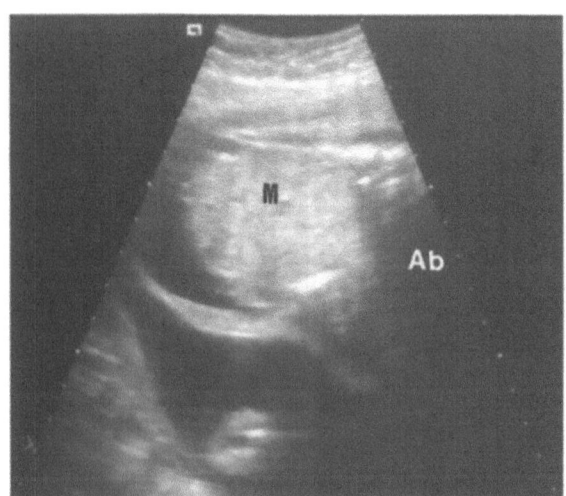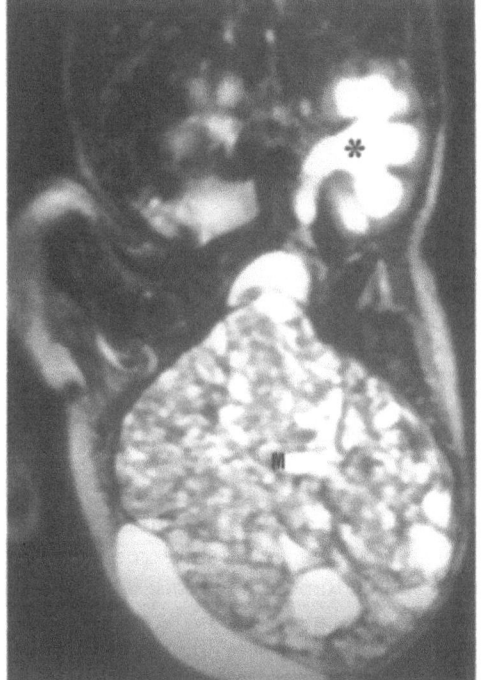

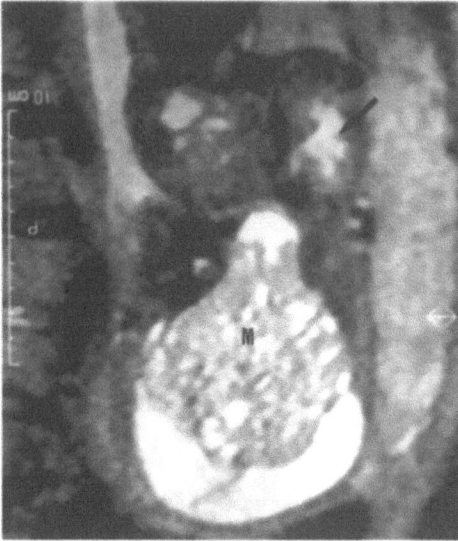

Fig. 13.17a–c. Sacro-coccygeal teratoma, microcystic pattern. Third trimester. **a** US through the mass. Sagittal scan of the lower spine demonstrating a highly echogenic mass (*M*). *Ab* abdomen. **b** Fetal MR imaging, T2-weighted sequence. Frontal scan of the mass (*M*) demonstrates a microcystic content and urinary tract dilatation (*arrow*). **c** MR imaging at birth demonstrating the extent of the mass (*M*) and the increasing urinary tract dilatation (*)

likely to be associated with hydrops. Other features associated with increased morbidity and mortality are placentomegaly, intra-abdominal extension, urinary tract dilatation and bladder compression as well as intratumoral bleeding (GOTO et al. 2000, HOLTERMAN et al. 1998, BRACE et al. 2000, CHRISHOLM et al. 1999). The extent of the mass is defined according to the classification of ALTMAN et al. into: grade I, completely extra-fetal mass; grade II, partially pelvic; grade III, abdomino-pelvic mass; and grade IV, completely intra-fetal mass (ALTMAN et al. 1974). MR imaging is more accurate than US in determining tumoral extent as well as defining tissue content, especially in non-cystic masses with possible hemorrhage (Figs. 13.17, 13.18) (QUINN et al. 1998, KIRKINEN et al. 1997, AVNI et al. 2002). The main differential diagnosis is meningocele, which is more likely to be associated with posterior vertebral defect. More difficult is the diagnosis of a grade IV SCT that has to be differentiated from the many possible intra-abdominal lesions (SHIPP et al. 1995).

After neonatal surgery, follow-up is mandatory in order to detect recurrences even if the entire tumor has been resected.

> Sacro-coccygeal teratoma is the commonest location for congenital teratoma. The extent of the mass is best assessed by fetal MR imaging.

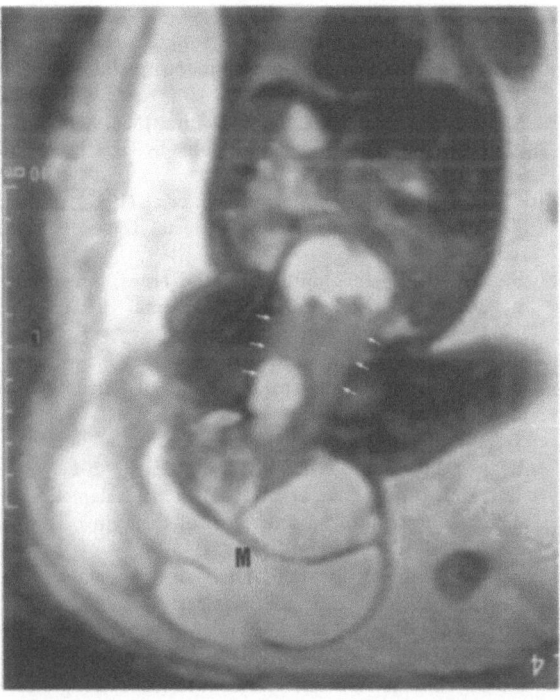

Fig. 13.18. Sacro-coccygeal teratoma, massive abdominopelvic extension. Third trimester. Fetal MR imaging clearly delineates the abdominal extension (*arrowheads*) of the mass (*M*)

13.10
Conclusion

Teratoma and cystic lymphangiomas are the most common tumors encountered in fetuses. Any organ or region can be affected; US allows the detection of most tumors but MR imaging determines more precisely the tumoral extent.

References

Abuhamad AZ, Lewis D, Inati MN, et al (1993) The use of color Doppler in the diagnosis of fetal hepatic hemangioma. J Ultrasound Med 12:223–226

Abramson SJ, Berdon WE, Ruzal-Shapiro C, et al (1993) Cervical neuroblastoma in eleven infants. Pediatr Radiol 23:253–257

Acharya S, Jayabose S, Kogan SJ, et al (1997) Prenatally diagnosed neuroblastoma. Cancer 80:304–3010

Adra A, Mejides AA, Salman FA, et al (1994) Prenatal US diagnosis of a third ventricle choroid plexus papilloma. Prenat Diagn 14:865–867

Altman RP, Randolph JG, Lilly JR (1974) Sacro-coccygeal teratoma. J Pediatr Surg 9:385–398

Ambrosio MM, Hernanz Schulman M, Horii SC, et al (1990) Prenatal diagnosis of nephroblastomatosis in two siblings. J Ultrasound Med 9:49–51

Applegate KE, Ghei M, Perez-Atayde AR (1999) Prenatal detection of a Wilms' tumor. Pediatr Radiol 29:65–67

Avni EF, Rodesch F, Vandemarckt C, Vermeylen D (1992) Detection and evaluation of fetal goitre by US. Br J Radiol 65:302–305

Avni EF, Guibaud L, Robert Y, et al (2002) The role of MR imaging for the assessment of fetal sacrococcygeal teratoma. AJR Am J Roentgenol (in press)

Bailey W, Freidenberg GR, James HE, et al (1990) Prenatal diagnosis of a craniopharyngioma using US and MRI. Prenat Diagn 10:623–629

Baker M (1988) Anechoic abdominal masses on US. Semin Roentgenol 33:143–144

Beckwith JB (1995) Certain conditions have an increased incidence of Wilms' tumors, AJR Am J Roentgenol 164:1294–1295

Beck JC, Devaney KD, Weatherly RA, et al (1999) Pediatric myofibromatosis of head and neck. Arch Otolaryngol Head Neck Surg 125:39–44

Beckwith JB (1999) Prenatal diagnosis of Wilms' tumor. Pediatr Radiol 29:64

Besscho T, Kubota K, Komori S, et al (1996) Prenatally detected hamartoma. Prenat Diagn 16:337–341

Brace V, Grant SR, Brackley KJ, et al (2000) Prenatal diagnosis and outcome in SCT. Prenat Diagn 20:51–55

Bove KE (1999) Wilms' tumor and related abnormalities in the fetus and newborn. Semin Perinatol 23:310–318

Bromley B, Frigoletto FD, Cramer D, et al. (1992) Fetal thyroid normal and abnormal measurements by US. J Ultrasound Med 11:25–28

Burbige KA (1993) Prenatal adrenal hemorrhage confirmed by postnatal surgery. J Urol 150:1867–1869

Burt TB, Condon VR, Matlak ME (1983) Fetal pancreatic hamartoma. Pediatr Radiol 13:287–289

Campagnola S, Fasoli L, Flessati P, et al (1998) Congenital cystic mesoblastic nephroma. Urol Int 61:254–256

Choi JM, Jaffe R, Maidman J, et al (2000) Multiple cardiac rhabdomyoma in utero. Fetal Diagn Ther 15:174–176

Chrisholm CA, Heider AL, Kuller JA, et al (1999) Prenatal diagnosis and perinatal management of fetal SCT. Am J Perinatol 16:47–500

Curros F, Brunelle F (2001) Prenatal thoraco-abdominal tumor mimicking pulmonary sequestration. Eur Radiol 11:167–170

Daneman A, Baunin C, Lobo E, et al (1997) Disappearing suprarenal masses in fetuses and infants. Pediatr Radiol 27:675–681

Davies RP, Ford WDA, Lequesne GW, et al (1989) US detection of subdiaphragmatic pulmonary sequestration in utero. J Ultrasound Med 8:47–49

De Bievre P, Dufour P, Lefebvre C, et al (1994) Diagnostic antenatal d'un hemangioendotheliome hepatique. J Gynecol Obstet Biol Reprod 23:435–439

De Bustamante TD, Azpeitia J, Miralles M, et al (2000) Prenatal US appearance of pericardial teratoma. J Clin Ultrasound 28:194–198

Deshpande P, Twinning P, O'Neill D (2001) Prenatal diagnosis of fetal lymphangioma by US. Ultrasound Obstet Gynecol 17:445–448

Devesa R, Munoz A, Torrents M, Carrera JM (1997) Prenatal US finding of intraabdominal cystic lymphangioma. J Clin Ultrasound 27:336–338

Dickinson JE, Knowles S, Philips JM (1999) Prenatal diagnosis of hepatic mesenchymal hamartoma. Prenat Diagn 19:81–84

Dreyfus M, Neuhart D, Baldauf JJ, et al (1994) Prenatal diagnosis of cystic neuroblastoma. Fetal Diagn Ther 94:269–272

Dreyfus M, Baldauf JJ, Dadoun K, et al (1996) Prenatal diagnosis of hepatic hemangioma. Fetal Diagn Ther 11:57–60

Duncan BW, Adzick NS, Erkalis A (1992) Retroperitoneal alimentary tract duplications detected in utero. J Pediatr Surg 27:1231–1233

Eich GF, Hoeffel JC, Tschappler H, et al (1998) Fibrous tumors in children. Pediatr Radiol 28:500–509

Fremond B, Poulain P, Odent S, et al (1997) Prenatal detection of a congenital pancreatic cyst. Prenat Diagn 17:276–280

Gallagher DM, Leiman S, Hux CH (1993) In utero diagnosis of a portal vein aneurysm. J Clin Ultrasound 21:147–151

Geipel A, Krapp M, Germer U, et al (2001) Perinatal diagnosis of cardiac tumors. Ultrasound Obstet Gynecol 17:17–21

Goncalves LF, Munoz Rojas MV, Vitorello D, et al (2000) Klippel Trenaunay Weber syndrome presenting as a massive lymphangiohemangioma of the thigh: prenatal diagnosis. Ultrasound Obstet Gynecol 15:337–341

Goto M, Makino Y, Tamura R, et al (2000) SCT with hydrops fetalis and bilateral hydronephrosis. J Perinat Med 28:414–418

Groves AMM, Fagg NLK, Cook A, et al (1992) Cardiac tumors in intrauterine life. Arch Dis Child 67:1189–1192

Grundy R, Anderson J, Gaze M, et al (2001) Congenital alveolar rhabdomyosarcoma. Cancer 91:606–612

Hackmon-Ram R, Wiznitzer A, Gohar J, Mazor M (2000) Prenatal diagnosis of fetal abdominal cyst. Eur J Obstet Gynecol 91:79–82

Haddad B, Haziza J, Touboul C, et al (1996) Congenital mesoblastic nephroma. Fetal Diagn Ther 11:61–66

Hanquinet S, Damry N, Heimann P, et al (1997) Association of a fetus in fetu and two teratomas: US and MRI, Pediatr Radiol 27:336–338

Heling KS, Chaoui R, Bollman R (2000) Prenatal diagnosis of an aneurysm of the Galen vein with 3D power angiography. Ultrasound Obstet Gynecol 15:333–336

Hirata GI, Matsunaga ML, Medaris AL, et al (1990) US diagnosis of a fetal abdominal mass: a case of mesenchymal hamartoma. Prenat Diagn 10:507–512

Holgerson LO, Subramanian S, Kirpekar M, et al (1996) Spontaneous resolution of antenatally diagnosed adrenal masses. J Pediatr Surg 31:153–155

Holterman A, Filiatrault D, Lallier M, Youssef S, et al (1998) The natural history of SCT diagnosed through routine obstetric US: a single institution experience. J Pediatr Surg 33:899–903

Ickowitz V, Eurin D, Rypens F, et al (2001) Prenatal diagnosis and postnatal follow-up of pericallosal lipoma. AJNR Am J Neuroradiol 22:767–772

Irsutti M, Puget C, Baunin C, et al (2000) Mesoblastic nephroma: prenatal US and MRI features. Pediatr Radiol 30:147–150

Jaffa AJ, Many A, Hartoov J, et al (1993) Prenatal US diagnosis of metastatic neuroblastoma. Prenat Diagn 13:73–77

Jennings RW, LaQuaglia MP, Leong K, et al (1993) Fetal neuroblastoma : prenatal diagnosis and natural history. J Pediatr Surg 28:1168–1174

Jung E, Won HS, Lee PR, et al (2000) The progression of mediastinal lymphangioma in utero. Ultrasound Obstet Gynecol 16:663–666

Katz VL, McCoy, McKuller JA, et al (1996) Fetal ovarian torsion cyst appearing as a solid type mass. J Perinatol 16:302–304

Kerner B, Flaum F, Mathews H, et al (1998) Cervical teratoma: prenatal diagnosis and long term follow-up. Prenat Diagn 18:51–59

Kesrouani A, Duchatel F, Seilaniain M, Muray JM (1999) Prenatal diagnosis of adrenal neuroblastoma by US. Ultrasound Obstet Gynecol 13:446–449

Kirkkinen P, Partanen K, Merikanto J, et al (1997) US and MR imaging of fetal SCT. Acta Obstet Gynecol Scand 76:917–922

Kueltuersay N, Gelal F, Mutluer S, et al (1995) Antenatally diagnosed neonatal craniopharyngioma. J Perinatol 15:426–428

Kurihara N, Tokieda K, Ikeda K, et al (2001) Prenatal MR findings in a case of aneurysm of the vein of Galen. Pediatr Radiol 31:160–162

Lee DY, Yoo SJ, Kim YM, et al (1999) Congenital glioblastoma diagnosed by fetal US. Child Nerv Syst 15:197–201

Lee TH, Shih JC, Peng SS, et al (2000) Prenatal depiction of angioarchitecture of an aneurysm of the vein of Galen. Ultrasound Obstet Gynecol 15:337–340

Levine D, Barnes P, Korf B, Edelman R (2000) TS in the fetus: second trimester diagnosis of subependymal tubers with ultrafast MR imaging. AJR Am J Roentgenol 175:1067–1069

Levine D, Jennings R, Barnewolt C, et al (2001) Progressive fetal bronchial obstruction caused by a bronchogenic cyst diagnosed using prenatal MR imaging. AJR Am J Roentgenol 179:49–52

Levy DA, Kay R, Elder JS (194) Neonatal testis tumors: a review of the prepubertal testis tumor registry, J Urol 151: 715–717

Liechtey KW, Crombleholme TM (1999) Management of fetal airway obstruction. Semin Perinatol 23:496–506

Lin JN, Lin GJ, Hung LJ, et al (1999) Prenatally detected tumor mass in the adrenal gland. J Pediatr Surg 34:1620–1623

Liyanage IS, Katoch D (1992) US prenatal diagnosis of liver metastases from adrenal neuroblastoma. J Clin Ultrasound 20:401–403

Lonergan JG, Martinez-Leon ML, Agron GA, et al (1998) Nephrogenic rests, nephroblastomatosis and associated lesions of the kidney. Radiographics 18:947–968

Lopez de Lacalle JM, Aguirre I, Irizabal JC, et al (2001) Congenital epulis: prenatal diagnosis by US. Pediatr Radiol 31:453–454

Macken MB, Wright JR, Lau H, et al (2000) Prenatal US detection of congenital hepatic cyst. J Clin Ultrasound 28:307–310

Magnus KG, Millar AJW, Sinclair-Smith CC, Rode H (1999) Intra-hepatic fetus in fetu. J Pediatr Surg 34:1861–1864

Markert DJ, Grumbach K, Haney PJ (1996) Thoraco-abdominal duplication cyst. J Ultrasound Med 15:333–336

McCauley RG, Beckwith JB, Elias ER, et al (1991) Benign hemorrhagic adrenocortical macrocysts in Beckwith-Wiedemann syndrome. AJR Am J Roentgenol 157:549–552

Meirowitz NB, Guzman ER, Underberg-Davis SJ, et al (2000) Hepatic hemangioendothelioma: prenatal US findings and evolution of the lesion. J Clin Ultrasound 28:258–263

Meizner (2000) Perinatal oncology the rôle of prenatal US diagnosis. Ultrasound Obstet Gynecol 16:507–509

Meizner I, Shalev J, Maschiach R, et al (2000) Prenatal US diagnosis of infantile myofibromatosis. Ultrasound Obstet Gynecol 16:84–86

Mejides AA ,Adra AM, O'Sullivan MJ, et al (1995) Prenatal diagnosis and therapy for a fetal hepatic vascular malformation Obstet Gynecol 85:850–853

Mernagh JR, Mohide PT, Lappalainen RE, Fedoryshin JG (1999) US assessment of the fetal head and neck. Radiographics 19:S229–S241

Morris J, Abbott J, Burrows P, Levine D (1999) Antenatal diagnosis of fetal hepatic hemangioma treated with maternal corticosteroids. Obstet Gynecol 94:813–815

Mitra AG, Dickerson C (2000) CNS tumor with associated unilateral ventriculomegaly. J Ultrasound Med 19:651–654

Morgan E (1995) Prenatal detection of neuroblastoma: a noninvasive approach. Pediatrics 95:161

Morganti VJ, Anderson NG (1991) Simple adrenal cysts in fetus, resolving spontaneously in neonate, J Ultrasound Med 10:521–524

Ogde RF, Jauniaux E (1999) Fetal scalp cysts: dilemmas in diagnosis. Prenat Diagn 19:1157–1159

Onderoglu LS, Yucel A, Yuce K (1999) Prenatal US features of embryonal rhabdomyosarcoma. Ultrasound Obstet Gynecol 13:210–212

Parkes SE, Muir KR, Southern L, et al (1994) Neonatal tumors: a thirty-year population based study. Med Pediatr Oncol 22:309–317

Patrick LE, O'Shea P, Simoneaux SF, et al (1996) Fibromatosis of childhood. AJR Am J Roentgenol 166:163–169

Patti G, Fiocca G, Latini T, et al (1993) Prenatal diagnosis of bilateral adrenal cysts. J Urol 150:1189–1191

Pilu G, Falco P, Perolo A, et al (1997) Differential diagnosis and outcome of fetal hypoechoic lesions. Ultrasound Obstet Gynecol 9:229–236

Pinto V Meo F, Loiudice L, D'Addario V (1999) Prenatal US diagnosis of an immature intracranial teratoma. Fetal Diagn Ther 14:220–222

Poutamo J, Vanninen R, Partanen K, et al (1999) MR imaging supplements US imaging of the posterior fossa, pharynx and neck in malformed fetuses. Ultrasound Obstet Gynecol 13:327–334

Quinn TM, Hubbard AM, Adzick NS (1998) Prenatal MR imaging enhances fetal diagnosis. J Pediatr Surg 33:553–558

Ranzini AC, Shen-Schwarz S, Guzman ER, et al (1998) Prenatal US appearance of hemorrhagic cerebellar infarction J Ultrasound Med 17:725–727

Reiss I, Gortner L, Moller J, et al (1996) Fetal intracerebral hemorrhage in the second trimester diagnosis by US and MR imaging. Ultrasound Obstet Gynecol 7:49–51

Rempen A, Feige A (1985) Differential diagnosis of US detected tumors in the fetal cervical region, Eur J Obstet Gynecol Reprod Biol 20:89–105

Richards DS, Langham MR, Anderson CD (1996) The prenatal US appearance of enteric duplication cysts. Ultrasound Obstet Gynecol 7:17–20

Roberts JA, Sepulveda W (1997) Prenatal US findings associated with lymphangioma of the chest wall. J Ultrasound Med 16:635–637

Rubenstein SC, Benaceraff BR, Retik AB, et al (1995) Fetal suprarenal masses: US appearance and differential diagnosis. Ultrasound Obstet Gynecol 5:164–167

Salim A, Wiknjosastro GH, Danukusuko D, et al (1998) Fetal retinoblastoma. J Ultrasound Med 17:717–720

Salloum E, Flamant F, Caillaud JM, et al (1990) Diagnostic and therapeutic problems of soft tissue tumors other than rhabdomyosarcoma in infants under 1 year of age. Med Pediatr Oncol 18:37–43

Saylors RL, Cohn SL, Morgan ER, Brodeur GM (1994) Prenatal detection of neuroblastoma by fetal US. Am J Pediatr Hemat Oncol 16:356–360

Schild RL, Plath H, Hofstaetter C, et al (2000) Diagnosis of fetal mesoblastic nephroma by 3D US. Ultrasound Obstet Gynecol 15:533–536

Sharony R, Kidron D, Aviram R, et al (1999) Prenatal diagnosis of fetal cerebellar lesions. Prenat Diagn 19:1077–1080

Shipp TD, Bromley B, Benacerraf B (1995) The US appearance and outcome for fetuses with masses distorting the face. J Ultrasound Med 14:673–678

Shipp TD, Shamberger RC, Benacerraf BR (1996) Prenatal diagnosis of a grade IV SCT. J Ultrasound Med 15:175–177

Schlembach D, Bornemann A, Rupperecht T, Beinder E (1999) Fetal intracranial tumors detected by US. Ultrasound Obstet Gynecol 14:407–418

Schwärzler P, Bernard JP, Senat MV, Ville Y (1999) Prenatal diagnosis of fetal adrenal masses: differentiation between hemorrhage and solid tumor by color Doppler US. Ultrasound Obstet Gynecol 13:351–355

Senoh D, Hanaoka U, Tanaka Y, et al (2001) Antenatal US features of giant fetal hemangiolymphangioma. Ultrasound Obstet Gynecol 17:252–254

Sepulveda WH, Dontsch G, Giuliano A (1993) Prenatal US diagnosis of fetal hepatic hemangioma. Eur J Obstet Gynecol Reprod Biol 48:73–76

Sepulveda W, Gomez E, Guttierez J (2000) Intrapericardial teratoma. Ultrasound Obstet Gynecol 15:547–548

284   F. E. Avni et al.

Sgro M, Barozzino T, Toi A, et al (1999) Prenatal detection
of cerebral lesions in a fetus with TS. Ultrasound Obstet
Gynecol 14:356–359

Shih HH, Teng RJ, Yau KI, et al (1997) Mature teratoma arising
from an intra-abdominal undescended testis. Ultrasound
Obstet Gynecol 10:209–211

Shih JC, Tsao PN, Huang SF, et al (2000) Antenatal diagnosis
of congenital hepatoblastoma in utero. Ultrasound Obstet
Gynecol 16:94–97

Shipp TD, Bromley B, Benaceraff B (1995) The US appearance
and outcome for fetuses with masses distorting the fetal
face. J Ultrasound Med 14:673–678

Shiraishi H, Nakamura M, Ichihachi K, et al (2000) Prenatal
MRI in a fetus with a giant neck hemangioma. Prenat
Diagn 20:1004–1007

Sonigo PC, Rypens FF, Carteret M, et al (1998) MR imaging of
fetal cerebral anomalies. Pediatr Radiol 28:212–222

Strouse PJ, Bowerman RA, Schlesinger AE (1995) Antenatal
US findings of fetal adrenal hemorrhage. J Clin Ultrasound
23:442–446

Suchet IB (1995) US of the fetal neck in the second and third
trimester. Can Assoc Radiol J 46:426–433

Suresh I, Suresh S, Arumugam R, et al (1997) Antenatal diagnosis of Wilms' tumor. J Ultrasound Med 16:69–72

Suzuki N, Tsuchida Y, Takahashi A, et al (1998) Prenatally
diagnosed cystic lymphangioma in infants. J Pediatr Surg
33:1599–1604

Tadmor OP, Ariel I, Rabinowitz R, et al (1998) Prenatal US

appearance of congenital fibrosarcoma. J Clin Ultrasound
26:276–279

Teinturier C, Kalifa C, Hartmann O, et al (1992) Tumeurs sol-
ides malignes néonatales. Arch Fr Pediatr 49:187–192

Toma P, Lucigrai G, Marzoli A, et al (1994) Prenatal diagnosis
of metastatic adrenal neuroblastoma with US and MR
imaging. AJR Am J Roentgenol 162:1183–1184

Tseng JJ, Chou MM, Lee YH, Ho ESC (1999) In utero diagnosis of cardiac hemangioma. Ultrasound Obstet Gynecol
13:363–365

Vadeyar S, Ramsay M, James D, O'Neill D (2000) Prenatal
diagnosis of congenital Wilms' tumor presenting as fetal
hydrops. Ultrasound Obstet Gynecol 16:80–83

Vanlieferinghen P, Lemery D, Sevely A, et al (1993) Diagnostic antenatal des tumeurs cerebrales congenitales. Arch Fr
Pediatr 50:39–41

Vergani P, Stroblet N, Locatelli A, et al (1996) Clinical significance of fetal intracranial hemorrhage. Am J Obstet Gynecol 175:536–543

Vollersen E, Hof M, Gembruch U (1996) Prenatal US diagnosis of fetal adrenal gland hemorrhage, Fetal Diagn Ther
11:286–291

Wang RM, Shih JC, Ko TM (2000) Prenatal US depiction of
fetal mediastinal immature teratoma. J Ultrasound Med
19:289–292

Yancey MK, Lasley D, Richards DS (1993) An unusual neck
mass in a fetus with Klippel Trenaunay Weber syndrome. J
Ultrasound Med 12:779–782

14 Fetal Hydrops

Françoise Rypens

CONTENTS

14.1   Introduction *285*
14.2   Pathophysiology *285*
14.3   Etiology *285*
14.3.1 Immune Hydrops Fetalis *285*
14.3.2 Nonimmune Hydrops Fetalis *286*
14.4   Ultrasound Diagnosis *289*
14.5   Management *290*
14.6   Prognosis *291*
14.6.1 Fetal Prognosis *291*
14.6.2 Maternal Prognosis *292*
        References *292*

14.1
Introduction

Hydrops fetalis is a nonspecific end stage of various fetal, placental and maternal diseases. It corresponds to excessive fluid accumulation in at least two fetal compartments, including the peritoneal, pleural and pericardial serous cavities, subcutaneous tissue, and placenta (GEMBRUCH and HOLZGREVE 2001). Isolated fluid accumulation (pleural effusion, ascites, pericardial effusion) is usually not considered as hydrops even if it may be the first sign of it.

14.2
Pathophysiology

Hydrops occurs when the rate of interstitial fluid production by capillary ultrafiltration exceeds the rate of interstitial fluid return to the circulation by the lymphatic vessels and the veins (APKON 1995). Six classical mechanisms are implicated in the development of hydrops: primary myocardial failure (myocarditis, malformation, metabolic disease, etc.),

F. RYPENS, MD
Department of Medical Imaging, Sainte-Justine Hospital, 3175 Côte-Sainte-Catherine, Montréal, Québec H3T 1C5, Canada

high-output cardiac failure (anemia, hemorrhage or arteriovenous fistula), low colloid oncotic plasma pressure due to renal protein loss or lack of hepatic protein production, increased capillary permeability (tissue hypoxia or sepsis), and obstruction of venous and/or lymphatic flow (thoracic and pulmonary disease) (APKON 1995, DE GROOT et al. 2000, GEMBRUCH and HOLZGREVE 2001). The development process of hydrops fetalis is different depending on the etiology (FOROUZAN 1997).

14.3
Etiology

The prevalence of the various etiologies of hydrops has evolved with time. It is strongly influenced by the population studied (GEMBRUCH and HOLZGREVE 2001). Hydrops is categorized into two types. The first type, immune hydrops (IHF), is due to the presence of circulating maternal antibodies directed against the fetal red blood cell antigens. The second type is nonimmune hydrops (NIHF), where there is no evidence of fetal-maternal blood group incompatibility (BULLARD and HARRISON 1995).

Since the introduction of efficient prevention of Rhesus incompatibility, the ratio between immune and nonimmune hydrops has inverted. In 1970, 82% of cases of hydrops were caused by immune disease; now over 92% have a nonimmunological origin (McCoy et al. 1995, BIANCHI et al. 2000a).

14.3.1
Immune Hydrops Fetalis

In IHF, maternal antibodies to some fetal blood group antigens cross the placenta, causing hemolysis of fetal blood and marked anemia. Most cases of IHF result from materno-fetal Rhesus blood group incompatibility (BIANCHI et al. 2000a). The stronger the obstetric history of Rhesus isoimmunization, the more likely the recurrence of severe disease in a future pregnancy (BIANCHI et al. 2000a). Even though non-Rhesus (D) blood group isoimmunization (Kell, ABO blood-groups, etc.) is becoming relatively more frequent than classical Rhesus isoimmunization, thanks to effective prevention programs, IHF secondary to ABO blood group incompatibility remains extremely rare (FOROUZAN 1997, McDONNELL et al. 1998, BIANCHI et al. 2000a).

14.3.2
Nonimmune Hydrops Fetalis

The prevalence of NIHF varies from 1/3800 to 1/830 deliveries (MACHIN 1989, BULLARD and HARRISON 1995, SWAIN et al. 1999, GEMBRUCH and HOLZGREVE 2001). The list of conditions associated with NIHF is long and continues to grow (Table 14.1) (MACHIN 1989, KEELING 1991, VAN MALDERGEM et al. 1992, KNISELY 1995, LALLEMAND et al. 1999, GEMBRUCH and HOLZGREVE 2001). It includes fetal, placental, and maternal causes (FOROUZAN 1997). Thanks to the progress of prenatal diagnosis, a cause or associated condition may be detected antenatally in up to 82% of cases (SOHAN et al. 2001). A precise diagnosis is useful in order to evaluate the prognosis and the risk of recurrence. Nevertheless, in some cases the etiology will remain uncertain despite extensive pathological analysis (JONES 1995).

The incidence and etiology of NIHF are strongly influenced by the gestational age, the patient population, and the pattern of referral (Table 14.2) (KNISELY 1995, McCOY et al. 1995, JAUNIAUX 1997). Karyotypic anomalies predominate in hydrops diagnosed early in pregnancy. Infections and anemias are rarely responsible for hydrops before 16 weeks of gestation due to the necessary delay before the manifestation of the disease (JAUNIAUX 1997, GEMBRUCH and HOLZGREVE 2001). (Evidence of recent maternal infection was only present in 1.4% in an early pregnancy group compared with 9.5% in later affected pregnancies: JAUNIAUX 1997). In midtrimester hydrops, chromosomal anomalies, fetal structural anomalies and infections are respectively responsible for 44.8%, 43.1% and 6.9% of cases of hydrops (HEINONEN et al. 2000). After 24 weeks of gestation, cardiothoracic anomalies, infections, and hematological etiologies predominate (McCOY et al. 1995, SOHAN et al. 2001).

Incidence and etiology are also strongly influenced by ethnic background: in South-East Asia, alpha-1-thalassemia is the main cause of hydrops, and is more frequent than cardiovascular and chro-

Table 14.1. Main circumstances associated with nonimmune hydrops fetalis

Aneuploidies:
  Trisomy 21
  Turner syndrome
  Trisomy 18
  Trisomy 13

Cardiac anomalies:
  Cardiac malformations:
    Atrioventricular septal defect
    Left heart hypoplasia
  Fetal arrhythmias:
    Tachyarrhythmias
    Supraventricular tachycardia
    Atrial flutter
    Ventricular tachycardia
    Bradyarrhythmias
    Complete heart block with structural defect
  Cardiac tumors:
    Rhabdomyoma
  Cardiomyopathy
  Myocarditis
  Idiopathic arterial calcifications

Infectious causes:
  Parvovirus B19
  Cytomegalovirus
  Bacteria
  Protozoans

Hematologic disorders causing fetal anemia:
  Alpha-1-thalassemia
  Hemorrhage
  Parvovirus B19 infection

Twin gestation:
  Twin-twin transfusion syndrome

Thoracic malformations:
  Primary unilateral or bilateral chylothorax
  Cystic adenomatoid malformation
  Sequestration
  Laryngeal atresia
  Diaphragmatic hernia

Gastrointestinal malformations

Renal anomalies:
  Nephrotic syndrome

Metabolic disorders

Vascular disorders:
  Arteriovenous malformations
  Idiopathic arterial calcifications

Tumors:
  Sacrococcygeal teratoma
  Hemangiom

Syndromes:
  Fetal akinesia syndrome
  Noonan
  Beckwith-Wiedemann

Skeletal dysplasias

Placental and umbilical cord anomalies:
  Chorioangioma

Maternal diseases (diabetes, Graves disease, etc.),
  medications

mosomal abnormalities (GHOSH et al. 1994, ANANDAKUMAR et al. 1996, GEMBRUCH and HOLZGREVE 2001). (Alpha-1-thalassemia is also observed in the Eastern Mediterranean region.) Cardiothoracic diseases, chromosomal anomalies and infections predominate in Caucasians (MCCOY et al. 1995, GEMBRUCH and HOLZGREVE 2001).

Fetal causes of NIHF in the Caucasian population usually fall into the following categories: chromosomal, cardiovascular, infection, hematological, twinning, and thoracic anomalies (MCCOY et al. 1995, FOROUZAN 1997, BIANCHI et al. 2000b). The other etiologies are rarer (metabolic, musculoskeletal diseases, etc.) (Table 14.2).

Table 14.2. Etiology of nonimmume hydrops fetalis according to the gestational age

First trimester	Second trimester	Third trimester
Aneuploidy	Aneuploidy	Cardiothoracic malformation
	Fetal malformation	Infection
	Infection	Hematological abnormality

Genetic causes account for 35% of cases of hydrops in fetal and neonatal autopsies and are detected in at least 10% of fetuses with hydrops (VAN MALDERGEM et al 1992, FOROUZAN 1997). The incidence of chromosomal anomalies is higher if hydrops is detected early during pregnancy (JAUNIAUX 1997, ISKAROS et al. 1997). (Before 18 weeks of gestation, the incidence of aneuploidy reaches 77.8%, and before 24 weeks of gestation 33–45% of fetuses with hydrops have an abnormal karyotype: MCCOY et al. 1995, ISKAROS et al. 1997, SOHAN et al. 2001). The most frequent anomalies are chromosomal: Turner syndrome is the main cause, being followed by trisomy 21 and then trisomy 18, 13 and 16, and triploidy (VAN MALDERGEM et al 1992, JAUNIAUX 1997). More than 64 different genetic etiologies are now described in association with hydrops: skeletal dysplasias, inborn errors of metabolism, hematological disorders (alpha-thalassemia), other autosomal recessive conditions (Pena-Shokeir and multiple pterygium syndromes), and dominant disorders have also been described in association with NIHF (VAN MALDERGEM et al 1992).

Cardiovascular anomalies are detected in 20–40% of cases of NIHF (KNILANS 1995, GEMBRUCH and HOLZGREVE 2001). Primary or secondary intrauterine cardiac failure is the most common mechanism of NIHF in the second and third trimesters of gestation (ISKAROS et al. 1997).

Structural malformations are the most common cardiovascular cause of NIHF (62%) (Fig. 14.1) (FOROUZAN 1997). All left-sided obstructive lesions that increase the right auricular pressure can be associated with hydrops. Among them, hypoplastic left heart syndrome is the main cause of hydrops (KNILANS 1995). Ventricular and atrioventricular septal defects, commonly reported in association with hydrops, are associated with 16–18% of chromosomal anomalies (ISKAROS et al. 1997). These malformations usually have a very poor prognosis when complicated by hydrops.

Tachyarrhythmia is the second most common cardiovascular abnormality associated with hydrops. Its prognosis is better because there exists an effective treatment. Bradyarrhythmia is less commonly associated with hydrops. Lastly, high-output heart failure (anemia or arteriovenous malformation), cardiac tumors, cardiomyopathy (metabolic or infectious), and idiopathic arterial calcification have been observed in association with hydrops (KNILANS 1995).

Hydrops resulting from atrioventricular valve insufficiency and/or supraventricular tachycardia can be successfully treated with antiarrhythmic medications administered to the mother (i.e., digoxin) (WY et al. 1999). The degree of pleural effusion in these cases may be predictive of survival (FOROUZAN 1997). The biventricular outer dimension of the heart is a good predictor for prognosis (FOROUZAN 1997).

Infections are responsible for up to 8% of cases of hydrops (BARRON and PASS 1995). Sepsis causes anoxia, endothelial cell damage, increased capillary permeability, and hepatic destruction (BARRON and

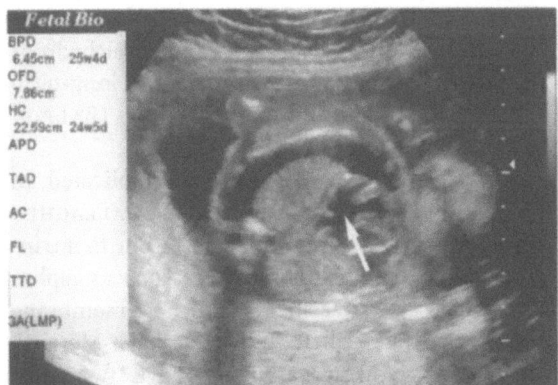

Fig. 14.1. A 22-week-old fetus with atrioventricular defect diagnosed at 18 weeks of gestation. Axial view of the chest shows skin edema and bilateral pleural effusion, diagnosing cardiac insufficiency and developing hydrops (*arrow*: atrial septal defect)

PASS 1995). The most frequent infectious agents reported are human parvovirus B19, cytomegalovirus (1–2% of NIHF), *Toxoplasma gondii*, and *Treponema pallidum*, but other agents have also been implicated including herpes simplex virus, coxsackievirus, adenovirus, rubella, polio, influenza B, various bacteria (*Listeria monocytogenes*), spirochetes, parasites (*Trypanosoma cruzi*), *Chlamydia*, *Ureaplasma*, etc. (BARRON and PASS 1995, FOROUZAN 1997).

In some series, B19 deoxyribonucleic acid is found in 18% of cases of idiopathic nonimmune hydrops fetalis (JORDAN 1996). Parvovirus B19 infection during pregnancy can be responsible for up to 27% of cases of nonimmune hydrops in anatomically normal fetuses (VON KAISENBERG and JONAT 2001). Approximately 40% of women of childbearing age are susceptible. Annual seroconversion rate varies from 1.5% to 10–15% during epidemics. Maternal infection in the first half of pregnancy is associated with 10% excess fetal loss and hydrops fetalis in 3% of cases (of which up to 60% resolve spontaneously or with appropriate management) (GILBERT 2000). The virus causes arrest of maturation of red blood cell precursors and a decrease in the number of platelets. Myocarditis and hepatitis are also observed. This infection may be responsible for hydrops during the first trimester of pregnancy (SOHAN et al. 2000). Fetal transfusion allows correction of the anemia until resolution of the infection. Usually, the average time from diagnosis to resolution is 6 weeks (range 2–12 weeks) (VON KAISENBERG and JONAT 2001).

Cytomegalovirus (CMV) is responsible for 1–2% of NIHF (BARRON and PASS 1995). The chances of survival are better than with other noninfectious causes of fetal hydrops, spontaneous resolution of hydrops being reported (MAZERON et al. 1994). Nevertheless, most surviving infants with congenital CMV disease severe enough to cause fetal hydrops will suffer neurological impairment, and long-term ophthalmological and auditory disabilities (BARRON and PASS 1995).

Hematological abnormalities are implicated in 10–27% of cases of NIHF (ARCASOY and GALLAGHER 1995, FOROUZAN 1997). Anemia may be due to intrinsic hemolysis (hemoglobinopathies such as alpha-thalassemia, rarer red cell enzymatic and membrane anomalies), extrinsic hemolysis (Kasabach-Merritt), hemorrhage (fetomaternal hemorrhage, twin-twin transfusion syndrome, etc.) or erythrocyte underproduction (in the case of fetal liver and bone marrow replacement syndromes, dyserythropoieses, infections, etc.) (ARCASOY and GALLAGHER 1995). Significant anemia leads to high-output heart failure when the hematocrit reaches 15% (ARCASOY and GALLAGHER 1995). This may be diagnosed with cardiac fetal ultrasound. This type of etiology must be kept in mind in the case of fetal or neonatal hemolysis, a previous history of NIHF, familial hematological anomaly or when extensive extramedullary erythropoiesis is discovered on pathological investigation (ARCASOY and GALLAGHER 1995).

Among the various possible causes of nonimmune anemic hydrops, homozygous alpha-thalassemia (Hb Bart), an autosomal recessive condition, is the main cause in South-East Asia.

Twin-twin transfusion syndrome complicates 5% of monochorionic twin pregnancies (FOROUZAN 1997). When hydrops happens in the second trimester of pregnancy, the prognosis is extremely poor (FOROUZAN 1997) (see Chap. 10).

Noncardiac thoracic abnormalities may cause hydrops by compression of the cardiac venous return and central venous hypertension (FOROUZAN 1997). Presence or absence of hydrops in fetuses with echogenic lung mass is a very important prognostic sign. In the absence of hydrops, provided there are no other anomalies, the survival rate may be as high as 90% (FOROUZAN 1997) (see Chap. 5).

Gastrointestinal anomalies are a rare cause of NIHF (FOROUZAN 1997). These anomalies are usually associated with isolated ascites, but secondary hepatic anomalies may lead to hydrops (GEMBRUCH and HOLZGREVE 2001).

Renal anomalies rarely cause hydrops except in cases of congenital nephrosis of the Finnish type (congenital nephrotic syndrome) (GEMBRUCH and HOLZGREVE 2001).

Metabolic anomalies (mostly lysosomal diseases) are seen in less than 5% of cases of hydrops (STEINER 1995). Ten different lysosomal storage disorders have been already described in association with hydrops: mucopolysaccharidosis VII and IVA, type 2 Gaucher disease, sialidosis, GM1 gangliosidosis, galactosialidosis, Niemann-Pick disease type C, Farber disease, infantile free sialic acid storage disease, and mucolipidosis (I-cell disease). A high index of suspicion is necessary in order to diagnose these diseases. Recurrence of hydrops must induce the search for a possible metabolic etiology (STONE and SIDRANSKY 1999). Genetic counseling is possible for some of these diseases (STONE and SIDRANSKY 1999).

Fetal tumors (teratoma, etc.) are exceptional causes of hydrops (VADEYAR et al. 2000, GRAF et al. 2000).

Placental chorioangioma is also rarely associated with hydrops. The vascularization of the tumor is a determinant factor of pregnancy outcome: if the tumor is hypervascularized, polyhydramnios, fetal growth restriction, hydrops, and premature labor may develop (JAUNIAUX and OGLE 2000).

Maternal causes, such as infections, diabetes or medication, are occasionally associated with NIHF (POESCHMANN et al. 1992, JONES 1995).

14.4
Ultrasound Diagnosis

Fetal hydrops may be diagnosed during routine fetal ultrasound (US) examination or after referral because increased fundal height measurement, preterm labor, maternal pre-eclampsia, vaginal bleeding, or a suspicious family history (MCCOY et al. 1995, GEMBRUCH and HOLZGREVE 2001).

The diagnosis of fetal hydrops relies upon US and is being done earlier and earlier during pregnancy (Figs. 14.2, 14.3) (JAUNIAUX 1997). Hydrops is diagnosed when abnormal fluid accumulation is detected in at least two different fetal compartments. There

is no agreement on the definition of hydrops in the medical literature (GEMBRUCH and HOLZGREVE 2001). The amniotic cavity is considered as a fetal compartment by some authors (including the presence of hydramnios in the definition of the syndrome) but not by others (JONES 1995, FOROUZAN 1997, GEMBRUCH and Holzgreve 2001). Polyhydramnios is associated with 30–75% of cases of hydrops, but in some circumstances (i.e., Turner syndrome, cytomegalovirus infection), oligohydramnios may be observed (GEMBRUCH and HOLZGREVE 2001).

US criteria of abnormal fluid accumulation vary according to the authors and the gestational age. Most authors diagnose subcutaneous edema when the cutaneous thickness is greater than 5 mm (skin edema must not be confused with increased body fat observed in macrosomic fetuses). Pericardial fluid effusion is diagnosed when an echolucent rim of at least 2 mm is observed around both ventricles (SHENKER et al. 1989). This abnormal effusion must be differentiated from the small amount of pericardial fluid observed normally and from the hypoechoic appearance of the peripheral myocardium in the case

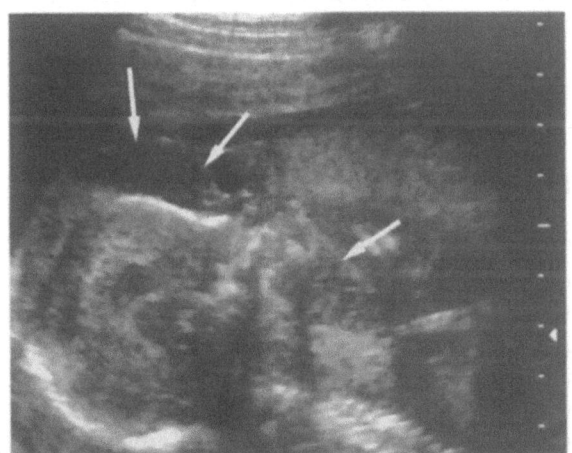
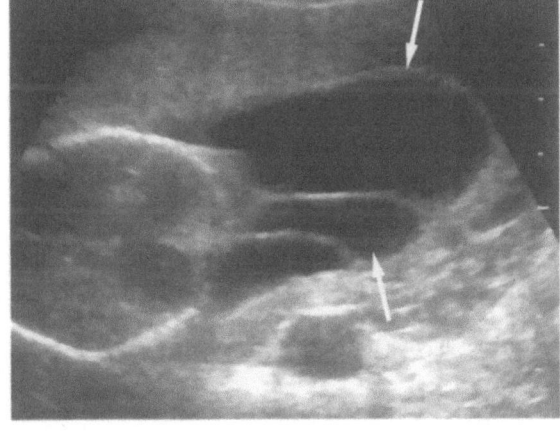
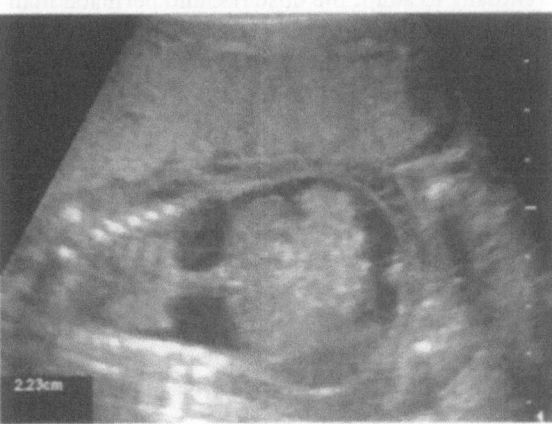

Fig. 14.2a–c. A singleton 17-week-old fetus. **a** Sagittal US view shows significant skin edema (*arrows*). **b** Axial view of the inferior part of the skull shows the typical appearance of a massive septated cystic hygroma (*arrows*). **c** Frontal view of the trunk shows bilateral pleural effusion, ascites, and skin edema: hydrops (*between crosses*: placenta)

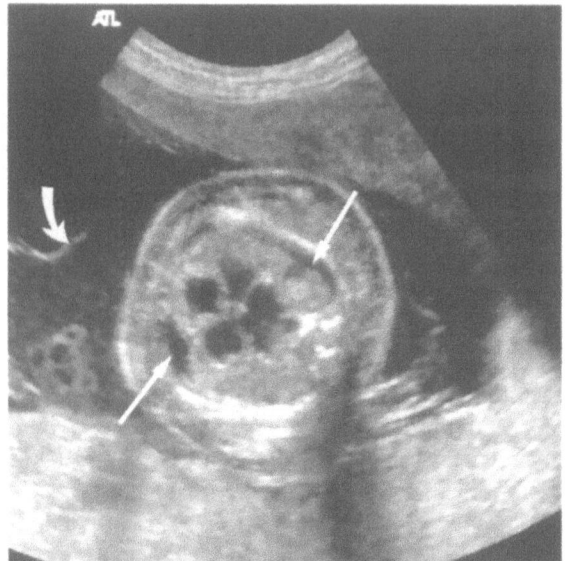

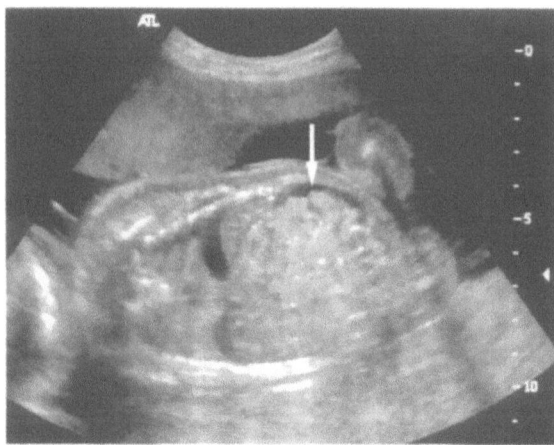

Fig. 14.3a, b. A 24-week-old fetus of a monochorionic diamniotic twin pregnancy complicated by twin-twin transfusion syndrome. **a** Axial view of the chest shows marked skin edema, and bilateral pleural effusion (*arrows*) (*curved arrow*: amniotic membrane). **b** Frontal view shows associated ascites (*arrow*)

of cardiac hypertrophy (WEIL and HUHTA 1993). M-mode echocardiography may be useful to detect a small amount of pericardial effusion (WEIL and HUHTA 1993). Ascites corresponds to the presence of fluid inside the peritoneal cavity. It should not be confused with the normal hypoechogenicity of abdominal or back musculature (JONES 1995, BIANCHI et al. 2000). Placental thickness increases linearly with gestational age and criteria for placental edema vary also according to the gestational age (ELCHALAL et al. 2000). Following the normograms recently published, a placenta is considered abnormal when its thickness is above the 90th percentile for the gesta-

tional age (ELCHALAL et al. 2000). At 18–21 weeks of gestation, the upper limit for a normal placenta seems to be 25–30 mm, and during the third trimester, placental thickness greater than 4 cm is considered as abnormal (JONES 1995, JAUNIAUX 1997, TONGSONG et al. 1999). Measurement of placental thickness is particularly useful for the precocious diagnosis of homozygous alpha-1-thalassemia in a high-risk population (GHOSH et al. 1994, KO et al. 1995, TONGSONG et al. 1999).

The location of fluid accumulation depends upon the gestational age and the underlying cause. In early pregnancy, generalized skin edema is often the first feature of fetal hydrops (JAUNIAUX 1997). Before 20 weeks, placental edema and generalized skin edema are commonly associated (JAUNIAUX 1997, ISKAROS et al. 1997). Ascites is also commonly found in early hydrops, but pleural and pericardial effusions are rarely observed before 15 weeks except in cases of Turner syndrome (JAUNIAUX 1997, ISKAROS et al. 1997). Pleural effusion predominates in abnormal lymphatic drainage or chromosomal anomalies (GEMBRUCH and HOLZGREVE 2001). In contrast, pleural effusion appears late in hydrops associated with anemia, tachyarrhythmia, or complete heart block (GEMBRUCH and HOLZGREVE 2001).

14.5
Management

The discovery of hydrops in a fetus represents an obstetric emergency and justifies early referral to a tertiary center (WY et al. 1999, SWAIN et al. 1999). A systematic approach (including fetal US, maternal and fetal blood testing, and amniocentesis or cordocentesis) is mandatory to narrow the etiology to a category of disorders, to discuss the prognosis, and eventually to adapt the obstetric and perinatal management (NORTON 1994, JONES 1995, MCCOY et al. 1995). The management depends on the etiology and the degree of fetal compromise (MCCOY et al. 1995). It is important to rule out potentially treatable conditions as well as genetic disorders with a risk of recurrence (NORTON 1994). The familial and obstetric history must be investigated (ARCASOY and GALLAGHER 1995). Not all possible complementary tests should be performed in each case, but should be selected according to the individual circumstances (JONES 1995). The major difficulty is to select those fetuses who may benefit from invasive procedures (WY et al. 1999).

The evaluation usually starts with US. A systematic US survey, including detailed fetal cardiac US examination, allows the detection of structural malformations or markers for karyotypic anomalies (JONES 1995). Further investigation of the hydropic fetus is largely based on the US findings and the resulting differential diagnosis.

In the case of hydrops where the etiology is not evident on US, the first step is to rule out immune hydrops with indirect Coombs testing. Maternal blood testing also includes blood grouping (ABO and Rh), screening for antibodies against TORCH agents (including parvovirus B19, CMV and syphilis), hemoglobin electrophoresis (for alpha-thalassemia), and Kleihauer-Betke preparation (to detect fetomaternal hemorrhage) (KNISELY 1995, JONES 1995, McCoy et al. 1995). Other rarer causes of anemia may be identified by means of maternal enzyme levels (glucose-6-phosphate dehydrogenase deficiency, pyruvate kinase deficiency).

Invasive testing of the fetus is reserved for identification of chromosomal and genetic diseases, fetal anemia, and fetal infection (JONES 1995). Fetal blood testing may include a complete blood count (hemoglobin, hematocrit, red cell indices, leukocyte count with differential platelet count), blood grouping with direct and indirect Coombs testing, screening for antibodies against TORCH agents including parvovirus B19 and syphilis, hemoglobin electrophoresis, karyotyping, and serum concentrations of albumin and hepatic enzyme activities (KNISELY 1995). Polymerase chain reaction on amniotic fluid or fetal blood is useful at all gestational ages for diagnosis of infection (JONES 1995). Metabolic analysis of the amniotic fluid may lead to diagnosis of metabolic diseases when a family history or specific US findings are detected (JONES 1995).

If all routine investigations rule out malformation and abnormal chromosomes, follow-up with US is useful since hydrops may sometimes be transient (SOHAN et al. 2001).

If an untreatable major fetal malformation (such as some cardiac structural malformations, skeletal dysplasias) is discovered, the prognosis is usually very poor and, depending on the gestational age and local practice, pregnancy termination or spontaneous evolution may be proposed. Detailed neonatal and pathological examination by an experienced geneticist and pediatric dysmorphologist, photography, skeletal survey, and biochemical investigations on body fluids and cultured fibroblasts are necessary to establish the precise diagnosis and the risk of recurrence (VAN MALDERGEM et al 1992, McCoy et al. 1995).

In contrast, some fetal anomalies are now potentially treatable. Therapeutic options remain limited and are clearly dependent on and directed towards the etiology. In the best circumstances, they can lead to significant improvement or even resolution of the hydrops (McCoy et al. 1995, ANANDAKUMAR et al. 1996). Treatment modalities are essentially limited to treatment of anemia (with fetal transfusions), pleural effusion (thoracocentesis or thoracoamniotic shunting), polyhydramnios, and cardiac rhythm disturbances (JONES 1995). Digoxin and other antiarrhythmic medications control most fetal arrhythmias (WY et al. 1999). Propylthiouracil in case of maternal Graves disease has been successfully used to treat fetal hyperthyroidism (TREADWELL et al. 1996). Intravenous maternal administration of penicillin seems to be efficient in cases of congenital syphilis (WY et al. 1999). In well-trained teams, fetal surgery has been used in specific circumstances for thoracic masses such as diaphragmatic hernia, cystic adenomatoid malformation, sequestration, and sacrococcygeal teratoma (BULLARD and HARRISON 1995). Fetoscopy may be useful in some cases of twin pregnancies complicated with twin-twin transfusion syndrome or in the presence of an acardiac twin (BULLARD and HARRISON 1995). For these fetuses, precise timing of the survey remain uncertain, as well as timing of delivery and optimal mode of delivery (BIANCHI et al. 2000b).

14.6
Prognosis

14.6.1
Fetal Prognosis

The prognosis for the fetus depends directly on the underlying etiology and the gestational age (JONES 1995, McMAHAN and DONOVAN 1995, JAUNIAUX 1997). The prognosis of hydrops is usually poor (McMAHAN and DONOVAN 1995). Tachyarrhythmia, and infection by parvovirus B19 complicated by NIHF, have a better prognosis because spontaneous resolution is observed and efficient treatment exist (JAUNIAUX 1997, GEMBRUCH and HOLZGREVE 2001). In the case of immune hydrops, the prognosis is related to the severity of hydrops (STEINER 1995).

Mortality statistics vary according to the series and the gestational age at diagnosis. Perinatal mortality reaches 86.6% in a series of nonimmune hydrops diagnosed after 20 weeks of gestation (McCoy et al.

1995). When diagnosed before 24 weeks, perinatal mortality may be as high as 95% (McCoy et al. 1995). Other authors have observed a similar survival rate before and after 24 weeks (Sohan et al. 2001). However, in some recent series the overall survival rate in midtrimester fetal hydrops remains lower than 10% (Heinonen et al. 2000). When diagnosed at birth, the reported mortality rate varies from 50% to 98%, depending on the severity of hydrops (McMahan and Donovan 1995, Wy et al. 1999). Although the use of surfactant, steroids, and high-frequency ventilation appear to prolong survival times in infants with hydrops, these treatments failed to alter overall survival outcome even with the best-trained teams (Wy et al. 1999).

No specific isolated US criteria exist to determine precisely an individual prognosis in cases of hydrops fetalis. Cardiomegaly and pulsatile umbilical venous flow (except if there is tachyarrhythmia) indicate cardiac dysfunction (Gembruch and Holzgreve 2001). A scoring system based on the number of serous spaces involved does not seem to be predictive of outcome (Forouzan 1997). However, the presence of a large pleural effusion (and associated pulmonary hypoplasia) and prematurity are significantly associated with perinatal mortality (Forouzan 1997, Wafelman et al. 1999). Recurrence risk depends on the specific etiological diagnosis.

14.6.2
Maternal Prognosis

Maternal complications are also more frequent in cases of hydrops. These include eclampsia, pregnancy-induced hypertension, theca lutein cysts, maternal hyperthyroidism, anemia, antepartum and postpartum hemorrhage, placentae abruptio, retained placenta, HELLP (hemolysis, elevated liver enzymes, low platelet count) syndrome, and preterm delivery (Ghosh et al. 1994, Forouzan 1997, Gembruch and Holzgreve 2001). A particular maternal complication may be observed in rare circumstances: the mirror syndrome (or Balantyne syndrome) which is a combination of fetal hydrops with generalized fluid overload and a pre-eclampsia-like state in the mother. In general, the maternal clinical features resolve only with delivery of the fetus and placenta; successful treatment of fetal disorder can rarely lead to resolution of the maternal disorder (Midgley and Harding 2000, Bianchi et al. 2000b).

References

Anandakumar C, Biswas A, Wong YC, et al (1996) Management of non-immune hydrops: 8 years' experience. Ultrasound Obstet Gynecol 8:196–200

Apkon M (1995) Pathophysiology of hydrops fetalis. Semin Perinatol 19:437–446

Arcasoy MO, Gallagher PG (1995) Hematologic disorders and nonimmune hydrops fetalis. Semin Perinatol 19:502–515

Barron SD, Pass RF (1995) Infectious causes of hydrops fetalis. Semin Perinatol 19: 493–501

Bianchi DW, Crombleholme TM, d'Alton ME (2000a) Immune hydrops. In: Bianchi DW, Crombleholme TM, d'Alton ME (eds) Fetology: diagnosis and management of the fetal patient. McGraw-Hill, New York, pp 953–958

Bianchi DW, Crombleholme TM, d'Alton ME (2000b) Nonimmune hydrops fetalis. In: Bianchi DW, Crombleholme TM, d'Alton ME (eds) Fetology: diagnosis and management of the fetal patient. McGraw-Hill, New York, pp 959–965

Bullard KM, Harrison MR (1995) Before the horse is out of the barn: fetal surgery for hydrops. Semin Perinatol 19:462–473

De Groot CJ, Oepkes D, Egberts J, Kanhai HH (2000) Evidence of endothelium involvement in the pathophysiology of hydrops fetalis? Early Hum Dev 57:205–209

Elchalal U, Ezra Y, Levi Y, et al (2000) Sonographically thick placenta: a marker for increased perinatal risk – a prospective cross-sectional study. Placenta 21:268–272

Forouzan I (1997) Hydrops fetalis: recent advances. Obstet Gynecol Surv 52:130–138

Gembruch U, Holzgreve W (2001) The fetus with nonimmune hydrops fetalis. In: Harrison MR (ed) The unborn patient: the art and science of fetal therapy, 3rd edn, WB Saunders, Philadelphia, pp 525–582

Ghosh A, Tang MH, Lam YH, Fung E, Chan V (1994) Ultrasound measurement of placental thickness to detect pregnancies affected by homozygous alpha-thalassaemia-1. Lancet 344:988–989

Gilbert GL (2000) Parvovirus B19 infection and its significance in pregnancy. Commun Dis Intell 24(Suppl):69–71

Graf JL, Albanese CT, Jennings RW, Farrell JA, Harrison MR (2000) Successful fetal sacrococcygeal teratoma resection in a hydropic fetus. J Pediatr Surg 35:1489–1491

Heinonen S, Ryynanen M, Kirkinen P (2000) Etiology and outcome of second trimester non-immunologic fetal hydrops. Acta Obstet Gynecol Scand 79:15–18

Iskaros J, Jauniaux E, Rodeck C (1997) Outcome of nonimmune hydrops fetalis diagnosed during the first half of pregnancy. Obstet Gynecol 90:321–325

Jauniaux E (1997) Diagnosis and management of early nonimmune hydrops fetalis. Prenat Diagn 17:1261–1268

Jauniaux E, Ogle R (2000) Color Doppler imaging in the diagnosis and management of chorioangiomas. Ultrasound Obstet Gynecol 15:463–467

Jones DC (1995) Nonimmune fetal hydrops: diagnosis and obstetrical management. Semin Perinatol 19:447–461

Jordan JA (1996) Identification of human parvovirus B19 infection in idiopathic nonimmune hydrops fetalis. Am J Obstet Gynecol 174:37–42

Keeling JW (1991) Hydrops fetalis and other forms of excess fluid collection in the fetus. In: Wigglesworth JS, Singer DB (eds) Textbook of fetal and perinatal pathology. Blackwell Scientific, Boston, pp 429–454

Knilans TK (1995) Cardiac abnormalities associated with hydrops fetalis. Semin Perinatol 19:483–492

Knisely AS (1995) The pathologist and the hydropic placenta, fetus, or infant. Semin Perinatol 19:525–531

Ko TM, Tseng LH, Hsu PM, Hwa HL, Lee TY, Chuang SM (1995) Ultrasonographic scanning of placental thickness and the prenatal diagnosis of homozygous alpha-thalassemia 1 in the second trimester. Prenat Diagn 15:7–10

Lallemand AV, Doco-Fenzy M, Gaillard DA (1999) Investigation of nonimmune hydrops fetalis: multidisciplinary studies are necessary for diagnosis – review of 94 cases. Pediatr Dev Pathol 2:432–439

Machin GA (1989) Hydrops revisited: literature review of 1,414 cases published in the 1980s. Am J Med Genet 34:366–390

Mazeron MC, Cordovi-Voulgaropoulos L, Perol Y (1994) Transient hydrops fetalis associated with intrauterine cytomegalovirus infection: prenatal diagnosis. Obstet Gynecol 84:692–694

McCoy MC, Katz VL, Gould N, Kuller JA (1995) Non-immune hydrops after 20 weeks' gestation: review of 10 years' experience with suggestions for management. Obstet Gynecol 85:578–582

McDonnell M, Hannam S, Devane SP (1998) Hydrops fetalis due to ABO incompatibility. Arch Dis Child Fetal Neonatal Ed 78:F220–F221

McMahan MJ, Donovan EF (1995) The delivery room resuscitation of the hydropic neonate. Semin Perinatol 19:474–482

Midgley DY, Harding K (2000) The mirror syndrome. Eur J Obstet Gynecol Reprod Biol 88:201–202

Norton ME (1994) Nonimmune hydrops fetalis. Semin Perinatol 18:321–332

Poeschmann RP, Verheijen RH, Van Dongen PW (1992) Differential diagnosis and causes of nonimmunological hydrops fetalis: a review. Obstet Gynecol Surv 46:223–231

Shenker L, Reed K, Anderson CF, Kern W (1989) Fetal pericardial effusion. Am J Obstet Gynecol 160:1505–1507

Sohan K, Carroll S, Byrne D, Ashworth M, Soothill P (2000) Parvovirus as a differential diagnosis of hydrops fetalis in the first trimester. Fetal Diagn Ther 15:234–236

Sohan K, Carroll SG, De La Fuente S, Soothill P, Kyle P (2001) Analysis of outcome in hydrops fetalis in relation to gestational age at diagnosis, cause and treatment. Acta Obstet Gynecol Scand 80:726–730

Steiner RD (1995) Hydrops fetalis: role of the geneticist. Semin Perinatol 19:516–524

Stone DL, Sidransky E (1999) Hydrops fetalis: lysosomal storage disorders in extremis. Adv Pediatr 46:409–440

Swain S, Cameron AD, McNay MB, Howatson AG (1999) Prenatal diagnosis and management of nonimmune hydrops fetalis. Aust NZ J Obstet Gynaecol 39:285–290

Tongsong T, Wanapirak C, Sirichotiyakul S (1999) Placental thickness at mid-pregnancy as a predictor of Hb Bart's disease. Prenat Diagn 19:1027–1030

Treadwell MC, Sherer DM, Sacks AJ, Ghezzi F, Romero R (1996) Successful treatment of recurrent non-immune hydrops secondary to fetal hyperthyroidism. Obstet Gynecol 87:838–840

Vadeyar S, Ramsay M, James D, O'Neill D (2000) Prenatal diagnosis of congenital Wilms' tumor (nephroblastoma) presenting as fetal hydrops. Ultrasound Obstet Gynecol 16:80–83

Van Maldergem L, Jauniaux E, Fourneau C, Gillerot Y (1992) Genetic causes of hydrops fetalis. Pediatrics 89:81–86

von Kaisenberg CS, Jonat W (2001) Fetal parvovirus B19 infection. Ultrasound Obstet Gynecol 18:280–288

Wafelman LS, Pollock BH, Kreutzer J, Richards DS, Hutchison AA (1999) Nonimmune hydrops fetalis: fetal and neonatal outcome during 1983–1992. Biol Neonate 75:73–81

Weil SR, Huhta JC (1993) Sonographic differential diagnosis of fetal cardiac abnormalities. Semin Ultrasound CT MR 14:298–318

Wy CA, Sajous CH, Loberiza F, Weiss MG (1999) Outcome of infants with a diagnosis of hydrops fetalis in the 1990s. Am J Perinatol 16:561–567

Subject Index

A

abdominal calcifications 146
– liver 146
– meconium peritonitis 147
– peritoneal tumors 147
– pseudocyst 147
– vascular calcifications 147
abnormal growth 235
acardius 240
achondrogenesis
– type I 204, 206
achondroplasia 206, 210
adrenal 183, 189, 190
– cysts 189
– hemorrhage 190
– masses 189
adreno-genital syndrome 183, 189
allantoid remnant cyst 174
ambiguous
– genitalia 183
amniotic
– band sequence 212
– Band Syndrome 135
– – associated anomalies 135
– – cause 135
– – definition 135
– – management 136
– – prognosis 136
– – US findings 135
– fluid 7
– membrane 7
anencephaly 46
anterior herniation 95
anorectal atresia 146
anterior herniation 95
antibiotic phrophylactic therapy 179
aortic arch view 108
aortic valvular stenosis 117
Apert's syndrome 219
arachnoid cysts 57
arrythmias 121
arthrogryposis 220
ascites 248
astrocytoma 268
atresia
– esophagia 139
– laryngeal 90
– tracheal 90
atrial
– ectopic beats 121
– septal defect 114

B

atrioventricular
– block 123
– septal defect 114
autosomal
– dominant polycystic kidney disease 169
– recessive polycystic kidney disease 168

B

Bardet-Biedl syndrome 158, 170, 219
Beckwith-Wiedemann syndrome 65, 91, 128, 272, 276
bladder 154
– exstrophy 136, 174
– – associated anomalies 136
– – cause 136
– – definition 136
– – prognosis 136
– – US findings 136
– outlet obstruction 174, 185
brachyphalangism 218
bradycardia 123
branchial cleft cysts 69, 272
bronchogenic cyst 88, 98
butterfly vertebra 221

C

calcifications 252
camptomelic dysplasia 216
candlestick appearance 251
cardiac
– failure 121
– pauses 121
– tumors 117
– – fibromas 117
– – intracardial teratomas 117
– – rhabdomyomas 117
cardiomegaly 247
cardiomyopathy 117
– dilated 117
– hypertrophic 117
cardiothoracic ratio 247
caudal regression syndrome 222
causes of NIHF 287
central nervous system 39
cephalocele 47
cerebellar hypoplasia 261
cerebral
– hemorrhage **53, 214**
– tumors 58
cerebriform pattern 189
cervical length 7, 10
childhood neoplasm 267

choledochal cyst 148, 274
chondrodysplasia 219
chorionic villous biopsy 255
chorioretinitis 251
choroid plexus cyst 57, 259
chylothorax 96
clavicles 200
cleft lip 65
cloacal exstrophy 136, 186
– associated anomalies 136
– cause 136
– definition 136
– management 137
– prognosis 137
– US findings 136
cloverleaf appearance 206
clubfoot 216, 262
clubhand 218, 262
– ulnar 218
– radial 218
coarctation of the aorta 115
color Doppler ultrasonography 110
common arterial trunk 119
compensatory hypertrophy 174
congenital
– CNS anomalies 44
– heart disease 103
– lobar emphysema 91
– nephrotic syndrome 158
conjoined twins 241
conotruncal anomalies 118
Conradi-Hünermann syndrome 204
constitutional shortness 210
cordocentesis 255
Cornelia de Lange syndrome 91
corpus callosum 57
– agenesis 57
– lipoma 271
– normal anatomy 42, 62
– partial agenesis 57
corrected transposition of the great arteries 120
co-twin demise 229
craniopharyngioma 268
cranosynostosis 50
crossed fused 156
CT 198
cyst
– arachnoid 57, 60, 268
– bronchogenic 88
– sub-arachnoid 57
– renal 147, 168
– thymic 97, 98
– thyroglossal 272
cystic 168
– adenomatoid malformation 83
– – Stocker's 83
– – classification 83
– – differential diagnosis 86
– hygroma 47, 69
– kidneys 262, 263
– lymphogiomas 273, 275
– masses 268
– neuroblastoma 190, 273

– obstructive dysplasia 158
– teratoma 273
cytomegalovirus 50, 246, 251

D
dacryocystocele 67, 272
Dandy-Walker
– malformation 54
– variant 54
daughter cyst sign 187
dextrocardia 104
dextroposition 104
diabetic mothers 198
diaphragmatic
– bilateral diaphragmatic 94
– eventration 94
– herniation 91
– hypoplasia 94
– left diaphragmatic hernia 92
– MRI 94
– prognosis 94
– right diaphragmatic hernia 93
diastermatomyelia 222
diastrophic dystrophy 219
DiGeorge syndrome 79, 265
ddizygotic 223
double-outlet right ventricle 119
Down's syndrome 210, 256, 272
ductal arch view 108
duodenal
– atresia 141
– obstruction 140
duplex kidney 164
dysrythmias 121

E
ear 65
Ebstein anomaly 112
echogenic
– dilated bowel loops 142
– – prognosis 142
– small bowel 141
– – management 142
– – prognosis 142
ectopic
– insertion 164
– kidney 156
– ureterocele 164
edema 249
Ehlers-Danlos syndrome 213
empty renal fossa 156
encephalocele 69
enlarged
– fetal bladder 161
– right atrium 112
epidermolysis bullosa 213
epispadias 183
equin-ovarus 217
esophageal
– atresia 139
– – associated anomalies 140
– – prognosis 140
– – US findings 139

– duplication 98
exencephaly 46
eyes 64

F
facial
– anatomy 62
– hemangioendothelioma 272
Fanconi anemia 214
femoral aplasia 213
fetal
– aorta 6
– abdomen 6
– abdominal circumference 3
– abdominal wall 6
– adrenals 189
– akinesia 220
– anemia 253
– biparietal diameter 3
– biometry 3
– bladder 6, 9
– brain 4, 42, 52, 246, 271
– – MR imaging 42
– calcaneum 10
– central nervous system 4
– cerebral sulci 9
– chest 5, 77
– choroids plexus 4
– colon 9
– diaphragm 79
– environment 7
– esophagus 79
– eyes 9, 64
– face 5, 59, 62
– falx cerebri 4
– femoral length 3
– gender 182
– growth 8
– – retardation 11, 97, 133, 140, 214, 219, 227, 257
– heart 6, 9, 79
– hydrops 97, 223, 248, 251, 263, 285
– – management 290
– – prognosis 291
– ultrasound diagnostic 289
– infection 245
– kidneys 6, 9
– lie 8
– lips 5, 9, 62
– liver 6
– lower extremities 7
– lungs 6, 79
– – development 78
– maxillary 5
– measurement 2
– meconium cells 10
– mediastinum 6
– MR imaging 247, 251
– MRI 81, 97, 198
– muscles 10
– neck 5
– normal anatomy 4, 9
– nose 5, 9
– orbits 5

– parovirus 253
– placenta
– – insertion 10
– – maturation 10
– posterior fossa 5
– profile 5, 65
– reflux nephropathy 180
– septum pellicidum 4
– sex 7, 10
– skeleton 199
– skull 4
– small bowel 9
– spinal cord 9
– spine 5
– stomach 6
– sylvian fissures 4
– testes 10, 183
– thymus 79
– thyroid 9
– trachea 9, 79
– upper extremities 7
– urinary tract 153
– uterus 10
– ventricle 4
– weight 8
– well-being 8, 10
fetal Growth restriction 13
– biophysic profile score 18
– definition 14
– diagnosis 13
– Doppler ultrasound 15
– middle cerebral artery 16
– "reversal of adaptation" 16
– ultrasound biometry 14
– umbilical artery 15
fibula
– agenesis 214
– hypoplasia 216
five-chamber view 107
foregut
– duplication cysts 274
– pathology 138
four chamber view 105
Fryns syndrome 91

G
gastric outlet obstruction 140
– US findings 140
gastroschisis 131
– associated anomalies 132
– cause 131
– definition 131
– prognosis 132
– US findings 131
– US follow-up 132
glioma 58
glomerulo-cystic
– kidneys 168
– type 170
goiter 71
growth-retarded fetus 210
gyration anomalies 50, 247

H

hamartoma 273
hemangioendothelioma 275
hemangioma 47, 147, 274
hemangiopericytoma 279
hemivertebrae 221
hemorrhage 52
hepatic cysts 274
hepatoblastoma 274
hepatomegaly 247
hepatosplenomegaly 248, 251
heterotopia 50
hitch-hiker thumb 219
holoprosencephaly 54
Holt Oram syndrome 214, 218
horseshoe 156
hydrocele 183
hydrocephaly 251
hydrocolpos 186
hydrops 248, 251, 263, 285
hyperechoic
– bowell 251, 260
– ependyma 251
– focus 105
hypokinesia deformation sequence 220
hypolasia of the fifth digit 260
hypophosphatasia 204
hypoplasia of the nasal bones 259
hypoplastic
– left heart Syndrome 111
– right heart Syndrome 111
hypospadias 183
hypothyroidism

I

idiopathic right atrial enlargement 113
iliac wings angle 202, 260
immune hydrops 285
imperforate hymen 186
inguino-scrotal hernia 278
intermediate-type malformation 213
intracardiac
– echogenic foci 259
– tumors 274
intracranial
– calcifications 246, 251
– teratoma 58
intrahepatic calcifications 248
intraperitoneal
– calcifications 146
– masses 146
intrascrotal hernia 183
intrauterine growth restriction 235
ischemia 52
isolated
– cortical cysts 168
– transposition of the great arteries 120
IUGR 249, 251

J

Jeune's syndrome 170

K

Kariotype 255
Kidneys 154, 252
– compensatory hypertrophy 174
– crossed fused 156, 157
– duplex kidney 162, 164, 167, 176
– ectopic kidney 156
– ectopic ureterocele 164, 167, 176, 179, 181
– hyperechogenicity 156
– horseshoe 156, 157
Klinefelter syndrome 262

L

labia 182
large bowell pathology 146
laryngeal atresia 90
left isomerism 105
levocardia 104
limb
– body wall complex 98, 134
– – associated anomalies 135
– – cause 134
– – definition 134
– – management 135
– – US findings 134
– deformities 253
– transverse distal amputations 212
lipoma 268
lips 63
liver
– hamartoma 274
– hemangioma 274
– metastasis 275
lobster claw hand 219
long axis view 108
long bone 203
– bowing 203
– angulas 203
– fracture 203
– shortening 260
longitudinal-type malformation 214
lung
– agenesis 97
– hypoplasia 97
– malformations 82
– tumors 273
lymphangioma 69, 279

M

M-mode echography 109
macroglossia 65, 272
macrosomia 18
– definition 18
– dystocia 20
– fetal weight 20
– ultrasound evaluation 18
mandible 199
maternal diabetes 222
maxilla 199
MDK 168, 181
– involution 181
Meckel-Gruber syndrome 171, 219

meconium
– peritonitis 145
– pseudocysts 275
mediastinal malformation 97
medical report 11
mega(poly)calycosis 161
megacystic-microcolon-hypoperistalsis syndrome 146, 164
megacystis-megaureter syndrome 161
megalo-urethra 185
metastasis 190
meningocele 47, 69
mesenchymal tumors 273
mesoblastic
– blastoma 171
– nephroma 276
mesocardia 104
metastasis
metatarsus adductus 217
microcephaly 47, 246, 250, 261
micrognathia 67
microphtalmy 67
monosomy 22, 265
monozygotic 224
morphologic examination 2
mouth 63
MR 80, 223
– imaging 146, 154, 171, 267, 271, 276
mucous plugs 91
multicystic dysplastic kidney (MDK) 161
multifetal gestations 230
– amniotic fluid 230
– biometry 230
– normal growth 230
myelomeningocele 47
– lemon-shaped 47
– banana sign 47
myocarditis 247

N
nasal
– bone 64
– bone hypoplasia 67
– teratoma 272
necrosis 249
nephroblastomatosis 171, 276
neural tube defects 45
neurenteric cyst 97
neuroblastoma 148, 189, 276
NIHF 287
– cardiovascular anomalies 287
– causes 287
– cytomegalovirus 288
– fetal tumors 288
   gastrointestinal anomalies 288
– generic causes 287
– haematological abnormalities 288
– infections 287
– maternal causes 289
– metabolic anomalies 288
– noncardiac thoracic abnormalities 288
– placental chorioangioma 288
– renal anomalies 288
– structural malformations 287

– tacyarrhythmia 287
– twin-twin transfusion syndrome 288
nonimmune hydrops 285
non-cystic tumors 268
Noonan syndrome 69
nuchal
– thickening 258
– translucency 255

O
obstructive cystic dysplasia 168
ocular retinoblastoma 272
oligohydramnios 249, 251
omphalocele 126, 262
– associated anomalies 128
– giant 127
– management 129
– ordinary 127
– prognosis 129
– typically 127
open spina bifida 47
– C-shaped 47
– vertebra 47
organomegaly 147
– cystic tumors 147
– mixed pattern tumors 147
osteogenesis imperfecta 204
– type 2 204
ovarian
– "cyst" 187
– torsion cysts 275
ovary 278

P
parenchymal liver calcifications 253
parvovirus fetal infection 253
patent urachus 37, 175
PCR 246
Pena-Shokeir syndrome 219, 220
penis 182
pentalogy of Candrell 98, 130
– associated anomalies 130
– definition 130
– prognosis 130
– US findings 130
pericallosal
– artery 251
– lipoma 57
pericardial
– effusion 98, 247
– teratoma 98
Perlmann syndrome 276
Pierre Robin sequence 67
placenta 249
– abruptia placentae 32
– accrete 30
– calcidications 28
– choriangioma 33
– circumvallate 26
– decidual septal cysts 29
– development 25
– environment 7
– infarct 29

– marginal hematoma 32
– position 30
– previa 30
– retroplacental area 31
– size 27
– shape 25
– succenturiate 26
– thick 27
– thin 27
pleural effusion 95
– primary 95
– secondary 95
– hydrothorax 95
– natural history 95
polydactyly 218, 262
polyhydramnios 249
posterior urethral valves 161, 185
pregnancy
– dating 2
proboscis 67
proximal femoral focal deficiency 213
Prune Belly sequence 174
Pterygia 220
pulmonary atresia with ventricular septal defect 118
pulsed Doppler ultrasonography 110
pyelectasis 260

R
radial hypoplasia 214
radiography 198
radius deficiency 214
renal
– agenesis 156
– – bilateral 156
– – unilateral 156
– cystic disease 168
– obstructive dysplasia 160
– tumors 171
– vein thrombosis 173
restrictive ductus arteriosus 116
rhabdomyomas 274
rhabdomyosarcoma 273, 279
right isomerism 105
routine echography 104
rubella infection 250

S
sacro-coccygeal teratoma 223, 279
sagittal sign 182
scalp cyst 47, 69
schizencephaly 50
second trimester 209
sequestration 86
– differential diagnosis 88
– extralobar 86
– intralobar 86
– pleural effusion 86
short femur 209
short-limb dwarfism 263
situs
– ambiguous 105
– solitus 105
skeletal dysplasias 198

small bowel
– atresia 143
– – US findings 143
– pathology 141
Smith-Lemli-Opitz syndrome 219
soft tissue neoplasm 279
spine 199
spontaneous involution 188
sternum 200
stippled epiphysis 204
stomach
– absence 139
strawberry-like cranium 261
Stuck-Twin syndrome 236
subependymal cysts 252
sylvian fissure 247
systematic examination 1
syndactyly 218, 219

T
tachycardias 122
– sinus 122
– supraventricular 122
– ventricular 123
tailored approach 203
TAR syndrome 214
teratoma 47, 69, 148, 268, 272, 273, 274, 276, 278
– cystic lesions 148
testicular tumors 183, 278
tetralogy of Fallot 118
thanatophoric dwarfism 204
three-dimensional US
thrombosis 249
thymic
– agenesis 265
– cysts 98
thyroglossal 272
tongue 63, 259
torsion 183
toxoplasmosis 50, 246, 251
tracheal atresia 90
transverse great vessels view 107
tricuspid valve dysplasia 112
trident hand 219
triploidy 263
trisomy
– 13 98, 219, 262
– 18 98, 219, 261
– 21 256
– – atrial ventricular defects 257
– – duodenal defects 257
– – fetal hydrops 257
– – major structural anomalies 257
– – minor structural anomalies 257
– scoring index 257
tuberous sclerosis 58
tubers 268
Turner syndrome 69, 262
twin 223, 224
– births 227
– discordance 234
– embolization syndrome 239
– monochorionic monoamniotic 240

– oligohydramnios-polyhydramnios sequence 237
– pregnancy 229
– reversal arterial perfusion 240
– type of 231
twin-twin transfusion syndrome 238
two-dimensional US 198

U

umbilical cord 7, 34
– anatomy 34
– coiling 35
– cysts 36, 262
– eccentric insertion 36
– enlarged cord 35
– insertion 35
– long umbilical cord 34
– nuchal cord 35
– persistence of the right umbilical vein 34
– prolapse 35
– short umbilical cord 34
– single umbilical artery 34
– vasa previa 36
– velamentous insertion 36
– Wharton's Jelly anomaly 35
univentricular heart 110
UPJ obstruction 160
urachal cyst
urachus 174
– cyst 174
– patent 174
uretero-vesical junction obstruction 161
urethral atresia 185
urinary tract dilatation 158
urinomas 168

uro-nephropathies 179
– treatment 179
uropathies 176
– investigation 176
– – neonatal 176
US
– Doppler 11
– safety 1
– technique 2
Uterus 182
UVJ obstruction 161

V

VACTERL association 218
vanishing twin 229
varicella 253
vascular malformations 274
VATER association 214
vena cava view 108
ventricular and atrial septal defects 247
ventricular Septal Defect 113, 261
ventriculomegaly 44, 246, 251, 259
– syndromic 45
– hydrocephaly 45
– hydranencephaly 45
vertebra 199
very short femur 203, 210
vesico-ureteric reflux 161
viral DNA 246
VUR 161

W

Wilm's tumor 171, 276

List of Contributors

FRED E. AVNI, MD, PhD
Professor, Department of Pediatric Imaging
University Children Hospital Queen Fabiola
Avenue J. J. Crocq 15
1020 Brussels
Belgium

MARIE CASSART, MD
Division of Perinatal Imaging
University Clinics of Brussels
Erasme Hospital
Route de Lennik 808
1070 Brussels
Belgium

CATHERINE CHRISTOPHE, MD
Department of Radiology
University Children Hospital
Avenue J.J. Crocq 15
1020 Brussels
Belgium

TERESA COS, MD
Department of Obstetrics and Gynecology
Brugmann Hospital
Place van Gehuchten 4
1090 Brussels
Belgium

CHRISTINE DEVALCK, MD
Department of Pediatric Oncology
University Children Hospital Queen Fabiola
Avenue J. J. Crocq 15
1020 Brussels
Belgium

CATHERINE DONNER, MD, PhD
Department of Obstetrics and Gynecology
University Clinic of Brussels
Erasme Hospital
Route de Lennik, 808
1070 Brussels
Belgium

JOSÉE DUBOIS, MD
Department of Medical Imaging
Sainte-Justine Hospital
Université de Montréal
3175 Côte-Sainte-Catherine
Montréal, Québec H3T 1C5
Canada

JUDY ESTROFF, MD
Department of Pediatric Radiology
Children's Hospital Medical Center
300 Longwood Ave.
Boston, MA 02115
USA

DANIÈLE EURIN, MD
Department of Pediatric Imaging
Charles Nicolle Hospital
1 rue de Germont
76031 Rouen Cedex
France

LAURENT GAREL, MD
Department of Medical Imaging
Sainte-Justine Hospital
3175 Côte-Sainte-Catherine
Montréal, Québec H3T 1C5
Canada

ANDRÉE GRIGNON, MD
Department of Medical Imaging
Sainte-Justine Hospital
3175 Côte-Sainte-Catherine
Montréal, Québec H3T 1C5
Canada

MICHELLE HALL, MD
Department of Pediatric Nephrology
University Children Hospital Queen Fabiola
Avenue J.J. Crocq 15
1020 Brussels
Belgium

ANNE MASSEZ, MD
Department of Pediatric Imaging
University Clinics of Brussels
Erasme Hospital
Route de Lennick 808
1070 Brussels
Belgium

YANN ROBERT, MD
Département d'Imagerie
Hôpital Jeanne De Flandre
CHRU Lille, Rue E. Avinée
59037 Lille Cedex
France

Françoise Rypens, MD
Department of Medical Imaging
Sainte Justine Hospital
3175 Côte-Sainte-Catherine
Montréal, Québec H3T 1C5
Canada

Pascale Sonigo, MD
Department of Pediatric Imaging
Enfants Malades Hospital
Rue de Sèvre, 149
75743 Paris Cedex
France

Guy Vaksmann, MD
Pediatric Cardiology Service
Hôpital de Cardiologie
CHRU Lille
2 Avenue Oscar Lambret
59037 Lille Cedex
France

Nicole Vanregemorter, MD
Department of Medical Genetics
University Clinics of Brussels
Erasme Hospital
Route de Lennick 808
1070 Brussels
Belgium

France Ziereisen, MD
Department of Pediatric Imaging
University Children Hospital Queen Fabiola
Avenue J.J. Crocq 15
1020 Brussels
Belgium

MEDICAL RADIOLOGY
Diagnostic Imaging and Radiation Oncology

Titles in the series already published

DIAGNOSTIC IMAGING

Innovations in Diagnostic Imaging
Edited by J. H. Anderson

Radiology of the Upper Urinary Tract
Edited by E. K. Lang

The Thymus - Diagnostic Imaging, Functions, and Pathologic Anatomy
Edited by E. Walter, E. Willich, and W.R. Webb

Interventional Neuroradiology
Edited by A. Valavanis

Radiology of the Pancreas
Edited by A. L. Baert,
co-edited by G. Delorme

Radiology of the Lower Urinary Tract
Edited by E. K. Lang

Magnetic Resonance Angiography
Edited by I. P. Arlart, G. M. Bongartz, and G. Marchal

Contrast-Enhanced MRI of the Breast
S. Heywang-Köbrunner and R. Beck

Spiral CT of the Chest
Edited by M. Rémy-Jardin and J. Rémy

Radiological Diagnosis of Breast Diseases
Edited by M. Friedrich and E.A. Sickles

Radiology of the Trauma
Edited by M. Heller and A. Fink

Biliary Tract Radiology
Edited by P. Rossi

Radiological Imaging of Sports Injuries
Edited by C. Masciocchi

Modern Imaging of the Alimentary Tube
Edited by A. R. Margulis

Diagnosis and Therapy of Spinal Tumors
Edited by P. R. Algra, J. Valk, and J. J. Heimans

Interventional Magnetic Resonance Imaging
Edited by J. F. Debatin and G. Adam

Abdominal and Pelvic MRI
Edited by A. Heuck and M. Reiser

Orthopedic Imaging
Techniques and Applications
Edited by A. M. Davies and H. Pettersson

Radiology of the Female Pelvic Organs
Edited by E. K.Lang

Magnetic Resonance of the Heart and Great Vessels
Clinical Applications
Edited by J. Bogaert, A. J. Duerinckx, and F. E. Rademakers

Modern Head and Neck Imaging
Edited by S. K. Mukherji and J. A. Castelijns

Radiological Imaging of Endocrine Diseases
Edited by J. N. Bruneton
in collaboration with B. Padovani and M.-Y. Mourou

Trends in Contrast Media
Edited by H. S. Thomsen, R. N. Muller, and R. F. Mattrey

Functional MRI
Edited by C. T. W. Moonen and P. A. Bandettini

Radiology of the Pancreas
2nd Revised Edition
Edited by A. L. Baert
Co-edited by G. Delorme and L. Van Hoe

Emergency Pediatric Radiology
Edited by H. Carty

Spiral CT of the Abdomen
Edited by F. Terrier, M. Grossholz, and C. D. Becker

Liver Malignancies
Diagnostic and Interventional Radiology
Edited by C. Bartolozzi and R. Lencioni

Medical Imaging of the Spleen
Edited by A. M. De Schepper and F. Vanhoenacker

Radiology of Peripheral Vascular Diseases
Edited by E. Zeitler

Diagnostic Nuclear Medicine
Edited by C. Schiepers

Radiology of Blunt Trauma of the Chest
P. Schnyder and M. Wintermark

Portal Hypertension
Diagnostic Imaging-Guided Therapy
Edited by P. Rossi
Co-edited by P. Ricci and L. Broglia

Recent Advances in Diagnostic Neuroradiology
Edited by Ph. Demaerel

Virtual Endoscopy and Related 3D Techniques
Edited by P. Rogalla,
J. Terwisscha Van Scheltinga, and B. Hamm

Multislice CT
Edited by M. F. Reiser, M. Takahashi, M. Modic, and R. Bruening

Pediatric Uroradiology
Edited by R. Fotter

Transfontanellar Doppler Imaging in Neonates
A. Couture and C. Veyrac

Radiology of AIDS
A Practical Approach
Edited by J.W.A.J. Reeders and P.C. Goodman

CT of the Peritoneum
Armando Rossi and Giorgio Rossi

Magnetic Resonance Angiography
2nd Revised Edition
Edited by I. P. Arlart, G. M. Bongratz, and G. Marchal

Pediatric Chest Imaging
Edited by Javier Lucaya and Janet L. Strife

Applications of Sonography in Head and Neck Pathology
Edited by J. N. Bruneton in collaboration with C. Raffaelli and O. Dassonville

Imaging of the Larynx
Edited by R. Hermans

3D Image Processing
Techniques and Clinical Applications
Edited by D. Caramella and C. Bartolozzi

Imaging of Orbital and Visual Pathway Pathology
Edited by W. S. Müller-Forell

Pediatric ENT Radiology
Edited by S. J. King and A. E. Boothroyd

Radiological Imaging of the Small Intestine
Edited by N. C. Gourtsoyiannis

Imaging of the Knee
Techniques and Applications
Edited by A. M. Davies and V. N. Cassar-Pullicino

Perinatal Imaging
From Ultrasound to MR Imaging
Edited by Fred E. Avni

Radiological Imaging of the Neonatal Chest
Edited by V. Donoghue

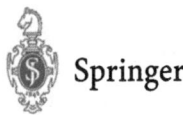 Springer

MEDICAL RADIOLOGY
Diagnostic Imaging and Radiation Oncology

Titles in the series already published

RADIATION
ONCOLOGY

Lung Cancer
Edited by C.W. Scarantino

Innovations in Radiation Oncology
Edited by H. R. Withers and L. J. Peters

Radiation Therapy of Head and Neck Cancer
Edited by G. E. Laramore

Gastrointestinal Cancer – Radiation Therapy
Edited by R.R. Dobelbower, Jr.

Radiation Exposure and Occupational Risks
Edited by E. Scherer, C. Streffer,
and K.-R. Trott

Radiation Therapy of Benign Diseases
A Clinical Guide
S.E. Order and S. S. Donaldson

**Interventional Radiation Therapy Techniques –
Brachytherapy**
Edited by R. Sauer

Radiopathology of Organs and Tissues
Edited by E. Scherer, C. Streffer,
and K.-R. Trott

**Concomitant Continuous Infusion
Chemotherapy and Radiation**
Edited by M. Rotman and C. J. Rosenthal

**Intraoperative Radiotherapy –
Clinical Experiences and Results**
Edited by F. A. Calvo, M. Santos,
and L.W. Brady

**Radiotherapy of Intraocular
and Orbital Tumors**
Edited by W. E. Alberti and R. H. Sagerman

**Interstitial and Intracavitary
Thermoradiotherapy**
Edited by M. H. Seegenschmiedt
and R. Sauer

Non-Disseminated Breast Cancer
Controversial Issues in Management
Edited by G. H. Fletcher and S.H. Levitt

**Current Topics in Clinical Radiobiology
of Tumors**
Edited by H.-P. Beck-Bornholdt

**Practical Approaches to Cancer Invasion
and Metastases**
A Compendium of Radiation
Oncologists' Responses to 40 Histories
Edited by A. R. Kagan with the
Assistance of R. J. Steckel

Radiation Therapy in Pediatric Oncology
Edited by J. R. Cassady

Radiation Therapy Physics
Edited by A. R. Smith

Late Sequelae in Oncology
Edited by J. Dunst and R. Sauer

Mediastinal Tumors. Update 1995
Edited by D. E. Wood and C. R. Thomas, Jr.

**Thermoradiotherapy
and Thermochemotherapy**

Volume 1:
Biology, Physiology, and Physics

Volume 2:
Clinical Applications
Edited by M.H. Seegenschmiedt,
P. Fessenden, and C.C. Vernon

Carcinoma of the Prostate
Innovations in Management
Edited by Z. Petrovich, L. Baert,
and L.W. Brady

Radiation Oncology of Gynecological Cancers
Edited by H.W. Vahrson

Carcinoma of the Bladder
Innovations in Management
Edited by Z. Petrovich, L. Baert,
and L.W. Brady

**Blood Perfusion and Microenvironment
of Human Tumors**
Implications for Clinical Radiooncology
Edited by M. Molls and P. Vaupel

Radiation Therapy of Benign Diseases
A Clinical Guide
2nd Revised Edition
S. E. Order and S. S. Donaldson

**Carcinoma of the Kidney and Testis, and Rare
Urologic Malignancies**
Innovations in Management
Edited by Z. Petrovich, L. Baert,
and L.W. Brady

**Progress and Perspectives in the Treatment
of Lung Cancer**
Edited by P. Van Houtte, J. Klastersky,
and P. Rocmans

**Combined Modality Therapy of
Central Nervous System Tumors**
Edited by Z. Petrovich, L. W. Brady,
M. L. Apuzzo, and M. Bamberg

**Age-Related Macular Degeneration
Current Treatment Concepts**
Edited by W. A. Alberti, G. Richard,
and R. H. Sagerman

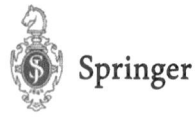 Springer